CRITICAL CARE MEDICINE
Just the Facts

Jesse B. Hall, MD

Professor of Medicine and Anesthesia & Critical Care
Section Chief, Pulmonary and Critical Care Medicine,
University of Chicago, Chicago, Illinois

Gregory A. Schmidt, MD

Professor of Medicine, Carver College of Medicine,
Division of Pulmonary Diseases, Critical Care, and Occupational Medicine
University of Iowa, Iowa City, Iowa

Associate Editor

D. Kyle Hogarth, MD

Assistant Professor, Section of Pulmonary and Critical Care Medicine,
University of Chicago, Chicago, Illinois

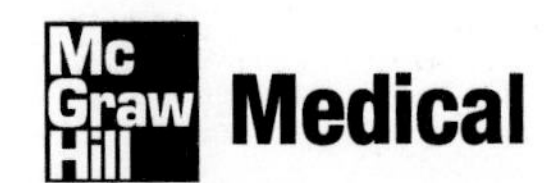

New York Chicago San Francisco Lisbon London Madrid
Mexico City Milan New Delhi San Juan Seoul
Singapore Sydney Toronto

The McGraw-Hill Companies

CRITICAL CARE MEDICINE

Just the Facts

1 2 3 4 5 6 7 8 9 0 QPD/QPD 0 9 8 7

ISBN 13: 978-0-07-144020-2
ISBN 10: 0-07-144020-8

This book was set in Times Roman by International Typesetting and Composition.
The editor was Ruth Weinberg.
The production supervisor was Catherine Saggese.
The production management was provided by International Typesetting and Composition.
The cover designer was Aimee Nordin.
Quebecor World Dubuque was printer and binder.

This book is printed on acid-free paper.

Library of Congress Cataloging-in-Publication Data

Critical care medicine : just the facts / [edited by] Jesse B. Hall and Gregory A. Schmidt ; associate editor, D. Kyle Hogarth.
p. ; cm.
"Represents the essential material contained in Principles of Critical Care, 3rd edition, published in 2005."
Includes bibliographical references and index.
ISBN 0-07-144020-8 (alk. paper)
1. Critical care medicine. I. Hall, Jesse B. II. Schmidt, Gregory A. III. Hogarth, D. Kyle.
[DNLM: 1. Critical Care. 2. Intensive Care Units. WX 218 C93385 2006]
RC86.8.C78 2006
616.02'8—dc22

2006042008

International Edition: ISBN 13: 978-0-07-110474-6; ISBN 10: 0-07-110474-7

To Nora, Daniel, Aaron, and Barbara, for helping me to edit my own life.

Jesse B. Hall, MD

To Karin for her consistent Unterstützung and to my three intensive-carelings, Lukas, Stefan, and Soren.

Gregory A. Schmidt, MD

To Krista, Conor, and Aidan for their patience, love, and continuous support. Also to Larry Wood, MD, PhD, for providing an amazing environment of learning and for setting a standard for Critical Care physicians.

D. Kyle Hogarth, MD

CONTENTS

Section 5
NEUROLOGIC DISORDERS

Section 6
HEMATOLOGY AND ONCOLOGY

Section 7
RENAL AND METABOLIC DISORDERS

CONTRIBUTORS

Timothy K. Baker, MD
Resident, Department of Internal Medicine
University of Chicago Hospitals
Chicago, Illinois
Acute-on-Chronic Respiratory Failure

George W. Bell, MD
Instructor of Medicine, Department of Medicine
University of Chicago Hospitals
Chicago, Illinois
Hypertensive Encephalopathy and Hypertensive Emergencies

Shashi Kiran Bellam, MD
Assistant Professor of Medicine, Feinberg School of Medicine, Northwestern University
Attending Physician, Division of Pulmonary and Critical Care, Evanston Northwestern Healthcare, Evanston, Illinois
Ventilator-induced Lung Injury and Acute Respiratory Distress Syndrome, Inhalation Injuries, Severe Community-Acquired Pneumonia, Thrombotic Thrombocytopenic Purpura, Acute Leukemia, Thyroid Disease, Adrenal Insufficiency, Pelvic and Extremity Trauma

John E. A. Blair, MD
Cardiovascular Fellow, Northwestern Memorial Hospital
Chicago, Illinois
Therapeutic Hypothermia

J. Matthew Brennan, MD
Fellow, Division of Cardiovascular Diseases
Department of Internal Medicine
Duke University Hospital
Durham, North Carolina
Care of the Postcardiac Surgery Patient, Pericardiocentesis

Melanie L. Brown, MD
Assistant Professor, Pediatric Critical Care
University of Chicago
Chicago, Illinois
Hypothermia, Near Drowning

David Brush, MD
Resident, Department of Internal Medicine
University of Chicago Hospitals
Chicago, Illinois
Botulism, Central Venous Catheter

Gordon E. Carr, MD
Resident, Department of Internal Medicine
University of Chicago Hospitals
Chicago, Illinois
Influenza

Steven Y. Chang, MD, PhD
Assistant Professor
MICU Director
Pulmonary and Critical Care Medicine
University of Medicine and Dentistry of New Jersey
Newark, New Jersey
Echocardiography in the Critically Ill Patient

Steven Q. Davis, MD
Fellow, Section of Pulmonary and Critical Care Medicine
University of Chicago Hospitals
Chicago, Illinois
Resuscitation, Acute Right Heart Syndromes, Acute-on-Chronic Respiratory Failure, Fungal Infections in the ICU, CNS Hemorrhage, Disseminated Intravascular Coagulation, Rhabdomyolysis, Electrical Trauma, Withholding and Withdrawing Life-Sustaining Therapy and Administering Palliative Care

Maria Dowell, MD
Assistant Professor, Section of Pediatric Pulmonary
University of Chicago
Chicago, Illinois
Status Asthmaticus, Hemoptysis and Pulmonary Hemorrhage, Restrictive Diseases of the Respiratory System, Anoxic Encephalopathy, Anemia, Transfusion, Massive Transfusion, Upper GI Hemorrhage, Lower GI Hemorrhage, Acute Pancreatitis, Burns

Jay Finigan, MD
Fellow, Pulmonary and Critical Care Medicine
Johns Hopkins University
5501 Hopkins Bayview Circle
Baltimore, Maryland
Ventricular Dysfunction in Critical Illness

Tim Floreth, MD
Critical Care Hospitalist
Macneal Hospital
Berwyn, Illinois
Interpretation of Hemodynamic Waveforms

Sascha Goonewardena, MD
Resident, Department of Internal Medicine
University of Chicago Hospitals
Chicago, Illinois
Noninvasive Assessment of Cardiac Output

Kevin Gregg, MD
Resident, Department of Internal Medicine
University of Chicago Hospitals
Chicago, Illinois
Empiric Antibiotic Selection in the Critical Care Setting

Ethan L. Gundeck, MD
Cardiologist
The Heart Center
Fishkill, New York
Mechanical Circulatory Assist Devices

D. Kyle Hogarth, MD
Assistant Professor
Section of Pulmonary and Critical Care Medicine
University of Chicago
Chicago, Illinois
Pain Management, Sedation Management in the ICU, Pericardial Disease, Sleep Disordered Breathing, Endocarditis, Ventilator-Associated Pneumonia, Viral Encephalitis, Viral Hemorrhagic Fevers, Status Epilepticus, Sickle Cell Disease, Acute Hepatic Failure, Spine Injuries, Pregnancy in the ICU, Chemical Weapons

Anna N. Kamp, MD
Research Fellow, Section of Pediatric Cardiology
University of Chicago Hospitals
Chicago, Illinois
Extracorporeal Membrane Oxygenation

Susan S. Kim, MD
Assistant Professor of Medicine
Section of Cardiology
University of Chicago
Chicago, Illinois
Rhythm Disturbances in the ICU

Brian Klausner, MD
Chief Resident, Internal Medicine
Macneal Hospital
Berwyn, Illinois
Acute Alcohol Withdrawal

Vidya Krishnan, MD, MHS
Fellow, Division of Pulmonary and Critical Care
Johns Hopkins University School of Medicine
Baltimore, Maryland
Assessment of the Critically Ill Patient, Infection Control In the ICU

Janelle C. Laughlin, MD
Rheumatology
Longmont Clinic
Longmont, Colorado
Rheumatology in the ICU

May M. Lee, MD
Fellow, Section of Pulmonary and Critical Care
University of Chicago Hospitals
Chicago, Illinois
Hyperbaric Oxygen Therapy

Jeremy Leventhal, MD
Fellow, Division of Nephrology
Department of Medicine
Mount Sinai School of Medicine
New York, New York
The eICU

Josh Levitsky, MD
Assistant Professor of Medicine
Section of Hepatology
Northwestern University
Chicago, Illinois
Chronic Liver Disease

Joseph Levitt, MD
Clinical Instructor of Medicine
Section of Pulmonary & Critical Care
Stanford University
Stanford, California
Monitoring the Cardiovascular System, Monitoring the Respiratory System, Nutrition in the Critically Ill, Soft Tissue Infections, Delirium in the Intensive Care Unit, Bone Marrow Transplantation, Mesenteric Ischemia, Dermatology in the ICU, Transporting the Critically Ill

Stephen C. Mathai, MD MHS
Fellow, Division of Pulmonary and Critical Care Medicine
Johns Hopkins University
Baltimore, Maryland
Using Respiratory Waveforms to Adjust Ventilator Settings

Meredith C. McCormack, MD, MHS
Fellow, Pulmonary and Critical Care Medicine
Johns Hopkins University
Baltimore, Maryland
Acid-Base Balance

Kristopher McDonough, MD
Fellow, Section of Pulmonary & Critical Care
Loyola University
Maywood, Illinois
Emergent Surgical Airway

Raina M. Merchant, MD
Resident, Department of Emergency Medicine
University of Chicago Hospitals
Chicago, Illinois
Therapeutic Hypothermia

Nuala J. Meyer MD
Fellow, Section of Pulmonary and Critical Care Medicine
University of Chicago
Chicago, Illinois
Airway Management, Neuromuscular Blockade, Pulmonary Embolism: Thrombus, Fat, Air, and Amniotic Fluid, Cardiovascular Diseases, Acute Respiratory Distress Syndrome, Life-Threatening Infections of the Head and Neck, Acute Spinal Cord Compression, Plasmapheresis in the ICU, Superior Vena Cava Syndrome

James K. Min, MD
Assistant Professor
Division of Cardiology
Weill Medical College of Cornell University
New York, New York
Myocardial Ischemia

E. Mirnalini Mohanraj
Chief Medical Resident, Department of Internal Medicine
John H. Stroger, Jr. Hospital of Cook County
Chicago, Illinois
Fluid Therapy

Michael J. Moore, MD
Assistant Professor of Medicine
Northwestern University
Feinberg School of Medicine
Division of Pulmonary and Critical Care Medicine
Chicago, Illinois
Assessment of Severity of Illness, Sepsis, Severe Sepsis, and Septic Shock, Drotrecogin Alfa (Activated), Urinary System Infections, Neuromuscular Weakness in the ICU, Bleeding Disorders in the ICU, Toxicities of Chemotherapy, Abdominal Compartment Syndrome, Toxicology in Adults

Sandy Nasrallah, MD
Resident, Department of Internal Medicine
University of Chicago Hospitals
Chicago, Illinois
Disseminated Intravascular Coagulation

Peter O'Donnell, MD
Fellow, Section of Hematology/Oncology
Department of Internal Medicine
University of Chicago Hospitals
Chicago, Illinois
Radiation Pneumonitis

Nina M. Patel, MD
Clinical Assistant Professor of Medicine
Columbia University Medical Center
New York, New York
Pulmonary Artery Catheter, Pathophysiology of Acute Respiratory Failure, Approach to Sepsis of Unknown Etiology, Gastrointestinal Infections, Cerebrovascular Accident, Head Trauma, Acute Renal Failure, Acute Abdomen, Anaphylaxis

Jonathan D. Paul, MD
Resident, Department of Internal Medicine
University of Chicago Hospitals
Chicago, Illinois
Early Goal-Directed Therapy for Sepsis

Mark C. Pohlman, MD
Fellow, Section of Pulmonary and Critical Care Medicine
University of Chicago
Chicago, Illinois
Liberation from Mechanical Ventilation

Daniel A. Pollyea, MD
Chief Medical Resident, Department of Internal Medicine
John H. Stroger, Jr. Hospital of Cook County
Chicago, Illinois
Thrombocytopenia in Critically Ill Patients

Amit Pursnani, MD
Resident, Department of Internal Medicine
University of Chicago Hospitals
Chicago, Illinois
Thrombolytic Therapy

Adam Ronan, MD
Resident, Department of Internal Medicine
University of Chicago Hospitals
Chicago, Illinois
Thoracentesis

Michael A. Samara, MD
Resident, Department of Internal Medicine
University of Chicago Hospitals
Chicago, Illinois
Carbon Monoxide Intoxication

Nathan Sandbo, MD
Fellow, Section of Pulmonary and Critical Care Medicine
University of Chicago
Chicago, Illinois
Aortic Dissection, Noninvasive Positive Pressure Ventilation, Neutropenic Patients, Severe Malaria, Coma and Persistent Vegetative State, Brain Death, Complications of Solid Organ Transplantation, Severe Hyperthermia

Jenny Sauk, MD
Resident, Department of Internal Medicine
New York Presbyterian Hospital—Weill Cornell Campus
New York, New York
Pulmonary Artery Catheter Insertion

John A. Schneider MD, MPH
Fellow, Section of Infectious Diseases
University of Chicago
Chicago, Illinois
Central Nervous System Infections

William Schweickert, MD
Fellow, Section of Pulmonary and Critical Care
University of Chicago
Chicago, Illinois
An Approach to Shock, Common Modes of Mechanical Ventilation, Managing the Ventilated Patient, Responding to Crises in the Ventilated Patient, AIDS in the ICU, Tetanus, Severe Electrolyte Disorders, Care of the Multisystem Trauma Patient

Shefali Shah, MD
Resident, Department of Internal Medicine
University of Chicago Hospitals
Chicago, Illinois
SARS

Stephen Skjei, MD
Naperville, Illinois
Diabetic Ketoacidosis in Adults, Intensive Insulin Therapy in the Critically Ill, Thyroid Disease

Sunanna Sohi, MD
Resident, Department of Internal Medicine
University of Chicago Hospitals
Chicago, Illinois
Bleeding Esophageal Varices and TIPS

Ignatius Y. Tang, MD, PharmD
Assistant Professor of Medicine
Section of Nephrology and Transplantation Medicine
University of Illinois—Chicago
Chicago, Illinois
Renal Replacement Therapy in the ICU

Samip Vasaiwala, MD
Fellow, Section of Cardiology
University of Illinois—Chicago
Chicago, Illinois
Plague: The Black Death

Kaveeta P. Vasisht, MD, PharmD
Clinical Instructor of Medicine
Department of Medicine
University of Chicago
Chicago, Illinois
Torso Trauma

Rekha Vij, MD
Resident, Internal Medicine
University of Chicago Hospitals
Chicago, Illinois
Inhalation Injuries

Ajeet Vinayak, MD
Assistant Professor of Medicine
MICU Medical Director
Department of Medicine
University of Virginia
Charlottesville, Virginia
Infectious Complications of Intravenous Devices, Anthrax and Smallpox

Timothy L. Zisman, MD
Fellow, Department of Gastroenterology
University of Chicago Hospitals
Chicago, Illinois
Inflammatory Bowel Disease

PREFACE

Just the Facts in Critical Care represents the essential material contained in Principles of Critical Care, 3rd Edition, published in 2005. Just the Facts was created to guide intensive care physicians, internists, anesthesiologists, surgeons, emergency physicians, and others who care for critically ill patients. Following roughly the framework of "Principles," this work provides essential information in a readily accessible format. Much of the background material and detail present in the larger text has been omitted in favor of facts vital to the clinician confronted with an acutely ill patient or the physician studying for board certification examinations. Just the Facts is not intended to be comprehensive or to replace the larger text, so each chapter refers the reader seeking additional detail to more complete information in "Principles."

In Critical Care, time is of the essence, a fact we took to heart in creating this work. Each chapter begins with a brief overview of the topic. The material is then divided into a highly organized structure, emphasized by a bullet-point style. Key points in recognition, diagnosis, evaluation, monitoring, therapy, and prognosis are clearly stated. Figures and tables, most created expressly for this work, serve to convey maximal information at a glance. Together, these features make for chapters that can be scanned quickly for maximum efficiency.

ACKNOWLEDGMENTS

We wish to articulate our thanks to the authors of the chapters in "Principles." That text served to inspire and guide the contributors of this work, who began by assimilating, trimming, and focusing those chapters. We will always be grateful for their collaboration. In addition, we are often reminded how much our careers have been enriched by our trainees over the past two decades: the students, residents, fellows, and practitioners who provoke us to organize our thoughts and motivate us to teach and write. Most of our enthusiastic contributors learned with us at some point in their training. The two senior editors of this text (GAS, JBH), also wish to thank their colleague Dr. Kyle Hogarth, who served as associate editor for this endeavor. His organization, enthusiasm, and skills in exhortation were essential elements in completing this work. Last, but not least, we acknowledge the guidance of a team of editors at McGraw-Hill who recognized the potential value of Just the Facts in Critical Care and assisted each in their own way to bring this work to completion.

Section 1
GENERAL MANAGEMENT OF PATIENTS

1 ASSESSMENT OF THE CRITICALLY ILL PATIENT

Vidya Krishnan

KEY POINTS

- Begin with a brief but careful history and directed examination, seeking acute life-threats.
- Vital signs, neck veins, oximetry, and chest radiography are particularly valuable diagnostic aids in the initial evaluation.
- Severity of illness scores may guide initial therapy and provide a rough guide to prognosis.
- Quickly liberate the patient from excessive early interventions so that there are not more treatments than diseases.
- Seek to identify the patient who may be dying and follow advance directives when available.

INITIAL ASSESSMENT

- Critical illness involves respiratory failure, hemodynamic instability, or other acute threat to life or limb. The initial assessment and management of the critically ill patient is crucial in the course of the patient's care. Exemplary critical care management involves the careful balance of the institution of rapid diagnostic and therapeutic interventions and development of a rational and compassionate management plan based on the therapeutic goals. The acquisition of the skills necessary to achieve this balance is a lifelong learning process.
- Advance directives. The formulation of a therapeutic plan should be guided by the patient's wishes for resuscitation and intubation. The presence of a "living will" does not obviate the need to discuss with the patient's significant others about the direction of therapy.
- Primary survey. Basic life support and advanced life support protocols provide a guide to initiating a patent airway, ensuring adequate ventilation, and managing circulation.

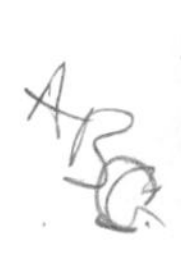

- Secondary survey. The role of clinical excellence, by obtaining a careful medical history, physical examination, and laboratory testing, is to elucidate the nature of the patient's current disease, and to formulate a rational diagnostic and therapeutic plan. A thorough compilation of the patient's medical history is often the most helpful information in directing further management of the critically ill patient.
  - Sources of information include the patient, his/her significant others, medical records, and prior radiologic studies and laboratory values.
  - Particular attention to the patient's health and activities preceding the acute event may contribute to defining the current pathophysiologic state.

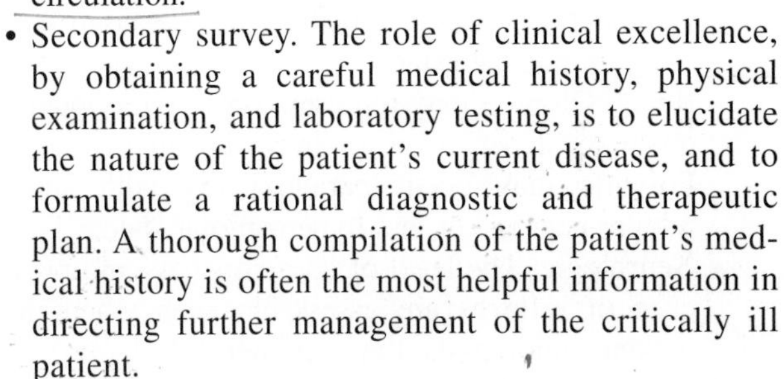

  - The physical examination will provide information regarding the patient's current condition. The following list is a guideline of physical findings to evaluate, and is by no means exhaustive:
    - Vital signs
      - Hypothermia and hyperthermia may be a sign of infection or inflammation.
      - Heart rate is usually elevated, but exceptions include beta-blocker use, hypoglycemia, and cardiac disease.
      - Blood pressure may be initially normal, due to compensatory mechanism, or deranged.
      - Respiratory rate abnormalities may reflect disturbances in acid-base status.
      - Pain ("the fifth vital sign") may direct medical attention to trauma or the source of infection.
    - Skin. Findings may include sweat, dry, altered temperature, decreased capillary refill, cyanosis, pale, duskiness, ecchymoses or purpura, erythema, or rash.

- Cardiovascular
    - Murmurs may represent valvular abnormalities, and should be compared to previous examinations for determination of whether this is a new finding.
    - Jugular venous distention may represent elevated right heart pressures. Flattened neck veins may signify hypovolemia.
    - Absence or reduced peripheral pulses may signify inadequate perfusion.
- Pulmonary
    - Rales could be a sign of an alveolar filling process (such as edema or infection).
    - Absence of breath sounds or wheezing may signify an obstruction or pneumothorax.
- Gastrointestinal
    - Shock may result in intestinal ileus or ischemia, pancreatitis, or acalculous cholecystitis.
    - Bleeding may occur anywhere along the intestinal tract, and when heme is present in gastric contents or feces, hemorrhage may be contributing to the acute state.
- Renal. Oliguria may represent obstruction, inadequate renal perfusion, or intrinsic renal disease. Polyuria may occur paradoxically with acute tubular necrosis or in a hyperosmolar state.
- Neurologic. The level of consciousness and presence of reflexes are assessable even when the patient cannot assist the examiner.

SCORING SEVERITY OF ILLNESS

- Severity-of-illness scoring systems (Table 1-1). Scoring systems give a quantification of the severity of illness that may assist in determining prognosis of individual patients in order to assist families and caregivers in making decisions about ICU care. However, in some studies the accuracy of prediction of outcomes from scoring systems is not greater than that of the individual clinician's judgment.

FORMULATE A WORKING DIAGNOSIS

- Based on the history and physical examination findings, hypotheses should be formulated concerning the mechanisms responsible for each main problem and a differential diagnosis should be generated. Laboratory testing and radiologic evaluations are tools to be used to confirm or refute the clinical hypotheses. Some common tools used in the evaluation of the critically ill patient include the following:
    - Arterial blood gas results can give insight into the patient's oxygenation, ventilation, and metabolic status.
    - Pulse oximetry will give an indication of oxygenation, but may be uninterpretable in the presence of poor peripheral circulation, deranged arterial hemoglobin-carrying capacity, or carbon monoxide poisoning.
    - Chest radiography is a useful tool to diagnose thoracic pathology and to confirm proper intervention techniques (e.g., endotracheal tubes and central venous access placement, development of pneumothorax or hemothorax).
    - Complete blood counts, basic chemistry panels, liver and renal function tests, cardiac enzymes, and coagulation pathway tests may all be helpful in the confirmation of clinical hypotheses.
    - Urinary analysis may reveal an active sediment consistent with acute tubular necrosis, hemorrhage, or infection.
    - Body fluid and tissue cultures assist in the diagnosis of infection and can direct therapy when specific pathogenic organisms are identified.
- Experienced critical care physicians recognize that the assessment and management of critically ill patients extend beyond the implementation of diagnostic and

TABLE 1-1 Comparison of Severity-of-Illness Scoring Systems

SCORING SYSTEM	DESCRIPTION	DISEASE-SPECIFIC	SIGNIFICANCE
Acute Physiology and Chronic Health Evaluation (APACHE)	It uses age, type of admission, chronic health evaluation, and 12 physiologic variables (Acute Physiology Score or APS) to predict hospital mortality. The 12 physiologic variables are defined as the most abnormal values during the 24 h after ICU admission	Yes	APACHE II is the most commonly used clinical severity-of-illness scoring system in North America
Mortality Probability Models (MPM)	It is the only scoring system that was derived at ICU admission and can therefore be used at ICU admission	No	Instead of a numeric score, the MPM II yields a direct probability of survival
Simplified Acute Physiology Score II (SAPS)	The probability of hospital mortality is calculated from the score	No	
Sequential Organ Failure Assessment (SOFA)		No	Independent of the initial values, an increase in the SOFA score during the first 48 h of ICU admission predicts a mortality rate of at least 50%

therapeutic interventions. Students of critical care management should keep in mind these additional clinical pearls.

- Liberate the patient from interventions, so that there are not more treatments than diagnoses. One of the consequences of protocol-driven resuscitations and fast-paced clinical decision processes observed in the management of ICU patients, is that the recovered patient has excessive and unnecessary treatments. Adverse events are associated with nearly all interventions, and the balance of positive and negative effects should be repeatedly evaluated. The approach of the critical care team should be frequent (at least daily) assessment of the need for interventions, and removal of unnecessary and potentially toxic interventions.
- Define therapeutic goals and seek the least intervention to achieve each. It is often helpful to concretely identify the therapeutic goals for a patient, so that the management plan will be focused to achieve these goals. Invasive and prolonged resuscitation efforts are inappropriate in a patient whose goals have been altered from cure to comfort.
- Communicate with the patient and his/her family. Family and patient meetings are necessary to introduce the critical care physician and the health care team, to communicate patient status, to obtain consent for anticipated interventions, and to answer questions and alleviate anxiety that naturally accompanies critical illness of one's self or significant others.

BIBLIOGRAPHY

Hall JB, Schmidt GA, Wood LDH. An approach to critical care. In: Hall JB, Schmidt GA, Wood LDH, eds., *Principles of Critical Care*, 3rd ed. New York, NY: McGraw-Hill; 2005: 3–9.

2 AIRWAY MANAGEMENT

Nuala Meyer

KEY POINTS

- Bag-mask ventilation is a life-saving skill.
- Prior to endotracheal intubation, the operator should assess the patient's disease, anatomy, and cardiovascular stability with particular attention to cervical spine stability, intracranial pressure, and drug contraindications.
- Esophageal intubation must be recognized promptly.
- Hypotension commonly complicates endotracheal intubation.
- A dislodged, freshly-placed tracheostomy tube should generally not be reinserted emergently—instead, insert an endotracheal tube through the mouth, then attempt open the tracheostomy wound.

BAG-MASK VENTILATION

- The first skill that any physician or respiratory therapist should master is the ability to successfully mask ventilate an awake or somnolent patient. When done correctly, mask ventilation can allow time for a more careful, well-planned intubation, and can avoid precipitating hemodynamic instability. The hallmarks of mask ventilation are:
  - Forming an adequate seal between the patient's skin and the Ambu-bag
  - Jaw-thrust maneuver to elevate the tongue away from the epiglottis
  - Steady breath support with 100% FiO_2, ideally augmenting the patient's own breathing efforts without hyperventilation
- Bag-mask ventilation can be performed either by a solo practitioner who can skillfully seal the mask and provide jaw thrust with one hand while delivering breaths with the other, or by two practitioners: one to control the mask and jaw, and another to deliver breaths.

INDICATIONS FOR INTUBATION

- The indications for intubation and mechanical ventilation are many and varied. They can be broadly categorized as involving one of the following four systems: airway disease, pulmonary disease, circulatory disease, and neurologic disease (Table 2-1).
  - *Airway disease* encompasses problems with airway support: for example, airway narrowing by edema or tumor; pharyngeal instability (e.g., facial fractures); depressed mental status causing inability to protect airway or clear secretions; or paralyzed vocal cords causing a functional airway obstruction.

TABLE 2-1 Indications for Intubation

INDICATION FOR INTUBATION	EXAMPLE
Airway disease	Tracheal obstruction with tumor, laryngeal edema
Pulmonary disease	Hypoxemia, chronic obstructive pulmonary disease (COPD) exacerbation, opioid overdose
Circulatory disease	Shock, sepsis, cardiac arrest
Neurologic disease	Loss of gag reflex, increased ICPs

  - *Pulmonary disease* refers to acute hypoxemic respiratory failure (low arterial oxygen saturation), ventilatory failure from an increased work of breathing or airway obstruction, or hypoventilation from weakness, drugs, or central nervous system (CNS) causes.
  - *Circulatory disease* can require intubation in cases of shock, sepsis, or cardiopulmonary arrest. In this instance, intubation and mechanical ventilation may decrease the proportion of cardiac output expended on the respiratory muscles, and decrease the body's oxygen consumption or VO_2.
  - *Neurologic disease*, such as elevated intracranial pressure (ICP) requiring hyperventilation or altered consciousness with loss of gag reflex, also benefits from elective intubation.
- Finally, intubation may be imperative in the transport of an unstable critically ill patient, for instance, to a radiologic procedure or between hospitals.

ASSESSMENT OF THE PATIENT PRIOR TO INTUBATION

- When called to intubate a critically ill patient, an expeditious but thorough assessment of the patient's underlying disease, airway anatomy, and cardiopulmonary status should be reviewed prior to intubation. Physicians should perform a risk assessment of the following conditions:
  - Anatomic impediments to intubation or to direct laryngoscopy; have a plan for urgent tracheostomy prior to attempting intubation.
    - Cervical instability, such as in rheumatoid arthritis or cervical fracture
    - Poor mouth opening
    - Short neck or large tongue
    - Tumor, edema, or infection encroaching on the airway
    - Mallampati classification
  - Neurologic factors which should necessitate IV general anesthesia for intubation.
    - Elevated ICP
    - Intracranial bleeding, arteriovenous malformation (AVM), or aneurysm
  - Aspiration risk—cricoid pressure (the Sellick maneuver) may be helpful.
    - NPO (nothing by mouth) status
    - Pregnancy
    - Gastroparesis
    - Obesity
  - Pulmonary risk—certain patients cannot be reliably bag-mask ventilated, and should have rapid intubation with institution of mechanical ventilation.
    - Bronchoconstriction
    - Severe refractory hypoxemia
  - Cardiovascular risk:
    - Ischemia risk—laryngoscopy and endotracheal intubation often produce myocardial ischemia in at-risk patients. Such patients may be best managed with awake intubation with aggressive topical anesthesia.
    - Hypovolemia—intubation and positive pressure ventilation will augment the hemodynamic effects of hypovolemia, and hypotension may be precipitated. Patients with suspected hypovolemia should be rapidly volume expanded with intravenous fluid once the decision is made to intubate.
    - Dysrhythmias may be observed in patients with structurally abnormal hearts.
  - Coagulation risk factors:
    - Thrombocytopenia or coagulopathy are relative contraindications to nasotracheal intubation, lest epistaxis be severe.
  - Contraindications to succinylcholine:
    - Hyperkalemia
    - Malignant hyperthermia
    - History of burns, crush injury, or spinal cord injury

EQUIPMENT AND PREPARATION

- When planning intubation of a critically ill patient, the following should be immediately available and ready for use by the anesthesiology team:
  - Functioning IV line
  - Monitors: pulse oximeter, blood pressure cuff or arterial line, ECG, and, if possible end-tidal CO_2 monitor/capnograph
  - Suction with Yankauer
  - Ambu-bag
  - Ventilator
- Establishment of an artificial airway is a skill obtained with significant amounts of training. Use of many of the drugs listed below should be reserved to physicians well versed in the management of a difficult airway. The physician or team performing intubation will need access to the following additional equipment:
  - Laryngoscope with functioning light × 2
  - Assortment of blades (Macintosh and Miller)
  - Variety of endotracheal tubes (ETT) of different sizes
  - Malleable metal stylet
  - Stethoscope
  - Drugs
    - Topical anesthetics: viscous lidocaine, benzocaine or lidocaine spray
    - Glycopyrrolate: dries the mouth to improve visualization
    - Paralytics: rocuronium or succinylcholine
    - IV anesthetic agents: lidocaine, midazolam, fentanyl, thiopental, etomidate, propofol, or ketamine

- A thorough review of intubation procedures is beyond the scope of this book, but can be found in numerous anesthesiology textbooks.

PHYSIOLOGIC CHANGES ASSOCIATED WITH INTUBATION

- The presence of an artificial airway and mechanical ventilation provokes certain predictable physiologic consequences (Box 2-1).
  - ETT cause increased airways resistance.
    - An 8.0 mm tube causes a 20% increase in airway resistance; a 7.0 mm tube has almost twice this resistance.
    - Inspissated mucus or respiratory secretions can further decrease the diameter of the ETT, causing increased resistance.
  - Tracheal intubation can trigger bronchospasm in certain individuals, especially patients with asthma.
  - Mechanical ventilation usually changes intrathoracic pressure from negative to positive, which may impair venous return and thus decrease cardiac output.
  - Mechanical ventilation may abolish stimuli such as hypoxia, hypercarbia, and dyspnea which may have contributed to an increased level of endogenous catecholamines; the abolition of these stimuli can sometimes cause a fall in blood pressure or heart rate commensurate with the fall in catechols.
  - Patients with small airways obstruction—asthma and emphysema—are at risk for auto-PEEP (positive end-expiratory pressure), in which the lungs are unable to return to their functional residual capacity (FRC), due to their need for a long expiratory time. Patients are especially prone to this phenomenon during vigorous Ambu-bag ventilation, where tidal volumes are not readily apparent. High levels of PEEP, whether from auto-PEEP or extrinsically from the ventilator, can increase the pulmonary vascular resistance and diminish versus return, thus producing hypotension.

BOX 2-1 Physiologic Changes Associated with Mechanical Ventilation

Increased airways resistance
Bronchospasm
Increased intrathoracic pressures
Decreased venous return
Decreased cardiac output
Hypotension
Auto-PEEP

COMPLICATIONS OF INTUBATION AND MECHANICAL VENTILATION

- Intubation of critically ill patients in the ICU is often necessary but can be fraught with danger. Some more common complications encountered, which should be fresh in one's mind when evaluating a patient postintubation, are:
  - Right mainstem intubation; all ETT placements must be confirmed by chest radiograph shortly after placement
  - Esophageal intubation
    - This can be minimized with the routine use of end-tidal CO_2 monitors to confirm gas exchange after intubation.
    - Breath sounds should always be confirmed once the ETT is in place.
    - End-tidal CO_2 monitoring is notoriously unreliable in the setting of cardiac arrest/absent circulation, and occasionally in children with severe bronchospasm.
  - Gastric aspiration
  - Dental injury and aspiration of teeth
  - Tracheal or esophageal lacerations
  - Vocal cord trauma
  - Impaired swallowing
  - Dysrhythmias
    - Premature ventricular contractions (PVCs), ventricular tachycardia, and ventricular fibrillation in patients susceptible to these rhythms.
    - Bradycardia can be observed in young patients with high vagal tone.
  - Death
    - Death occurs around the time of intubation in approximately 3% of critically ill patients.
    - Death may be a consequence of airway manipulation, or may speak to the severity of illness in patients requiring intubation.

TRACHEOSTOMY

- Tracheostomy may be indicated in evolving upper airway obstructions such as angioedema, epiglottitis/supraglottic abscess, bilateral vocal cord paralysis, or tumor encroachment on the trachea. It is also the preferred route to provide long-term mechanical ventilation. Tracheostomy is used to treat patients who are unable to handle their airway secretions, and finally, may be the best method to liberate patients from protracted mechanical ventilation.
- Benefits of tracheostomy include:
  - Easier and safer access to the mouth than patients with orotracheal tubes; this allows better oral hygiene.

  - More comfortable than orotracheal intubation; facilitates eventual phonation and eating.
  - Less airway trauma over time; in general, patients who will require mechanical ventilation for more than 2 weeks will benefit from tracheostomy.
  - Reduces anatomic dead space, thus increasing the alveolar ventilation for every given minute ventilation. This allows patients with chronic weakness or chronically high ventilatory demand to have effective ventilation with a decreased workload.

COMPLICATIONS OF TRACHEOSTOMY

- Immediate:
  - Hemorrhage—neck hematomas can compress or deviate the trachea
  - Malpositioning
  - Pneumothorax/pneumomediastinum
- Long-term:
  - Irritation or erosion of trachea into esophagus (tracheoesophageal fistula)
  - Tracheal stenosis/tracheal malacia
- In the event that a freshly placed tracheostomy becomes dislodged, *do not attempt to replace the tracheostomy!* Doing so carries great risk of dissecting into the soft tissues of the neck, and failing to adequately ventilate the patient. Instead, mask-ventilate the patient while you *call anesthesia or reintubate the patient endotracheally.*
- Airway management skills take a great deal of time and practice to master. The optimal place for training in this regard is in the operating room, guided by experienced anesthesiologists. Because critically ill patients do not tolerate multiple attempts at establishing adequate ventilation, these skills are best learned in the elective setting and then translated to the ICU.

BIBLIOGRAPHY

Gaj TJ. Pulmonary mechanics in normal subjects following endotracheal intubation. *Anesthesiology* 1980;52:27–35.

Jardin F, Farcot J-C, Boisante L, et al. Influence of positive-end expiratory pressure on left ventricular performance. *N Engl J Med* 1981;304:387–392.

Marsh HM, Gillespie DJ, Baumgartner AE. Timing of tracheostomy in the critically ill patient. *Chest* 1989;96:190–193.

O'Connor MF, Ovassapian A. Airway management. In: Hall JB, Schmidt GA, Wood LDH, eds., *Principles of Critical Care*, 3rd ed. New York, NY: McGraw-Hill; 2005: 465–480.

Schwartz DE, Matthay MA, Cohen NH. Death and other complications of emergency airway management in critically ill adults. *Anesthesiology* 1995;82:367–376.

3 RESUSCITATION

Steven Q. Davis

KEY POINTS

- Survival to discharge after cardiac arrest is still an uncommon event.
- Early response and use of ACLS protocols is the key to patient survival.
- Patients at risk for sudden cardiac death should be evaluated for automatic internal cardiac defibrillators (AICDs).

EPIDEMIOLOGY

- Overall, 44% of 14,720 adult in-hospital cardiac arrest victims had a return of spontaneous circulation, but only 17% survived to hospital discharge.
- Ventricular fibrillation (VF) was the initial lethal rhythm in 16% of victims, of whom 34% survived to discharge.
- The survival numbers for out-of-hospital arrests are much lower.

PREVENTION

- Patients frequently exhibit signs and symptoms of deterioration up to 12 hours before they suffer an arrest.
- These may include:
  - Vital sign changes
    - Progressive hypotension
    - Tachycardia
    - Hypothermia
    - Hypoxemia
    - Tachypnea
  - Mental status changes
  - Progressive dyspnea

PROGNOSIS

- The most important intervention is the rapid application of advanced cardiac life support (ACLS) protocols, particularly early defibrillation.
- Time from notification of the arrest to first shock ideally should be <5 minutes.
- This principle has lead to the development and public availability of automatic external defibrillators (AEDs) for first responders.

TREATMENT

- Treatment of an arrested patient begins with the ABCs (Airway, Breathing, and Circulation). A practitioner of critical care should be familiar with all ACLS guidelines for cardiac arrest and resuscitation.
- Calling for immediate assistance is very important. A successful resuscitation is usually a team effort.
- A clear "leader" or "runner" for the code needs to be established. One person is in charge of orders and directing the team, while other members of the team focus on the needed activities.
  - Airway management
  - Intravenous access
  - Chest compressions
  - Drug administration
  - Transcribing and recording
  - Family counseling
- Initially, the airway should be managed with a bag-valve-mask to ensure the airway is patent. A skilled operator well versed in bagging while maintaining a patent airway should perform this. The airway should then be secured with an endotracheal tube as soon as is feasible.
- 100% FiO_2 should be delivered via either the bag-valve-mask or the endotracheal tube.
- As a general rule, the radial pulse disappears at a pressure of 80 mmHg, the femoral at 70, and the carotid at 60. If the carotid pulse cannot be felt, compressions should be initiated at a rate of 100 beats per minute with a depth of 1–2 in. Attention should be paid to the quality of compressions as they are often inadequate.
- End-tidal carbon dioxide measurement (capnography) can be used to assess the adequacy of the circulation (either native or via compressions). A low (<10 mmHg) end-tidal carbon dioxide level portends a dismal prognosis.
- Large bore IV access should be obtained as soon as possible.
  - If a large bore central catheter is chosen, the optimal site is the femoral vein, since other sites will be difficult due to chest compressions and airway management.
  - A triple lumen catheter is not a large bore catheter.
  - If a central catheter is not possible, 14–18 gauge peripheral IV access is acceptable.
- Once an IV access is established, the patient should receive at least 500–1000 cc of normal saline or lactated Ringer over a few minutes (wide open, not on an infusion pump).
- If an intravenous catheter is placed during a resuscitation attempt, it should be considered a nonsterile line and removed no later than 8 hours after successful resuscitation.
  - As the patient is stabilized, sterile insertion of any monitoring devices should be obtained. It is a "general rule" that any device inserted during a patient resuscitation is contaminated.
- ACLS protocols should be followed throughout the resuscitation event, realizing that different algorithms will be employed as the patient moves though various arrhythmias.
- Particular attention should be given to finding a cause for pulseless electrical activity (PEA). These include: cardiac tamponade, drug overdose, hyperkalemia, hypothermia, hypovolemia, hypoxia, massive pulmonary embolism, myocardial infarction, and tension pneumothorax. Hypovolemia and hypoxemia are the most likely etiologies for inpatients (Box 3-1).
- When making the decision to terminate resuscitation efforts, the team leader should verbally summarize efforts so far, and ask for any further suggestions from other members of the team.
- A debriefing session should occur shortly after the resuscitation attempt, preferably while every member of the team is still near the location of the resuscitation. If applicable, records should be forwarded to the hospital's cardiopulmonary resuscitation (CPR) committee for quality review.
- Biphasic defibrillators are becoming more prevalent. Hospital personnel involved in resuscitation will need to become familiar with them.
- AEDs are becoming more prevalent in the community, and significantly reduce the time to first shock.

BOX 3-1 Causes of PEA Arrest: The Differential Diagnosis for PEA

Mechanical
Pulmonary embolism (e.g., clot, air, and amniotic fluid)
Pericardial tamponade
Tension pneumothorax
Myocardial infarction
Auto-PEEP

Systemic
Drug overdose
Hyperkalemia
Hypothermia
Hypovolemia
Hypoxemia

OTHER CONCERNS AND INTERVENTIONS

- A new model has emerged for cardiac arrest, breaking it down into three core components:
  - Electrical (first 4 minutes)
  - Circulatory (4–10 minutes)
  - Metabolic phase (after 10 minutes)

- The most important therapeutic intervention during the electrical phase is defibrillation for VF/ventricular tachycardia (VT).
- Somewhat in discord with the American Heart Association guidelines, the circulatory phase appears to be treated most effectively initially with CPR and ventilation, then defibrillation several minutes later.
- Ischemia and reperfusion injury become apparent during the metabolic phase. Induced hypothermia may have a role in the treatment of this phase of arrest.
  - Subjects cooled to 32–34°C after their arrest had a survival benefit (see Chap. 69 on therapeutic hypothermia).
- Resuscitation personnel must stay current with resuscitation protocols (i.e., ACLS, pediatric advanced life support [PALS], and neonatal advanced life support [NALS]). Recommendations for pharmacologic intervention change at regular intervals.
- Thrombolytic therapy should be considered if there is a strong suspicion for pulmonary embolism as the etiology for cardiac arrest.
- When having end-of-life discussions with patients and their family, it is of paramount importance to remember that "do not resuscitate" does NOT mean "do not treat."

BIBLIOGRAPHY

ACLS Guidelines: The American Heart Association.

Peberdy MA, Kaye W, Ornato JP. Cardiopulmonary resuscitation of adults in the hospital. *Resuscitation* 2003;58:297–308.

4 FLUID THERAPY

E. Mirnalini Mohanraj

KEY POINTS

- The need for intravenous fluids should be judged initially and reassessed frequently.
- In severe sepsis, urgent fluid resuscitation may reduce subsequent mortality.
- Right atrial and pulmonary wedge pressures are poor predictors of fluid responsiveness.
- Dynamic indicators, such as the inspiratory fall in right atrial pressure (in the spontaneously breathing patient) or the arterial pulse pressure variation (in the passively ventilated patient), are superior to static pressure measurements.
- Maintenance fluids are rarely appropriate, given the large volume of obligatory fluids infused into most critically ill patients.
- Colloids offer no advantage over crystalloids.

INTRAVENOUS FLUID THERAPY

- Several considerations should enter into every decision to employ intravenous (IV) fluid therapy in critically ill patients.
- Initially, the patients' intravascular volume state and their likelihood of responding to IV fluid therapy should be assessed.
- Secondly, both the type of fluid to be used and the rate at which the infusion occurs should be determined.
- These decisions are highly dependent on the underlying disease process and severity of illness. As with all therapies, IV fluid therapy should be individualized on a case-by-case basis.

ASSESSMENT OF INTRAVASCULAR VOLUME

- Historical data, physical examination, and laboratory data should be used as the initial means of assessing volume status. The following factors should be addressed when performing an initial history and physical examination:
- Historical data
  - Decrease in oral intake
  - Dizziness
  - Syncope
  - Confusion or change in mental status
  - Vomiting or diarrhea
  - Polyuria
  - Bleeding (hematemesis, hematochezia, melena, other)
  - Recent change or noncompliance with medications
- Physical examination findings
  - General appearance
  - Altered mental status
  - Vital signs with attention to orthostatics and tachycardia
  - Oliguria or anuria
  - Skin turgor
  - Mucous membranes
  - Jugular venous pressure
  - Cardiac examination (tachycardia, murmurs, extra heart sounds)
  - Pulmonary examination (crackles, effusion)

- Peripheral perfusion (capillary refill, peripheral pulses)
- Peripheral edema
- Evidence of bleeding (gross blood on rectal examination, hematemesis, hemoptysis)

- Laboratory data
  - An increased blood urea nitrogen (BUN) to creatinine ratio of >20 may suggest acute renal insufficiency that is secondary to volume depletion. This finding, however, is not specific as there are other causes for an elevation of the BUN that is out of proportion to the creatinine.
  - A decreased hematocrit may be an indicator of bleeding as a cause of volume depletion. Such a finding should prompt re-evaluation of the patient's intravascular volume status and the need for transfusion.
  - An elevated hematocrit may be a sign of hemoconcentration, but this finding is not specific to volume depletion and should not be used alone as a reliable indicator of intravascular volume.
- Central venous pressure (CVP)
  - The CVP as a surrogate for right atrial pressure is frequently used as an estimate for intravascular volume. The relationship is poor, however, perhaps reflecting the vagaries of ventricular dysfunction, pericardial disease, pulmonary disease, and the effects of positive pressure ventilation.
  - Changes in the right atrial pressure may be used during resuscitation to assess adequacy of volume expansion (e.g., increased CVP indicates improved intravascular status).
  - A study of 33 spontaneously breathing patients looked at the ability of the inspiratory fall in CVP to predict fluid responsiveness. An inspiratory fall in right atrial pressure of >1 mmHg indicated that the patient would likely have an increase in perfusion in response to rapidly infused saline. Those whose CVP did not fall during inspiration did not respond to fluid.
- Pulmonary artery catheters (PACs) have been used to measure pulmonary capillary wedge pressure (PCWP) as an estimation of left atrial pressure and left ventricular end-diastolic volume and subsequently as an estimate of intravascular volume.
- There are limitations to this practice, causing PACs to be used less frequently as the standard for assessing volume status. Limitations to use of PACs include the following:
  - Technical (zero, level).
  - Inappropriate interpretation (i.e., failure to read at end-expiration)
  - PEEP (end-expiratory pressure) and auto-PEEP (positive end-expiratory pressure) may alter the true value.
  - PCWP represents a pressure not a volume.
  - PCWP is a very poor predictor of patient responsiveness to volume.
  - Recent studies of patients with sepsis, acute respiratory distress syndrome (ARDS), or undergoing high-risk operative procedures have failed to confirm earlier concerns about harm due to the catheter, but also, without exception, have shown that patients do not benefit from PAC-derived information.
  - While further studies are underway to assess the benefits and risks of using PACs, the current data indicate that alternate measures of intravascular volume may be necessary.
- Many of these traditional methods for assessing intravascular volume are unreliable measures that do not reflect true intravascular volume and do not indicate a patient's potential responsiveness to volume resuscitation.
- Dynamic measures, such as the change in arterial pulse pressure or systolic pressure during passive ventilator breaths, seem much more reliable than static measures such as the CVP or wedge pressure.

MAINTENANCE FLUIDS

- Traditionally, the continuous infusion of IV fluids was thought to be a relatively benign intervention.
- Maintenance fluid therapy has been routinely advocated for pre- and postoperative treatment as well as for empiric treatment for patients with poor to little oral intake while in the hospital.
- More recent data reveal that empiric use of maintenance fluids without clinical evidence of intravascular depletion puts patients at risk for multiple complications as well as increasing their mortality.
- Inappropriate volume expansion in an intravascularly replete patient can lead to volume overload and secondary complications including third-spacing of fluid, pulmonary edema, myocardial dysfunction, and limited diffusion of oxygen to tissues.
- Studies on surgical patients have shown that there are correlations between postoperative weight increases and mortality.
  - A multicenter trial evaluated postoperative complications and mortality in patients randomized to either a standard IV fluid regimen or a restricted IV fluid regimen (aimed to maintain preoperative weight).
  - There were significantly fewer cardiopulmonary and tissue-healing complications in the restricted group.
- This and additional studies advocate a more cautious approach to IV fluids and the avoidance of routine use of maintenance fluids.
- Each patient should receive at minimum a daily assessment of his or her intravascular and total body

volume status and IV fluid therapy for the purposes of volume expansion should be only administered when there is true evidence for volume depletion.
- IV maintenance fluids should not be used as a surrogate for enteral or parenteral nutrition.

FLUIDS IN THE CRITICALLY ILL PATIENT

- Clinically significant volume depletion often develops when large amounts of volume are lost via gastrointestinal tract, skin (burn patients), hemorrhage, or third-space sequestration. Signs and symptoms of serious volume loss and possible tissue ischemia may include:
  - Hypotension
  - Oliguria or anuria
  - Altered mental status
  - Renal dysfunction
  - Cardiac ischemia
  - Other organ system failure
  - Decreased peripheral perfusion
- Rapid assessment of intravascular volume status and rapid fluid resuscitation is necessary to avoid progression toward acute ischemic injuries and hypovolemic shock.
- While the usefulness of traditional methods for volume assessment (see above) should not be minimized, data suggest these measures may be inadequate.
- An alternate technique using pulse pressure variation (PPV) has been proposed as a means to assess intravascular volume status.
  - In intubated patients, the PPV with each ventilator breath is a superior measure of intravascular volume and a better predictor of responsiveness to fluid therapy than right atrial pressure, systolic blood pressure, or PCWP.
  - The PPV can be easily and accurately measured in patients with an indwelling arterial catheter.
  - A study of 40 mechanically ventilated patients with circulatory failure secondary to sepsis presented the PPV as a simple and effective means of predicting clinical responsiveness to fluid resuscitation.
  - A PPV value of 13% or greater allowed reliable discrimination between patients who would and would not respond to fluid resuscitation.
  - Reliable prediction of responsiveness to IV fluid therapy is essential for rapid resuscitation of patients with true volume depletion.
  - PPV is an equally important predictor of nonresponders to volume expansion.
  - Identifying nonresponders prevents unnecessary resuscitation that may result in volume overload and secondary complications including third-spacing of fluid, pulmonary edema, myocardial dysfunction, and limited diffusion of oxygen to tissues.

CRYSTALLOID FLUIDS

- Crystalloid fluids are primarily composed of sodium chloride (NaCl) and pass readily between the intravascular and extravascular compartments.
- Administration of IV crystalloid follows the same bodily distribution as interstitial fluids, with 75% of the infused water and electrolytes passing to the interstitial space and 25% remaining in the intravascular space.
- Given this pattern of distribution, patients undergoing large volume fluid resuscitation are at high risk for developing pulmonary and generalized interstitial edema, particularly with a preexisting state of fluid overload (e.g., congestive heart failure and renal failure).
  - Isotonic saline (0.9% NaCl) is the most commonly used crystalloid fluid. It is actually slightly more tonic and acidic than plasma; these variations are clinically negligible. The high chloride content may induce a hyperchloremic metabolic acidosis with infusion of large volumes of isotonic saline.
  - Lactated Ringer solution has an electrolyte composition which mimics the ionic concentrations of calcium, potassium, and chloride in plasma more closely than isotonic saline. The added lactate is converted to bicarbonate by the liver. The intention was for the bicarbonate to act as a buffer in patients with metabolic acidosis; however, this effect is not a clinically significant one. Furthermore, the added calcium may act as a binder for many drugs and impair both bioavailability and efficacy.
  - Normosol/Plasmalyte are solutions supplemented with magnesium and altered with buffering agents that mimic the pH of plasma. They are not readily available and are not superior to unbuffered solutions. Similarly, IV or oral magnesium supplementation is preferred as it is more readily titratable to individual patient laboratory abnormalities. These solutions are contraindicated in patients with renal failure due to the risk of causing hypermagnesemia.
  - Dextrose solutions were previously used frequently as a source of nonprotein caloric intake for critically ill patients. Complete enteral or parenteral feeding is now the "standard of care" for providing adequate nutrition in the intensive care unit. While IV dextrose solutions are still beneficial in the management of glucose-deficient states, it is the least potent volume expander of the crystalloid solutions. Additionally, there are several adverse effects including increased production of carbon dioxide,

increased lactate production, and cell dehydration due the infusion of a hypertonic solution.

COLLOID FLUIDS

- Colloid fluids contain large molecules that do not diffuse as readily between the intravascular and extravascular compartments.
- Colloid solutions are assigned a colloid oncotic pressure (COP) based on molecular weight and ability to draw fluid into the intravascular space.
  - Albumin is a physiologic transport protein that is responsible for the major oncotic pressure in plasma. A 5% albumin solution has a COP of 20 mmHg, similar to plasma. Approximately 50% of this solution will remain in the intravascular compartment. A 25% albumin solution has a COP of 70 mmHg and may transiently increase the plasma volume by up to five times the amount of volume infused. However, due to the mechanism of expansion, the added volume is drawn from the interstitial space and is not recommended for volume resuscitation purposes, particularly in hypovolemic patients.
  - Hetastarch (6% hetastarch in isotonic saline) is a synthetic colloid solution composed of amylopectin molecules of varying sizes. Its COP of 30 mmHg is slightly higher than that of 5% albumin and theoretically causes a greater volume expansion. While its half-life is 17 days, its oncotic effects last no longer than 24 hours. Elevated amylase levels may be expected after infusion as the enzyme is responsible for cleavage of amylopectin prior to renal excretion. This should resolve within 1 week. Other documented side effects include rare episodes of anaphylaxis and prolonged partial thromboplastin time without associated bleeding.
  - The dextrans are hyperoncotic solutions composed of glucose polymers diluted in isotonic saline. Their high COP (40 mmHg) was thought to induce a larger plasma volume expansion than crystalloid solutions, 5% albumin or hetastarch. However, the effects are short-lived and associated with multiple side effects including anaphylaxis, increased risk of bleeding due to impaired platelet aggregation, reduced activation of factor VIII, and increased fibrinolysis, elevated ESR, and rare renal failure.

CRYSTALLOID vs. COLLOID

- While both crystalloid and colloid solutions are used frequently for volume resuscitation, there has been longstanding controversy regarding the effects of these solutions on morbidity and mortality.
- One of the strongest arguments against the use of crystalloid fluids has been that they cause a dilutional hypoalbuminemia that puts patients at increased risk for developing pulmonary edema. Physiologically speaking, this is not the case.
  - Alveolar capillaries have a high permeability to albumin and as a patient becomes hypoalbuminemic, there is concomitant loss of protein from the lung interstitium.
  - The oncotic pressure gradient of the alveoli and subcutaneous tissue decrease in parallel and infusion of crystalloid solutions does not pose a higher risk of developing pulmonary edema.
- Multiple studies now indicate that there are no benefits from using colloid rather than crystalloid solutions.
  - The *SAFE (Saline vs. Albumin Fluid Evaluation) Study* was a multicenter, randomized, double-blind trial that compared mortality outcomes of medical and surgical ICU patients. All patients were hypovolemic and received either 4% albumin or isotonic saline. There was no significant differences at 28 days in all-cause deaths, single-organ or multiple-organ failure, duration in the ICU or hospital, days of renal-replacement therapy or days of mechanical ventilation.
  - A meta-analysis of 55 randomized-controlled trials compiled data on 3504 patients treated with either albumin or crystalloid solutions for volume expansion. There was no significant difference in outcomes or mortality.
- Given these data, crystalloid solutions are generally the preferred agent for initial volume expansion in patients who are not bleeding. There is no mortality benefit to using colloid solutions and crystalloid solutions are readily accessible and markedly less expensive.

BIBLIOGRAPHY

Brandstrup B, Tonnesen H, Beier-Holgersen R, et al. Effects of intravenous fluid restriction on postoperative complications: comparison of two perioperative fluid regimens. *Ann Surg* 2003;238:641–648.

Connors AF Jr, Speroff T, Dawson NV, et al. The effectiveness of right heart catheterization in the initial care of critically ill patients. SUPPORT Investigators. *JAMA* 1996;276:889–897.

Finfer S, Bellomo R, Boyce N, et al. SAFE Study Investigators. A comparison of albumin and saline for fluid resuscitation in the intensive care unit. *N Engl J Med* 2004;250:2247–2256.

Guyton AC, Hall JE, eds., *Textbook of Medical Physiology*, 11th ed. Philadelphia, PA: W.B. Saunders; 2005.

Kramer A, Zygun D, Hawes H, et al. Pulse pressure variation predicts fluid responsiveness following coronary artery bypass surgery. *Chest* 2004;126:1563–1568.

Marino PL. *The ICU Book*, 2nd ed. Philadelphia, PA: Lippincott Williams & Wilkins; 1998: 228–241.

Michard F, Boussat S, Chemla D, et al. Relation between respiratory changes in arterial pulse pressure and fluid responsiveness in septic patients with acute circulatory failure. *Am J Respir Crit Care Med* 2000;162:134–138.

Michard F, Teboul JL. Predicting fluid responsiveness in ICU patients: a critical analysis of the evidence. *Chest* 2002;121: 2000–2008.

Raper R, Sibbald WJ. Misled by the wedge? The Swan-Ganz catheter and left ventricular preload. *Chest* 1986;89:427–434.

Richard C, Warszawski J, Anguel N, et al. Early the pulmonary artery catheter and outcomes in patients with shock and acute respiratory distress syndrome: a randomized controlled trial. *JAMA* 2003;190:2713–2720.

Rose BD, Post TL. *Clinical Physiology of Acid-Base and Electrolyte Disorders*, 5th ed. New York, NY: McGraw-Hill; 2001:441–442.

Sandham JD, Hull RD, Brant RF, et al., for the Canadian Critical Care Clinical Trials Group. A randomized, controlled trial of the use of pulmonary-artery catheters in high-risk surgical patients. *N Engl J Med* 2003;348:5–14.

5 PAIN MANAGEMENT

D. Kyle Hogarth

KEY POINTS

- Almost all patients admitted to an ICU will experience some form of pain.
- Causes include any underlying disease process, trauma, a surgical incision, an invasive procedure, the presence of the endotracheal tube, and airway suctioning.
- The Joint Commission for Accreditation of Health Care Organizations (JCAHO) has mandated the monitoring of pain in all patients.
- Surveys of patients indicate recall of significant unrelieved pain in the ICU.

PAIN AND CARDIAC MORBIDITY

- The stress response from pain causes activation of the sympathetic nervous system with increases in heart rate, blood pressure, myocardial contractility, and myocardial oxygen consumption.
- The stress response to pain may be enough to induce cardiac ischemia or infarction depending on limits of oxygen supply to the myocardium (e.g., hypotension, anemia, and hypoxemia).
- Opioid medications can lower blood pressure and afterload via venous and arterial dilation and can diminish oxygen consumption by the myocardium via a decreased heart rate through a direct sinoatrial node effect and through sympatholysis.

PAIN AND RESPIRATORY DYSFUNCTION

- Major abdominal and thoracic surgeries will result in abnormal pulmonary function.
- A general rule is the closer the surgery to the diaphragm, the more likely the pulmonary dysfunction.
- These abnormalities result from spasm and splinting of abdominal and intercostal muscles, limited diaphragm movement, and pain.
- Forced expired volume in one second (FEV_1) and forced vital capacity (FVC) can decline by 60% of their preoperative level, and functional residual capacity (FRC) can decline by 30% in thoracic and upper abdominal procedures. Lower abdominal procedures will result in 30% and 10% declines in FVC and FEV_1, respectively.

VENTILATED PATIENTS AND PAIN CONTROL

- In ventilated patients, a frequently overlooked cause of agitation is pain, and assessing adequacy of analgesia is an important part of the continuous assessment of a patient. Remember, the patient "bucking the vent" may be in pain.
- None of the drugs commonly used for sedation provide analgesia.
- Opioid medications have demonstrated synergistic effects with sedative drugs, particularly benzodiazepines, and combined use of an analgesic and sedative often results in lesser doses of each.
- In some patients, an opioid analgesic alone will achieve both pain control and tranquility.
- Almost every patient admitted to an ICU on a ventilator should receive opioid medications.

ASSESSMENT OF PAIN

- Pain should be assessed and managed in all patients.
- Rating Scales for pain assessment are most often employed as they are easy to use and have been shown to be very reliable.
- The Visual Analog Scale is most often used, ranking pain from extremes of "no pain" to "worst pain I have ever had" along a horizontal scale.
- Pain can be difficult to assess in the ICU, especially if patients are being sedated for ventilation.

COMPLICATIONS OF PAIN CONTROL

- Ensuring the control of pain for the patient may result in some complications. While the goal is to provide adequate pain relief, too much opioid may increase the likelihood of complications. For this reason, the pain of the patient should be continuously assessed so that the patient may remain on the optimal dose of opioid.
- The principal concern arising from the administration of opioids is the effect these drugs have on central respiratory drive. If the patient is not being mechanically ventilated, these drugs should be administered in a controlled setting by experienced personnel.
- Naloxone needs to be available for emergency administration in any patient receiving narcotics. However, naloxone administration can result in pulmonary edema, hypertension, and tachycardia.
- The continuous infusion of opioids often results in decreased gastrointestinal motility and may interfere with the administration of enteral nutrition. Opioids often cause nausea as well. The use of promotility agents, antinausea medications, and bowel stimulants may be able to overcome these effects.
- The continuous infusion of opioids raises the possibility of a patient developing a physical addiction to these medications.
- The agitation and restlessness of a ventilated patient during liberation from mechanical ventilation may relate in large part to withdrawal symptoms. This problem can affect patient populations of all ages.
- The majority of patients exhibiting withdrawal from opioids will either have had significant exposure prior to their critical illness, or will have received high doses of drugs for more than 3–5 days during their ICU management.
- The incidence of withdrawal symptoms has been shown to increase with concurrent use of neuromuscular blockade and prolonged use of sedatives and analgesics.
- Concern for the development of possible addiction should not result in the under dosing of narcotic for pain.

METHODS OF PAIN CONTROL

- *Intravenous opioids*. This allows titration of the medication to the desirable level that provides adequate analgesia. Medication can be administered via as-needed boluses or as a continuous infusion. A continuous infusion often provides more relief and fewer side effects as it avoids the peaks and troughs of drug levels associated with boluses.
- *Patient controlled analgesia (PCA)*. If a patient is conscious and able to manipulate the PCA machine, this method of analgesia is superior for pain relief. Besides the potential psychological effect of the patient "being in control," the PCA has been shown to be superior to other methods of pain control in some studies. Overdoses are rare and are usually associated with machine or physician errors.
- *Intramuscular opioids*. This is not a desirable way to administer pain medications as the absorption of drug can be extremely variable.
- *Epidural anesthesia*. It can provide complete thoracic, abdominal, and lower extremity pain relief while minimizing the risk of respiratory suppression.
- Epidural anesthesia can cause hypotension, urinary retention, and motor blockade. Rarely, spinal or epidural hematomas can form that may lead to irreversible neurologic injury. Muscle weakness, pain, and sensory deficits are usual symptoms. Hematomas occur more often in patients with coagulation abnormalities.
- Intercostal blockade is best employed for localized pain involving thoracic dermatomes, such as lateral thoracotomies and rib fractures. Injection of bupivacaine into the intercostal space can provide relief for 6–12 hours. Pneumothorax is a rare complication of intercostal blockade.

MEDICATIONS FOR PAIN CONTROL

- Morphine is the most commonly used medication for pain control in the ICU. It is relatively inexpensive and most physicians are comfortable with the drug.
- Morphine is highly soluble in water, resulting in slower membrane penetration. Therefore, the peak onset of morphine is around 30 minutes with effects lasting 2–4 hours.
- Other commonly used opioid drugs include fentanyl and hydromorphone.
- Fentanyl has a rapid onset of action, within 2–5 minutes with an effect lasting 30–45 minutes. Fentanyl does not cause the release of histamine.
- Meperidine should not be used in the ICU. The prodrug and active metabolite accumulate in patients with renal dysfunction, a common occurrence in the critically ill. The accumulation may result in prolonged opioid effect as well as neurotoxicity which may manifest as delirium, myoclonus, and seizures (Table 5-1).

BIBLIOGRAPHY

Gehlbach B, Kress JP. Pain control, sedation, and use of muscle relaxants. In: Hall JB, Schmidt GA, Wood LDH, eds., *Principles of Critical Care*, 3rd ed. New York, NY: McGraw-Hill; 2005: 139–163.

TABLE 5-1 Comparison of Commonly Used Intravenous Opioid Medications in the ICU

DRUG	PEAK EFFECT	ELIMINATION HALF-LIFE	MINIMAL SUGGESTED DOSE
Morphine	30 min	2–4 h	1–4 mg bolus 1–10 mg/h infusion
Fentanyl	3 min	1–2 h	25–100 μg bolus 25–200 μg/h infusion
Hydromorphone	20 min	2–4 h	0.2–1 mg bolus 0.2–2 mg/h infusion
Pentazocine	3 min	2–3 h	30 mg bolus, no infusion
Butorphanol	5 min	3–4 h	1 mg bolus, no infusion
Ketorolac (nonsteroidal anti-inflammatory drug [NSAID])	2 h	6–8 h	30 mg bolus, no infusion

SOURCE: Modified from Liu LL, Gropper MA. Postoperative analgesia and sedation in the adult intensive care unit: a guide to drug selection. *Drugs* 2003;63:755–767.

Hogarth DK, Hall JB. Management of sedation in mechanically ventilated patients. *Curr Opin Crit Care* 2004;10:40–46.
Liu LL, Gropper MA. Postoperative analgesia and sedation in the adult intensive care unit: a guide to drug selection. *Drugs* 2003;63:755–767.

6 SEDATION MANAGEMENT IN THE ICU

D. Kyle Hogarth

KEY POINTS

- Most critically ill patients can be assumed to experience pain: analgesics should often be given before sedatives.
- Sedative use is often complicated by prolonged depression of consciousness.
- Sedative choice depends on goals, drug half-life, cardiovascular stability, and organ (especially liver and renal) dysfunction.
- A daily sedative interruption reduces time on the ventilator and duration of ICU stay.
- The depth of sedation should be monitored objectively and documented frequently.

INTRODUCTION

- The need for mechanical ventilation is one of the principal reasons a patient is admitted to the intensive care unit (ICU).
- No matter what the indication for intubation, providing the patient adequate comfort while being mechanically ventilated is imperative.
- Many patients have memory of being uncomfortable while in the ICU, but this may in part relate to inadequate analgesia as opposed to inadequate sedation.
- The majority of patients admitted to an ICU for mechanical ventilation will receive one or more sedative medications.
- The drugs used for sedation and analgesia in the ICU have a broad range of half lives. Metabolism of these drugs can be impaired as there is frequent organ failure associated with critical illness.

WHY SEDATE?

- Adequate sedation to facilitate care by the ICU team is imperative to ensure the patient receives safe and proper care.
- Being on a ventilator can be very anxiety provoking, and patients on mechanical ventilation can be confused and delirious, and sometimes combative and violent.
- A patient's need for sedating medication can be high, depending on the indication for intubation. For example, a patient in acute respiratory distress syndrome (ARDS) undergoing a strategy of permissive hypercapnia during mechanical ventilation may require more sedative to overcome the respiratory drive from a climbing CO_2 while a long-term emphysema patient may require little or no sedation for ventilatory failure.
- The traumatic self-removal of an endotracheal tube puts the patient at risk for vocal cord trauma, aspiration, bleeding, hypoxia, and can be life threatening.

- Unintended removal of arterial and venous catheters can result in bleeding, interruption of medications, and require additional procedures to replace these catheters.
- Ensuring patient comfort can minimize the need for physical restraints. Restraints can have a negative impact on post-ICU psychological recovery and family members are often concerned about physical restraints.
- While some physicians advocate complete amnesia as a goal of sedation, this may carry adverse consequences. Lack of memory of a critical illness may predispose patients to long-term psychological problems.
- In all patients receiving neuromuscular blockade (NMB), complete and deep sedation is mandatory.

COMPLICATIONS OF SEDATION

- A common complication of sedation is drug accumulation with protracted depression of central nervous system function.
- Continuous infusion of sedation has been associated with prolonged time on the ventilator, prolonged ICU stays, prolonged hospital stays, increased utilization of diagnostic procedures and imaging modalities, and difficulty in adequately monitoring a patient's neurologic function.
- The continuous infusion of opioids and benzodiazepines can cause a physical addiction to these medications. This problem can affect patient populations of all ages. The majority of patients exhibiting withdrawal from opioids and benzodiazepines will either have had significant exposure prior to their critical illness, or will have received high doses of drugs for more than 3–5 days during their ICU management.

MEDICATIONS FOR SEDATION

- Pain should always be assessed before the use of sedatives. A common cause of patient agitation and "bucking the vent" is inadequate analgesia. Opioids and benzodiazepines have synergistic effects allowing for lower doses of both drugs to be used.
- Opioid drugs (morphine, methadone, hydromorphone, fentanyl) are used in most critically ill patients. Meperidine should not be used as the prodrug and active metabolite accumulate in patients with renal dysfunction. This can result in prolonged opioid effect as well as neurotoxicity, including delirium, myoclonus, and seizures.
- Benzodiazepines (diazepam, lorazepam, midazolam) are frequently used to provide anxiolysis. These drugs provide no pain relief. Drug metabolism kinetics and the volume of distribution of benzodiazepine drugs change during critical illness, especially in patients with impaired renal and hepatic function. Even drugs considered "ultra-short-acting" when given as a single bolus (such as midazolam) may accumulate when given by continuous infusion or repeated bolus in the critically ill patient.
- Propofol is an alkylphenol anesthetic that provides *no analgesia*. When used concurrently with opioids, patients may require higher analgesic dosing than with benzodiazepines. It has a short half-life and a rapid onset of action, but has not been shown to be superior to other sedating agents.
- The ventilatory depression of propofol can be profound, and it should only be used in a patient with a secured airway or with staff immediately available to intubate.
- Propofol is insoluble in water, so it is delivered in a lipid emulsion, which can lead to elevated triglyceride levels. Patients on TPN must have their lipid infusion adjusted if receiving propofol and all patients receiving propofol should have baseline, 72 hours, and then weekly triglyceride levels measured and if significant elevations occur, the infusion should be stopped.
- A dose of 75 μg/kg/min is a recommended maximum to minimize the possibility of a Propofol Infusion Syndrome: profound myocardial failure and severe lactic acidosis.
- Haloperidol has no analgesic or amnesic properties, and has a long half-life. Patients receiving haloperidol demonstrate indifference to their surrounding environment, and may even have cataleptic immobility, making it difficult to perform pain and sedation assessment. Haloperidol is useful for acute agitation and treating patients with psychotic behavior, but should not be used as a primary agent for sedation.
- Extrapyramidal effects, hypotension, and prolongation of the QT-interval limit the usefulness of haloperidol in the ICU. In one study, an incidence of torsades de pointes of 3.6% was seen with haloperidol use.
- Gas anesthesia (e.g., isoflurane) is a very effective sedative. For practical reasons related to maintaining a closed inhalation-exhalation circuit, its use is not routine in the ICU.
- Dexmedetomidine is a lipophilic derivative of imidazole, recently approved for use in the United States that has a high affinity for α_2-adrenoreceptors, with sedative, analgesic, and sympatholytic effects.
- In early studies in the ICU and the operating room, dexmedetomidine has been shown to reduce the quantity of IV sedation, inhalation anesthesia, and IV opioid administered, while also providing anxiolysis, improved perioperative hemodynamic stability, and no suppression of respiratory drive.

TABLE 6-1 Comparison of Commonly Used Medications for Sedation in the ICU

DRUG	PEAK EFFECT	ELIMINATION HALF-LIFE	MINIMAL SUGGESTED DOSE
Diazepam	3–5 min	20–40 h	5–10 mg bolus Infusion not recommended
Midazolam	2–5 min	3–5 h	1–2 mg bolus 0.5–10 mg/h infusion
Lorazepam	2–20 min	10–20 h	1–2 mg bolus 0.5–10 mg/h infusion
Propofol	90 s	20–30 h	Bolus not recommended 25–100 mg/kg/min infusion
Dexmedetomidine	60 s	2 h	1 mg/kg bolus over 10 min 0.2–0.7 mg/kg/min infusion

SOURCE: Modified from Liu LL, Gropper MA. Postoperative analgesia and sedation in the adult intensive care unit: a guide to drug selection. *Drugs* 2003;63:755–767.

- While initial data regarding dexmedetomidine are promising, the lack of large randomized trials demonstrating decreased mechanical ventilation time precludes recommending the routine use of this medication at present (Table 6-1).

MONITORING OF SEDATION

- Early use of a spontaneous breathing trial (SBT) reduces time spent on the ventilator. However, in order to perform a SBT, the patient should be awake and interactive with care providers. Patients often receive continuous infusions of sedative medications in the ICU, but this has been shown to lead to prolonged intubation and mechanical ventilation.
- Various scales to assess level of sedation have been developed, all with the goal of permitting the bedside clinician to adjust sedative dose to achieve adequate but not excessive sedation. A majority of the literature regarding sedation has used the Ramsay Sedation Scale, developed in 1974. However, the Ramsay scale was not originally intended to be used as a tool for clinical monitoring, and has not been rigorously tested for reliability and validity.
- Recently, The Richmond Agitation and Sedation Scale (RASS) was introduced and has proven to be a useful bedside tool in the management of sedation (Table 6-2). This is a 10-point scale that is rated using three well-defined steps. RASS has been validated and shown to be reliable across multiple different observers.

MANAGEMENT OF SEDATION

- A protocol-driven approach to mechanical ventilation and SBTs leads to reduced time on the ventilator, but over-sedation remained a principal reason for failure to implement successful weaning.
- Kress and colleagues clearly demonstrated that the daily interruption of continuous sedation decreased the length of time on the ventilator, the time in the ICU, and diminished the number of diagnostic tests performed to evaluate why a patient was not waking up once sedatives had been discontinued.

TABLE 6-2 Richmond Agitation–Sedation Scale

SCORE	TERM	DESCRIPTION
+4	Combative	Overtly combative/violent. Danger to staff
+3	Very agitated	Pulls/removes tubes or catheters. Aggressive
+2	Agitated	Nonpurposeful movement. Not synchronous with ventilator
+1	Restless	Anxious, but movements not aggressive/violent
0	Alert and calm	
−1	Drowsy	Sustained awakening (>10 s) with eye contact, to voice
−2	Light sedation	Briefly awakens (<10 s) with eye contact, to voice
−3	Moderate sedation	Movement to voice, but no eye contact
−4	Deep sedation	No response to voice. Movement to physical stimulation
−5	Unarousable	No response to voice or physical stimulation

Procedure:

1. Observe patient. Calm (score zero). Do they have restless or agitated behavior (1–4)
2. If not alert, speak name in loud clear voice, and direct them to look at speaker. Repeat once if necessary. Gauge response (−1 to −3)
3. If no response to voice, then physically stimulate patient. Gauge response (−4 to −5)

SOURCE: Adapted from Sessler CN, Gosnell MS, Grap MJ, et al. The Richmond Agitation-Sedation Scale: validity and reliability in adult intensive care unit patients. *Am J Respir Crit Care Med* 2002;166:1338–1344.

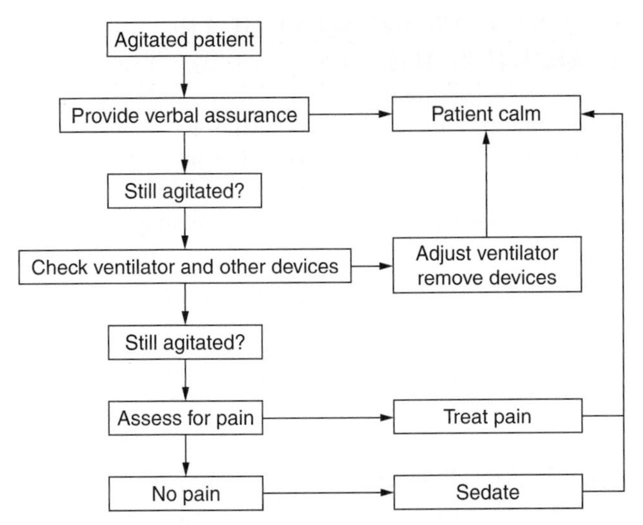

FIG. 6-1 Algorithm for assessing agitated patient on the ventilator.

- The daily interruption protocol involved the daily stopping of the continuous drug infusion (including opiates) and monitoring the patient until they started to show signs of awakening. The drugs were then restarted at half the previous dose and were titrated at the discretion of the bedside nurse to achieve a Ramsay sedation score of 3–4. In comparison to routine management, the daily cessation of drug infusions significantly reduced time on the ventilator and in the ICU, and provided a valuable window of opportunity for assessment of the patient's neurologic function (Fig. 6-1).

BIBLIOGRAPHY

Gehlbach B, Kress JP. Pain control, sedation, and use of muscle relaxants. In: Hall JB, Schmidt GA, Wood LDH, eds., *Principles of Critical Care*, 3rd ed. New York, NY: McGraw-Hill; 2005:139–163.

Hogarth DK, Hall JB. Management of sedation in mechanically ventilated patients. *Curr Opin Crit Care* 2004;10:40–46.

Kress JP, Pohlman AS, O'Connor MF, et al. Daily interruption of sedative infusions in critically ill patients undergoing mechanical ventilation. *N Engl J Med* 2000;342: 1471–1477.

Liu LL, Gropper MA. Postoperative analgesia and sedation in the adult intensive care unit: a guide to drug selection. *Drugs* 2003;63:755–767.

Sessler CN, Gosnell MS, Grap MJ, et al. The Richmond Agitation-Sedation Scale: validity and reliability in adult intensive care unit patients. *Am J Respir Crit Care Med* 2002;166:1338–1344.

7 NEUROMUSCULAR BLOCKADE

Nuala J. Meyer

KEY POINTS

- Neuromuscular blocking drugs are used less often in ICUs due to the frequent complication of acquired weakness
- Neuromuscular blockers can facilitate mechanical ventilation and improve gas exchange in some patients
- Sedatives must always be given along with neuromuscular blockers
- The depth of neuromuscular blockade should be monitored with a peripheral nerve stimulator

MECHANISM OF ACTION

- Neuromuscular blocking agents (NMBs) block transmission of acetylcholine (ACh) at the neuromuscular junction, resulting in the abolition of voluntary muscle control or, in simpler terms, paralysis. At the neuromuscular junction, arrival of a nerve impulse causes the release of ACh from presynaptic terminals, which then crosses the junctional cleft and stimulates the postsynaptic ACh receptors. These postsynaptic receptors allow ions to flow through them and depolarize the motor end plate, resulting in muscle contraction.

NEUROMUSCULAR BLOCKADE IN THE INTENSIVE CARE UNIT

- Neuromuscular blocking agents are commonly used to induce a brief paralysis of the patient for intubation, both for critically ill patients as well as those undergoing elective intubation.
- NMBs are helpful in the management of tetanus, when chest wall rigidity limits adequate ventilation. They are also used to prevent shivering in patients in whom therapeutic cooling is indicated (e.g., following cardiac arrest).
- Use of NMBs in the intensive care unit (ICU) is limited by the frequently reported side effects and complications of such therapy, and by the need to

continuously and carefully monitor the depth of sedation and paralysis. Rarely, NMBs are used to improve ventilation or oxygenation of patients in respiratory failure in the ICU.
- NMBs must be used in conjunction with sedative hypnotic medications with both analgesic and amnestic qualities, and should never be used without deep sedation.
- In the case of severe ventilatory failure, such as status asthmaticus, paralysis with NMBs in conjunction with heavy sedation may allow time for bronchodilator and anti-inflammatory therapy to begin to take effect, while improving lung compliance and allowing a strategy of permissive hypercapnia. Neuromuscular blockade may also distribute blood away from the muscles of respiration—which in respiratory failure can be an enormous source for oxygen consumption—and decrease shock associated with respiratory failure. However, as discussed below, patients who receive both NMBs and corticosteroids, as is often the case in obstructive lung disease, are at an extremely high risk for neurologic complications.
- In hypoxemic respiratory failure such as acute respiratory distress syndrome (ARDS), NMBs may be employed to decrease oxygen consumption, facilitate "lung-protective" ventilation which is often uncomfortable to the patient, and to improve venous oxygen saturation.

COMPLICATIONS OF NEUROMUSCULAR BLOCKADE

- The principal complication of NMBs as used in the ICU is prolonged muscular weakness. Patients may remain partially paralyzed for weeks despite the cessation of NMBs, and may necessitate prolonged rehabilitation or mechanical ventilation.
- Paralysis can be due to the abnormal metabolism of NMBs, or, more commonly, due to the effect of the drug on the neuromuscular unit.
- Asthmatic patients receiving concomitant therapy with NMBs and corticosteroids are at extremely high risk for myopathy and polyneuropathy. Aminoglycoside antibiotics may also confer a higher risk of myopathy.
- NMBs can produce adverse effects at both nicotinic and muscarinic ACh receptors other than those of the neuromuscular junction. Muscarinic blockade may produce tachycardia and hypotension. Histamine release may also occur, causing vasodilation, hypotension, and reflex tachycardia.

SPECIFIC NEUROMUSCULAR BLOCKING AGENTS

- The bulk of clinically useful NMBs act by interfering with the postsynaptic action of ACh on ACh receptors, thereby abolishing the electrical signal from the motor nerve to the muscle. These medicines may be further categorized as the depolarizing blocking agents—medicines which have agonist activity at the ACh receptor and the nondepolarizing agents—those which act by antagonizing or blocking ACh receptors. Both forms of NMBs are discussed here.

SUCCINYLCHOLINE

- Succinylcholine is the one depolarizing NMB agent currently available. As mentioned, it binds to the ACh receptor and causes muscle contraction, similar to ACh. However, unlike ACh, it is very slowly broken down by acetylcholinesterase, and thus causes a persistent depolarization and blockade of the neuromuscular junction.
  - In patients with normally functioning pseudocholinesterase, it causes a brief paralysis, for 2–8 min. Patients with a homozygous deficiency of pseudocholinesterase (approximately 1 in 3200 patients) may be paralyzed for up to 8 hours.
  - For intubation, a dose of 1.0–1.5 mg/kg is typically used.
  - Potential side effects of succinylcholine include elevated intracranial pressure, bradycardia (severe), malignant hyperthermia, and severe hyperkalemia. These limitations make succinylcholine relatively contraindicated for patients with crush injuries, spinal cord injuries or brain injuries, renal insufficiency, muscular dystrophies, and burns.
- Nondepolarizing NMBs compete with ACh for binding at the ACh receptor. Once bound, nondepolarizing agents inhibit the ion flux through ACh receptor, thus prohibiting membrane depolarization and causing a flaccid paralysis. This class has a slower onset of action compared to succinylcholine, and a longer duration of action. Nondepolarizing NMBs can be reversed by the administration of an acetylcholinesterase drug such as neostigmine or edrophonium, which allows ACh to accumulate and thus compete with the NMB for binding to the ACh receptor.

PANCURONIUM

- Pancuronium is typically dosed as 0.08 mg/kg and has an onset of action within 3 minutes, with a duration of approximately 80 minutes. For maintenance, a drip beginning at 0.025 mg/kg/h is appropriate. Excretion of pancuronium is both renal and biliary; its duration of action is prolonged in patients with either renal or hepatic insufficiency.

VECURONIUM

- Vecuronium also has a short onset of action, and a slightly shorter duration of action, of approximately 40 minutes. It is dosed initially as 0.1 mg/kg for induction of paralysis, followed by a drip of 0.07 mg/kg/h if a maintenance dosing schedule is necessary. Vecuronium has minimal cardiovascular effects. Its excretion is mainly biliary, so its elimination is prolonged with hepatic insufficiency or biliary obstruction. A smaller fraction of excretion is renal, so that occasionally vecuronium's action is prolonged in patients with renal failure.

CISATRACURIUM

- Cisatracurium, an isomer of atracurium, is among the most frequently used NMBs in the ICU. The onset of action for the drug is approximately 8 minutes, and its duration of action is between 40 and 60 minutes after one dose. Cisatracurium is typically dosed as a 0.1 mg/kg loading dose followed by a 2–3 μg/kg/min continuous infusion. Advantages of cisatracurium over older nondepolarizing blockers include its lack of histamine release and its decreased production of the metabolite laudanosine, which has been proven to provoke seizures in animals at high doses. Cisatracurium is degraded by ester hydrolysis in the plasma (Hofmann degradation), and therefore does not require dose adjustment in renal failure.

MONITORING THE DEPTH OF NEUROMUSCULAR BLOCKADE

- When using any NMB agent in a maintenance fashion, depth of paralysis should be monitored with the use of a peripheral nerve stimulator to obtain a "train of four." In this setup, the nerve stimulator is set to deliver four impulses sequentially, each at 2 Hz. Without paralysis, four twitches of the nerve being studied—typically the ulnar nerve—would be observed. With 90% blockade of ACh receptors by the NMB, only one in four twitches is visible. With 70% ACh receptor occupancy, two to three twitches are visible.
- The goal of neuromuscular blockade is to maintain a depth which produces two to three twitches for a train of four.
- The use of such monitoring decreases the amount of drug used; the recovery time after neuromuscular blockade; and the incidence of postparalytic weakness.

BIBLIOGRAPHY

Bowman WC, Neuromuscular-blocking agents. In: *Pharmacology of Neuromuscular Function*, 2nd ed. London: Butterworth-Heinemann; 1990:134–230.

Gehlbach B, Kress JP. Pain control, sedation, and use of muscle relaxants. In: Hall JB, Schmidt GA, Wood LDH, eds., *Principles of Critical Care*, 3rd ed. New York, NY: McGraw-Hill; 2005:139–163.

Hunter JM. New neuromuscular blocking drugs. *N Engl J Med* 1995;332:1691–1699.

Murray MJ, Cowen J, DeBlock H, et al. Clinical practice guidelines for sustained neuromuscular blockade in the adult critically ill patient. *Crit Care Med* 2002;30:142–156.

Wiklund RA, Rosenbaum SH. Anesthesiology: first of two parts. *N Engl J Med* 1997;337:1132–1141.

8 MONITORING THE CARDIOVASCULAR SYSTEM

Joseph Levitt

KEY POINTS

- Multiple prospective trials, in several patient subsets, have failed to reveal any benefit to a pulmonary artery catheter
- Early therapy of sepsis, directed towards normalizing the central venous oxygen saturation, improves outcome
- The adequacy of perfusion can be judged by central venous oximetry. This method has limitations, but these are fewer than with thermodilution cardiac output measurement
- Fluid responsiveness is best predicted by pulse pressure variation (for passively ventilated patients) and right atrial pressure variation (during spontaneous breathing).
- Combined with echocardiography, these dynamic measures can supplant the pulmonary artery catheter
- Recommendations for optimal monitoring of the cardiovascular system remain controversial and the subject of ongoing investigation. At the center of the controversy lie two fundamental issues:
  - First is the lack of consistent evidence documenting safety and efficacy of invasive monitoring.

A retrospective analysis of the network fluid and catheters treatment pulmonary artery catheter (PAC) suggested a detrimental effect. Subsequent prospective analyses have demonstrated safety, but failed to show a beneficial effect.

- Second, guidelines for monitoring hemodynamics are incomplete without recommendations for how to respond to the obtained data. Great variability in fluid and vasoactive drug therapy exists, with little evidence to guide current recommendations. Utility of PACs and a liberal versus conservative fluid strategy in acute respiratory distress syndrome (ARDS) are the subjects of the recent ARDS network Fluid and Connector Treatment Trial. An aggressive diuretic regimen reduced time on the ventilator, but the PAC was no better than a CVC.

MONITORING THE SEPTIC PATIENT

- Despite the existing uncertainties, early recognition and treatment of inadequate circulation remains imperative. Results of a recent trial of early goal-directed therapy in sepsis suggest a role for routine and prompt placement of a central venous catheter (CVC) in the superior vena cava. In this trial, patients randomized to protocol-driven therapy (goals of achieving a CVP of 8–12, MAP > 65, and urine output > 0.5 cc/kg, with red cell transfusions and dobutamine used to raise central venous oxygenation > 70%) in the first 6 hours had a significantly improved survival compared to patients receiving standard care.
- This study highlights the importance of the two main components of invasive monitoring: measuring venous oxygen saturation (SVO_2) and assessing intravascular volume. The mixed venous oxygen content (and, proportionately, the saturation) is related to oxygen transport and consumption by $VO_2 = (CaO_2 - CVO_2) \times Qt$ (where V_2 = oxygen consumption, CaO_2 = arterial oxygen content, CVO_2 = venous oxygen content, and Qt = cardiac output). When oxygen delivery is appropriate for demand, SVO_2 is 70–75%.
- Lower values of SVO_2 suggest impaired oxygen delivery and a quick assessment of arterial-venous oxygen content difference can easily distinguish decreased CaO_2 (hypoxemia or anemia) from low cardiac output. A level >75% suggests an increased ratio of oxygen delivery to demand and while it is important in identifying the etiology of hypotension (i.e., sepsis and liver failure), it is probably not useful as a therapeutic endpoint. A large multicentered randomized-controlled trial failed to show benefit in clinically relevant endpoints in patients randomized to have a supranormal SVO_2. While measuring SVO_2 requires a PAC, a central venous saturation appears to be a reliable substitute and requires only placement of a CVC into the superior vena cava. Thus, CVC sampling of the $SCVO_2$ allows qualitative assessment of cardiac output which, unless future studies identify an optimal cardiac output, may be just as useful as the quantitative information obtained from a PAC.

ALTERNATINGS TO THE PAC

- The second component of invasive monitoring, assessing intravascular filling pressures, has long been the realm of the PAC. PACs allow measurement of the pulmonary artery occlusion pressure (PAOP) and thus estimation of the left ventricular end-diastolic filling pressure, which, for many practitioners, has been the "holy grail" of hemodynamic monitoring. However, this focus on the PAOP as the major determinant of cardiac output lacks appreciation of Guyton's early studies on the determinants of cardiac output. His work described a cardiovascular system where the heart serves primarily as a passive pump, with the gradient between mean systemic pressure and right atrial pressure (RAP) serving as the driving force for venous return and thus cardiac output. Again, the additional information derived from a PAC may not provide a benefit over a CVC in the superior vena cava for optimizing cardiac output. A PAC with a PAOP may be useful diagnostically to more readily distinguishing between left (acute myocardial infarction [MI], acute mitral insufficiency, decompensated congestive heart failure [CHF], and so forth) and right (pulmonary embolism [PE], pulmonary hypertension, right ventricular (RV) infarct, and so forth) heart failure. However, combining a noninvasive transthoracic echocardiogram with a CVC may provide equivalent data.
- Both PACs and CVCs suffer the same limitation when attempting to assess intravascular volume: they only measure intravascular filling pressure when what is really needed is volume. While pressure is a reliable surrogate for volume in most conditions, it can be misleading in states of increased intrathoracic or intracardiac pressure (i.e., mechanical ventilation with high positive airway pressures, tension pneumothorax, cardiac tamponade, and abdominal compartment syndrome). In such cases, recognition of variation in intravascular pressure with the respiratory cycle may be more important than absolute values. In the ventilated patient, the rise in pleural pressure with inspiration raises RAP impeding venous return and thus (with a short lag time to allow for transit time through the pulmonary circulation) impeding left ventricular preload and stroke volume. The magnitude of this effect is dependent on the relative position on the Starling curve at which the heart is operating and is reflected in the arterial pulse pressure (PP). A recent study compared

the PAOP, RAP, change in arterial systolic pressure, and change in PP with inspiration in passive mechanically ventilated patients for utility in predicting fluid responsiveness. A change in arterial pulse pressure $[\Delta PP(\%) = (PP_{max} - PP_{min})/((PP_{max} + PP_{min})/2)]$ of >13% reliably predicted fluid responsiveness. PAOP was the least reliable, followed closely by RAP. A second study in ventilated but spontaneously breathing patients found a fall of >1 cmH_2O in RAP predicted fluid responsiveness.

- The growing recognition of the importance of assessing intravascular volumes as opposed to pressures has also led to increased use of echocardiography in the critical care setting. Transthoracic echocardiography (TTE) has sensitivity and specificity for diagnosing hemodynamically significant pulmonary emboli and is safer to perform on the hemodynamically unstable patient. RV dysfunction on TTE with acute PE may also have important prognostic and therapeutic implications.
- In summary, optimal monitoring of hemodynamics in the critically ill remains controversial. With many old and new technologies to choose from, more studies demonstrating therapeutic efficacy are needed. Strict guidelines for monitoring hemodynamics also await future studies documenting the optimal response to the obtainable data. For now, the early and routine placement of a CVC with judicious interpretation of the RAP and $SCVO_2$ seems reasonable. Addition of TTE to evaluate for coexisting intrinsic cardiac dysfunction may also be prudent. Recommendations regarding routine use of a PAC are pending results of the ongoing ARDS-NET FACCT trial.

BIBLIOGRAPHY

Connors AF Jr, Speroff T, Dawson NV, et al. The effectiveness of right heart catheterization in the initial care of critically ill patients. SUPPORT Investigators. *JAMA* 1996;276:889–897.

Faber T. Central venous versus mixed venous oxygen content. *Acta Anaesthesiol Scand* 1995;107(Suppl):33–36.

Guyton AC, Richardson TQ, Langston JB. Regulation of cardiac output and venous return. *Clin Anesth* 1964;3:1–34.

Magder S, Lagonidis D, Erice F. The use of respiratory variations in right atrial pressure to predict the cardiac output response to PEEP. *J Crit Care* 2001;16:108–114.

Michard F, Boussat S, Chemla D, et al. Relation between respiratory changes in arterial pulse pressure and fluid responsiveness in septic patients with acute circulatory failure. *Am J Respir Crit Care Med* 2000;162:134–138.

Rhodes A, Cusack RJ, Newman PJ, et al. A randomised, controlled trial of the pulmonary artery catheter in critically ill patients. *Intensive Care Med* 2002;28:256–264.

Rivers E, Nguyen B, Havstad S, et al., for the Early Goal-Directed Therapy Collaborative Group. Early goal-directed therapy in the treatment of severe sepsis and septic shock. *N Engl J Med* 2001;345:1368–1377.

Sandham JD, Hull RD, Brant RF, et al. A randomized, controlled trial of the use of pulmonary-artery catheters in high-risk surgical patients. *N Engl J Med* 2003;348:5–14.

9 MONITORING THE RESPIRATORY SYSTEM

Joseph Levitt

KEY POINTS

- Impending respiratory failure is often better judged at the bedside than through blood gas measurement.
- In mechanically ventilated patients it is often not necessary to normalize pH and PCO_2: it may even be harmful.
- Ventilator displays of pressure and flow can guide ventilator settings and judgments regarding the progress of lung function.
- A daily trial of spontaneous breathing speeds liberation from the ventilator.

INTRODUCTION

- The first and most important component of monitoring the respiratory system is recognition of impending respiratory failure.
- Evaluating for the presence of crackles, wheezing, egophony, dullness to percussion, and so forth, may assist in elucidating the etiology of respiratory distress, but is not necessary in diagnosing respiratory failure. Pulse oximetry and blood gas sampling are often redundant or misleading.
- Simple bedside observations can typically identify a patient in extremis. This is often signaled by the "tripod" position (bending forward with hands braced on thighs), accessory muscle use, thoraco-abdominal dyssynchrony, rapid respiratory rates (>40), and inability to speak in short sentences. Confusion and agitation, often with removing of oxygen mask and IVs, are late findings. Agonal respirations are a very late finding and predict immediate respiratory arrest.

ARTERIAL BLOOD GAS ANALYSIS

- Blood gas sampling allows accurate measurement of the arterial pH, PaO_2, and $PaCO_2$.

- While it remains essential in evaluating the gas exchange properties of the lung (severity of lung injury is often determined by the PaO_2/FiO_2 ratio) and acid-base status, it is often overutilized.
- Pulse oximetry provides accurate noninvasive measurements of the arterial oxygen saturation in most situations.
- Normalization of the pH and $PaCO_2$ are often overemphasized in the management of respiratory failure and should not be the primary endpoints of mechanical ventilator settings. Furthermore, a rising $PaCO_2$ and a falling PaO_2 are often very late findings in respiratory failure and of limited utility in guiding therapy.

PULSE OXIMETRY

- Continuous pulse oximetry allows early detection of hypoxemia in at-risk patients. However, despite near ubiquitous use in ICUs and operating room, the clinical benefit of routine continuous monitoring has not been clearly established.
- Pulse oximetry is found to be accurate ± 4% at saturations >90%. Accuracy at saturations below 80% is less established. Also, distinguishing arterial blood from venous or tissue blood requires a clear pulsatile signal and is therefore impaired by poor perfusion states in critically ill patients.

CAPNOMETRY

- Capnometry is defined as the measurement of expired CO_2, usually by infrared absorption. Graphic representation of expired CO_2 (capnography) allows estimation of end-tidal CO_2 ($PetCO_2$) which should approximate $PaCO_2$. This technology can be used in measuring respiratory quotients to determine adequacy of nutritional supplementation, calculations of pulmonary dead space, and estimations of cardiac output using the Fick equation. However, variations in ventilation-perfusion ratios in the critically ill can lead to unreliable relationships between $PetCO_2$ and $PaCO_2$.
- Capnometry is widely used to reliably differentiate endotracheal from esophageal intubations.

AIRWAY PRESSURE MONITORING DURING MECHANICAL VENTILATION

- When endotracheal intubation and mechanical ventilation are required, the ventilator can provide valuable information in both diagnosis and management of respiratory failure.
- Graphic display of pressure versus time and flow versus time waveforms give vital information about patient-ventilator interaction.
- Readings of tidal volumes and peak and plateau pressures should not be made without simultaneous confirmation of patient-ventilator synchrony.
- Peak airway pressure is a function of static compliance of the lung and chest wall plus the resistive component of the airway. In volume control modes, an end-inspiratory pause briefly ceases flow after delivering the tidal volume, eliminating the resistive component of the airway pressure. This plateau or occlusion pressure thus reflects only the compliance of the respiratory system (lung and chest wall) independent of airway resistance (and any positive end-expiratory pressure [PEEP] or auto-PEEP).
- Large gradients between peak and plateau pressures suggest high airway resistance which could be occurring at any level from the ventilator tubing, through the endotracheal tube to large and small airways of the bronchial tree and should help to guide therapy (i.e., suctioning vs. steroids and bronchodilators).
- Elevated plateau pressures suggest a noncompliant or overdistended respiratory system, including lungs (i.e., pulmonary edema and fibrosis), chest wall (i.e., pneumothoraces and circumferential burns), and abdomen (i.e., obesity and abdominal compartment syndromes).
- Similarly, an expiratory pause ceases flow at end-expiration and allows detection of auto or intrinsic PEEP above set levels, although this maneuver requires a very passive patient.
- Flow versus time waveforms provide readily available information on airway resistance even in less passive patients. Coving or scooping of the expiratory flow suggests increased airway resistance. Failure of expiratory flow to return completely to zero prior to the subsequent breath implies at least some degree of auto-PEEP.
- Pressure-volume curves are the subject of much debate because of speculation that the lower inflection point of the inspiratory limb represents the dynamic recruitment of alveolar lung units and an upper inflection point implies overdistention of the lung in acute respiratory distress syndrome (ARDS). Setting PEEP to the lower inflection point may prevent derecruitment of alveoli during expiration and thus decrease shear forces experienced by alveoli during repeated collapse and re-expansion. However, difficulties in reliably determining the lower inflection point and lack of clinical trials demonstrating a clinical benefit with titrating PEEP to this point limit the use of pressure-volume curves in routine practice.

MONITORING FOR LIBERATION FROM MECHANICAL VENTILATION

- Once an intubated patient's condition has stabilized, he or she should be screened daily for suitability for liberation. Patients who are arousable, with adequate cough and gag, without high minute ventilations, can tolerate FiO_2 levels that can be safely delivered noninvasively at a PEEP ≤ 5, and are stable hemodynamically should undergo a spontaneous breathing trial.
- Spontaneous breathing trials can be performed on a T-piece, continuous positive airway pressure (CPAP), or CPAP with minimal pressure support (5–7 cmH_2O depending on endotracheal tube size) and last for 30–120 minutes. Patients able to maintain a frequency to tidal volume (in liters) ratio < 105 throughout the trial without other signs of distress or instability should proceed to a trial of extubation.

RESPIRATORY DRIVE AND MUSCLE STRENGTH

- Although not routinely done, patients with unexplained respiratory failure or failure to liberate from mechanical ventilation should be considered for testing of respiratory drive and muscle strength.
- A negative inspiratory pressure (NIP) >30 cmH_2O and a forced vital capacity (FVC) >1 L are generally adequate to maintain a safe minute ventilation, however, in an individual patient, trends over time are far more important than absolute values.
- Respiratory drive can be evaluated by measuring an airway occlusion pressure in the first 100 ms of inspiration (P 0.1). While the peak negative airway pressure a patient can generate is a function of respiratory muscle strength, the P 0.1 is thought to be determined by central respiratory drive and be independent of muscle strength.
- Finding a normal or even elevated magnitude of P 0.1 may point to unrecognized neuromuscular weakness in a patient previously thought to have central respiratory failure.

BIBLIOGRAPHY

Caples SM, Hubmayr RD. Respiratory monitoring tools in the intensive care unit. *Curr Opin Crit Care* 2003;9:230–235.

Sevransky JE, Levy MM, Marini JJ. Mechanical ventilation in sepsis-induced acute lung injury/acute respiratory distress syndrome: an evidence-based review. *Crit Care Med* 2004;32:S548–S553.

10 ASSESSMENT OF SEVERITY OF ILLNESS

Michael Moore

KEY POINTS

- Severity-of-illness scoring systems have been developed to predict and evaluate the outcomes of groups of critically ill patients admitted to ICUs.
- Most scoring systems have been developed using multivariate regression analysis of large clinical databases to identify the most relevant variables related to mortality with subsequent prospective validation in other patient populations.
- The value of a predictive score in an individual patient is limited and such scores should never be the sole basis for recommendations regarding withdrawal of life-sustaining treatments
- Scoring systems are most useful compared to clinicians' predictions of outcomes in patients who are neither gravely ill nor have an excellent prognosis.

CHARACTERISTICS OF SCORING SYSTEMS

- All critical care predictive scoring systems utilize numerical values to describe the severity of a patient's illness.
- Scores are then assigned predicted mortalities using a mathematical formula.
- Important principles in assessing outcome instruments:
  - Scoring systems should measure an important outcome.
    - Most ICU scoring systems predict hospital mortality.
    - Interest has developed in assessing long-term mortality and functional status.
  - Scoring instruments should be easy to use.
    - Data collected during the routine care of the critically ill.
    - Data points should be easily measured, objective, and reproducible.
  - The usefulness of any system depends on its predictive accuracy.
- Characteristics used to judge the value of a predictive system:
  - Discrimination:
    - Describes the accuracy of a given prediction.
    - Considered discriminant if the area under the Receiver Operating Characteristic (ROC) curve > 0.8.

- Illustrates the discriminating ability over the entire range of prediction scores.
- Example: Area of 0.9 means that a randomly selected nonsurvivor will have a more severe score than a randomly selected survivor 90% of the time.

- Calibration:
  - Compares the observed mortality to the predicted mortality within a stratum of severity.
  - Example: A predictive instrument would be highly calibrated if it were accurate at mortalities of 90%, 50%, and 20%.
- Reliability:
  - Refers to the inter- and intraobserver agreement when calculating a severity of illness score.
  - A scoring system that is more subjective will be less reliable.
- Content validity:
  - Reflects the comprehensiveness of the model.
  - In general, more variables in the model increase the content validity but may decrease the reliability and ease of use.
- Methodological rigor:
  - Refers to the avoidance of bias in the development of the model.

- All scoring systems have limitations:
  - Outcomes can only be predicted in populations that were included in the derivation data set.
  - Poor application of a rigorously developed and validated scoring system will decrease its usefulness.

ACUTE PHYSIOLOGIC AND CHRONIC HEALTH EVALUATION II

- Acute physiologic and chronic health evaluation (APACHE) II is the most widely used scoring system.
- Validated in 5813 ICU admissions from 13 U.S. hospitals.
- APACHE II scoring:
  - Disease specific.
  - Score is derived from points given for age, type of admission, chronic health evaluation, and 12 physiologic variables.
  - The 12 physiologic variables are defined as the most abnormal during the first 24 hours after admission.
- Predicted death rate is computed form the weighted sum of the APACHE II score, a variable determined by need for emergency surgery, and the specific diagnostic category.
- APACHE II flaws:
  - Predicted mortality is less than that observed among patients transferred from other inpatient facilities.
  - Cannot accurately predict outcome for specific patient subgroups, for example, liver failure and sepsis.

ACUTE PHYSIOLOGIC AND CHRONIC HEALTH EVALUATION III

- Designed to correct many of the flaws in APACHE II.
- Derived from 17,440 admissions in 40 U.S. hospitals.
- New variables include prior treatment location and disease requiring ICU admission.
- APACHE III score:
  - Sum of 17 physiologic variables, age, and 7 potential comorbid conditions.
  - Final score can vary between 0 and 300.
- Predicted death rate:
  - Computed from the weighted sum of disease category, a coefficient related to prior treatment location, and the APACHE II score.
  - 78 diagnostic categories are included.
  - Requires a proprietary logistic regression equation.
- Clinical information can be updated daily to provide a dynamic predicted mortality score.
- Limitations:
  - Underestimates mortality in less severely ill and overestimates it in more severely ill patients.
  - Requires a large amount of detailed physiologic data.
  - Requires proprietary computer technology.

SIMPLIFIED ACUTE PHYSIOLOGIC SCORE II

- A non-disease-specific system intended to streamline data collection and analysis without compromising diagnostic accuracy.
- Developed from a sample of 13,152 admissions in 12 countries.
- Score is derived from 17 variables selected by logistic regression:
  - 12 categorical physiologic variables
  - Age
  - Type of admission
  - Underlying disease
    - Acquired immune deficiency syndrome
    - Metastatic cancer
    - Hematologic malignancy
- Predicted hospital mortality is calculated from the simplified acute physiologic score (SAPS) II.
- Excellent discrimination and calibration.
- May be suitable for use in the intermediate care unit setting.

- May be less accurate in predicting mortality when patients are admitted to the ICU for noncardiovascular disease.

MORTALITY PREDICTION MODEL II

- Developed from a sample from 19,124 ICU admissions in 12 countries.
- A non-disease-specific scoring system that excluded burn, coronary care, and cardiac surgery patients.
- Model uses 15 variables to derive a direct probability of survival:
  - Age
  - Three physiologic variables
  - Five acute and three chronic diagnoses
  - Type of admission
  - Use of cardiopulmonary resuscitation (CPR)
  - Use of mechanical ventilation
- All of the variables are dichotomous (i.e., present or absent) except for age.
- Each variable is assigned a coefficient and the sum is entered into a published mathematical formula to calculate the predicted hospital mortality.
- Excellent calibration and discrimination.
- Timing of mortality prediction model (MPM) score:
  - MPM_0 is calculated on ICU admission
  - MPM_{24}
    - Recalculated after 24 hours by updating five admission variables and including eight additional variables.
    - Allows comparison to other scoring systems where the score is calculated after 24 hours in the ICU (SAPS, APACHE).

COMPARISON OF SYSTEMS

- APACHE II, SAPS II, and MPM II all have excellent discrimination and calibration.
- APACHE II and APACHE III have been compared in 1144 patients from the United Kingdom.
  - APACHE II had better calibration and APACHE III had better discrimination.
  - Both underestimated hospital mortality with APACHE III underestimating by a greater degree.
- Differences and limitations:
  - Variables used in the models
    - APACHE II variables were selected by committee based on which variables were thought to be important to patient outcome.
    - MPM II, SAPS II, and APACHE III variables were chosen using statistical techniques to identify variables that were independently associated with death.
  - Data collection
    - APACHE and SAPS use the worst physiologic values measured within 24 hours of admission.
    - MPM data are collected immediately on ICU admission and can be modified after 24 hours of hospitalization.
    - APACHE III requires precise physiologic measurements.
    - SAPS and MPM use broader physiologic categories simplifying data collection.
  - Timing of score
    - APACHE II, MPM, and SAPS can only estimate mortality on admission (MPM_0) or after 24 hours in the ICU.
    - APACHE III can recalculate estimated mortality on a daily basis.
      - May have greater predictive power versus a single projection.
      - However, at least one study that provided intermittently updated likelihood estimates for patient death and disability failed to change physician behavior or improve patient outcomes.
  - Mortality calculation
    - APACHE III uses proprietary computer software to calculate predicted mortality.
    - SAPS and MPM use published equations in which the severity score is entered into equations whose solutions provide the predicted mortalities.
  - Cost
    - APACHE III requires proprietary computer technology and substantial data collection.
    - APACHE II score calculators are available to the public.
    - MPM and SAPS require somewhat less data and no additional computer investment.

USE OF SEVERITY SCORES IN THE ICU

- Severity scoring is ideally suited to the ICU:
  - The ICU population is well-defined and care is well-circumscribed.
  - Evidence suggests that ICU severity of illness is the major determinant of hospital mortality.
  - There is a large range of applications in health care management and research.
- Scoring systems in clinical research:
  - Allows comparison between studies that include heterogenous samples of critically ill patients.

- Allow clinicians to compare the studied population to their practice.
- Scoring systems in randomized-controlled trials have multiple functions:
  - Describe severity of illness
  - Assess comparability of control and treatment groups at baseline
  - Determine sample size
  - Perform stratified randomization
  - Determine success of randomization
- Scoring systems in ICU administration:
  - Describe acuity of illness
  - Assess the quality of ICU care
    - APACHE scores have been used to compare open and closed ICUs with respect to patient outcomes.
  - Compare interhospital ICU mortality as an indicator of quality
    - A study using APACHE III suggested that teaching hospitals have higher ICU severity and somewhat better risk-adapted patient outcomes.
    - APACHE, SAPS, and MPM have been used to identify ICUs that have higher than predicted mortality.
  - Manage some hospital resources
    - Assigning severity scores to ICU patients may identify those patients who can be placed in less expensive settings.
- Limitations:
  - ICU scoring systems are powerful research tools but the value of a predictive score in an individual patient or ICU may be limited.
  - The databases used to derive most scoring systems do not have sufficient statistical power to study most disease subsets in critical care, for example, liver failure, obstetrics, and AIDS.
  - Lead time bias is well described in APACHE II (patients transferred from other hospitals and ICUs have a higher than predicted mortality) and may be important in scoring systems other than APACHE III.

BIBLIOGRAPHY

Auriant I, Vinatier I, Thaler F, et al. Simplified Acute Physiology Score II for measuring severity of illness in intermediate care units. *Crit Care Med* 1998;26:1368–1371.

Beck DH, Taylor BL, Millar B, et al. Prediction of outcome from intensive care: a prospective cohort study comparing Acute Physiology and Chronic Health Evaluation II and III prognostic systems in a United Kingdom intensive care unit. *Crit Care Med* 1997;25:9–15.

Capuzzo M, Valpondi V, Sgarbi A, et al. Validation of severity scoring systems SAPS II and APACHE II in a single-center population. *Intensive Care Med* 2000;26: 1779–1785.

Castella X, Artigas A, Bion J, et al., for the European/North American Severity Study Group. A comparison of severity of illness scoring systems for intensive care unit patients: results of a multicenter, multinational study. *Crit Care Med* 1995;23:1327–1335.

Cowen JS, Kelley MA. Errors and bias in using predictive scoring systems. *Crit Care Clin* 1994;10:53–72.

Escarce JJ, Kelley MA. Admission source to the medical intensive care unit predicts hospital death independent of APACHE II score. *JAMA* 1990;264:2389–2394.

Glance LG, Osler TM, Dick A. Rating the quality of intensive care units: is it a function of the intensive care unit scoring system? *Crit Care Med* 2002;30:1976–1982.

Hall JB, Schmidt, GA, Wood LDH. *Principles of Critical Care*, 3rd ed. New York, NY: McGraw-Hill; 2005:1123–1136.

Knaus WA, Draper EA, Wagner DP, et al. APACHE II: a severity of disease classification system. *Crit Care Med* 1985;13: 818–829.

Knaus WA, Wagner DP, Draper EA, et al. The APACHE III prognostic system: risk prediction of hospital mortality for critically ill hospitalized adults. *Chest* 1991;100:1619–1936.

Kollef MH, Schuster DP. Predicting intensive care unit outcome with scoring systems: underlying concepts and principles. *Crit Care Clin* 1994;10:1–18.

Le Gall JR, Lemeshow S, Saulnier F. A new Simplified Acute Physiology Score (SAPS II) based on a European/North American multicenter study [published correction appears in *JAMA* 1994;271:1321]. *JAMA*. 1993;270: 2957–2963.

Lemeshow S, Teres D, Klar J, et al. Mortality probability models (MPM II) based on an international cohort of intensive care unit patients. *JAMA* 1993;270:2478–2486.

Metnitz PG, Valenti A, Vesely H, et al. Prognostic performance and customization of the SAPS II: results of a multicenter Austrian study. Simplified Acute Physiology Score. *Intensive Care Med* 1999;25:192–197.

Multz AS, Chalfin DB, Samson IM, et al. A "closed" medical intensive care unit (MICU) improves resource utilization when compared with an "open" MICU. *Am J Respir Crit Care Med* 1998;157:1468–1473.

The SUPPORT Principal Investigators. A controlled trial to improve care for seriously ill hospitalized patients: the study to understand prognoses and preferences for outcomes and risks of treatments (SUPPORT). *JAMA* 1995;274:1591–1598.

Wagner DP, Knaus WA, Harrell FE, et al. Daily prognostic estimates for critically ill adults in intensive care units: results from a prospective, multicenter, inception cohort analysis. *Crit Care Med* 1994;22:1359–1372.

Zimmerman JE, Shortell S, Knaus WA, et al. Value and cost of teaching hospitals: a prospective, multicenter, inception cohort study. *Crit Care Med* 1993;21:1432–1442.

Zimmerman JE, Wagner DP, Draper EA, et al. Evaluation of acute physiology and chronic health evaluation III predictions of hospital mortality in an independent database. *Crit Care Med* 1998;26:1317–1326.

11 PULMONARY ARTERY CATHETER

Nina M. Patel

KEY POINTS

- The PA catheter is a flow-directed catheter used to measure intravascular pressures and oxyhemoglobin saturations and to calculate cardiac output and various additional hemodynamic values.
- Six randomized controlled trials in varied populations have failed to demonstrate any benefit to the use of the PA catheter. These devices should not be used routinely.
- The decision to pursue invasive hemodynamic monitoring with a PA catheter is a clinical judgment based on potential risks of the procedure for each individual patient weighed against availability of noninvasive means of hemodynamic assessment (e.g., echocardiography) and results and risks of empiric trials of therapy (e.g., diuresis or volume challenge).
- Complications of a PA catheter include thrombosis, embolism, knotting of the catheter, pulmonic valve insufficiency, arrhythmias, endocarditis, catheter-related sepsis, pulmonary infarction (due to persistent wedging), and arterial rupture. Data from a PA catheter can offer valuable clinical information, yet is often misinterpreted. Proper use of a PAC depends on complete understanding of the data obtained.

EPIDEMIOLOGY

- 1.5 million pulmonary artery (PA) catheters are placed per year in North America.

FORM AND FUNCTION

- The PA catheter is a flexible, flow-directed, balloon-tipped catheter that has been utilized since the 1970s to directly measure intravascular pressures and guide hemodynamic assessment.
- The catheter (7 French [F]) consists of a proximal lumen (30 cm), distal lumen (tip of catheter), thermistor (to calculate cardiac output [CO]), and a 1.5 mL inflatable balloon.
- It is inserted through an introducer (8.5 F) placed in either the internal jugular or subclavian veins. (The femoral and axillary veins can also be used under special circumstances.) The distal port is connected to a pressure transducer which records pressure waveforms throughout catheter insertion. The transducer is "zeroed" at the level of the phlebostatic axis (midaxillary line, 4th intercostal space). This step is essential as deviation of the transducer above or below the phlebostatic axis will under- or overestimate pressures.
- Initially, the catheter is advanced to the level of the right atrium (RA, approximately 10–15 cm), at which point the balloon is inflated. The catheter is subsequently "floated" through the RA, right ventricle (RV), and finally to the PA. When an adequate PA pressure tracing is achieved, the balloon is deflated and the catheter locked into position (Fig. 11-1).

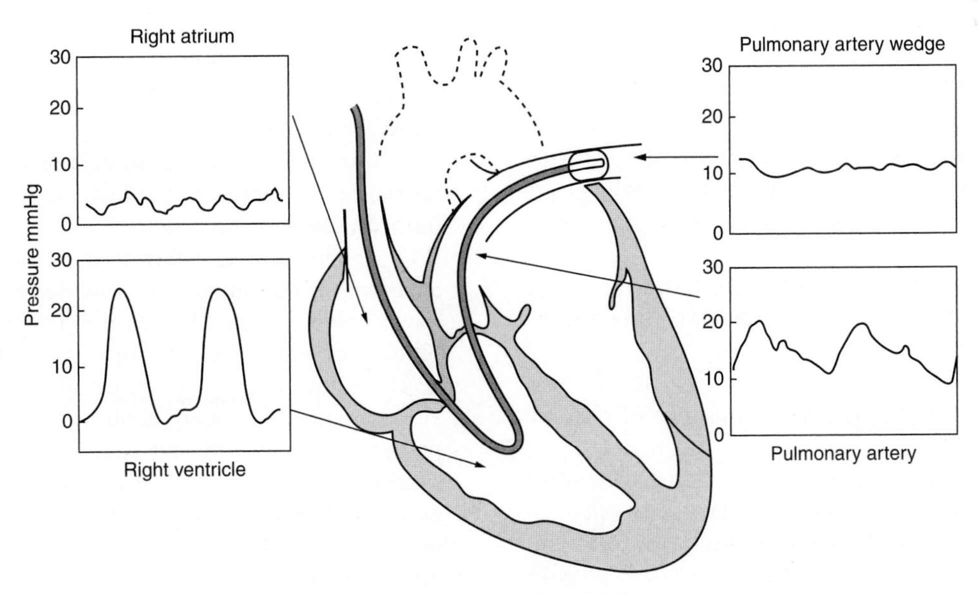

FIG. 11-1. Waveforms as shown during right heart catheterization.
SOURCE: Adapted from Marino PL. The ICU Book. Baltimore, MD: Williams & Wilkins; 1998:157.

- Passage of the catheter through each chamber is identified by a characteristic pressure waveform.
- During catheter insertion, patients may experience arrhythmias. In general, these arrhythmias are transient and will resolve if the catheter is withdrawn to the superior vena cava (SVC). In rare cases, complete heart block or ventricular tachycardia will persist and necessitate intervention with placement of a transvenous pacemaker and administration of appropriate antiarrhythmic agents (e.g., amiodarone).

INDICATIONS

- The data procured from a PA catheter: right atrial pressure (RAP), right ventricular end-diastolic pressure (RVEDP), pulmonary artery pressure (PAP), pulmonary artery wedge pressure (PAWP), CO, and mixed venous oxygen saturation (SvO_2), are utilized diagnostically to differentiate among various etiologies of shock, respiratory failure, cardiovascular failure, and renal failure.
- In addition, the PA catheter is employed to guide patient management through real time evaluation of intravascular volume status and effectiveness of therapeutic interventions (e.g., change in CO or SvO_2 with addition of inotrope).
- The decision to pursue invasive hemodynamic monitoring with a PA catheter is a clinical judgment based on potential risks of the procedure for each individual patient weighed against availability of noninvasive means of hemodynamic assessment (e.g., echocardiography) and/or results and risks of empiric trials of therapy (e.g., diuresis or volume challenge).

WAVEFORMS

- Pressure waveforms transduced from the PA catheter, in conjunction with simultaneous ECG recordings, are valuable in characterizing normal versus pathologic cardiac states.
- A normal atrial pressure waveform is characterized by two ascents, the *a* and *v* waves and two descents, the *x* and *y* descents.
- Distinctive alterations in the normal atrial pressure waveform characterize a number of cardiac disorders:
  - "Cannon" *a* waves: atrioventricular dissociation; atrial contraction against a closed atrioventricular valve
  - Large *v* waves: acute mitral regurgitation, ventricular septal defect, hypervolemia
  - Broad *v* wave + a rapid *y* descent: tricuspid regurgitation
  - Blunted *x* and *y* descent: pericardial tamponade; impaired cardiac filling in diastole with subsequent equalization of diastolic pressures
  - Rapid *x* and *y* descent: constrictive pericarditis and RV infarction; rapid ventricular filling in early diastole
- Overdamping of the catheter, catheter whip, incomplete wedging, and overwedging can hinder acquisition of accurate waveforms.

DATA ACQUISITION—PRESSURES, CARDIAC OUTPUT, AND MIXED VENOUS OXYGEN SATURATION

- The PA catheter confers ability to directly measure or derive a number of critical hemodynamic variables. These include: (a) intravascular pressures, (b) CO, and (c) SvO_2.

INTRAVASCULAR PRESSURES

- Respiratory variations in intrathoracic pressure are transmitted to the vasculature and resultantly alter intravascular pressure measurements. By convention, measurements are taken at end-expiration at which time the pleural pressure is least perturbed by respiration. Even at end-expiration, however, the pleural pressure may be far from its baseline value, as seen in patients on positive end-expiratory pressure (PEEP) (or having auto-PEEP) or when the expiratory muscles are active at end-expiration as in many patients with airflow obstruction.
- Normal ranges of intravascular pressures are:
  - RA pressure: 2–8 mmHg
  - RV pressure: 15–25/2–8 mmHg
  - PA pressure: 15–30/4–12 mmHg
  - PAWP: 2–12 mmHg
- RA pressure is equivalent to central venous pressure (CVP) and is frequently used as a surrogate marker of intravascular volume status.
- $PA_{diastolic}$ pressure is determined by flow (Q), resistance within the pulmonary vascular circuit, and the downstream (left atrial) pressure. Under normal conditions, in which the pulmonary vascular resistance (PVR) is low, $PA_{diastolic}$ pressure approximates PAWP. However, in situations of abnormally high PVR (e.g., pulmonary embolism and acute respiratory distress syndrome [ARDS]) or Q (e.g., sepsis) through the pulmonary circuit, $PA_{diastolic}$ may exceed PAWP significantly.
- The PAWP offers valuable clinical information, yet is often misinterpreted and as such can lead to errors in patient management.

- Advancing the inflated PA catheter through the PA until complete occlusion of blood flow is achieved derives PAWP. This creates a static column of blood among the pulmonary arteriole, pulmonary venule, and the left atrium. Thus, pressure transduced at the tip of an inflated PA catheter represents pressure transmitted from the pulmonary venule immediately downstream of the catheter.
- PAWP is often equated with left atrial pressure or left ventricular end-diastolic volume (LVEDV)/preload. This is an erroneous practice; particularly in critically ill patients, as it does not take into account LV compliance and/or the presence of mitral valvular abnormalities.
- PAWP is measured in West's zone 3 lung, in which pulmonary arterial pressure (Ppa) exceeds pulmonary venous (Ppv) and pulmonary alveolar pressures (Palv). These conditions (Ppa > Ppv > Palv) ensure that the catheter is truly measuring intravascular, as opposed to alveolar pressure. If PAWP exceeds $PA_{diastolic}$, it is likely that the PA catheter is not in zone 3 lung.
- PAWP reflects pulmonary venous pressure rather than pulmonary capillary hydrostatic pressure.

CARDIAC OUTPUT

- Cardiac output calculated by thermodilution is another hemodynamic variable derived from the PA catheter.
  - The Stewart Hamilton equation utilizes the area of decay under the temperature-time curve between cold injectate infused at the proximal port of the PA catheter and blood withdrawn at the distal port to calculate flow or CO.
  - Cardiac arrhythmias, tricuspid regurgitation, and shunts can introduce significant variability into this measurement.

MIXED VENOUS OXYGEN SATURATION

- SvO_2 is the oxygen saturation of blood aspirated from the distal port of the PA catheter.
- The normal difference between arterial oxygen saturation (SaO_2) and venous oxygen saturation (SvO_2) is related to oxygen consumption and CO, and normally is 20–25%.
- SvO_2 reflects roughly the adequacy of oxygen delivery to peripheral tissues.
- Decreases in SvO_2 suggest either increased peripheral oxygen consumption or decreased rate of oxygen delivery (e.g., reduced CO, anemia, or decreased SaO_2) with subsequently increased oxygen extraction.

- One of the most essential features in using a PA catheter is to integrate the numerous data points derived from it to achieve an understanding of the hemodynamic status of the patient. This is particularly useful in classic presentations of shock:

TYPE OF SHOCK	CO	SVR	PAWP	SvO_2
Cardiogenic	Decreased	Increased	Increased	Decreased
Septic	Increased	Decreased	Decreased	Increased
Hypovolemic	Decreased	Increased	Decreased	Decreased

COMPLICATIONS

- Thrombosis, embolism, knotting of the catheter, pulmonic valve insufficiency, endocarditis, catheter-related sepsis, pulmonary infarction (due to persistent wedging), and PA rupture are all rare complications that may develop while a PA catheter is in place.
- PA rupture is reported to occur infrequently at a rate of 0.06–0.2% of PA catheter placements. However, when this complication does occur, consequences are severe with an estimated mortality rate of 50%.
- Catheter whip, overdamping of the system, over-wedging, and incomplete wedging are commonly encountered problems that can impede the acquisition of accurate PA pressure and PAWP.

CLINICAL APPLICATIONS/ CONTROVERSIES

- The appreciable margin for error in interpretation of PA catheter data as well as potential for complications during placement and use of the catheter have raised concern regarding the efficacy, morbidity, and mortality associated with PA catheter use. Three recent randomized prospective trials have all failed to demonstrate any benefit attributable to the catheter.
- These data suggest that the PA catheter is not useful when applied to general categories of patients with shock, ARDS, or high-risk surgical status. It is unknown whether this is related to failings of the PA catheter or simply to the useful role of complementary means of assessing volume state and perfusion, as discussed in other chapters, but including echocardiography and pulse pressure variation. It also remains possible that some subsets of patients or unusual individual patients might benefit from the PA catheter even though populations of patients do not.

BIBLIOGRAPHY

Sandham JD, Hull RD, Brant RF, et al. A randomized, controlled trial of the use of pulmonary-artery catheters in high-risk surgical patients. *N Engl J Med* 2003;348:5–14.

Leatherman JW, Marini JJ. Clinical use of the pulmonary artery catheter. In: Hall JB, Schmidt GA, Wood LDH, eds., *Principles of Critical Care*, 2nd ed. New York, NY: McGraw-Hill; 1992/1998:155–176.

Connors AF Jr, Speroff T, Dawson NV, et al. The effectiveness of right heart catheterization in the initial care of critically ill patients. *JAMA* 1996;276(11):889–897.

Rivers E, Nguyen B, Havstad S, et al. Early goal-directed therapy in the treatment of severe sepsis and septic shock. *N Engl J Med* 2001;345:1368–1377.

12 NUTRITION IN THE CRITICALLY ILL

Joseph Levitt

KEY POINTS

- Critical illness is often associated with hypermetabolism, increased insulin resistance, accelerated lipolysis, and net protein catabolism. In combination with prolonged bedrest, these derangements can result in severe depletion of lean body mass, impaired immune function, impaired ventilatory reserve, and increased infectious morbidity and mortality.
- Malnutrition is present in up to 40% of intensive care unit (ICU) patients and is associated with an increased mortality. Nutritional support cannot fully prevent or reverse the metabolic alterations associated with critical illness.
- Nutritional support can improve wound healing, decrease catabolic response to injury, improve gastrointestinal (GI) function, and improve clinical outcomes.
- Despite these benefits and the widespread use of nutritional support, much controversy and variation in practice exists over what, when, and how to feed critically ill patients.
- While many trials have addressed these questions, significant heterogeneity in results, feeding strategies (e.g., enteral vs. parenteral, early vs. late, positioning of feeding tube, and content of diet), and patient enrollment (e.g., surgical, medical, burn, trauma, obese, and malnourished) make definitive recommendations difficult.

ENTERAL VERSUS PARENTERAL FEEDING

- While significant debate exists even over this most fundamental question, the bulk of evidence and practice guidelines support early enteral feeding over parenteral feeding whenever possible. While a clear mortality benefit has not been established by meta-analysis, infectious complications are clearly lower with enteral feeding.
- Potential benefits of enteral feeding include preservation of gut structure and function with reduced translocation of bacteria, as well as avoidance of increased risks of line sepsis, immunosuppression, hepatobiliary dysfunction, hyperglycemia, and increased cost associated with parenteral nutrition.
- However, enteral feeding carries an increased risk of aspiration and inability to achieve target rates of supplementation due to displacement of feeding tubes, high residuals or GI symptoms, and invasive procedures or road trips from the ICU leading to frequent interruption of feeding.
- Although not rigorously studied, generally accepted contraindications to enteral feeding include bowel perforation/fistula, obstruction, bowel ischemia, severe exacerbations of inflammatory bowel disease, high nasogastric losses, and imminent bowel resection or endoscopy. Uncomplicated bowel anastomosis is not a clear contraindication.
- Importantly, nasojejunal feeding improves outcome in cases of severe pancreatitis compared to parenteral nutrition. It is unclear if similar benefit exists for more proximal forms of enteral nutrition but some evidence suggests even gastric feeding is safe and is probably preferable to parenteral nutrition if jejunal positioning is not available.

EARLY VERSUS LATE FEEDING

- It is unclear how long critically ill patients can survive without food. Surgical literature suggests morbidity and mortality increase significantly with >2 weeks of glucose infusion alone. Meta-analysis of randomized trials show a trend toward improved mortality and infectious complications with early (<24 or 48 hours) enteral nutrition compared to delayed (either enteral or parenteral) feeding. However, it is unclear how long it is safe to withhold enteral feeding when contraindicated before starting parenteral feeding.
- While, some authors, in nonrandomized trials have found increased harm associated with early aggressive feeding, the Canadian Clinical Practice Guidelines recommend starting enteral feeding within 24–48 hours

of admission in all mechanically ventilated patients without contraindications.

WHERE AND HOW MUCH TO FEED

- Many small clinical trials have found mixed results of the benefit of small bowel versus gastric feeding. However, meta-analyses suggest a trend toward increased caloric intake and fewer infectious complications with small bowel feeding, which is generally recommended when feasible.
- Importantly, even small bowel feeding dramatically increases gastric secretions and may not significantly reduce aspiration events. Also the association of high gastric residual volumes and aspirations events is not clearly established. Some authors even recommend tolerating residual volumes up to 400–500 mL. If these recommendations were widely followed, the increased caloric intake associated with small bowel feeding may diminish.
- Early achievement of target rates of enteral feeding improved outcomes in a study of critically brain-injured patients. While not directly translatable to other critically ill patients, these results suggest that strategies to maximize delivery, for example, starting at goal rates, tolerating higher residual volumes, and use of promotility agents (metoclopramide preferable to erythromycin due to concerns over bacterial resistance) should be considered.
- The addition of parenteral nutrition to enteral feeding to improve caloric intake has generally been associated with worsened outcomes. However, many of these findings may be the result of overfeeding, and the effect of adding parenteral nutrition when enteral feeding is poorly tolerated, is unclear. Nonetheless, starting parenteral nutrition, before all measures to optimize enteral feeding have been exhausted, is not recommended.
- When parenteral nutrition is deemed necessary, short-term (<10 days) use of hypocaloric, lipid-free formulas may reduce infectious complications. However, safety in malnourished patients and longer-term use has not been established.
- Instituting detailed nutritional protocols may also increase rates of achieving nutritional goals and improve clinical outcomes.

WHAT TO FEED

- In general, specialized or enhanced formulas, for example, arginine supplemented or peptide instead of whole protein-based diets, are expensive and have not been shown to be beneficial in most critically ill patients. However, small clinical trials suggest possible benefit in some areas:
    - Enteral fish oils and other antioxidants may improve outcomes in acute respiratory distress syndrome (ARDS).
    - Enteral glutamine may benefit burn and trauma patients, while glutamine-enhanced parenteral nutrition may be superior to standard formulas for critically ill patients.
    - Fat-free parenteral nutrition for <10 days may reduce infectious complications compared to standard formulas.

TIGHT GLUCOSE CONTROL

- A single large randomized prospective trial found a significant mortality benefit with tight glucose control (80–110 mg/dL vs. 180–200 mg/dL) in surgical ICU patients. However, patients consisted predominantly of elective cardiothoracic patients with low acuity (acute physiologic and chronic health evaluation [APACHE] II scores of 7–13) and many received early parenteral nutrition.
- Concern exists for increased complications due to hypoglycemia if these strict targets are extended to more labile patients outside of a study setting. It is also unclear if a similar benefit would be found in nonsurgical patients not receiving parenteral nutrition.
- Nonetheless, good glycemic control should be emphasized in all critically ill patients, but optimal target levels remained to be established.

BIBLIOGRAPHY

Heyland DK, Dhaliwal R, Drover JW, et al. Canadian clinical practice guidelines for nutrition support in mechanically ventilated, critically ill adult patients. *JPEN J Parenter Enteral Nutr* 2003;27:355–373.

Klein S, Kinney J, Jeejeebhoy K, et al. Nutrition support in clinical practice: review of published data and recommendations for future research directions. Summary of a conference sponsored by the National Institutes of Health, American Society for Parenteral and Enteral Nutrition, and American Society for Clinical Nutrition. *Am J Clin Nutr* 1997;66:683–706.

Marik PE, Zaloga GP. Meta-analysis of parenteral nutrition versus enteral nutrition in patients with acute pancreatitis. *BMJ* 2004;328:1407–1410.

Metheny NA, Schallom ME, Edwards SJ. Effect of gastrointestinal motility and feeding tube site on aspiration risk in critically ill patients: a review. *Heart Lung* 2004;33:131–145.

Section 2
CARDIOVASCULAR DISORDERS

13 AN APPROACH TO SHOCK

William Schweickert

KEY POINTS

- Shock is a physiologic state characterized by a significant reduction in tissue perfusion with resultant oxygen deprivation. Progressive, untreated hypoperfusion leads to the loss of cell membrane integrity, intracellular edema, loss of intracellular contents, inadequate pH regulation, and eventually cell death—manifesting as end-organ damage or failure. Early recognition and prompt treatment is necessary to prevent this cascade of damage.
- Shock is almost always signaled by systemic hypotension (defined as a systolic blood pressure ≤ 90 mmHg or a mean arterial pressure ≤ 60 mmHg) and tachycardia, with commonly associated clinical features of multiple organ system hypoperfusion including tachypnea, oliguria, mental status changes, diaphoresis, and metabolic acidosis.
- Three primary types of shock states are typically recognized: hypovolemic, cardiogenic, and septic. A brief, directed physical examination will help to recognize these most common etiologies of shock.
- Less commonly, shock may be attributed to another etiology, almost universally recognized by accompanying historical details and adjunctive tests (beyond complete blood counts and chemistries) which elevate the clinical suspicion. These can be categorized under three broad headings: high output hypotension, high right atrial pressure hypotension, and nonresponsive hypovolemia.
    - *Historical clues*: food and medicine allergies, recent changes in medications, potential acute or chronic drug intoxication, preexisting diseases, immunosuppressed states, and hypercoagulable conditions.
    - *Important adjunctive tests*: LFTs, pancreatic enzymes, arterial lactate, cardiac enzymes, arterial blood gas, toxicology screen, ECG, and urinalysis.

BEDSIDE ASSESSMENT OF SHOCK: WHAT TYPE OF SHOCK IS IT?

- *Step one*: Is the cardiac output reduced or elevated (Table 13-1)?
    - *Septic shock* is strongly suggested by high cardiac output hypotension, mediated by a primary decrease in systemic vascular resistance (SVR) which is frequently signaled by a widened pulse pressure (with marked diastolic reduction relative to systolic pressure), a strong apical cardiac impulse, warm extremities with brisk nail bed return, fever or hypothermia, and leukocytosis or leukopenia (for more details, see Chap. 43).
    - Low cardiac output indicates cardiogenic or hypovolemic shock. A narrow pulse pressure, reduced apical cardiac impulse, and cool extremities with poor nail bed return signal low cardiac output.
- *Step two*: If the cardiac output is low, is the heart empty or too full (Table 13-2)?
    - *Cardiogenic shock* is most commonly signaled by volume overload. Findings include a large heart with gallops or murmur, crackles on lung auscultation, elevated jugular venous pressure (JVP), and peripheral edema. The electrocardiogram may demonstrate ischemic changes and a chest x-ray (CXR) may show a large cardiac silhouette with a widened vascular pedicle, prominent azygos vein, pulmonary edema, and upper lobe pulmonary vasculature. A broad differential must be entertained,

TABLE 13-1 Shock Algorithm: Is the Cardiac Output Low?

	YES	NO
Pulse pressure	Decreased	Increased
Peripheral pulse	Decreased	Increased
Extremity warmth	Decreased	Increased
Nail bed return	Decreased	Increased
Heart sounds	Muffled	Crisp
Clinical clues	Angina	Increased WBC
	ECG change	Liver function
Working diagnosis	Cardiogenic	Sepsis
	Hypovolemic	Sepsis
		Sepsis
		Liver disease
		Beriberi
		Paget disease
		Aortic insufficiency

including systolic dysfunction (best represented by the above findings), diastolic dysfunction, valvular disease, and arrhythmia (for more details, see Chap. 14).

- *Hypovolemic shock* may be obvious intravascular depletion, including blood loss (indicated by hematemesis, tarry stool, abdominal distention, reduced hematocrit, or trauma) and dehydration (indicated by decreased skin turgor, vomiting, diarrhea, or a negative fluid balance). Less commonly, it may be the result of "central hypovolemia" or elevated right atrial pressure-mediated hypotension (see "Recognizing the less common causes," below).

TABLE 13-2 Shock Algorithm: Is the Heart Too Full?

	YES	NO
Examination	S_3	Dry mucous membrane (MM)
	JVD increased	Decrease skin turgor
	Cardiomegaly	
Setting	Angina	Hemorrhage
	Dyspnea	Dehydration
Data	ECG	BUN/creatinine
	Echo	Hgb
	CXR	
Working diagnosis	Cardiogenic	Sepsis
		Hypovolemic

ABBREVIATIONS: JVD, jugular venous distention; BUN, blood urea nitrogen.

RECOGNIZING THE LESS COMMON CAUSES

- High output hypotension (distributive shock)
  - This situation involves escalated cardiac output in the presence of reduced vascular tone and reactivity, often associated with abnormal distribution of blood flow. Most commonly this is the result of septic shock; however, the differential also includes the following:
    - *Liver failure:* most commonly the end result of acute decompensation (occasionally superimposed on a chronic hepatic insufficiency), this shock is recognized quickly by deranged liver function tests (LFTs), and mandates testing for infectious (viral) processes, medication/toxin abuse, and vascular phenomena.
    - *Severe pancreatitis*: similar to liver failure, this is usually recognized by historical survey and screening serology (pancreatic enzyme levels, LFTs).
    - *Thyroid storm* should be considered in anyone with proptosis, goiter, recent iodine load, or access to synthetic thyroid hormone. A screening TSH and free thyroxine index are indicated, and early endocrinology consultation is warranted.
    - *Trauma* with significant systemic inflammatory response.
    - *Anaphylaxis* requires the appropriate clinical context: drug or contact exposure, ingestion, or insect bite. Signs and symptoms may include wheezing, stridor, skin rash, and cyanosis.
    - *Others*: arteriovenous fistula, Paget disease, beriberi.
- High right atrial pressure hypotension
  - In this situation, the left ventricle experiences functional hypovolemia mediated by the circulatory obstacle(s) of pulmonary hypertension and/or right ventricular failure. The pulse pressure is narrow, dependent edema is present; however, the lungs are not congested.
  - Pulmonary hypertension
    - *Pulmonary embolus* suggested by the clinical scenario (perioperative state, immobilization, thrombophilia), symptoms (dyspnea, chest pain, hemoptysis), and physical examination (loud P2 with a widened and fixed split of the second heart sound), new hypoxemia without obvious parenchymal disease, right heart strain on ECG.
    - *Acute-on-chronic pulmonary hypertension* causes shock in the setting of prior primary pulmonary hypertension, recurrent pulmonary emboli, progression of collagen-vascular disease, or chronic respiratory failure (e.g., chronic obstructive pulmonary disease [COPD] or pulmonary fibrosis) aggravated in part by hypoxic pulmonary vasoconstriction.

The resultant right ventricular overload impairs left ventricular filling, and similar to the above "cardiogenic" shock, pulse pressure is small and extremities are cool with peripheral edema. Oxygen therapy, inotropic agents, and possible pulmonary vasodilator therapy can reduce pulmonary hypertension and increase cardiac output in a small but significant proportion of patients.

  - *Right ventricular infarction*: rarely occurs in the absence of left ventricular injury, but may be signaled by conduction disturbances (AV block), right precordial ECG lead findings, and cardiac enzyme elevation.
  - *Cardiac tamponade*: the pericardial effusion is suggested by the clinical setting (renal failure, malignancy, chest pain), physical examination (distant heart sounds, elevated neck veins, pulsus paradoxus), and routine investigations (CXR with "water bottle" heart, ECG with low voltage or electrical alternans). Echocardiography is a necessity—in the interim, intravenous fluids may help to mediate small improvements in blood pressure, while reductions in effective circulating blood volume can be catastrophic. Tamponade physiology requires urgent evacuation of the pericardial space (catheter or surgical drainage).
  - *Other etiologies*: constrictive pericarditis, tension pneumothorax, massive pleural effusion, positive pressure ventilation with high positive end-expiratory pressure (PEEP), and very high intra-abdominal pressure.
- Nonresponsive hypovolemia
  - In this clinical scenario, large volumes of fluid may be necessary to replete circulating volume, and hypotension may persist despite such measures.
  - *Adrenal insufficiency*: considered in patients with history of steroid exposure (especially, recent withdrawal), adrenal infarction or infection (e.g., meningococcemia and tuberculosis). Establish the diagnosis by measuring serum cortisol and conduct a corticotrophin stimulation test.
  - *Spinal shock (neurogenic shock)*: considered in the setting of spinal injury with the absence of hemorrhage. Its hallmark is decreased vascular tone, particularly venous capacitance. Therapy is volume and catecholamines.

BIBLIOGRAPHY

Walley KR. Shock. In: Hall JB, Schmidt GA, Wood LDH, eds., *Principles of Critical Care*, 3rd ed. New York, NY: McGraw-Hill;2005:249–265.

14 VENTRICULAR DYSFUNCTION IN CRITICAL ILLNESS

Jay Finigan

KEY POINTS

- Cardiac dysfunction is a common complication of critical illness.
- Disturbances of cardiac function in the ICU include those of rate, rhythm, afterload, preload, valves, systolic pump function, and diastolic filling.
- While hypotension in the ICU, particularly in the setting of sepsis, is often a problem of refractory decreases in systemic vascular resistance (SVR), ventricular disturbances are common and can contribute to increased morbidity and mortality.
- The causes of ventricular dysfunction in the ICU are myriad and rapid identification and correction of ventricular derangements is crucial to improved mortality in critical care.

CARDIAC FUNCTION

- Cardiac output (CO) is the product of heart rate and ventricular stroke volume (CO = HR × SV).
- In most critically ill patients, CO is controlled largely by the systemic vessels, not the heart, and determined by the mean systemic pressure, the resistance to venous return, and the right atrial (RA) pressure. In those with severe ventricular dysfunction, however, it may be more helpful to consider the cardiac determinants of SV, including *contractility*, *preload*, and *afterload*. Alterations in any of these can result in decreased ventricular performance.
  - Note that the right (RV) and left ventricle (LV) each have a preload and afterload: RV preload is RA pressure and afterload is pulmonary vascular impedance while LV preload is LV end-diastolic pressure and afterload is a function of outflow tract pressure and ventricular volume.
- Contractility represents inotropic capability of the ventricle independent of preload and afterload.
- Insufficient or excessive preload can depress ventricular performance.

ASSESSMENT OF VENTRICULAR FUNCTION

- History and physical examination can identify clues of ventricular dysfunction.
  - Distended neck veins, presence of an S_3, and crackles suggest a failing ventricle.
  - Echocardiography can rapidly and accurately assess systolic function, diastolic function, wall motion abnormalities, valves, and the pericardium.
- Central access can be used to measure central venous pressure (CVP) which is a measure of RV preload. CVP is *not* a measure of LV preload.
- Pulmonary artery catheters (PACs) can be used to assess several cardiac parameters including RA pressure (which represents RV preload), RV pressure, pulmonary artery pressure (which represents RV afterload), and pulmonary capillary wedge pressure (PCWP) which represents LV preload.
  - Early studies suggested that PACs might cause harm, but this has not been confirmed in more recent, randomized trials. On the other hand, PACs also do not improve outcome. Multiple studies have shown that the measured wedge pressure is a very poor predictor of whether a patient will respond to a fluid challenge.

CAUSES OF VENTRICULAR DYSFUNCTION

- *Chronic* ventricular dysfunction secondary to ischemia, alcohol, or viral myocarditis.
- *Acute* ventricular dysfunction in the ICU has several causes:
  - *Ischemia*: Global or localized myocardial ischemia, particularly resulting in infarction, can depress ventricular function. Even in the setting of normal coronary arteries, low oxygen tension can lead to decreased contractility, CO, and coronary artery perfusion.
  - *Hypocalcemia*: Calcium homeostasis is critical to cardiac function. Low serum ionized calcium leads to decreased cardiac myocyte calcium flux and subsequent depressed contractility. Causes of decreased ionized calcium include red cell transfusions (red cells stored in citrate which can bind calcium), lactic acid, and bicarbonate infusion.
  - *Acidosis*: Respiratory acidosis ($PCO_2 > 60$ mmHg) can result in decreased contractility and CO, while metabolic acidosis seems to have less of an effect on LV function.
  - *Drugs*: Toxins such as alcohol as well as drugs such as beta-blockers, calcium channel blockers, disopyramide, and procainamide can depress contractility.
- *Sepsis*: Ventricular dysfunction, specifically decreased contractility, occurs early in patients with sepsis, even those who maintain normotension. However, after volume loading CO is often maintained or even increased in sepsis. This has been referred to as "warm shock" and is marked by warm extremities and moist skin.
  - Septic patients initially manifest a depressed ejection fraction (EF) which increases over 7–10 days. Interestingly, *survivors* present with ventricular dilation and a low EF (~0.32) which increases over time while *nonsurvivors* present with a higher EF (~0.55) which remains high until death indicating that depressed LV contractility in sepsis might be protective.
  - The cause of sepsis-induced myocardial depression is believed to be secondary to circulating myocardial depressants such as tumor necrosis factor (TNF), nitric oxide (NO), and interleukin (IL)-6, among others. Evidence demonstrates that coronary hypoperfusion and ischemia are not sources of decreased EF in sepsis.

TREATMENT

- Identify and treat reversible causes.
  - Use of supplemental oxygen and red cell transfusion to prevent or treat ischemia.
  - Intravenous calcium can correct hypocalcemia. Many measure ionized calcium levels after large red cell transfusions (≥6 units), although it is not clear whether calcium administration during critical illness is helpful or harmful.
  - Replete other electrolytes (potassium, magnesium) as needed.

MANAGEMENT

- Key to managing ventricular pump function in critical illness, especially in sepsis, is to optimize preload. In general, in the absence of cardiogenic shock, hypotension and ventricular dysfunction should be managed first with the institution of fluids.
  - According to Starling Law of the Heart, contractile strength is a function of muscle fiber length, that is, other things being equal, a stretched ventricle (by increased volume) will contract more forcefully than an unstretched ventricle. Normal end-diastolic LV filling pressure is in the range of 10 mmHg but a heart with depressed contractility requires higher filling pressures to increase SV (Fig. 14-1).

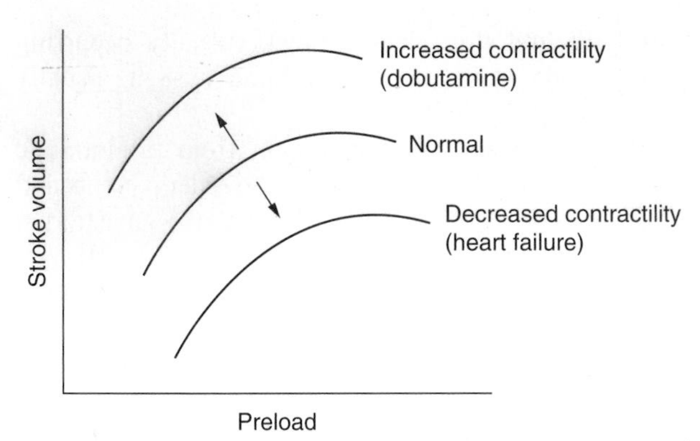

FIG. 14-1 Frank-Starling curve. Three different curves of contractility, normal, heart failure and use of the inotropic agent such as dobutamine. At a given level of contractility, increasing preload will increase stroke volume (until the systolic function of the heart is overwhelmed). Heart failure and inotropes cause a shift of the curve down and to the right or up and to the left to a new curve of contractility.

  - Major limitation to volume loading is creation of pulmonary edema which, in patients with normal albumin concentrations and endothelial cells, forms at PCWP ≥ 20–25 mmHg. In patients with decreased serum albumin and/or endothelial cell disruption (e.g., acute respiratory distress syndrome [ARDS]), pulmonary edema can form at lower wedge pressures.
- *Afterload reduction* with vasodilators (angiotensin converting enzyme inhibitors [ACE-I], nitrates), blood pressure permitting, will further improve ventricular systolic function.
- *Inotropic agents*, such as dobutamine can boost contractility and are effective adjuncts in patients with a low CO despite adequate resuscitation. In patients with hypotension it occasionally causes hypotension, prompting the addition of a vasopressor.
- In cases of severe, refractory heart failure from damaged myocardium, support using *intra-aortic balloon counterpulsation* (IABC) can serve as a bridge to recovery or corrective surgery. IABC aids a failing heart in both diastole, via increased diastolic coronary filling pressure and in systole, by decreasing cardiac afterload.

DIASTOLIC DYSFUNCTION

- Diastolic dysfunction (DD) is a condition of decreased SV marked by increased diastolic stiffness.
- Abnormal diastolic filling of the LV has been observed by echocardiography in patients with hypotensive and normotensive sepsis.
- In contrast to systolic function (see above), more severe DD is associated with worse outcomes in sepsis.
- Therapy of DD is limited and includes identifying and treating reversible causes (ischemia, excessive tachycardia) as well as initiating standard treatment for heart failure: afterload reduction and achieving an appropriate end-diastolic volume with the judicious use of fluids and diuretics. In addition, treating supraventricular tachycardias can be important as patients with DD have an increased reliance on the atrial contribution to end-diastolic volume.

RIGHT VENTRICULAR DYSFUNCTION

- It is a given that the input and output of the RV and LV must be equal and that alterations in either side can result in clinically apparent heart failure.
- RV dysfunction is a common finding in critical care as well as sepsis.
- In sepsis, especially if there is acute lung injury, pulmonary vascular resistance may be elevated contributing to RV dysfunction.
- Decreased intrinsic RV contractility also contributes to RV dysfunction in sepsis.
- Low RV EF has been associated with worse outcomes. Similar to the situation regarding the LV, survivors often present with lower RV EFs than nonsurvivors.

BIBLIOGRAPHY

Kumar A, Krieger A, Symeoneides S, et al. Myocardial dysfunction in septic shock. Part I: clinical manifestations of cardiovascular dysfunction. *J Cardiothorac Vasc Anesth* 2001;15:364–376.
Vincent JL. Cardiovascular alterations in septic shock. *J Antimicrob Chemother* 1998;41:9–15.
Walley KR. Ventricular dysfunction in critical illness. In: Hall JB, Schmidt GA, Wood LDH, eds., *Principles of Critical Care*, 3rd ed. New York, NY: McGraw-Hill; 2005:267–282.

15 RHYTHM DISTURBANCES IN THE ICU

Susan S. Kim

KEY POINTS

- Rhythm disturbances are common in the ICU.
- In medical and surgical ICUs, dysrhythmias are markers of critical illness more often than signals of organic heart disease.

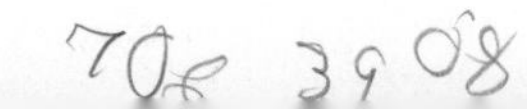

- A 12-lead electrocardiogram, long rhythm strip, and a systematic approach aid the diagnosis of rhythm disturbances. Cardiologic consultation may be appropriate in some cases.
- Tachyarrhythmias should always prompt a search for underlying precipitants, such as hemorrhage or hypoxemia, which might have specific remedies. ST should almost never be treated directly.
- Unstable patients with nonsinus tachyarrhythmias should be electrically cardioverted.
- Bradyarrhythmias may follow vagal stimulation.
- Transcutaneous and transvenous pacing, as well as therapy delivered through an existing ICD, can be considered in appropriate patients.

EPIDEMIOLOGY

- In a single-center study of 756 medical, cardiac, or postoperative ICU patients, roughly one in five patients developed a significant arrhythmia during their ICU stay.
- Tachyarrhythmias accounted for 90% of rhythm disturbance episodes.
- Atrial fibrillation (AF) affected the highest proportion of patients (47% of patients).
- Ventricular tachycardia (VT) accounted for the highest proportion of arrhythmia episodes (52% of episodes).

PATHOPHYSIOLOGY

- Rhythm disturbances can be divided into tachyarrhythmias and bradyarrhythmias.
- Tachyarrhythmias can be further divided into narrow-complex (usually supraventricular in origin [SVT]) and wide-complex (usually either supraventricular with aberrant conduction or ventricular [VT]) tachycardias.
  - Tachyarrhythmia mechanisms include re-entry, triggered activity, increased automaticity, or a combination of these factors.
  - Regardless of mechanism, both SVTs and VTs may be stimulated by factors such as cardiac ischemia, a hyperadrenergic state, sympathomimetic medications, other medication toxicity, hypotension, hypoxemia, electrolyte abnormality, catheter irritation, and acid-base disturbance.
- Bradyarrhythmias represent sinus node dysfunction (SND), atrioventricular block (AVB), or both.
  - SND may manifest as inappropriate sinus bradycardia, sinus pause, or sinus arrest.
  - AVB may take the form of first-degree or type I second-degree block (usually occurring at the level of the AV node, usually benign) or type II second-degree and third-degree block (usually occurring infranodally in the His-Purkinje system, usually pathologic).
  - Both SND and AVB can stem from (a) intrinsic nodal pathology such as is seen in older patients and those with cardiovascular disease, (b) an external insult such as an acid-base disturbance, electrolyte abnormality, hypoxemia, hypotension, medication toxicity, or increased vagal tone, or (c) a combination of intrinsic and extrinsic factors.
  - AVB may also result from erosion into the AV node by a focus of infectious endocarditis.
  - Junctional rhythm is a secondary or "escape" rhythm that occurs in response to a primary bradyarrhythmia such as any form of SND or AVB.
  - Asystole (ventricular) represents either sinus arrest or complete heart block with no escape rhythm.

CLINICAL FEATURES

- Tachyarrhythmias
  - Sinus tachycardia (ST) is a very common rhythm in the ICU. It is characterized by upright P waves in lead II and gradual (vs. abrupt, such as in SVT) rises and falls in the heart rate. ST frequently occurs in response to a hemodynamic insult such as low stroke volume (SV) or low systemic vascular resistance (SVR). ST may also reflect fever, pain, or anxiety.
  - Narrow-complex tachycardias (nonsinus) are usually supraventricular in origin and can represent AF, atrial flutter (AFl), a paroxysmal supraventricular tachycardia (PSVT, such as atrioventricular nodal tachycardia [AVNRT], orthodromic re-entry tachycardia [ORT], or atrial tachycardia [AT]), multifocal atrial tachycardia (MAT), or junctional ectopic tachycardia (JET).
  - Not uncommonly, the appearance of a wide-complex tachycardia is generated by artifact (caused by motion, poor lead contact, chest physical therapy, and so forth).
  - Wide-complex tachycardias can represent artifact, supraventricular tachycardia with aberrant conduction, antidromic re-entry tachycardia, drug or electrolyte imbalance, VT, or ventricular fibrillation (VF).
- Bradyarrhythmias
  - In the ICU, heightened vagal tone is a common cause of bradycardia (both SND and AVB). Factors such as nausea, vomiting, pain, coughing, and undergoing suctioning can cause heightened vagal tone. This autonomic input can slow or even halt sinus node or atrioventricular nodal function. In most instances, these episodes are self-limited and carry a benign prognosis.

- Bradycardia due to increased vagal tone is usually episodic (lasting on the order of several seconds), is gradual in onset and resolution, and is usually associated with one of the conditions noted above. For example, vagally mediated bradycardia may manifest as gradual sinus slowing or gradual prolongation of the PR interval with eventual AVB (AV nodal Wenckebach).
- SND may manifest as sinus arrest, sinus pause, or inappropriate sinus bradycardia.
- With AVB, prolonged or blocked conduction is occurring either at the level of the AV node or infranodally in the His-Purkinje system. This distinction is important as the level of block frequently correlates with the likelihood of long-term loss of AV conduction (low and high, respectively).
- In most cases, first-degree and type I second-degree AVB (AV nodal Wenckebach) occur at the level of the AV node and do not lead to long-term loss of AV conduction. A common cause of first-degree or type I second-degree AV block is increased vagal tone causing slowed conduction through the AV node.
- Similarly, in most cases, type II second-degree AVB and third-degree AVB occur at the level of the His-Purkinje system and represent fixed, structural conduction system disease. These forms of AVB are associated with a high likelihood of long-term loss of AV conduction.

DIAGNOSIS AND DIFFERENTIAL

- Whenever possible, obtain a formal 12-lead electrocardiogram and follow this protocol:
  1. Is it a tachyarrhythmia? If yes, then proceed to #2. If not, then go to #5
  2. Rule out ST. If not ST, then go to #3
  3. Rule out narrow-complex tachycardias. If not, then go to #4
  4. Wide-complex tachycardias
  5. Bradyarrhythmias
- Permanent pacemakers and implantable cardioverter-defibrillators (ICDs) may be programmed to store supraventricular or ventricular arrhythmia events. As such, interrogation of these devices and extraction of those event data may assist in diagnosis.

INTENSIVE CARE UNIT CARE

- Tachyarrhythmias
  - ST is frequently a compensatory hemodynamic response; therefore, it should rarely be treated. Rather, the underlying disorder promoting the ST should be addressed (e.g., hypotension and fever).
  - Look for an underlying trigger of the tachyarrhythmia.
  - Follow advanced cardiac life support (ACLS) guidelines.
  - Cardiovert the patient if unstable.
  - Adenosine at 6 and 12 mg IV doses can cause AV block. Its half-life is a few seconds and so it should be administered with rapid IV push followed by a rapid flush. It may cause transient shortness of breath and chest pressure. It is contraindicated in asthma patients.
  - Adenosine may terminate rhythms that depend on the AV node (atrioventricular nodal re-entrant tachycardia [AVNRT], atrioventricular re-entrant tachycardia [AVRT]) or simply block conduction of supraventricular input to the ventricles.
  - Most ICDs and some pacemakers can be programmed to deliver commanded antitachycardia pacing. ICDs can deliver commanded internal shocks. Thus, these implanted devices may be programmed by qualified personnel to deliver commanded therapy to treat tachyarrhythmias.
- Bradyarrhythmias
  - Medication toxicity should start with cessation of the offending agent and continuous cardiac telemetry monitoring.
  - In more extreme cases with significant bradycardia or hypotension, therapies directed at reversing toxic effects may be applied. Beta-blocker toxicity may be treated effectively with glucagon, calcium channel blocker toxicity with intravenous calcium, and digoxin toxicity with digoxin-specific antibody infusion.
  - Look for extrinsic, reversible factors.
  - Temporary pacing can take one of several forms: transcutaneous pacing, transvenous pacing with an isolated temporary pacing wire, transvenous pacing through a pacer-port pulmonary artery catheter, and epicardial pacing.
  - Transcutaneous pacing allows for immediate, noninvasive pacing. However, it can be painful; may not be effective, especially in obese patients; and has less long-term reliability than does invasive pacing. It is useful as a short-term, temporizing measure. Pacing pads should be placed to maximize energy delivery to the left ventricle. Conscious patients should be sedated.
  - Transvenous pacing through a pacer-port pulmonary artery catheter can be a convenient option in a patient with a preexisting pacer-port pulmonary artery catheter. Because the wire is threaded through the catheter (exiting at a port 20 cm from the catheter tip), this method allows for more guided placement of the wire tip into the right ventricle—an advantage, especially, when fluoroscopy is not available. Wire positioning, though, is subject to the stability of catheter position.

- Transvenous pacing with an isolated temporary pacing wire allows for more stable positioning over time, but is most safely placed under fluoroscopic guidance. Balloon-tipped wires are available and are safer to place without fluoroscopy than are non-balloon-tipped wires.
- Any transvenous pacing wire carries the risk of myocardial perforation and consequent tamponade as well as the risk of introducing endocardial infection.
- Patients with transvenous pacing wires should have daily chest roentgenograms and 12-lead electrocardiograms to monitor positioning.
- Epicardial temporary pacing is another option, but is mostly limited to postcardiac surgery patients who have had epicardial wires placed intraoperatively. Thresholds rapidly increase with these types of wires so that by 3 days, about half no longer capture.
- Pacing is effective only if it results in myocardial depolarization or "capture." Capture is affected by the vector of energy delivery (as with transcutaneous pad placement), transvenous wire contact with the myocardium, and amount of programmed energy delivery. The ability to capture with pacing may change over time due to wire malpositioning or may be affected by hypoxemia, hypotension, and acid-base status.

BIBLIOGRAPHY

Artucio H, Pereira M. Cardiac arrhythmias in critically ill patients: epidemiologic study. *Crit Care Med* 1990;18(12):1383–1388.

Drew BJ, Califf RM, Funk M, et al. Practice standards for electrocardiographic monitoring in hospital settings. *Circulation* 2004;110(17):2721–2746.

Reinelt P, Karth GD, Geppert A, et al. Incidence and type of cardiac arrhythmias in critically ill patients: a single center experience in a medical-cardiological ICU. *Intensive Care Med* 2001;27:1466–1473.

16 NONINVASIVE ASSESSMENT OF CARDIAC OUTPUT

Sascha Goonewardena

KEY POINTS

- Cardiac output is one of the most important hemodynamic variables for the assessment of cardiac function and for the guidance of therapy in the intensive care setting (Table 16-1).

TABLE 16-1 Uses of CO Measurement

Determination of etiologies of shock
Targeting treatment strategies
Risk stratification and prognostication

- The gold standard for measurement of CO is the thermodilution technique that involves invasive monitoring with a pulmonary artery catheter. However, the use of invasive methods to determine CO has associated risks and potential adverse outcomes. The use of noninvasive methods to determine CO provides intensivists with the necessary clinical information without the potential risks associated with invasive devices.
- Even the thermodilution technique for CO determination is susceptible to inaccuracies; intracardiac shunts, tricuspid regurgitation, and inaccurate measurements are the major sources of error when determining CO using the thermodilution technique.
- Noninvasive methods to determine CO include echocardiography with Doppler ultrasound, thoracic bioimpedance, and the indirect Fick method.
- Each method has inherent advantages and disadvantages (Table 16-2). Because of the noninvasive nature of each method, certain assumptions are required when utilizing each method.
- Proper utilization of noninvasive methods of CO assessment can enable intensivists to more appropriately diagnose, risk stratify, and titrate specific therapies to the patient's clinical situation.
- A major advantage of continuous CO monitoring is that important physiologic alterations can be detected that may not be evident with intermittent monitoring.

ECHOCARDIOGRAPHY WITH DOPPLER ULTRASOUND

- Echocardiography relies on high-frequency sound waves that penetrate body tissues. As these sound waves encounter tissues of different acoustic densities, a fraction of the emitted sound wave is reflected.
- When an ultrasound beam is directed toward a moving target, the reflected sound wave changes its frequency; this phenomenon is known as *Doppler shift*. The magnitude of this Doppler shift is directly proportional to the velocity of the blood flow.
- The Doppler shift equation is $Fd = 2\ fo/CV \cos\theta$, where Fd represents the Doppler shift, fo is the transmitted frequency, V is the velocity of the moving blood, C is the velocity of the ultrasound in blood

TABLE 16-2 Comparison of Noninvasive CO Determination Techniques

METHOD	ADVANTAGE	DISADVANTAGE
Echocardiography with Doppler ultrasound	Noninvasive, can assess large number of cardiac and hemodynamic variables in addition to CO	Operator dependent, poor image quality in certain patient populations, and relies on mechanical assumptions for heart and vasculature
Thoracic bioimpedance	Noninvasive, only requires minimal equipment	Less reliable in critically ill patients, highly dependent on lead position and other mechanical variations, susceptible to inaccuracies when ventricular arrhythmias present
Indirect Fick method	Noninvasive, continuous CO determination	Less accurate at high CO, susceptible to small variations in VO_2 and VCO_2 measurements, requires steady state conditions

(constant), and the angle θ is the angle between the direction of the moving blood and the transmitted ultrasound beam.

- Echocardiography can measure ascending aortic flow velocity and cross-sectional diameter of aortic root to calculate cardiac output (CO).
- The velocity time integral (VTI) of blood flow is the area under the velocity-time curve.
- Stroke volume (SV) = cross-sectional area of aortic root × VTI. Then, by using the equation, CO = SV × heart rate (HR), the approximate CO can be calculated.
- Accurate estimates of CO are dependent on the accurate alignment of Doppler signal with aortic blood flow, the assumption that the aortic dimensions can be estimated, and the assumption that aortic blood flow is laminar.
- Deviations from these assumptions can lead to errors of CO estimation by up to 15%.
- Transesophageal echocardiography (TEE) has improved accuracy over transthoracic echocardiography because of decreased deviations from the assumptions mentioned above.
- TEE also enables intensivists to record CO continuously.
- Echocardiography can provide information on a host of hemodynamic variables in addition to CO including an estimation of left ventricular filling pressures, atrial interactions, and pulmonary pressures.
- Up to 25% of patients cannot be adequately imaged using echocardiography.

THORACIC BIOIMPEDANCE

- Thoracic bioimpedance technology utilizes continuous electric current stimulation to determine impedance variations that are associated with physiologic changes in the body. These variations can be utilized to estimate the SV and CO.
- Two methods exist for performing bioimpedance analysis of CO: thoracic electrical bioimpedance and whole body electrical bioimpedance.
- According to Kirchov law, electric current passes preferentially through vessels of higher conductance. Consequently, when alternating currents of 20–100 kHz are applied to the thorax, the currents are primarily distributed via the extracellular fluid and the blood vessels. Thus, with each systolic increase in the aortic blood volume, there is a proportional increase in the aortic electrical conductance.
- The relation between these two changes is expressed as: $\Delta V/V = \Delta R/R$, where change in V equals the stroke volume, V is the aortic volume immediately preceding systole, and change in R is the systolic electrical resistance to change, and R is the baseline resistance of the electrical field involved.
- A potentiometer is the device used for measuring body resistance or impedance. It is composed of two bipolar electrodes that can be applied to any accessible part of the body.
- The Sramek-Bernstein method is the most frequently used impedance cardiographic method since 1986.
- In general, most trials have demonstrated significant correlation between CO with impedance cardiography and other diagnostic methods including thermodilution; the results, however, have not always been consistent. Meta-analysis of the studies in cardiac patients comparing bioimpedance to thermodilution shows a correlation coefficient of 0.77 (0.71–0.82).
- Most clinical trials suggest that electrical bioimpedance is feasible and reliable in healthy volunteers; however, the reliability and accuracy decreases in intensive care patients.
- Limitations of thoracic electrical bioimpedance include hemodynamically significant aortic valve insufficiency, significant aortic dilation, aneurysm and coarctation, significant intracardiac shunts, significant ventricular arrhythmias, and significant pulmonary edema.

- Limitations for whole body electrical bioimpedance include hemodynamically significant aortic valve insufficiency; significant aortic dilation; aneurysm or coarctation; peripheral artery disease; intracardiac shunts; restless patients, significant ventricular arrhythmias; and peripheral edema.
- In addition to the above limitations, lead placement and estimates of the volume of electrically participating tissue (VEPT) are crucial to accurate determination of CO using electrical bioimpedance technology.

INDIRECT FICK METHOD

- The Fick principle is based on the conservation of mass. This principle states that blood flow through the pulmonary artery is equal to the ratio of the uptake or elimination of a gas and the difference in concentration of that gas in the blood flowing into and out of the lungs.
- The components of the Fick principle can be determined invasively (direct method) and noninvasively (indirect calorimetry and modified CO_2 Fick method).
- The major limitations of the direct method are related to errors in sampling and analysis, difficulty in obtaining oxygen uptake continuously and reliably, and the inability to maintain and record consistent hemodynamic states.
- Indirect calorimetry measures O_2 consumption as the amount of O_2 taken up from the respiratory gases. This is assessed within a breathing circuit whereby inspired and expired flow rates of O_2 are measured relative to one another, usually by means of an insoluble gas marker like nitrogen.
- The discrepancies between indirect calorimetry and more invasive methods of CO determination are attributed to O_2 consumption by lung tissue. In addition, very precise calibration of measurement devices is necessary to minimize variability of measured variables.
- The CO_2 Fick method is noninvasive and relies on the determination of CO_2 delivery and elimination.
- Fick equation using CO_2 is: $Q = VCO_2/CvCO_2 - CaCO_2$, where Q is cardiac output, VCO_2 is the CO_2 elimination, and $CvCO_2$ and $CaCO_2$ are the mixed venous and arterial CO_2 blood contents.
- The indirect Fick method that utilizes CO_2 is advantageous because CO_2 elimination is more easily measured than O_2 uptake and estimates of arterial CO_2 concentration can be made from the gas exhaled by the lungs.
- Monitoring the CO_2 partial pressure in the expired gas and relating this measurement to the CO_2 dissociation curve can noninvasively estimate the CO_2 concentration in the alveolar end-capillary blood.
- For all assessments of CO utilizing Fick principle or a variation of the general principle require that the patient be in a relatively steady hemodynamic state. The patient's being cared for in the intensive care setting often violates this prerequisite.

BIBLIOGRAPHY

Botero M, Lobato EB. Advances in noninvasive cardiac output monitoring: an update. *J Cardiothorac Vasc Anesth* 2001;5: 631–640.

Brandi LS, Bertolini R, Pieri M, et al. Comparison between cardiac output measured by thermodilution technique and calculated by O_2 and modified Fick methods using a new metabolic monitor. *Intensive Care Med* 1997;23:908–915.

Dhingra VK, Fenwick JC, Walley KR, et al. Lack of agreement between thermodilution and Fick cardiac output in critically ill patients. *Chest* 2002;122:990–997.

Moshkovitz Y, Kaluski E, Milo O, et al. Recent developments in cardiac output determination by bioimpedance: comparison with invasive cardiac output and potential cardiovascular applications. *Curr Opin Cardiol* 2004;19:229–237.

Peyton PJ, Robinson GJB. Measured pulmonary oxygen consumption: difference between systemic oxygen uptake measured by the reverse Fick method and indirect calorimetry in cardiac surgery. *Anesthesia* 2005;60:146–150.

17 INTERPRETATION OF HEMODYNAMIC WAVEFORMS

Tim Floreth

KEY POINTS

- Knowledgeable interpretations of pressure waveforms allows critical evaluation of cardiopulmonary status.
- Vascular pressures are recorded by fluid-filled plastic tubes connecting the patient's intravascular device to external pressure transducers. Ensuring that the system is working properly is of paramount importance before clinical decisions are made.
- The mean arterial pressure is superior to the systolic pressure as an indicator of the true driving force of blood to vital organs and, unlike the systolic pressure, is unchanged throughout the arterial tree.

- The pulmonary artery catheter measures pressure and can sample blood from the right atrium, right ventricle (RV), and PA. It provides an estimate of the end-diastolic pressure of the left ventricle (LV) via the pulmonary venous system and the left atrium. No randomized trial has proven a beneficial effect of PACs using a clinically meaningful endpoint.

INTRAVASCULAR PRESSURES

- Direct invasive monitoring is necessary in patients in which a clinical determination of volume status is difficult to assess by examination or a specific goal of treatment must be reached.
- Vascular pressures are recorded by fluid-filled plastic tubes that connect the patient's internal pressures via catheters to the external pressure transducers.
- The Flush test (a brief flush to the catheter tubing system) gives data to indicate whether the transducer to recording system is intact.
- Systems can be overdamped due to bubbles in the line and the system must be flushed. Systems can be underdamped by the excessive length of connecting tubing, connecting tubing with stopcocks, and high output cardiac states.

THE ARTERIAL PRESSURE WAVEFORMS

- The contour of the arterial pressure changes from the proximal aorta to the distal femoral artery. As such, the absolute systolic pressure increases and the waveform narrows.
- The mean arterial pressure is superior to the systolic pressure as an indicator of the true driving force of blood to vital organs and, unlike the systolic pressure, is unchanged throughout the arterial tree.
- Measured mean arterial pressures are more accurate than estimated pressures (calculated as $[2 \times BP_{diast} + BP_{syst}]/3$) especially when the pulse pressure is >60.

THE PULMONARY ARTERY CATHETER

- The pulmonary artery (Swan-Ganz) catheter (PAC) measures pressures and can sample blood from the right atrium, right ventricle (RV), and PA. It is able to provide an estimate of the pressure of the left ventricle (LV) via the pulmonary venous system and the left atrium.
- The catheter is inserted into the circulation of the superior vena cava (SVC) in which pressures are similar to the right atrium and advanced gently, allowing the normal blood flow to guide the catheter into the correct location. Differences in waveforms and pressures allow the operator to know where the catheter is currently located during the insertion. Figure 17-1 shows waveform examples. In general, the right atrial (RA) pressures and waveforms will be similar to the SVC. Once the catheter advances to the RV, the diastolic pressure will not change, but the systolic pressure will increase. Visually, the waveform increases in size due to the increased pulse pressure of the RV. As the catheter advances into the PA, the diastolic pressure increases and the waveform narrows. The systolic pressure of the PA typically equals the systolic pressure of the RV. The catheter is then advanced until the mean pressure falls and (usually) the waveform dampens to resemble an atrial waveform. This is the PA occlusion (or "capillary wedge") pressure (Ppw) that typically is the same as the PA diastolic pressure (6–12 mmHg).
- Knowledgeable interpretations of the pressure waveforms allows critical evaluation of cardiopulmonary status via estimation of the atrial and ventricular pressures. Multiple randomized trials have demonstrated that this catheter has no impact on meaningful outcomes (neither harmful nor helpful). For this and other reasons, such as the ready availability of echocardiography, use of the catheter is in substantial decline. The many clinical uses and the primary data used to determine various cardiopulmonary states are outlined in Table 17-1.

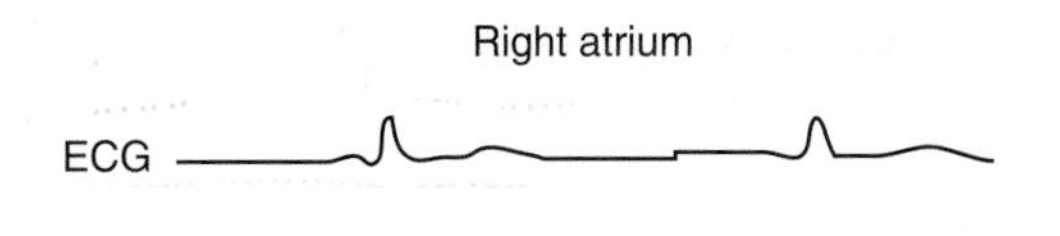

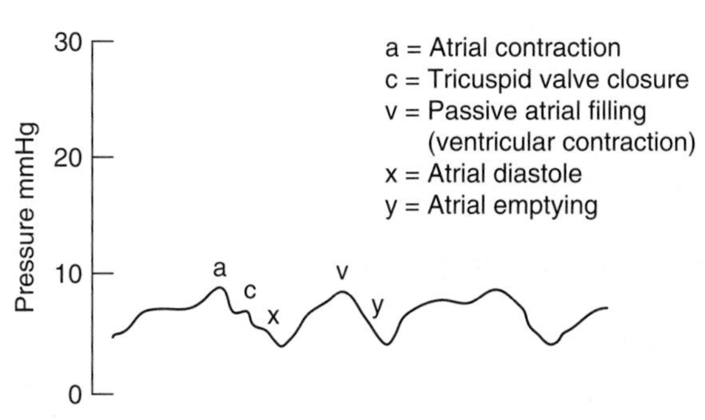

FIG. 17-1 RA pressure tracing. This schematic diagram shows the different components of the RA pressure tracing. A simultaneous ECG is shown to demonstrate the timing of the different components.

SOURCE: Silvestry, F.E., Swan-Ganz catheterization interpretation of tracings. Up to date online 14.3.

TABLE 17-1 Clinical Uses of PA Catheterization

Diagnostic uses	Data sought
Pulmonary edema	Ppw
Shock	Qt and SVR; Ppw; Svo_2
Oliguric renal failure	Ppw, Qt
Perplexing lactic acidemia	Qt, Svo_2
Pulmonary hypertension	Ppa, Ppad, Ppw
Cardiac disorders	
Acute mitral insufficiency	V wave
Ventricular septal defect	O_2 sat RA vs. PA
RV infarction	Pra, RVEDP, Ppw
Pericardial tamponade	Pra, RVEDP, Ppad, Ppw
Narrow complex tachyarrhythmias	RA waveform (flutter waves)
Wide complex tachyarrhythmias	RA waveform (cannon A waves)
Monitoring uses	
Assess volume	
Hypotension	
Oliguria	
High-risk surgical pt	
Assess the effect of Ppw on pulmonary edema	
Assess therapy for shock	
Cardiogenic (vasodilator, inotrope)	
Septic (volume, vasopressor, inotrope)	
Hypovolemic (volume)	
Assess effects of PEEP on DO_2 in ARDS	

ABBREVIATION: Ppw, pulmonary wedge pressure; Qt, cardiac output; SVR, systemic vascular resistance; Svo_2, mixed venous O_2 saturation; Ppa, pulmonary artery pressure; Ppad, Ppa diastolic; Pra, right atrial pressure; RVEDP, right ventricular end-diastolic pressure; Do_2, oxygen delivery; RV, right ventricle; RA, right atrium.
SOURCE: Adapted from Principles of Critical Care., Hall, J. et al. 3rd edition.

- The waveforms and data can be used to help differentiate between left and right heart failure. In right heart failure the RA pressures (Pra) will be high and the cardiac output (Qt) will be low. Left heart dysfunction will demonstrate elevated left ventricular end-diastolic pressures (LVEDP) as estimated by the Ppw and diminished cardiac output. The systemic vascular resistance (SVR) will be elevated.
- The three classic types of hypotension can also be differentiated based on PAC data. In hypovolemic shock, Pra is low, Qt is low, and SVR is high. In cardiogenic shock, Pra is high, Qt is low, and SVR is high. In vasogenic shock, Pra is low, Qt is high, and SVR is low. Table 17-2 compares types of shock and their PAC data.

TABLE 17-2 Typical PAC Data for Different Types of Shock

	HYPOVOLEMIC	CARDIOGENIC	VASOGENIC (SEPSIS)
RA pressure	Low	High	Low
Cardiac output	Low	Low	High
SVR	High	High	Low

SOURCES OF VARIABILITY

- "Zeroing" the catheter is performed by opening the system to establish atmospheric pressure as zero. The zero reference point is the intersection of the midaxillary line and the fourth intercostal space and corresponds to the right and left atrium in a supine patient. Therefore, patient and bed position are also important variables in determining correct pressure information.

WEDGE TRACING

- The wedge pressure is assumed to reflect the pressure in the left atrium and, by inference, the LVEDP since balloon occlusion creates a static column of blood from the tip of the catheter, through the pulmonary capillaries, postcapillary venules, veins, left atrium, and to the LV. It is important to understand that Ppw is a pressure, not a volume, and that there is a poor correlation between measured Ppw and LVEDV, in part because of the unpredictable compliance of the LV.
- Like all hemodynamic pressures, Ppw should be read at end-expiration, since this minimizes the likelihood that respiratory muscle activity is raising or lowering pressures from their passive values. Even at end-expiration, however, respiratory muscles may be active, especially in the sickest patients, further complicating the assessment of ventricular preload by the Ppw.

CARDIAC OUTPUT MEASUREMENT

- The PAC can also give measurements of cardiac output via the indicator thermodilution method (via thermal depression or "cold") or the assumed Fick method.
- In this process, cold saline is injected through the proximal lumen into the RA, travels through the RV, and finally passes into the PA where the thermistor at the end of the catheter senses the dynamic temperature

change over time. The area under this curve is inversely proportional to the flow rate or the cardiac output.

- Cases where the cardiac output is inherently inaccurate are tricuspid regurgitation (Qt is variably under- or overestimated) and intracardiac shunts (Qt is overestimated).
- Systemic and pulmonary vascular resistance can also be calculated based on the fact that resistance is equal to pressure change divided by flow. These are both indirect and often inaccurate data.

RIGHT ATRIAL WAVEFORMS

- There are normally three positive and two negative deflections in the RA waveforms of a competent tricuspid valve.
- The "a" wave represents contraction during atrial systole, the "c" wave represents the small deflection during closure of the tricuspid valve, and the "x" descent represents the decrease in RA pressure following the atrial systolic contraction (Fig. 17-1).
- The "v" wave represents ventricular systole and passive filling of the atrium. The "y" descent occurs after the opening of the tricuspid valve in which the RV passively fills until the next "a" wave.
- Normal RA pressures range from 0 to 7 mmHg. Elevations can be seen in any condition that produces a back up of pressure due to obstruction of flow or decrease in forward flow such as tricuspid valve disease, pulmonic stenosis, pulmonary hypertension, RV dysfunction, pericardial disease, or left heart dysfunction.
- Tricuspid regurgitation produces elevated "v" waves as blood is regurgitated into the RA during ventricular systole.
- RA pressures can be elevated and approach those of the Ppw in cardiac tamponade ("equalization of pressures").
- Disturbances in cardiac rhythm can also be seen on RA waveforms. Atrial fibrillation is associated with a loss of normal "a" waves while atrial flutter may produce sawtooth "f" waves. Ventricular tachycardia, complete heart block, and supraventricular tachycardias may produce cannon "a" waves due to contractions of the atria and ventricle simultaneously against a closed tricuspid valve.

RIGHT VENTRICULAR WAVEFORMS

- Two pressures are typically measured in the RV: the peak right ventricular systolic pressure (15–25 mmHg) and the right ventricular end-diastolic pressure (0–12 mmHg).
- Elevated RV systolic pressures can be seen in pulmonary hypertension, pulmonic stenosis, and acute pulmonary embolism. Increase in RV end-diastolic pressure is seen in cardiomyopathy, right ventricular ischemia, infarction, and tamponade.

PULMONARY ARTERY WAVEFORM

- The main components of the PA tracing are the systolic (15–25 mmHg) and diastolic pressures (8–15 mmHg) and the dicrotic notch which correlates with the closure of the pulmonic valve.
- Elevated PA pressures occur in conditions associated with volume overload or elevated pulmonary vascular resistance such as left heart failure, mitral valve disease, primary lung disease, pulmonary hypertension, or primary pulmonary hypertension.

PULMONARY ARTERIAL OCCLUSION WAVEFORM

- PA occlusion waveforms are similar to those of the right atrium but with slightly higher pressures due to the lower compliance of the LV compared to the RV (6–12 mmHg).
- The "a" wave reflects atrial systole and the "x" descent represents the fall in left atrial pressure after the contraction. The "c" wave that would reflect mitral closure is not visualized (Fig. 17-2)

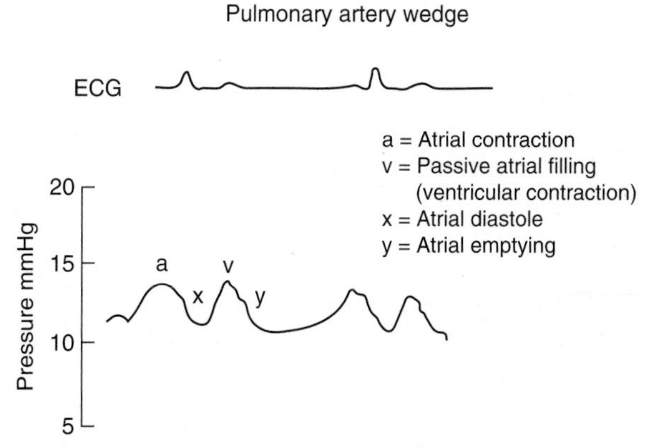

FIG. 17-2 Pulmonary artery wedge pressure tracing. This schematic diagram shows the different components of the pulmonary artery wedge pressure tracing. A simultaneous ECG is shown to demonstrate the timing of the different components. The peak of the "v" wave falls outside the peak of the electrocardiographic T wave. SOURCE: Adapted from Gore JM, Alpert JS, Benntti JR, et al. *Handbook of Hemodynamic Monitoring*. Boston, MA: Little, Brown & Co;1985.

- The "v" wave represents ventricular systole and atrial filling. The "y" descent reflects the fall in left atrial pressure after mitral valve opening.
- Elevations in the "a" wave of the Ppw are due to resistance of flow into the LV such as with mitral stenosis, volume overload, decreased compliance due to myocardial infarction, or left ventricular diastolic or systolic dysfunction. Elevations of the "v" wave of the Ppw tracing represent mitral regurgitation.
- The Ppw is an accurate reflection of the left atrial pressure if the tip is in zone 3 of the lungs, the area of the lungs (below the left atrium) where the pulmonary capillary pressure is higher than the mean alveolar pressure. Signs that the catheter site is not in zone 3 include significant respiratory variation in the tracing, and increases in Ppw of more than 50% of the applied positive end-expiratory pressure (PEEP).
- When PEEP is applied, the end-expiratory lung volume rises above functional residual capacity, raising the pleural pressure. The effect of this on the Ppw is variable, depending on the compliance of the lungs and chest wall, as well as the degree of lung recruitment. It is generally not advised to reduce or remove PEEP while measuring Ppw since this may precipitate life-threatening hypoxemia.

BIBLIOGRAPHY

Gore JM, Alpert JS, Benntti JR, et al. *Handbook of Hemodynamic Monitoring*. Boston, MA: Little, Brown & Co; 1985.

Hall JB, Schmidt GA, Wood LDH, eds., *Principles of Critical Care*, 3rd ed. New York, NY: McGraw-Hill; 2005.

Marino P. *The ICU Book*, 2nd ed. Philadelphia, PA: Lippincott Williams & Wilkins; 1998.

Silvestry F. Swan-Ganz catheterization: interpretations of tracings. *UpToDate*; 2007.

18 MYOCARDIAL ISCHEMIA

James K. Min

KEY POINTS

- Many patients in the ICU for noncardiac causes are also at risk for acute myocardial ischemia complicating their critical illness.
- The 12-lead electrocardiogram is invaluable in the assessment of both silent and symptomatic myocardial ischemia.
- Measurement of cardiac-specific enzymes is essential in the diagnosis of myocardial ischemia. Creatinine kinase (CK) with MB fraction and troponin levels will be elevated in the setting of NSTEMI or STEMI. Troponin T is more sensitive than CK and becomes elevated more quickly.
- Myocardial ischemia should be initially managed with antiplatelet agents, beta blockade, nitrates, pain control, anticoagulation, ACE inhibition, and statins.
- A cardiologist should be consulted urgently to consider interventions, such as thrombolytic drugs and cardiac catheterization.

BACKGROUND

- There are 13 million U.S. adults with a history of symptomatic coronary artery disease (CAD; history of myocardial infarction or angina pectoris). Moreover, 70 million U.S. adults have some form of cardiovascular disease.
- Many critically ill patients in the intensive care unit (ICU) are at risk for acute myocardial ischemia.

PATHOPHYSIOLOGY

- Myocardial ischemia may occur as a manifestation of impaired coronary blood flow or from a supply-demand imbalance of myocardial oxygen. Acute coronary syndromes—including unstable angina, non-ST-elevation myocardial infarction (NSTEMI), or ST-elevation myocardial infarction (STEMI)—may result as a manifestation of myocardial ischemia, either as result of partial or complete occlusion of an epicardial coronary artery. Acute coronary syndromes may also occur as a result of epicardial coronary vasospasm.

CLINICAL FEATURES OF MYOCARDIAL ISCHEMIA

- Myocardial ischemia may be symptomatic or asymptomatic. Symptomatic myocardial ischemia is most characteristically manifested as substernal chest pain or pressure. The location of the pain is typically on the left side of the chest and often radiates to the left arm, shoulder, or jaw. Less typical forms of presentation include right-sided chest pain, epigastric discomfort, or interscapular soreness. Myocardial ischemia is often associated with diaphoresis or dyspnea.

- Myocardial ischemia must be differentiated from other syndromes that may mimic angina. These states include dissecting aortic aneurysm, pulmonary embolism, pericarditis, pleurisy, gastroesophageal reflux, or costochondritis.
- The physical examination, while typically insensitive, may be helpful in diagnosing myocardial ischemia. If the acute coronary syndrome precipitates new left ventricular systolic dysfunction, the physical examination may reveal the presence of lung crackles, increased jugular venous pressure (JVP), and an S_3 or S_4 heart sound. The presence of a new murmur may signal mitral regurgitation or ventricular septal defect formation as a complication of myocardial infarction.
- Silent myocardial ischemia—which is not accompanied by signs and symptoms of angina—must not be overlooked. It is diagnosed by electrocardiography and associated with ST-segment depression.

DIAGNOSIS OF MYOCARDIAL ISCHEMIA

- The 12-lead electrocardiogram is invaluable in the assessment of both silent as well as symptomatic myocardial ischemia. Ischemia may manifest with ST-segment depression, T-wave alterations (flattening or inversion), or pseudonormalization of T waves (previously inverted T waves becoming upright).
- ST-segment depression and dynamic T-wave changes may occur in response to a host of other states unrelated to myocardial ischemia, including drug-related causes (such as digoxin or other vasoactive drugs), electrolyte disturbances (such as hyperkalemia), and supraventricular tachycardia (in the absence of significant CAD).
- If total epicardial artery occlusion occurs, ST segments typically elevate. ST elevation may also occur in pericarditis. However, in this state, the ST elevation is typically more diffuse. Also, PR depression is often seen during pericarditis.
- Other electrocardiographic abnormalities include QT prolongation, Q-wave development, and poor R-wave progression. Evolution of Q waves occurs hours after the onset of a total epicardial coronary artery occlusion.

LABORATORY ANALYSIS OF MYOCARDIAL ISCHEMIA

- Measurement of cardiac-specific enzymes is essential in the diagnosis of myocardial ischemia. Creatinine kinase (CK) with MB fraction and troponin levels will be elevated in the setting of NSTEMI or STEMI. Troponin T is more sensitive than CK and becomes elevated more quickly.
- Cardiac-specific enzymes should be measured in the critically ill patient suspected to have myocardial ischemia and should be repeated every 6–8 hours for 24–36 hours.
- A B-type natriuretic peptide (BNP) may be useful for determining whether symptoms are related to left ventricular volume overload.
- A complete blood count is useful. An elevated white blood cell count is sometimes seen during myocardial ischemia, though it is relatively insensitive. Significant anemia may be a cause of impaired myocardial supply versus demand in the critically ill patient. Severe thrombocytopenia (e.g., $<30\ mm^3$) may preclude the use of certain agents such as glycoprotein IIb/IIIa inhibitors or clopidogrel or aspirin.
- A complete metabolic panel will be useful to rule out any significant electrolyte abnormalities. An elevated creatinine has been associated with a poorer prognosis and may be useful to help stratify risk of cardiac-related mortality. Elevated aminotransferases may preclude the use of statin medications.

THERAPEUTIC APPROACH TO THE PATIENT WITH MYOCARDIAL ISCHEMIA

- Antiplatelet agents are critical for the treatment of myocardial ischemia. Aspirin (325 mg) should be administered immediately. If bleeding contraindications are not present, clopidogrel (300 mg initially) should be administered.
- Beta-blockade is useful for its negative chronotropic and inotropic properties as heart rate and contractility are two essential characteristics of myocardial oxygen consumption. IV metoprolol (5 mg IV initially) may be readministered to achieve a heart rate of approximately 60 beats per minute. Beta-blockers should be discontinued in the setting of severe hypotension.
- Nitrates are a mainstay of therapy for myocardial ischemia. They are coronary vasodilators and reduce preload in patients with left ventricular volume overload. Sublingual nitroglycerin (0.4 mg) may be administered every 5 minutes (× three times) to reduce anginal symptoms. If angina persists, intravenous nitroglycerin may be initiated at a dose of 10–20 μg/min. Nitrates should be discontinued in the setting of severe hypotension.
- Narcotic therapy is useful to reduce anginal pain. IV morphine can be particularly helpful as it also favorably affects myocardial oxygen supply.
- Intravenous heparin infusion is standard therapy for the high-risk individual with myocardial ischemia (in

the absence of bleeding contraindication). Heparin may be given IV initially as a bolus (5000–10,000 U) and then continuously (1000 U/h or using a weight-based nomogram) to achieve an activated partial thromboplastic time (PTT) 1.5–2.5 times normal.

- High-dose statin medications have been shown to positively affect outcomes in patients with myocardial ischemia. Atorvastatin (80 mg) can be administered immediately during the ischemic episode.
- Angiotensin-converting enzyme (ACE) inhibitors have also been shown to positively affect outcomes in patients with STEMI. Intravenous or oral enalapril may be utilized providing that significant hypotension is not present.
- Glycoprotein IIb/IIIa inhibitors may be useful in the high-risk individual with NSTEMI or STEMI without bleeding contraindication. Abciximab, tirofiban, or eptifibatide may be administered as a bolus and then as a continuous infusion. Consultation with a cardiologist may be prudent before administering these agents.
- Thrombolytic therapy is beneficial in the STEMI patient. Consultation with a cardiologist should be obtained before administration of these agents.
- Early intravenous coronary angiography is essential in the high-risk individual with myocardial ischemia. Consultation with a cardiologist should be obtained immediately to determine whether a critically ill patient should be further evaluated with angiography and possible intervention in the cardiac catheterization laboratory.

REFERENCES

Hollenberg SM, Parrillo JE. Myocardial Ischemia, Ch 25. In: Hall JB, Schmid GA, Wood LDH, *Principles of Critical Care*, 3rd ed., New York, NY: McGraww-Hill;2005.

19 ECHOCARDIOGRAPHY IN THE CRITICALLY ILL PATIENT

Steven Y. Chang

KEY POINTS

- Echocardiography allows non-invasive data to be quickly assessed at the patient bedside. Given limitations in moving critically ill patients, echocardiography has quickly become a useful tool in the management of ICU patients.
- Echocardiography allows evaluation of cardiac size, function, structure, and disease of the pericardium.
- Echocardiography can provide real-time clinical assessment of intravascular volume, response to fluids or inotropic agents, and help manage acute right heart syndromes.

DATA OBTAINED BY ECHOCARDIOGRAPHY

- Cardiac chamber size and function
- Valvular structure and function
- Pericardial fluid collection
- Intracardiac masses
- Semiquantitative or qualitative information about hemodynamics
- Directionality of blood flow

TRANSTHORACIC ECHOCARDIOGRAPHY AND TRANSESOPHAGEAL ECHOCARDIOGRAPHY

- Both transthoracic echocardiography (TTE) and transesophageal echocardiography (TEE) employ ultrasound to examine the structure and function of the heart, its valves, and associated great vessels.
- TTE examines the heart from the surface of the thoracic wall.
- TEE examines the heart from the esophagus and stomach. Because of the proximity of the esophagus to the posterior heart, the cardiac chambers and aorta can be well visualized.
- Advantages of TTE include: noninvasive and relatively easy to perform.
- Disadvantages of TTE include: poor visualization of heart under certain circumstances including severe obesity, end-stage lung disease, chest wall deformities, and mechanical ventilation.
- Advantages of TEE include: improved image quality, ability to image certain structures that cannot be visualized with TTE including the left atrial appendage, pulmonary veins, and descending aorta.
- Disadvantages of TEE include: invasive and uncomfortable, need for conscious sedation or intubation, aspiration, small but real likelihood of esophageal perforation.

ECHO TECHNIQUES AND MODALITIES

- Motion (M-) mode—gives a view of structures along a single line. It is especially useful for looking at moving structures. The changes in movement of structures are plotted as a linear graph.

- Two-dimensional (2-D)—gives a cross-sectional view of the heart.
- Doppler—gives information about directionality and velocity of blood flow. It can be used to grade the severity of valvular disease, shunts, and even to extrapolate hemodynamic information.

SELECT TWO-DIMENSIONAL TRANSESOPHAGEAL ECHOCARDIOGRAPHY VIEWS

- Orientation is determined by the position of the ultrasound probe (parasternal, apical, subcostal) and view (long axis, four-chamber, five-chamber, and short axis).
- *Parasternal long axis* views allow for visualization of the left atrium (LA), right ventricle (RV), left ventricle (LV), left ventricular outflow tract, aortic valve, mitral valve, and interventricular septum.
- Depending on the level of visualization (at the aortic valve, the mitral valve, or the papillary muscles), multiple structures can be evaluated with the *parasternal short axis* view. This view is useful for comparing the relationship of the RV and LV.
- *Apical long axis* views allow visualization of the LV and its outflow tract, the ascending aorta, the aortic valve, the mitral valve, the interventricular septum, and the LA.
- *Apical four-chamber* views allow for visualization of the four cardiac chambers, the interventricular septum, the tricuspid valve, and the mitral valve.
- In addition to the structures mentioned for the four-chamber view, the *apical five-chamber* view also allows for visualization of the left ventricular outflow tract, aortic valve, and proximal ascending aorta. Occasionally, the LA appendage can be seen.
- *Subcostal four-chamber* views allow for examination of the RV. Additionally, the other three chambers can be visualized along with the interatrial septum, the interventricular septum, the tricuspid and mitral valves.
- *Subcostal short axis* views are useful for comparing the relationship of the two ventricles.
- These different views are complementary and should be considered together.

SELECT TRANSESOPHAGEAL ECHOCARDIOGRAPHY VIEWS

- Similar to the TTE, orientation is determined by the position of the ultrasound probe (transesophageal and transgastric).
- *Transesophageal four-chamber* views are useful for examining the four cardiac chambers, and the mitral and tricuspid valves. Slight changes in position allow for visualization of the LV outflow tract and aortic valve.
- *Transgastric* views allow for imaging similar to apical four- and five-chamber views.

REASONS FOR PERFORMING ECHOCARDIOGRAPHY IN THE CRITICALLY ILL

- It can change care in a substantial number of patients.
- Cardiovascular monitoring including cardiac output and preload (can be used independently of, or in complementary fashion with information from a right atrial or pulmonary artery catheter). For example, a hypovolemic patient will manifest reduced ventricular volumes and a hypercontractile state. Septic patients may manifest reduced ejection fractions despite a hyperdynamic state.
- Titration of medicines, especially vasoactive agents. For example, the response to the addition of an inotrope can be directly visualized.
- Suspected ventricular dysfunction (e.g., cardiomyopathies and sepsis).
- Myocardial ischemia and infarction which results in wall motion abnormalities.
- Suspected mechanical complications after myocardial infarction such as ventricular free wall rupture.
- Evaluation of right heart syndromes such as massive pulmonary embolism or RV infarct. Echocardiography can aid in determining if the RV is overfilled resulting in an interventricular shift into the LV with resultant poor cardiac output.
- Suspected valvular dysfunction.
- Evaluation of prosthetic valve structure and function.
- Suspected endocarditis.
- Suspected congenital or structural heart disease.
- Suspected aortic dissection.
- Exclusion of thrombus for cardioversion in atrial fibrillation.
- Diagnoses of right-to-left and left-to-right shunting in the setting of septal defects.
- Suspected extracardiac shunting (e.g., hepatopulmonary syndrome).
- Suspected pericardial tamponade.
- Suspected hemodynamically compromising intracardiac masses.
- Evaluation of cerebrovascular accidents (CVAs) and transient ischemic attacks (TIAs).
- Aid in evaluation of dysrhythmias.

SPECIFIC INDICATIONS FOR TRANSESOPHAGEAL ECHOCARDIOGRAPHY

- Suspected endocarditis (87–93% sensitive and 91–96% specific for left-sided lesions).
- Evaluation of mitral valve disease.
- Perivalvular abscess.
- Evaluation of septal defects.
- Stratification of risk of embolism prior to cardioversion for atrial fibrillation and atrial flutter.
- Diagnosis and evaluation of suspected aortic dissection (95% sensitive and 98% specific).
- Inadequate TTE (often a problem in hyperinflated, mechanically ventilated patients).

BIBLIOGRAPHY

Kaddoura S. *Echo Made Easy*, 7th ed. New York, NY: Churchill Livingstone; 2002.

Milani RV, Lavie CJ, Gilliland YE, et al. Overview of transesophageal echocardiography for the chest physician. *Chest* 2003;124:1081–1089.

Voga G, Krivec B. Echocardiography in the intensive care unit. *Curr Opin Crit Care* 2000;6:207–213.

20 ACUTE RIGHT HEART SYNDROMES

Steven Q. Davis

KEY POINTS

- Acute increases in PA pressures can lead to rapid right ventricular dysfunction and decreased RV contractility and ejection.
- Acute decompensation of the right ventricle can lead to acute diastolic dysfunction of the left ventricle (e.g., "right heart failure causing left heart failure").
- Clinical signs of acute right heart syndromes include elevated neck veins, a pulsatile liver, peripheral edema, a right-sided S_3, and tricuspid regurgitation.
- Diagnosis of right heart dysfunction can be confirmed quickly with bedside echocardiography.
- Therapy is directed at the underlying cause (e.g., treatment of the pulmonary embolism) while optimizing preload, supporting contractility, and minimizing right ventricular afterload.

PHYSIOLOGY

- Right ventricular function deteriorates in the face of elevated pulmonary vascular resistance or pulmonary arterial hypertension.
- Right ventricular oxygen consumption increases significantly with increased workload, but when coupled with systemic hypotension, coronary perfusion to the right ventricle will fall.
- The resultant right heart ischemia leads to decreased right ventricular contractility and systolic ejection.
- As right heart pressures increase, the intraventricular septum may shift to the left causing left ventricular diastolic dysfunction, which will in turn further reduce the coronary perfusion pressure to the right heart.

DIAGNOSIS

- A previous history of pulmonary hypertension should alert the clinician to the possibility of acute-on-chronic right heart dysfunction.
- Clinical signs include: elevated neck veins, a pulsatile liver, peripheral edema, a right-sided S_3 or tricuspid regurgitation.
- Radiologic features include an enlarged pulmonary artery or right ventricle, a Westermark sign (oligemia of a lobe or entire lung), or a plump azygous vein.
- The electrocardiogram may show a rightward axis or right axis deviation, right atrial enlargement, right ventricular hypertrophy, right bundle branch block, right precordial T-wave inversions, and an S1-Q3-T3 pattern.
- Echocardiographic findings may include a normally functioning left ventricle (often with end-systolic obliteration of the cavity), a thin-walled and poorly contracting right ventricle, right atrial enlargement, tricuspid insufficiency, increased pulmonary arterial pressures, leftward shift of the intraventricular septum, right pulmonary artery dilation, and/or loss of respiratory variation in the inferior vena cava.
- Echocardiography should be obtained as soon as the diagnosis of acute right heart syndrome is entertained.

SPECIFIC ETIOLOGIES

- The classic etiology of acute pulmonary hypertension is acute pulmonary embolism. Other etiologies include acute respiratory distress syndrome (ARDS), drug effect, and inflammation, including sepsis.
- Chronic pulmonary hypertension may be exacerbated by any critical illness that requires an increase in cardiac output.
- Right ventricular infarction occurs as a result of an inferior myocardial infarction or, less commonly, an anterior myocardial infarction. Echocardiography can

readily distinguish between right ventricular infarction and acute pulmonary artery hypertension.

THERAPY

- Other than therapy directed at the underlying condition (i.e., thrombolysis for pulmonary embolism), the goals of therapy are to reduce systemic oxygen demand while improving delivery.
- Oxygen therapy should be used to avoid alveolar hypoxic vasoconstriction as well as to enhance arterial saturation.
- While fluids are first-line therapy for shock in general, they may prove detrimental for patients suffering from right heart syndrome. Additional fluid may move the intraventricular septum further into the left ventricular cavity. Since some patients may be volume depleted at the time of presentation, a closely monitored fluid challenge may be considered, paying close attention to markers of end-organ perfusion.
- When vasoactive agents are needed, dobutamine and norepinephrine appear to be the most effective.
- Inhaled nitric oxide may be used as a pulmonary vasodilator.
- Ventilator management should employ the following general strategies: give sufficient oxygen to avoid hypoxic vasoconstriction; avoid hypercapnia; maintain positive end-expiratory pressure (PEEP) at the lowest level needed for adequate alveolar recruitment and oxygenation; and minimize auto-PEEP, and using the lowest tidal volume necessary to maintain an acceptable PCO_2.

BIBLIOGRAPHY

Douglas IS, Schmidt GA. Acute right heart syndromes. In: Hall JB, Schmidt GA, Wood LDH, eds., *Principles of Critical Care*, 3rd ed. New York, NY: McGraw-Hill; 2005:353–346.

21 PULMONARY EMBOLISM: THROMBUS, FAT, AIR, AND AMNIOTIC FLUID

Nuala J. Meyer

KEY POINTS

- Pulmonary Embolism causes approximately 25,000 deaths each year.
- Risk factors for PE include Virchow's triad of stasis, hypercoagulability, and vascular injury.
- PE disrupts gas exchange by creating dead space in alveoli which are ventilated but not perfused.
- Mechanical obstruction of the pulmonary artery as well as humoral factors released in response to pulmonary artery thrombus increase right ventricular (RV) afterload and right ventricular oxygen consumption, which can precipitate right ventricular ischemia.
- Clinically, patients may present with nonspecific symptoms of dyspnea, chest pain, and apprehension. Tachypnea and tachycardia are the most common clinical signs of PE. Hypoxemia is present in approximately two-thirds of patients, so the lack of hypoxemia cannot be relied on to exclude disease. Fever is present in up to half of patients with PE, but is typically below 38.5°C.
- Diagnosing PE relies on one's clinical judgment, and diagnostic tests should be pursued either until a firm diagnosis is reached or PE is judged to be clinically unlikely. These tests include D-dimer, Doppler venous ultrasound, V/Q scans, CT angiography, and PA angiography. Each test has its own strengths and weaknesses.
- Treatment for pulmonary embolism includes anticoagulation and sometimes thrombolytics. Vena cava interruption with a filter can be considered for those unable to receive anticoagulation.
- Air embolism occurs when a gas (typically air) enters the vasculature and travels to the pulmonary circulation, where it causes either circulatory or respiratory distress. The most common causes include trauma, surgery, and intravascular catheters.
- Like PE, air embolism can acutely raise the pulmonary arterial pressure, causing right ventricular strain and potentially impeding venous return to the left ventricle. In the pulmonary circulation, air emboli cause endothelial injury, often triggering alveolar flooding as well as bronchoconstriction.
- Treatment of Air Embolism focuses on preventing further embolization and supporting the patient's cardiopulmonary circulation.
- The fat embolism syndrome (FES) occurs when fat particles enter the circulation, typically from long bone fracture, and cause lung dysfunction, neurologic changes, and petechiae.
- Like other emboli, fat emboli may raise pulmonary artery pressures, and cause right heart strain or failure. Treatment is supportive.
- Amniotic fluid embolism (AFE) is thought to occur with a frequency of 1 in approximately 30,000 births.
- Amniotic fluid embolism is typically a dramatic presentation of abrupt dyspnea, hypoxemia, and hypotension, often with rapid progression to heart failure. Pulmonary edema is common. Disseminated intravascular coagulopathy (DIC) may also be present.

- Diagnosis is clinical; sampling of pulmonary arterial fluid for fetal tissue is neither sensitive nor specific. Treatment is supportive.

PULMONARY THROMBOEMBOLISM

EPIDEMIOLOGY

- Pulmonary embolism (PE), whereby a thrombus fragments from a deep venous thrombus and travels to the pulmonary circulation, prompts hospitalization at a frequency of approximately one case per 1000 persons per year, or 200,000–300,000 U.S. annual hospitalizations. PE causes approximately 25,000 deaths each year.

PATHOPHYSIOLOGY

- Thrombus formation begins with microthrombi at the site of venous stasis or injury, typically in the lower extremity. Because thrombosis impedes venous flow and contributes to further stasis, clots may enlarge and propagate.
- Clots which propagate into proximal deep veins in the legs and pelvis have an increased risk of embolization, and are responsible for the majority of significant PE. As central venous catheterization becomes more frequent, however, a small but significant proportion of PE may be due to upper extremity thrombi.
- PE exerts its greatest effect on gas exchange and the circulation. Gas exchange is deranged by the creation of dead space in alveoli which are ventilated but not perfused due to the emboli occluding pulmonary arterial flow. At the same time, V/Q mismatch causes a widening of the alveolar to arterial gradient for oxygen ($[A\text{-}a]PO_2$), and thus hypoxemia is present in approximately 60% of patients. Gas exchange may also be impaired by atelectasis.
- PE can also affect the circulation. Both the mechanical obstruction of the pulmonary artery as well as humoral factors released in response to pulmonary artery thrombus tend to increase right ventricular (RV) afterload and right ventricular oxygen consumption, which can precipitate right ventricular ischemia. In the most extreme cases, PE can induce *cor pulmonale*, or acute right heart failure.

CLINICAL FEATURES

- Risk factors for PE include Virchow's triad of stasis, hypercoagulability, and vascular injury, as well as certain clinical situations such as pregnancy/peripartum status, orthopedic surgery (especially hip fractures or hip or knee replacements), malignancy (especially adenocarcinoma), and indwelling central venous lines. Pulmonary artery catheterization was found to be a risk factor for PE in at least one study.
- PE is famous for its varied presentation among different patients. Dyspnea, chest pain, and apprehension are the most common symptoms, affecting 80%, 70%, and 60% of patients, respectively. Symptoms of deep vein thrombosis (DVT) are present in only one-third of patients.
- Tachypnea and tachycardia are the most common clinical signs of PE. Hypoxemia is present in approximately two-thirds of patients, so the lack of hypoxemia cannot be relied on to exclude disease. Fever is present in up to half of the patients with PE, but is typically below 38.5°C.

DIAGNOSIS

- In many ways, diagnosing PE relies on one's clinical judgment, and diagnostic tests should be pursued either until a firm diagnosis is reached or PE is judged to be clinically unlikely.
- Pulmonary angiography has long been considered the gold standard for diagnosing PE. A positive study is one in which a filling defect of a 2 mm or larger vessel is noted on more than one view. However, pulmonary angiography is invasive, has a reported mortality rate of 0.2%—potentially higher in patients with pulmonary hypertension—and necessitates intravenous contrast.
- D-dimer, a degradation product of cross-linked fibrin, is highly sensitive (95%) though not specific for DVT and PE. Very low levels of D-dimer strongly argue against PE. Unless one's pretest probability of PE is very high, a negative D-dimer assay should end the workup for PE.
- Helical computed tomography (CT) angiography, sometimes called "PE-protocol CT," has a sensitivity for PE ranging from 50 to 100%, and a specificity of 81 to 100%. Helical CT angiography performs better at detecting clots larger than the subsegmental level, as does pulmonary angiography. It seems to be as safe to withhold anticoagulation based on a negative helical CT angiogram as based on a negative pulmonary angiogram.
- Ventilation-perfusion scanning can be helpful, but again the test result can only be viewed in the context of one's clinical pretest probability. The test is helpful when read as normal or high probability, in which case the test can dictate therapy. Difficulties arise in the majority of cases, however, if the reading is either

low or intermediate probability, the rate of PE varies between 16 and 40%. Thus, a V/Q scan can beget additional testing. V/Q scanning can be technically challenging from the ICU due to a higher probability of underlying cardiopulmonary disease.

- Chest x-ray is frequently abnormal in PE, but many potential patterns, including atelectasis, pleural effusion, or pulmonary infarction, can be seen. Two classic but rare findings include "Hampton hump," a wedge-shaped, pleural-based opacity representing pulmonary infarction, and "Westermark sign," detailing relative oligemia of one lung compared to its counterpart.
- ECG, another nonspecific test, most commonly shows sinus tachycardia. Other possible findings include right axis deviation, right ventricular strain, or right bundle branch block (RBBB).
- Lower extremity venous duplex studies perform exceptionally well in patients with symptoms of proximal DVT. In asymptomatic patients, Doppler studies perform less well, and since less than half of patients with PE have a distinct DVT at the time of PE diagnosis, lower extremity Doppler cannot exclude the possibility of PE. Noninvasive leg studies may diagnose DVT and thus provide grounds for anticoagulation, which may render inconsequential the question of PE.

INTENSIVE CARE UNIT MANAGEMENT

- Anticoagulation is the mainstay of treatment for PE.
- Traditionally, unfractionated heparin has been used at a dose sufficient to keep the activated partial thromboplastin time (aPTT) equal to or greater than 1.5 times the patient's baseline aPTT. It is more important to reach this threshold (≥1.5 aPTT) than to prevent the aPTT from getting too high, as bleeding has not been correlated with supratherapeutic levels. A typical dosing regimen would be a bolus of heparin at 80 units/kg of body weight, followed by a continuous infusion at 18 units/kg/h. Many weight-based dosing nomograms are widely available. Heparin use mandates repeat testing of the aPTT.
    - Common complications of unfractionated heparin include serious bleeding (approximately 3% of patients) and thrombocytopenia (1–3%). Hyperkalemia, osteoporosis, and hypersensitivity are less common reactions.
- Low-molecular weight heparins (LMWH) are smaller fragments of heparin which preserve heparin's active site. This family of medicines can be dosed once or twice subcutaneously per day, have a more reliable dose-response relationship compared to heparin, and have a trend toward fewer DVT/PE recurrences and less hemorrhage when compared to heparin. In an uncomplicated patient with PE, LMWH should be given first consideration.
    - LMWH are cleared by renal metabolism, and dose adjustments for renal impairment are not well-tested. Therefore, LMWH should be reserved for those with normal renal function.
    - Complications observed with LMWH include hemorrhage and thrombocytopenia (<1% of patients), but at rates lower than with heparin.
    - ICU patients may be unsuitable for LMWH if they have renal failure, morbid obesity, or a need for ongoing invasive or urgent procedures.
- Direct thrombin inhibitors such as lepirudin or argatroban are not well tested in PE, but are approved for use in patients with a history of heparin-induced thrombocytopenia. Newer anticoagulants such as ximelagatran and fondaparinux may be used in the future.
- Risk stratification for patients is appropriate, as patients with PE may range from asymptomatic to overt shock. Echocardiography, while neither sensitive nor specific enough for diagnosis of PE, can be helpful in determining those at highest risk for mortality and shock, and determining which patients may require intensive care monitoring. Echocardiographic data such as right heart strain indicate a poorer prognosis.
- When patients with PE present with hypotension or hypoperfusion, treatment with thrombolytic medicines—streptokinase, urokinase, or alteplase—is warranted. The risk of hemorrhage with these medications is as high as 22%, and intracerebral hemorrhage may complicate 3% of patients receiving thrombolysis. Absolute contraindications to thrombolytic therapy include hemorrhagic stroke, active intracranial hemorrhage, recent intracranial surgery, or recent internal bleeding. Other bleeding risks may be compelling relative contraindications.
- Vena caval interruption devices (VCI), such as the Greenfield filter, may be helpful when patients have compelling contraindication to anticoagulation or if embolization continues despite anticoagulation. Because much of the benefits of VCI appear to be in the early weeks following a DVT or PE, much interest has been given to temporary VCI, which could be removed after 1–6 months. More data will be helpful in this regard.

AIR EMBOLISM

PATHOPHYSIOLOGY

- Air embolism occurs when a gas (typically air) enters the vasculature and travels to the pulmonary circulation, where it causes either circulatory or respiratory distress.

- Air embolism results from the communication of air with a blood vessel while there is a pressure gradient favoring the movement of air into the vessel. The most common etiologies are trauma, surgery, and intravascular catheters, but the syndrome has been reported following positive pressure ventilation or SCUBA diving.
- Like PE, air embolism can acutely raise the pulmonary arterial pressure, causing right ventricular strain and potentially impeding venous return to the left ventricle. In addition to the mechanical phenomena, air embolism may also trigger cytokine release leading to further increase in the pulmonary vascular resistance.
- In the pulmonary circulation, air emboli cause endothelial injury, often triggering alveolar flooding as well as bronchoconstriction.

CLINICAL FEATURES

- Air embolism typically causes acute hypoxemic respiratory failure and presents radiographically as diffuse alveolar filling.
- Patients have increased ventilatory dead space, and are dyspneic with high minute ventilation and low PCO_2.
- Diagnosis is clinical, and relies on a high level of suspicion, especially in high-risk situations. Air embolism should be strongly considered when other causes of noncardiogenic pulmonary edema have been excluded.
- Once further air embolization is prevented, resolution is often swift.

INTENSIVE CARE UNIT MANAGEMENT

- Treatment focuses on preventing further embolization and supporting the patient's cardiopulmonary circulation.
  - The source of air entry should be identified and reversed.
  - Raising the intravascular pressure (e.g., with volume resuscitation) can lessen the gradient favoring air entry.
  - If positive pressure ventilation may be the source of air entry, the plateau and airway pressures should be reduced, with low tidal volumes and lower positive end-expiratory pressure (PEEP).
  - Oxygen speeds the reabsorption of air from bubbles, so patients should receive 100% O_2.
  - When mechanical ventilation is necessary, management should be similar to patients with acute respiratory distress syndrome (ARDS): low tidal volumes and plateau pressures.
  - Corticosteroids may be prophylactic for air embolism in humans, however, as the syndrome is rare and tends to resolve rapidly, there is no role for the routine use of steroids.

FAT EMBOLISM

PATHOPHYSIOLOGY

- The fat embolism syndrome (FES) occurs when fat particles enter the circulation and cause lung dysfunction, neurologic changes, and petechiae.
- FES can result from trauma—especially long bone fracture or orthopedic surgery which exposes bone marrow to the circulation—or atraumatic, with fat particles likely arising from lipids in the blood.
- Like other emboli, fat emboli may raise pulmonary artery pressures, and cause right heart strain or failure.

CLINICAL FEATURES

- Classically, patients are asymptomatic for approximately 12–72 hours after the embolization occurs, and then present similar to ARDS with a diffuse lung lesion. In addition, there is often confusion or mental status changes, petechiae, thrombocytopenia, and anemia.
- Retinal examination may reveal embolized fat in retinal vessels (Purtscher retinopathy).
- Diagnosis is clinical, based on the presence of an at-risk scenario with ARDS and neurologic manifestations.
- Fat globules in the urine, bronchoalveolar lavage fluid, or serum are not reliably sensitive or specific.

INTENSIVE CARE UNIT MANAGEMENT

- To help prevent the FES, long bone fractures are reduced early.
- Corticosteroids may be useful, as transthoracic echocardiography performed in patients undergoing specific orthopedic procedures found fewer echo-detected emboli and less hypoxemia in patients receiving steroids. However, as the syndrome is more commonly mild than severe, and as steroids may increase infection or delay wound healing, many clinicians argue against the use of prophylactic steroids.
- Once ARDS has developed, treatment of the FES is identical to that of all other forms of ARDS.

AMNIOTIC FLUID EMBOLISM

PATHOPHYSIOLOGY

- Amniotic fluid embolism (AFE) is thought to occur with a frequency of 1 in approximately 30,000 births, and when severe causes high maternal and fetal mortality.
- AFE occurs when amniotic fluid, typically confined to the fetal placenta, crosses the placental membrane. For this to happen, there must be disruption of fetal membranes, open or disrupted maternal circulation, and a gradient favoring the entry of material from the amnion to the mother's veins.
- Early on, AFE is thought to cause right heart strain and hypoxemia, much like other embolic phenomena. However, AFE often progresses to left ventricular dysfunction, with cardiogenic pulmonary edema. Almost certainly, the interaction of amniotic fluid with maternal vessels incites a humoral response which intensifies any mechanical phenomena.

CLINICAL FEATURES

- Amniotic fluid embolism is typically a dramatic presentation of abrupt dyspnea, hypoxemia, and hypotension, often with rapid progression to heart failure. Pulmonary edema is common.
- Disseminated intravascular coagulopathy (DIC) occurs in approximately 40% of cases, and may be the presenting symptom in up to 15%.
- Neurologic manifestations are common, and may progress to seizures or cerebrovascular accident.
- Diagnosis is clinical; sampling of pulmonary arterial fluid for fetal tissue is neither sensitive nor specific.

INTENSIVE CARE UNIT MANAGEMENT

- Treatment of AFE is symptomatic, with careful monitoring of coagulation parameters to exclude DIC, and close attention to volume management and cardiac function.

BIBLIOGRAPHY

Clark SL. New concepts of amniotic fluid embolism: a review. *Obstet Gynecol Surv* 1990;45:360–468.

Goldhaber SZ. Pulmonary embolism. *Lancet* 2004;363:1295–1305.

Jerjes-Sanchez C, Ramirez-Rivera A, Garcia M, et al. Streptokinase and heparin versus heparin alone in massive pulmonary embolism: a randomized controlled trial. *J Thromb Thrombolysis* 1884;2:227–229.

Marini JJ, Culver BH. Systemic gas embolization complicating mechanical ventilation in the adult respiratory distress syndrome. *Ann Intern Med* 1989;110:699–703.

Meyer NJ, Schmidt GA. Pulmonary embolic disorders: thrombus, air, and fat. In: Hall JB, Schmidt GA, Wood LDH, eds., *Principles of Critical Care*, 3rd ed. New York, NY: McGraw-Hill; 2005:347–372.

PIOPED investigators. Value of the ventilation/perfusion lung scan in the diagnosis of pulmonary embolism. *JAMA* 1990;263:2753–2759.

Schonfeld SA, Ploysongsang Y, DiLisio R, et al. Fat embolism prophylaxis with corticosteroids: a prospective study in high-risk patients. *Ann Intern Med* 1983;99:438–443.

22 PERICARDIAL DISEASE

D. Kyle Hogarth

KEY POINTS

- Pericardial disease does not always lead to altered physiology in the patient.
- The dominant physiologic effect of significant pericardial disease is lowered cardiac output. The effects of pericardial disease on the heart result from impaired cardiac filling, thus pericardial disease per se does not affect systolic function. A low cardiac output state requires prompt attention; understanding the role pericardial disease may or may not play in the patient's condition can allow the clinician to properly focus care.
- Patients with increasing effusions become "dependent" on atrial systole in order to fill the ventricles. Atrial flutter and fibrillation can be deadly in a patient with a significant pericardial effusion.
- Tamponade is characterized by elevated diastolic pressures, equal end-diastolic pressures across chambers, and the absence of early filling of the ventricle during diastole.
- Treatment of Tamponade includes fluid resuscitation and immediate drainage of the fluid. Inotropic support can be initiated, but there is little evidence to support this. Mechanical ventilation can further reduce cardiac output by impeding venous return due to the positive thoracic pressures, but may be needed if there is impending cardiopulmonary collapse.

HEMODYNAMIC EFFECTS OF PERICARDIAL DISEASE

- The effects of pericardial disease on the heart result from impaired cardiac filling, thus pericardial disease per se does not affect systolic function.
- Compliance of the heart is partly determined by the pericardial tissue and the amount of pericardial fluid.
- The process causing the disease may progress rapidly (e.g., effusion) or slowly (e.g., constriction), but the decompensation by the patient can be acute in both examples.

PERICARDIAL EFFUSIONS AND TAMPONADE

- Pericardial fluid distributes evenly, and pericardial pressure is distributed evenly across all chambers.
- As pericardial fluid accumulates, pericardial pressure increases in relation to pericardial compliance.
- Ventricular filling occurs during late diastole in pericardial effusion patients.
- Patients with increasing effusions become "dependent" on their atrial systole in order to fill their ventricles. Atrial flutter and fibrillation can be deadly in a patient with a significant pericardial effusion.
- Cardiac compression by the pericardial space occurs at 15–20 mmHg.
- In cardiac tamponade, the external pericardial pressure exceeds the pressures acting to distend the cardiac chambers. When the pressure external to the heart is greater than the internal pressures, flow cannot occur. As the pressure is equally distributed, an increase in the pericardial pressure above the right atrial (RA) pressure will result in no passive filling of the right ventricle (RV) during diastole.
- Tamponade is characterized by elevated diastolic pressures, equal end-diastolic pressures across chambers, and the absence of early filling of the ventricle during diastole.

CLINICAL FINDINGS IN TAMPONADE

- Sinus tachycardia.
- *Elevated jugular venous pressure (JVP)*: The "x" descent will be maintained. However, the "y" descent will become absent due to limited early diastolic filling of the ventricle.
- *Pulsus paradoxus*: normally, systolic blood pressure decreases <10 mmHg on inspiration. In pulsus paradoxus, this change is >10 mmHg on inspiration.
- *Kussmaul sign*: lack of decline in JVP during inspiration.
- *Pericardial rub*: may be present in inflammatory causes of pericardial fluid.

DIAGNOSIS OF TAMPONADE

- Usually made clinically, especially in acute cases, but the diagnosis is aided with various diagnostic modalities.
  - *ECG*: will have tachycardia and low voltage, and may have electrical alternans (beat-to-beat alteration in the QRS complex).
  - *Chest x-ray (CXR)*: can show enlarged cardiac silhouette.
  - *Echocardiography*: can show volume of fluid, cardiac chamber collapse (especially diastolic collapse of the right side), and "swinging" of the heart within the large volume of fluid.
  - *Cardiac catheterization*: pulmonary artery catheter will show equalization of the diastolic pressures across all chambers.

TREATMENT OF TAMPONADE

- Fluid resuscitation.
- Immediate drainage of the fluid via percutaneous approach or surgical approach.
- Inotropic support (e.g., dobutamine), but little evidence to support this.
- Mechanical ventilation should be avoided as this will further reduce cardiac output by impeding venous return due to the positive thoracic pressures (see Chap. 135).

CONSTRICTIVE PERICARDITIS

- The characteristic presentation of constrictive pericarditis is severe right heart failure, without another apparent cause.
- In constrictive pericarditis, the pericardial tissue has become thickened or calcified and therefore is less compliant.
- There is no effect on diastolic filling at low cardiac volumes. Consequently, early filling during diastole is not impaired. However, as filling continues and the maximum volume allowed by the pericardial constriction is reached, pressures in the chambers equalize and filling stops. Filling is early in diastole for constrictive pericarditis patients.
- Observing when the ventricle fills during diastole allows one to differentiate between tamponade and constrictive pericarditis.

- Echocardiography may be helpful, as there are several echocardiographic findings associated with constrictive pericarditis, but none are pathognomonic.
- Pericardial thickening can be detected easily by computed tomography (CT) and magnetic resonance imaging (MRI) but is not always present, and may be absent in 20% of patients.
- Left and right cardiac catheterization is needed for simultaneous measurement of filling pressures in order to aid in the diagnosis.
- Pericardiectomy is the only effective treatment.

CLINICAL FINDINGS IN CONSTRICTIVE PERICARDITIS

- Increased JVP.
- Signs of right heart failure (peripheral edema, ascites, hepato-jugular reflex).
- A pericardial knock may be present (essentially, an S_3).

DIAGNOSTIC FINDINGS IN CONSTRICTIVE PERICARDITIS

- No specific ECG findings, though low-voltage may be present.
- CXR may show calcification around the heart or the pericardium.
- Echocardiography will demonstrate increased pericardial thickness and abnormal ventricular filling. The inferior vena cava (IVC) will usually be dilated and will not have respiratory variation in diameter. Atria typically will be dilated.
- CT scan can demonstrate increased pericardial thickness and calcification.
- MRI can demonstrated increased pericardial thickness.
- Cardiac catheterization will demonstrate:
  - Increased RA pressures
  - Increased "x" and "y" descents
  - Increased RV diastolic pressures
  - The "dip and plateau" or "square-root sign" on left ventricle (LV) and RV diastolic tracings, which show an early diastolic decrease followed by a plateau

ACUTE PERICARDITIS

- Pericarditis commonly presents with a characteristic syndrome that includes central, pleuritic chest pain that is worse supine and improves some with upright positioning or leaning forward.
- A pericardial friction rub is not always present.
- The ECG is often normal or not diagnostic; diffuse ST elevation is often not present.
- PR segment depression is very suggestive of pericarditis.
- The primary concern is always to distinguish pericardial pain from myocardial ischemia.
- The classical symptoms of pericarditis, unassociated with symptoms, signs, or ECG changes suggesting ischemia or infarction, can be confidently attributed to acute pericarditis.
- Minor elevations in cardiac enzymes, including troponin T or I, can occur in acute pericarditis.
- Treatment is with nonsteroidal anti-inflammatory drugs (NSAIDs). If the cause of the pericarditis is known, then specific therapy directed at that disease should be initiated.

PURULENT PERICARDITIS

- Purulent pericarditis is a rare disease, often presenting in the immunocompromised patient.
- It is highly fatal and requires emergent drainage.
- Purulent pericarditis is most often the result of local spread from empyema, mediastinitis, pneumonia, endocarditis, prior pericardiotomy, or burn injury.
- The diagnosis is made with pericardial fluid sampling.

BIBLIOGRAPHY

Belenkie I, Tyberg J. Pericardial disease. In: Hall JB, Schmidt GA, Wood LDH, eds., *Principles of Critical Care*, 3rd ed. New York, NY: McGraw-Hill; 2005:373–384.

23 CARDIOVASCULAR DISEASES

Nuala J. Meyer

KEY POINTS

- There are three major etiologies of noninfectious valvular dysfunction: (1) congenital malformations of the valve, typically seen in young patients; (2) rheumatic heart disease following acute rheumatic fever, classically involving the mitral valve prior to the aortic; and (3) calcific or degenerative valvular disease, usually involving the aortic valve of older individuals.
- Echocardiography is a useful bedside tool to evaluate valvular abnormalities.

- Acute valvular abnormalities often require urgent surgical intervention.
- Critical AS exists when the mean transvalvular pressure gradient exceeds 50 mmHg, or when the calculated valve area is 0.75 cm^2 or less.
- Aortic stenosis may be asymptomatic until late in its course, but early symptoms of AS—angina and syncope—relate to left ventricular hypertrophy.
- Aortic Insufficiency can present two ways: Acute AI typically causes a patient to present critically ill, with pulmonary edema, diaphoresis, cyanosis, and cardiogenic shock. Chronic AI, in contrast, generally presents with a gradual onset of congestive heart failure.
- Mitral stenosis occurs when the valve area is 2 cm^2, and critical MS when the valve area is 1 cm^2 or less.
- To maintain normal cardiac output in the face of a narrowed mitral valve area, a higher transvalvular pressure gradient must be generated. Over time this leads to chronically elevated left atrial pressure, and eventually to elevated pulmonary venous and pulmonary arterial pressures.
- In acute MR, for instance with rupture of the chordae, the left atrial size is unchanged but LA pressure is significantly and abruptly increased, resulting in pulmonary edema.

VALVULAR HEART DISEASE

EPIDEMIOLOGY

- Valvular heart disease is a common cause of morbidity and mortality in the United States.
- Recognition of the potential complications for a patient with disordered valves is essential when caring for such a patient in the ICU.
- Once the most common cause for valvular heart disease, rheumatic heart disease has become relatively rare in the western world with the routine use of antibiotic therapy for recognized bacterial pharyngitis and impetigo.
- Patients may still present with symptoms from valvular disease which they acquired many years earlier.
- In addition, as the population ages, degenerative valvular problems are becoming increasingly common.

AORTIC STENOSIS

ETIOLOGY

- There are three major etiologies of valvular dysfunction: (1) congential malformations of the valve, typically seen in young patients; (2) rheumatic heart disease following acute rheumatic fever, classically involving the mitral valve prior to the aortic; and (3) calcific or degenerative valvular disease, usually involving the aortic valve of older individuals.

PATHOPHYSIOLOGY

- 1–2% of aortic valves are estimated to be bicuspid, making this the most common congenital heart disease.
- Bicuspid valves are subject to more stress than normal tricuspid aortic valves, and thus are prone to earlier calcification.
- Older adults may have senile calcification of otherwise normal, tricuspid aortic valves.
- In either congenital or senile aortic stenosis (AS), progression of the calcification reduces valve opening, causing an increased resistance to blood flow along the aortic outflow tract.
- Critical AS exists when the mean transvalvular pressure gradient—that is, the gradient between pressure on the ventricular versus the aortic side of the aortic valve—exceeds 50 mmHg, or when the calculated valve area is 0.75 cm^2 or less.
- In response to the elevated pressure gradient across the aortic valve, the left ventricle (LV) hypertrophies, usually causing first diastolic and later systolic dysfunction.

CLINICAL FEATURES

- Aortic stenosis may be asymptomatic until late in its course.
- Early symptoms of AS—angina and syncope—relate to left ventricular hypertrophy (LVH).
- Angina may occur from either decreased coronary arterial perfusion during diastole due to the outflow tract obstruction, or from coronary arterial disease.
- Syncope may result when an increase in LV pressure with exertion is not accompanied by an increase in aortic pressure, due to the fixed obstruction.
- Late in AS, LV dysfunction may occur, causing pulmonary edema and dyspnea.
- The typical murmur of AS is a loud crescendo/decrescendo systolic murmur heard at the base of the heart radiating to the carotids, with a soft or absent S_2 component. Carotid upstrokes may be weak and delayed, *pulsus parvus et tardus.*

DIAGNOSTIC EVALUATION

- ECG typically shows LVH with repolarization abnormalities.

- Chest x-ray (CXR) may show a calcified aortic valve, and, in severe or advanced cases, an enlarged cardiac silhouette.
- Echocardiogram reliably diagnoses AS and provides the clinically relevant transvalvular gradient and aortic valve area by Doppler flow. Echo is also critical in determining the LV function for patients with AS.
- Cardiac catheterization may confirm the severity of AS and allow measurement of the left ventricular end-diastolic pressure, or LVEDP, often elevated in patients with AS. In addition, patients who may undergo surgical correction of their valves should be evaluated for coronary artery disease prior to undergoing surgery.

INTENSIVE CARE UNIT MANAGEMENT

- Definitive treatment of AS requires surgery to correct the mechanical obstruction.
- Patients with AS and decreased LV function have a high mortality, with an estimated survival of just 1 year. Thus, development of LV dysfunction in a patient with critical AS is an indication for surgery as soon as medically stable.
- In treating ill ICU patients with comorbid AS, the clinician faces a difficult challenge. Recent evidence supports the use of careful afterload reduction with nitroprusside as a bridge to surgical repair in patients with AS and decreased LV function. Dobutamine, a positive inotrope, may also be helpful in optimizing LV function whilst avoiding hypotension. Limited experience with angiotensin-converting enzyme inhibitors (ACEI) and digitalis suggest they may also have a role in the medical management of AS.
- Percutaneous balloon aortic valvotomy, where a balloon is inflated across the stenosed aortic valve to force the leaflets apart, may be a temporizing measure for a patient in cardiogenic shock or with need for noncardiac surgery, but the high rate of restenosis within 6 months precludes its recommendation as a definitive procedure.

AORTIC INSUFFICIENCY

ETIOLOGY

- Aortic insufficiency (AI) may result from problems with the aortic valve leaflets or from diseases of the aortic root.
- AI can be classified as chronic or acute; acute AI can be a life-threatening emergency.
- The most common etiologies of AI are: (1) infective endocarditis, (2) aortic dissection, and (3) rupture or prolapse of the aortic valve leaflet.
- The aortic valve can also be injured following blunt chest trauma or deceleration injury.

PATHOPHYSIOLOGY

- In chronic AI, the LV gradually dilates in response to the chronic volume overload of regurgitant flow back into the LV during diastole. Dilation alters the usual pressure-volume relationship of the LV, so that for any change in volume, the pressure increase is less. Chronic AI can thus remain compensated for some time, until an additional strain such as ischemia or decreased LV function causes rapid deterioration.
- In acute AI, there has been no time for the LV to dilate. A small change in LV volume therefore causes a large change in LVEDP, and therefore acute pulmonary venous hypertension and congestion.

CLINICAL FEATURES

- Acute AI typically causes a patient to present critically ill, with pulmonary edema, diaphoresis, cyanosis, and cardiogenic shock. Patients are tachycardic, low or normotensive with a normal pulse pressure, and a short diastolic murmur over the base with a soft S_1 and loud P_2.
- Chronic AI, in contrast, generally presents with a gradual onset of congestive heart failure.

DIAGNOSTIC EVALUATION

- In acute AI, ECG may be normal with the exception of sinus tachycardia. Clues to acute AI on CXR may include pulmonary edema in the presence of a normal heart silhouette, or a widened mediastinum if the etiology of AI was aortic dissection.
- In chronic AI, ECG tends to show LVH, and the CXR often shows an enlarged cardiac silhouette with a prominent LV, and an unfolded or dilated aorta.
- Echocardiogram, either transthoracic (TTE) or transesophageal (TEE), is quite helpful in the detection and evaluation of AI, as Doppler techniques can estimate the severity of regurgitant flow and LV function can be simultaneously assessed. TEE can also provide clues to the etiology of valvular disease, demonstrating for example aortic dissection, vegetation, or abscess on a valve leaflet.
- Cardiac catheterization allows evaluation of the degree of regurgitant flow, the status of the aortic root, and the status of the coronary arteries if surgery is planned.

INTENSIVE CARE UNIT MANAGEMENT

- Acute AI is a medical emergency, and often presents in dramatic fashion with severe pulmonary edema. A rapid investigation into the cause of the insufficiency—particularly looking for aortic dissection or aortic valve endocarditis—should be sought.
- Early valve replacement should be considered when the regurgitation is severe, and when the resultant heart failure cannot be managed medically.
  - Loop diuretics and venodilators such as sodium nitroprusside are the mainstay of therapy, as inotropes are typically not helpful in the setting of an already hyperdynamic LV, and vasoconstricting medications are relatively contraindicated as they tend to increase the amount of regurgitation.
  - Intra-aortic balloon pumps are absolutely contraindicated, as they worsen insufficiency.
  - In aortic valve endocarditis causing severe AI, early valve replacement has shown a decreased mortality. However, if the heart failure can be successfully managed medically, and if the patient is responding to antibiotic therapy, surgery may be delayed while the infection is treated.
- Chronic AI can be treated with long-term afterload reduction, using medicines such as hydralazine, ACEI, and calcium channel blockers.
- To optimize the patient's heart function, surgery for AI should occur before any decrement in LV function can be demonstrated.

MITRAL STENOSIS

ETIOLOGY

- Rheumatic disease following rheumatic fever remains the most common reason for mitral stenosis (MS), particularly in the developing world. Rarely, MS results from severe calcification of the mitral annulus, typically in the elderly or in patients with renal failure.

PATHOPHYSIOLOGY

- In rheumatic MS, inflammation following rheumatic fever causes fusion of the mitral commissures, the chordae tendinae, or both. The valve gradually degenerates, resulting in a narrowed valve area.
  - Normally, the mitral valve area is 4–6 cm^2.
  - Mild MS occurs when the valve area is 2 cm^2, and critical MS when the valve area is 1 cm^2 or less.
- To maintain normal cardiac output in the face of a narrowed valve area, a higher transvalvular pressure gradient must be generated. Over time this leads to chronically elevated left atrial pressure, and eventually to elevated pulmonary venous and pulmonary arterial pressures.
- MS patients are especially challenged by any increase in heart rate, which shortens diastolic filling time and further elevates the transvalvular gradient, thus further exacerbating left atrial pressure overload. The left atrium tends to dilate—placing patients at high risk for atrial fibrillation—and its chronically elevated pressure often causes pulmonary edema.
- Tachycardia in any form exacerbates left atrial pressure overload, as diastolic filling time is shortened, and worsens pulmonary edema.
- Eventually, long-standing MS with high left atrial pressures will result in pulmonary hypertension, which in turn leads to right ventricular (RV) failure.

CLINICAL FEATURES

- While patients with MS may remain asymptomatic for many years after their acute rheumatic fever, eventually they tend to present with dyspnea on exertion, atrial fibrillation, or acute pulmonary edema.
- Hemoptysis from disruption of bronchial veins—a complication of pulmonary hypertension—may be dramatic, and may also be precipitated by exertion.
- The dilated left atrium with atrial fibrillation is particularly prone to clot formation, and results in many strokes in patients with MS.
- On examination, one may hear an opening snap prior to S_1, followed by a diastolic rumble at the apex. As MS worsens, the murmur becomes louder toward end-diastole and closer to S_2.
- When pulmonary hypertension is present, the examination can reveal fixed splitting of the second heart sound with a loud P_2, RV heave, and even the Graham Steele murmur of pulmonic insufficiency.

DIAGNOSTIC EVALUATION

- Electrocardiogram often reveals atrial fibrillation and right ventricular hypertrophy (RVH). If sinus rhythm is present, left atrial enlargement may be suggested by a tall P wave.
- The CXR often shows splaying of the carina, as the left mainstem bronchus is driven cephalad by the dilated left atrium. The left atrial shadow is prominent in the aortopulmonary window, and pulmonary arteries are frequently enlarged. The mitral annulus is often calcified and easily visible, and pulmonary edema may be present.

- Echocardiogram with Doppler flow is useful to study the valve anatomy and to noninvasively obtain the transvalvular gradient, thus judging the severity of the lesion.
- Cardiac catheterization may confirm the severity of the valve gradient, and right heart catheterization can estimate the left atrial pressure, although a more accurate technique is transseptal puncture of the interatrial septum, with direct measurement of left atrial pressure.

INTENSIVE CARE UNIT MANAGEMENT

- When patients with MS present in pulmonary edema, they should be managed with careful diuretic therapy and aggressive rate control with either beta-blockers or calcium channel blockers. Digoxin is considered second-line therapy.
- Anticoagulation is essential for patients with MS and atrial fibrillation, with a goal international normalized ratio (INR) of 2 to 3.
- Once symptoms of MS are present, surgical or procedural therapy is indicated.
  - In pure rheumatic MS, the procedure of choice is catheter balloon commissurotomy. Via a right heart catheterization, a catheter is placed transseptally in the left atrium and a balloon passed across the mitral valve.
  - Contraindications to balloon commissurotomy are significant mitral regurgitation, left atrial thrombus, or unfavorable valve morphology.
  - Balloon commissurotomy is successful and has low mortality. When the procedure is contraindicated, surgical commissurotomy or valve replacement is indicated.

MITRAL REGURGITATION

ETIOLOGY

- Mitral regurgitation (MR) can result from damage to the valve leaflets, the mitral annulus, the chordae tendinae, or the papillary muscles.
- The mitral valve leaflets can be damaged by rheumatic heart disease, trauma, infective endocarditis, Libman-Sacks endocarditis from lupus, or myxomatous degeneration from mitral valve prolapse.
- The mitral annulus suffers from either dilation—for example, in dilated cardiomyopathies—or from calcification, usually age-related.
- Ischemic heart disease, particularly acute MI, can cause disruption of either papillary muscles or chordae tendinae, and can result in acute MR. The chordae are also occasionally damaged by infective endocarditis or by mitral valve prolapse.

PATHOPHYSIOLOGY

- When regurgitant blood flows into the left atrium during systole, the early response of the LV is to augment its cardiac output, due to increased diastolic filling and decreased systolic pressure and volume. However, over time the LV dilates and is subjected to higher systolic wall tension. This in turn reduces LV performance; when the ejection fraction has fallen to just mild LV dysfunction, a significant decrement in LV contractility has already occurred.
- In acute MR, for instance with rupture of the chordae, the left atrial size is unchanged but LA pressure is significantly and abruptly increased, resulting in pulmonary edema. In this setting, a large V wave might be observed on pulmonary arterial catheter tracings.
- In chronic MR, by contrast, the left atrium accommodates to its increased volume with dilation, and thus avoids significant elevations in left atrial pressures. Atrial fibrillation is common due to the massively dilated chamber size.

CLINICAL FEATURES

- In acute MR, patients often present in florid pulmonary edema and with low cardiac output. Frequently, ischemia is present, and has resulted in chordae or papillary muscle rupture.
- In chronic MR, symptoms often are absent until either atrial fibrillation occurs or the LV function is compromised.
- Critical illness, or any process elevating the systemic vascular resistance, will dramatically worsen the regurgitant flow, and may precipitate congestive heart failure (CHF).
- On examination, the LV impulse is frequently laterally displaced.
  - An S_3 is often present.
  - A blowing, high-pitched holosystolic murmur is heard loudest at the apex and radiates to the axilla. The murmur typically obliterates S_1 and S_2.
  - MR murmurs can be distinguished from tricuspid regurgitation (TR) in that they tend to decrease slightly in intensity with inspiration, while the murmur augments in TR. Dynamic LV outflow murmurs such as idiopathic hypertrophic subaortic stenosis are also holosystolic, but these tend to be harsher than MR murmurs and will soften with maneuvers that increase afterload/decrease preload (e.g.,

standing), whereas MR murmurs are louder with such maneuvers.

DIAGNOSTIC EVALUATION

- Unless it shows evidence of myocardial ischemia, the ECG in acute mitral regurgitation is typically normal. In chronic MR, the ECG may show left atrial enlargement, RVH, or atrial fibrillation.
- On CXR, patients with MR have an enlarged cardiac silhouette with LV prominence, left atrial enlargement and, at times, mitral annular calcification.
- Echocardiogram often elucidates the etiology of mitral regurgitation in addition to grading its severity.
- Cardiac catheterization with left ventriculogram can effectively demonstrate MR severity and estimate LV ejection fraction. Right heart catheterization may also be helpful, in showing a prominent V wave which represents simultaneous filling of the left atrium by both the pulmonary veins and by the regurgitant LV during ventricular systole.
- Exercise testing can be an important adjunct to evaluate the asymptomatic patient with chronic MR, as it may precipitate symptoms and thus indicate a need for surgical intervention.

INTENSIVE CARE UNIT MANAGEMENT

- Patients presenting with acute MR can be treated identically to patients with acute heart failure, with afterload reduction (ACEI, nitroprusside, or hydralazine), diuresis, and positive inotropes as necessary. Noninvasive positive pressure ventilation (NIPPV) is frequently extremely effective in treating pulmonary edema and for further afterload reduction.
- Acute mitral regurgitation carries a high mortality; patients should be treated aggressively and early consideration for surgical intervention—for example, for chord rupture with flail valve leaflet, papillary muscle rupture, or valve vegetation causing acute MR—is appropriate.
- In chronic MR, surgery for either valve repair or valve replacement should be considered when a patient is symptomatic. Exercise testing may elucidate an otherwise asymptomatic patient's complaints. In addition, asymptomatic patients should be considered for surgery when their ejection fraction falls below 50%, their end-systolic volume index exceeds 50 mL/m^2, or when pulmonary hypertension develops.
- The decision to replace versus repair a valve often depends on the underlying etiology of the valve dysfunction and on the valve structure.

BIBLIOGRAPHY

Bellone A, Barbieri A, Ricci C, et al. Acute effects of non-invasive ventilatory support on functional mitral regurgitation in patients with exacerbation of congestive heart failure. *Intensive Care Med* 2002;28:1348–1350.

Carroll JD, Feldman T. Percutaneous mitral balloon valvotomy and the new demographics of mitral stenosis. *JAMA* 1993;270: 1731–1736.

Khot UN, Novaro GM, Popovic ZB, et al. Nitroprusside in critically ill patients with left ventricular dysfunction and aortic stenosis. *N Engl J Med* 2003;348:1756–1763.

Sorrentino MJ. Valvular heart disease. In: Hall JB, Schmidt GA, Wood LDH, eds., *Principles of Critical Care*, 3rd ed. New York, NY: McGraw-Hill; 2005:385–400.

Zile MR, Gaasch WH. Heart failure in aortic stenosis—improving diagnosis and treatment. *N Engl J Med* 2003;348:18–19.

24 AORTIC DISSECTION

Nathan Sandbo

KEY POINTS

- Risk factors include hypertension, Marfan syndrome, and congenital aortic anomalies.
- Aortic dissection typically presents with intense, sharp chest pain combined with hypertension, but symptoms can be subtle.
- Diagnosis rests on echocardiography, helical CT angiography, or magnetic resonance imaging, and sometimes requires aortography.
- Treatment involves urgent pain and blood pressure control, using drugs that blunt the systolic rise in aortic pressure (such as labetalol), followed by surgery for dissections involving the ascending aorta (type A dissection).
- Careful monitoring is required to detect complications such as vascular occlusion, pericardial tamponade, aortic rupture, or aortic valve insufficiency.

EPIDEMIOLOGY

- Most common emergent condition involving the aorta with an incidence of 5–30 cases per million per year, making it two to three times as common as rupture of abdominal aortic aneurysm.

- Men have two to three times greater risk of developing aortic dissection than women. Peak age of incidence is 50–55 years old.
- Up to 90% of patients have hypertension at time of presentation, with 62–78% having a history of chronic systemic hypertension.
- Marfan syndrome is present in the majority of patients presenting with aortic dissection under the age of 40.

TABLE 24-2 Classification of Aortic Dissections

- Daily (or Stanford) classification system
  - Type A: dissection of the ascending aorta, regardless of site of initial tear
  - Type B: dissection of the descending aorta
- DeBakey classification system
  - Type 1: dissection of the ascending and descending aorta
  - Type 2: dissection of the ascending aorta
  - Type 3: dissection of the descending aorta

PATHOPHYSIOLOGY

- A dissecting hematoma that separates the intima and inner layers of the media from the outer medial and adventitial layers. Most commonly initiated via a tear in the intima that precedes either anterograde or retrograde, creating a false lumen. Tear is due to weakening of the wall of the aorta (most often the medial layer), increased shear stress, or both.
- May be complicated by rupture into the pericardial space, or pleural space, occlusion of branching arteries with consequent ischemic symptoms, or involvement of the aortic valve commissures with subsequent insufficiency.
- Table 24-1 shows dissection risk factors.
- Connective tissue diseases such as Marfan syndrome or Ehlers-Danlos syndrome predispose to medial degeneration.
- Secondary causes of reduced wall strength include annuloaortic ectasia, bicuspid aortic valve, coarctation, and pregnancy. Other causes of increased shear stress include instrumentation of the aorta, deceleration injury from blunt trauma, cocaine use, and abrupt discontinuation of a beta-blocker.
- Classified by:
  - Timing: acute (<2 weeks) or chronic (>2 weeks)
  - Location: type A (60%), ascending aorta is involved (independent of site of intimal tear), or type B (40%), only descending aorta (beyond left subclavian artery)
- Mortality is highest for type A dissections.
- See Table 24-2 for classification schemes.

TABLE 24-1 Risk Factors for Dissection

- Systemic hypertension
- Connective tissue disease
  - Marfan syndrome
  - Ehlers-Danlos syndrome
  - Vasculitis
    - Takayasu arteritis
    - Giant-cell arteritis
  - Rheumatoid arthritis
- Congenital defects
  - Annuloaortic ectasia
  - Bicuspid aortic valve
  - Coarctation of aorta
  - Turner syndrome
- Acquired risk factors
  - Preexisting aortic aneurysm
  - Syphilis
  - Pregnancy
  - Previous aortic valve replacement
  - Coronary artery bypass grafting (CABG)
  - Trauma
  - Cocaine

CLINICAL PRESENTATION

- Presentation can be subtle (diagnosis is missed in up to 38% of patients).
- Pain is most consistent presenting complaint (95%), located anteriorly, where it is most often retrosternal, but occasionally epigastric, or posteriorly, when it is usually interscapular. Almost always described as sharp, tearing, or knifelike, with a sudden onset. It is usually extremely intense, and may be difficult to control with opiates.
- Patients may present with evidence of shock, with cool, clammy periphery, ashen coloring, and depressed level of consciousness. Elevated blood pressure (>200 mmHg systolic) is usually present, but may be absent if dissection results in tamponade, aortic rupture, or severe aortic regurgitation.
- A new murmur of aortic insufficiency is present in 50–66% of type A dissections and 25% of all patients.
- One-third of patients will present with compromised flow to a major branch of the aorta, with the innominate artery (resulting in reduced right carotid and right subclavian flow) being the most often affected. This can result in the presence of a blood pressure differential between left and right brachial arteries (present in 38% of patients), focal neurologic signs associated with differential cerebral hypoperfusion (5–10% of patients), and a spectrum of peripheral sensory and motor neuropathies due to involvement of arterial branches supplying the spinal cord.

- Aortic rupture is the most common cause of early mortality with severe aortic regurgitation, the second most common cause.

DIAGNOSIS

- A high clinical suspicion is necessary to establish the diagnosis in many patients.
- Laboratory data are usually within normal limits in patients with acute dissection, although leukocytosis is sometimes seen.
- ECG is most often normal or shows left ventricular hypertrophy, but may mimic a myocardial infarction, especially in type A dissection if there is involvement of one of the cusps of the coronary arteries.
- Chest x-ray may show widened mediastinum (absent in up to 40% of type A dissections), or pleural effusion (left > right, with associated apical cap).
- Appropriate diagnostic imaging is the key to diagnosis, but some controversy exists over the best diagnostic test to most effectively diagnose aortic dissection. Aortic angiography, computed tomography (CT) aortic imaging, magnetic resonance imaging (MRI), and echocardiography are all viable options.
  - Echocardiography is a diagnostic modality of choice, with transesophageal imaging superior to transthoracic with sensitivity and specificity of >95% and >90%, respectively.
  - CT scanning is noninvasive, but is less sensitive (83%) than angiography, but has excellent (up to 100%) specificity. Advantages include widespread availability, noninvasiveness, and cost.
  - Aortic angiography is most invasive, with sensitivity and specificity of 85–90% and 75–95%, respectively.
  - MRI is still investigational, but some studies suggest it may have sensitivities and specificities rivaling transesophageal echo, however, its widespread application is limited by lack of immediate availability. Difficulty in adequately monitoring a potentially critically ill patient while getting an MRI may also limit its use.

TREATMENT

- Cardiac monitoring, with intra-arterial monitoring of blood pressure.
- Adequate central venous access should be obtained.
- Surgical consultation is required for emergent reparative surgery, which is indicated in all type A dissections, and type B dissections with rapid expansion, impending rupture, uncontrollable pain, or evidence of end-organ/limb ischemia. Mortality is up to 50% at 72 hours for untreated type A dissection, and 90% at 3 months, while operative mortality is 5–21%. Early surgical management is desirable with both longer time to operation and development of complications leading to a worse prognosis.
- Immediate initiation of blood pressure control and pain control with intravenous medications. Medications that reduce the pulse pressure are preferred (labetalol, esmolol, propranolol), but often combination therapy with a direct-acting arterial vasodilator (nitroprusside) is required for adequate control. Target systolic blood pressure should be as low as 90–100 mmHg as long as organ perfusion is maintained.
- Uncomplicated type B dissections are most often managed medically with aggressive blood pressure control (survival of 80%). Endovascular stent placement may be a less invasive alternative to surgery in select patient populations.
- Frequent monitoring of parameters of end-organ perfusion such as pulse checks, urine output, mental status, bowel sounds, and complete neurologic checks in an intensive care environment allow for early detection of progression of dissection.
- Long-term control of blood pressure is crucial to decrease the risk of subsequent aneurismal complications.

BIBLIOGRAPHY

Austin JJ. Aortic dissection. In: Hall JB, Schmidt GA, Wood LDH, eds., *Principles of Critical Care*, 3rd ed. New York, NY: McGraw-Hill; 2005:401–413.

Khan IA, Nair CK. Clinical, diagnostic, and management perspectives of aortic dissection. *Chest* 2002;122:311–328.

Kouchoukos NT, Dougenis D. Surgery of the thoracic aorta. *N Engl J Med* 1997;336:1876–1888.

Nienaber CA, Fatttori R, Lund G, et al. Nonsurgical reconstruction of thoracic aortic dissection by stent-graft placement. *N Engl J Med* 1999;340:1539–1545.

Pretre R, Von Segesser LK. Aortic dissection. *Lancet* 1997;349: 1461–1464.

25 MECHANICAL CIRCULATORY ASSIST DEVICES

Ethan L. Gundeck

KEY POINTS

- Intra-aortic balloon pumps and ventricular assist devices are being used increasingly.
- IABPs inflate in diastole and deflate in systole, unloading the left ventricle.

- IABP is generally used for patients in cardiogenic shock or at high-risk during cardiac catheterization; vascular complications should be sought regularly.
- VAD can unload either the right or left ventricle, generally as a bridge to definitive treatment or to allow the heart to improve (acutely or in the long-term).
- Hemorrhage is the most frequent complication of VAD.

INTRODUCTION

- Due to the aging of the U.S. population and improved therapies for patients with heart disease, heart failure is increasing in frequency.
- Mechanical circulatory assist devices, specifically intra-aortic balloon pumps (IABP) and ventricular assist devices (VAD), can offer significant benefit to patients with (or at high-risk for) cardiogenic shock.

INTRA-AORTIC BALLOON PUMP

INTRODUCTION

- An IABP is a helium-filled balloon generally placed in the descending aorta.
- It inflates during diastole, displacing between 30 and 50 mL of blood into the proximal aorta, and deflates at the start of systole.
- The predominant effect is to reduce afterload, although it may directly improve flow to the coronaries as well.

INDICATIONS

- Most common indications are to provide hemodynamic support during or after cardiac catheterization and for the treatment of cardiogenic shock.
- May also be used for weaning from cardiopulmonary bypass, preoperative stabilization of high-risk patients (left main disease, severe aortic stenosis), and treatment of refractory unstable angina.
- Has been used successfully for intractable ventricular arrhythmias and mechanical complications after myocardial infarction (post-MI ventricular septal defect or mitral regurgitation).

CONTRAINDICATIONS

- The major contraindication to use is aortic insufficiency (balloon inflation during diastole can greatly exacerbate this valvular abnormality).
- Other contraindications include abdominal aortic aneurysm or dissection; severe, bilateral peripheral vascular disease; uncontrolled bleeding; or sepsis.

PRACTICAL CONSIDERATIONS

- May be placed through an arterial sheath (generally requires anticoagulation) or without a sheath (the sheathless device can be used without anticoagulation).
- Chest radiography confirms proper placement in the descending aorta: the tip of balloon should be at the level of the tracheal carina.
- The balloon inflates during diastole (should be timed to the dichrotic notch of the intra-arterial wave form displayed on the IABP console), and deflates during the isovolumic phase of systole (generally timed to the R wave on the ECG).
- Improper timing can cause suboptimal or even deleterious hemodynamic effects.
- The pump can be set to inflate in a fixed relationship to the cardiac cycle. For example, with 1:1 timing, the IABP synchronizes with each heartbeat, whereas with 1:3 timing, the balloon inflates only every third heartbeat.
- Use 1:2 or 1:3 frequency when adjusting the timing of balloon inflation. Look for diastolic augmentation of pressure during inflation and reduced systolic and diastolic pressures during the subsequent beat.
- Look for decrease in systolic pressure, increase in diastolic pressure, decrease in heart rate, decrease in wedge pressure, and increase in cardiac output (or surrogates such as central venous oxyhemoglobin saturation) as indicators that the IABP is having a positive effect.

COMPLICATIONS

- Complications are divided into vascular and nonvascular.
- Vascular complications include limb ischemia, vascular laceration, hemorrhage, arterial dissection, spinal cord ischemia, and visceral ischemia.
- Vascular complications are more likely in patients with peripheral vascular disease, older age, female gender, diabetes, hypertension, prolonged use of the device, larger catheter size, body surface area <1.8 m^2, or cardiac index <2.2 L/min.
- Nonvascular complications include cholesterol embolization, stroke (rare if placed properly), sepsis if in place more than 7 days, rupture of balloon with subsequent thrombosis, thrombocytopenia, hemolysis, groin infection, and peripheral neuropathy.
- Limb ischemia and other complications generally warrant prompt removal of the device.
- Lower mortality rates in IABP patients have been seen in centers which use them more frequently.

VENTRICULAR ASSIST DEVICE

INTRODUCTION

- These mechanical pumps take over some of the function of a failing ventricle to improve hemodynamics and end-organ perfusion.
- Can assist a failing right ventricle (RVAD), left ventricle (LVAD), or both (BiVAD).
- For RVAD, blood is removed from the right atrium and returned to the main pulmonary artery.
- For LVAD, blood is removed from either the left atrium or apex of the left ventricle, and returned to the ascending aorta.
- Types of VADs are divided into centrifugal, pneumatic pulsatile, and electric pulsatile.
- Centrifugal pumps provide nonpulsatile flow and require anticoagulation and continuous monitoring. These pumps are generally used only for short-term cardiopulmonary bypass.
- Pneumatic pulsatile pumps provide pulsatile flow with minimal trauma to blood cells. After the first few days of placement, minimal supervision is required for these devices, but they are somewhat bulky and limit patient mobility.
- Electric pulsatile pumps are similar to the pneumatic pulsatile pumps, except that they may only be used for the left ventricle. The bulky drive console of the pneumatic device is replaced with a small, portable external controller and battery pack. These devices allow for increased patient mobility, and the possibility for discharge to home with the device in place.

INDICATIONS AND EFFECTS

- Indications for these devices fall into three categories: (1) temporary assistance for a failing ventricle that is expected to recover (e.g., postcardiotomy shock); (2) as a bridge to transplant in a ventricle that is failing to provide adequate end-organ perfusion; or (3) for permanent use (so-called, "destination" therapy).
- Patients stabilized on these devices have improved 6-minute walk times and improved oxygen consumption. Improved histopathologic findings with long-term use have been described as well (regression of hypertrophy, improved fiber orientation, reversal of dilatation). Reports exist of cardiac function improving to the point that the device may be removed.

CONTRAINDICATIONS

- Contraindications to placement: Aortic insufficiency of any significant degree, and severe, unrepaired mitral stenosis. Mitral regurgitation is eliminated by a functioning LVAD (since ventricular afterload is completely reduced) and is not a contraindication, nor is aortic stenosis. Atrial and ventricular arrhythmias are generally well tolerated. Congenital defects should be corrected prior to VAD placement as left ventricular unloading may uncover right-to-left shunt and hypoxemia. Bad obstructive pulmonary disease and neurologic impairment are considered contraindications as well.

COMPLICATIONS AND PRACTICAL MATTERS

- Echocardiographic findings of a functioning LVAD include a completely decompressed left ventricle, no aortic insufficiency, and a closed aortic valve throughout the cardiac cycle.
- Hemorrhage is the most common major complication, occurring in up to 30% of patients. Coagulopathies need to be aggressively corrected.
- Right-sided failure from LVAD placement, thromboembolism, infection, device malfunction, and hemolysis are other complications.

BIBLIOGRAPHY

Laham RJ, Aroesty JM. Intraaortic balloon pump counterpulsation, 2003. Available at: http://www.uptodateonline.com/application/topic.asp?file=chd/24375&type=A&selectedTitle=1~15. Accessed 11/27/05.

Richenbacher WE, Pierce WS. Treatment of heart failure: assisted circulation. In: Braunwald E, Zipes DP, Lippy P, eds., *Heart Disease: A Textbook of Cardiovascular Medicine.* Philadelphia, PA: W.B. Saunders; 2001:600–614.

26 HYPERTENSIVE ENCEPHALOPATHY AND HYPERTENSIVE EMERGENCIES

George W. Bell

KEY POINTS

- Hypertension is an extremely common diagnosis. Elevated blood pressure can progress beyond stage 3 hypertension to accelerated-malignant hypertension as well as hypertensive encephalopathy.

TABLE 26-1 Hypertensive Emergencies

Cardiac
Aortic dissection
Left ventricular failure
Myocardial infarction

Drug-related
MAOI interactions
Cocaine
Antihypertensive withdrawal

Surgical
Postoperative management (coronary artery bypass graft [CABG], kidney transplant, vascular)
Prior to emergent surgery

Neurologic
Hypertensive encephalopathy
Intracerebral hemorrhage
Subarachnoid hemorrhage

Renal
Glomerulonephritis
Collagen vascular

Other
Pheochromocytoma
Eclampsia
Burns
Epistaxis

- In addition, a wide range of other disease processes can require urgent and even rapid correction of elevated blood pressure (Table 26-1).
- At a given threshold, elevated blood pressure can cause end-organ damage that may or may not be reversible.
- The rate of increase in blood pressure is often the determining factor of disease severity, but all patients with a sustained diastolic blood pressure of 130 mmHg or higher should be considered for immediate treatment.
- Persistently elevated blood pressure can precipitate aggravating local and systemic effects.
- Because of its deleterious effects urgent and sometimes rapid correction of blood pressure may be required.
- Intensive monitoring and treatment options are available depending on the clinical situation.
- Better outpatient control of hypertension likely decreases the incidence of hypertensive emergencies.

EPIDEMIOLOGY

- Hypertension is highly prevalent in the U.S. population, and the number of affected patients increases with age.
- After adolescence, blacks are more likely to have hypertension with more severe complications when compared to income-matched whites.
- Although <1% of patients with primary hypertension will develop accelerated-malignant phase hypertension, more patients with primary hypertension than secondary hypertension will present in a hypertensive crisis.
- Some causes of secondary hypertension, including pheochromocytoma and renovascular hypertension, are more likely to proceed to a hypertensive crisis than primary hypertension.

CAUSES OF HYPERTENSIVE CRISES

- There are many causes of hypertensive crises, including medical nonadherence, acute glomerulonephritis, renal artery stenosis, pheochromocytoma, monoamine oxidase inhibiter (MAOI) interactions, sympathetically driven drug use (cocaine), myocardial infarction, and eclampsia.
- Previously normotensive individuals may experience hypertensive encephalopathy at moderate blood pressures if the change in pressure was acute. Such examples include eclampsia and cocaine use.
- Myocardial ischemia, regardless of its progression to myocardial infarction or not, often increases the patient's blood pressure.

PATHOPHYSIOLOGY OF HYPERTENSIVE ENCEPHALOPATHY

- Patients can suffer acute vascular damage at different levels of blood pressure elevation. Vascular damage may be secondary to abnormal endothelial function and platelet activation, as seen by elevated levels of endothelial microparticles and circulating platelet microparticles in severely hypertensive patients.
- Chronic hypertensive patients withstand higher pressures than normotensive patients. This is due to the fact that, over time, arterioles of hypertensive patients respond to chronically high blood pressure by remodeling and developing greater wall thickness.
- In an effort to maintain constant cerebral perfusion, arterioles adjust to the current level of blood pressure. When blood pressure is acutely elevated, arterioles constrict. When blood pressure acutely decreases, arterioles dilate. Together, these ensure steady cerebral perfusion (autoregulation), a phenomenon well studied in animal models and believed to be true in humans as well.
- However, above a certain cut-off point, arterioles can no longer respond to elevated pressure. At this cut-off

blood pressure, arterioles dilate. The arteriole dilation starts in areas of less muscular vessels but progresses globally.

- Once cerebral arterioles dilate as a result of elevated blood pressure, cerebral hyperperfusion and extravasation of fluid into the perivascular tissue occurs. Consequently, cerebral edema, which is a hallmark of hypertensive encephalopathy, follows.
- This cut-off point in which elevated blood pressure causes breakthrough cerebral hyperperfusion has been evaluated in humans. When studying cerebral perfusion as a reflection of varying levels of blood pressure, researchers identified a mean arterial pressure cut-off value in normotensive patients of 120 mmHg. In hypertensive patients, the mean arterial pressure that resulted in cerebral hyperperfusion was 180 mmHg.
- Typically, acute vascular damage correlates with a diastolic blood pressure of 130 mmHg or higher. However, hypertensive encephalopathy can be seen in normotensive patients with an acute rise in their blood pressure to as low as 150/100 mmHg.

DIAGNOSIS AND CLINICAL FEATURES

- Patients will often present in a hypertensive crisis with a diastolic blood pressure >140 mmHg. However, varying levels of hypertension can cause neurologic deficits and other end-organ damage, so it is important to recognize the clinical features of a patient in a hypertensive crisis.
- Patients are said to have accelerated-malignant hypertension when an acute rise in blood pressure causes retinal hemorrhage, exudates, or papilledema.
- Hypertensive encephalopathy is marked by cerebral edema secondary to hypertension-induced cerebral hyperperfusion.
- Patients with hypertensive encephalopathy can present with neurologic findings of an altered level of consciousness, headache, and irritability. In addition to the global findings of confusion, somnolence, and stupor, patients can have focal neurologic deficits as well. Untreated hypertensive encephalopathy can progress to coma or seizure.
- Additional organ systems affected during a hypertensive crisis include the cardiac, gastrointestinal, renal, and hematologic systems. Congestive heart failure can occur, while the gastrointestinal involvement includes nausea and vomiting. Renal involvement includes oliguria and azotemia. Occasionally, hemolysis or thrombocytopenia is seen.
- Some patients do not present with the above constellation of symptoms despite being in a hypertensive crisis with end-organ damage. Specifically, young black men may not have any signs or symptoms other than marked renal insufficiency.
- In patients with a blood pressure elevated enough to cause hypertensive encephalopathy or accelerated-malignant hypertension there exist other markers that represent end-organ damage.
    - Renal insufficiency can develop, marked by proteinuria and red cells in the urine. Both azotemia and acute oliguric renal failure can develop.
    - At such high blood pressures there is also risk of diffuse intrarenal ischemia. This diffuse intrarenal ischemia can cause elevated plasma renin and subsequent secondary aldosteronism, presenting as hypokalemia. Besides hypokalemia, elevated renin levels and secondary aldosteronism can exacerbate the patient's already high blood pressure.
    - Accelerated-malignant hypertension can cause microangiopathic hemolytic anemia with subsequent schistocytes and intravascular coagulation.

NATURAL HISTORY

- Because of the vast amount of damage caused by such elevated blood pressure, treatment should be instituted immediately.
- Likely causes of death in the short-term include central nervous system dysfunction, while those who survive the acute setting are more likely to later die from renal failure or stroke.
- Prior to more effective therapy the 1-year survival of accelerated-malignant hypertension was <25%. At that same time the 5-year survival of poorly treated accelerated-malignant hypertension was 1%.
- Fortunately, newer treatment options have significantly reduced the mortality associated with accelerated-malignant hypertension. The 1-year survival rate has increased to 90%, while the 5-year survival rate has increased to 80%.

TREATMENT OPTIONS

- With newer medications available and the appropriate utilization of hemodialysis, patients presenting in a hypertensive crisis have a greater chance of survival.
- Although the etiology of the hypertensive crisis is important, treatment must often be swift even without a known etiology. However, certain illnesses that mimic the signs and symptoms of a hypertensive crisis require alternative therapy and should thus be recognized (Table 26-2).
- It is important to remember that the neurologic findings of hypertensive encephalopathy can be reversed

TABLE 26-2 Hypertensive Scenarios That Should be Differentiated From Hypertensive Crises

Acute left ventricular failure
Renal failure
Collagen vascular diseases
Subarachnoid hemorrhage
Intracerebral hemorrhage
Thromboembolic stroke

with early detection and appropriate treatment. Persistently high diastolic blood pressures above 140 mmHg often require parenteral treatment. Signs of hypertensive encephalopathy should also prompt parenteral treatment.

- Parenteral agents include the vasodilators nitroprusside, nitroglycerin, nicardipine, hydralazine, enalapril, and fenoldopam. The parenteral adrenergic inhibitors include phentolamine, esmolol, and labetalol. In these circumstances, patients often require parenteral furosemide to prevent sodium and water retention, which if left untreated will cause a recurrent rise in blood pressure. Furosemide should only be considered in the euvolemic or hypervolemic patient, and it often helps lower the blood pressure even further. Special care must be taken not to give furosemide to the hypovolemic patient with hypertensive crisis.
- Initially, blood pressure should be lowered by no more than 25% to protect against cerebral ischemia. When using parenteral agents, intra-arterial blood pressure monitoring should be considered.
- Patients who do not appear in acute danger and who are cognitively intact may be considered for oral therapy.
- Those who have suffered a stroke should not have their blood pressure lowered too rapidly, or ischemia can develop.

NITROPRUSSIDE

- Nitroprusside likely acts similarly to endogenous nitric oxide with venous and arterial dilation. It has a rapid onset and is considered first-line treatment in severe hypertensive crises. It is especially indicated in aortic dissection, but a drug to blunt the aortic pressure rise, such as propranolol, must be used concomitantly (Table 26-3).
- Its venous dilation properties can decrease cardiac preload and cardiac output with subsequent tachycardia.
- When treating hypertension in patients with acute systolic dysfunction and pulmonary edema, nitroprusside can be efficacious when used with a loop diuretic.

TABLE 26-3 Preferred Treatment Options Directed at Specific Clinical Hypertensive Situations

First-line treatment
Nitroprusside
Aortic dissection
Nitroprusside Trimethaphan camsylate Propranolol Labetalol
Myocardial ischemia
Nitroprusside Nitroglycerine
Preeclampsia/eclampsia
Hydralazine Labetalol Nicardipine Nifedipine
Pheochromocytoma
Phentolamine
Cocaine-induced
Labetalol

- Nitroprusside may increase intracranial pressure by raising cerebral blood flow, especially when intracranial compliance is reduced.
- Side effects include nausea, vomiting, and diaphoresis. Muscle twitching has been noted as well.
- Thiocyanate intoxication must be monitored when administering nitroprusside.
- The dose ranges from 0.25 to 10 μg/kg/min by intravenous infusion. Onset of action is nearly instantaneous and intra-arterial blood pressure monitoring is required.

NITROGLYCERIN

- Nitroglycerin is another effective vasodilator especially useful during periods of coronary ischemia.
- The side effects include flushing, headache, tachycardia, and vomiting.
- Like the vasodilator nitroprusside, nitroglycerin coupled with a loop diuretic can be effective in treating hypertension in patients with systolic dysfunction and pulmonary edema.
- Patients must be monitored for methemoglobinemia.
- The dose is 5–100 μg/min intravenously, and its onset is between 2 and 5 minutes.

NICARDIPINE

- This calcium antagonist is useful in preserving tissue perfusion in patients experiencing ischemia. Nicardipine offers a controllable reduction in blood pressure with little chance of overcorrection and hypotension.

- Side effects include flushing, headache, and tachycardia. Local phlebitis has been seen.
- The dose is 5–15 mg/h intravenous infusion with an onset of 5–10 minutes.

HYDRALAZINE

- This medication remains the treatment of choice for preeclampsia and eclampsia.
- It can be dosed intravenously with 5 mg boluses repeated every 20 minutes for a total of 20 mg, and its onset is 10–20 minutes when given IV. Intramuscular dosing at 10–50 mg IM with an onset of 20–30 minutes is also available for hypertensive crises when intravenous access cannot be secured rapidly.
- Patients may experience flushing, headache, tachycardia, vomiting, or worsening angina.

ENALAPRIL

- Enalapril is the only angiotensin-converting enzyme (ACE) inhibitor available intravenously and may be especially beneficial in hypertensive patients with heart failure.
- Enalapril can be given at a range of 1.25–5 mg intravenously every 6 hours with onset by 15 minutes.
- Hypovolemic patients and those with renal artery stenosis or a high renin state must be monitored closely for dangerous decreases in blood pressure. Patients must be monitored closely due to the variable response of intravenous enalapril.

FENOLDOPAM

- Fenoldopam acts as a selective dopamine agonist at the DA_1 receptor. It can improve renal blood flow and natriuresis.
- Patients may experience flushing, headache, nausea, and tachycardia with fenoldopam administration.
- Fenoldopam should not be used for >48 hours.
- The dose of fenoldopam ranges from 0.1 to 0.3 μg/kg/min with an onset of action in <5 minutes.

PHENTOLAMINE

- This alpha-1 antagonist is first-line therapy for treatment of hypertension associated with pheochromocytoma.
- Flushing and tachycardia can be seen with phentolamine use.
- Its dose is 5–15 mg intravenously, with a quick onset in 1–2 minutes.

ESMOLOL

- Esmolol is indicated in aortic dissection. It is given at 500 μg/kg/min for 4 minutes then dosed at 150–300 μg/kg/min intravenously. Onset of action is between 1 and 2 minutes, and hypotension must be monitored for closely.

LABETALOL

- This adrenergic antagonist (alpha- and beta-blocker) can be used as an adjunct in treating preeclampsia and eclampsia. Labetalol is useful as an addition to nitroprusside when treating aortic dissection. It is also used when treating hypertension during periods of acute increased sympathetic activity such as MAOI interaction, pheochromocytoma, and cocaine use (although its use here is controversial due to the concern for myocardial ischemia).
- Selective beta-blockade only without alpha-receptor antagonism should be avoided in instances of increased sympathetic activity due to the subsequent rise in blood pressure from unopposed alpha-receptor stimulation absent of beta-receptor-induced vasodilation.
- Labetalol should only be used with caution in acute heart failure.
- A bolus of 20–80 mg should be given intravenously every 10 minutes followed by a 2 mg/min intravenous infusion.
- Onset of activity is typically 5–10 minutes, and patients may experience dizziness, orthostatic hypotension, scalp tingling, throat burning, and vomiting.

ORAL THERAPY

- Oral agents can be considered for asymptomatic patients who are cognitively alert and in no acute danger. Most short-acting medications can be considered, including captopril, felodipine, furosemide, and propranolol.
- Resuming a patient's prior oral regimen is reasonable if the elevated blood pressure is secondary to medication withdrawal and if the prior oral regimen offered adequate blood pressure control.
- Ischemia can result from an excessively rapid decrease in blood pressure. For this reason liquid and sublingual nifedipine preparations should be avoided.

BIBLIOGRAPHY

Kaplan NM. Management of hypertensive emergencies. *Lancet* 1994;344:1335–1338.

Kaplan NM. Systemic hypertension: mechanisms and diagnosis. In: Braunwald E, Zipes DP, Libby P, eds., *Heart Disease: A Textbook of Cardiovascular Medicine*, 6th ed. St. Louis, MO: W.B. Saunders; 2001:966–971,991–992.

Preston RA, Jy W, Jimenez JJ. Effects of severe hypertension on endothelial and platelet microparticles. *Hypertension* 2003;41: 211–217.

Sibai BM. Treatment of hypertension in pregnant women. *N Engl J Med* 1996;335:257–265.

Tuncel M, Ram VC. Hypertensive emergencies: etiology and management. *Am J Cardiovasc Drugs* 2003;3:21–31.

Section 3
RESPIRATORY DISORDERS

27 PATHOPHYSIOLOGY OF ACUTE RESPIRATORY FAILURE

Nina M. Patel

KEY POINTS

- Acute respiratory failure results from an abnormality in gas exchange that is associated with an inability to maintain adequate oxygenation and/or ventilation, resulting in hypoxia and at times, hypercapnia.
- The four major classes of ARF are:
  1. Type I: shunt
  2. Type II: hypoventilatory
  3. Type III: perioperative/atelectasis
  4. Type IV: shock/hypoperfusion

OXYGEN TRANSPORT

- The movement and uptake of oxygen from lung to tissues can be described by four major variables:
  1. Arterial O_2 content (CaO_2)
  2. Oxygen delivery (DO_2)
  3. Oxygen consumption (VO_2)
  4. Oxygen extraction ratio (O_2ER)
- There are four major derangements which lead to arterial hypoxemia:
  1. Shunt, which is generally alveolar
  2. Alveolar hypoventilation
  3. Ventilation/perfusion (V/Q) mismatch
  4. Decreased mixed venous PO_2, which becomes relevant when there is shunt or V/Q mismatch

ARTERIAL OXYGEN CONTENT (CaO_2)

- $CaO_2 = 1.39$ mL O_2/g Hgb × [Hgb] × SaO_2 + 0.003 mL/ O_2/mmHg × (PaO_2).
- This equation highlights a number of important aspects of oxygen transport. First, hemoglobin (Hgb) is a principal determinant of oxygen-carrying capacity of blood. Second, due to the poor solubility of oxygen in blood, PaO_2 has a significantly more limited capacity than Hgb to impact arterial O_2 content.
- These principles are demonstrated graphically by the Hgb-oxygen dissociation curve (see Fig. 27-1). As PO_2 values rise to ≥60 mmHg, the Hgb saturation curve reaches a plateau. After this point, further increases in PaO_2 minimally impact CaO_2 because Hgb is already fully saturated.

OXYGEN DELIVERY (DO_2)

- DO_2 (mL O_2/min) = cardiac output (Q, L/min) × CaO_2 (mL/O_2/dL).
- O_2 delivery depends on both cardiac output and arterial O_2 content.
- Normal values for DO_2: 520–570/mL/min/m.

OXYGEN CONSUMPTION (VO_2)

- VO_2 (mL O_2/min) = Q (L/min) × 10 (dL/L) × 1.39 mL O_2/g Hgb × Hgb (g/dL) × (SaO_2 − SvO_2) (expressed as fractions, not %).
- VO_2 reflects peripheral oxygen uptake. This value is relatively constant under normal conditions. Conversely, in situations of increased metabolic demand (e.g., fever, seizures), VO_2 rises.

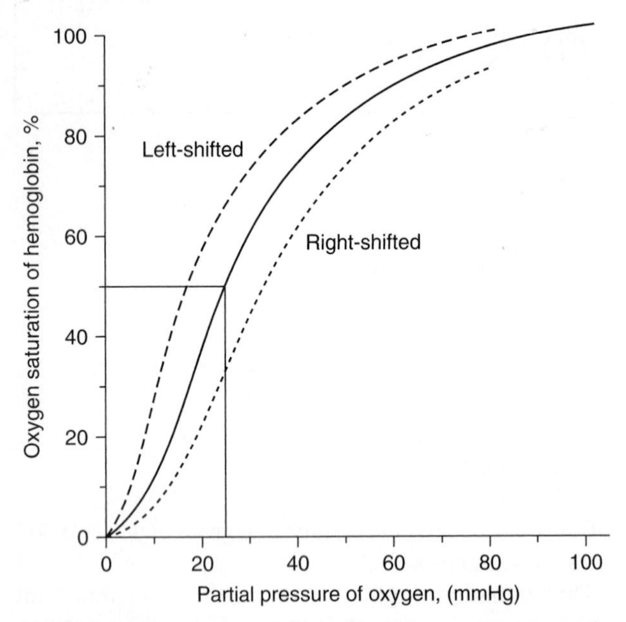

FIG. 27-1 Hgb-oxygen dissociation curve. Depicted here is the oxyhemoglobin dissociation curve for normal adult hemoglobin (hemoglobin A, solid line). Note that hemoglobin is 50% saturated with oxygen at a partial pressure of 27 mmHg (i.e., P50 is 27 mmHg) and is 100% saturated at a PO_2 of approximately of 100 mmHg. Depicted here are curves that are "left-shifted" (dotted line, representing increased oxygen affinity) and "right-shifted" (dotted line, decreased oxygen affinity). The effect of right- or left-shifting of the curve is most pronounced at low oxygen partial pressures. In the examples shown, the right-shifted curve means that hemoglobin can deliver approximately 70% of its attached oxygen at a PO_2 of 27 mmHg. In contrast, the left-shifted hemoglobin can deliver only about 35% of its attached oxygen at this PO_2. A high proportion of fetal hemoglobin, which has high oxygen affinity, shifts this curve to the left in newborns.

OXYGEN EXTRACTION RATIO (O_2ER)

- $O_2ER = VO_2/DO_2$.
- Under basal conditions, $O_2ER = 0.20–0.25$, signifying that 20–25% of delivered O_2 is being consumed by peripheral tissues. O_2ER can increase to as high as 0.5–0.6 to either (a) meet oxygen requirements in face of increased peripheral oxygen consumption (e.g., exercise) or (b) compensate for decreased oxygen delivery (e.g., low output heart failure).
  - A point of "critical oxygen delivery" arises when peripheral tissues can no longer increase oxygen extraction sufficiently to maintain VO_2. When DO_2 falls below the critical value, anaerobic metabolism ensues as peripheral tissues attempt to meet energy requirements.
- Endotracheal intubation or noninvasive ventilation (NIV) should be considered early in all patients with acute respiratory failure (ARF). Normally, VO_2 related to work of breathing is low. In ARF, however, VO_2 can increase substantially. Endotracheal intubation serves to concurrently decrease VO_2 related to work of breathing and continuously deliver supplemental oxygen at an increased FiO_2.
- Optimization of CaO_2 and DO_2 with supplemental O_2, augmentation of cardiac output (e.g., use of inotropic agents or crystalloid infusion), or packed red blood cell transfusion are essential components in the management of ARF.

MECHANISMS OF HYPERCAPNIA

- The major etiologies of hypercapnia are:
  1. Increased metabolic CO_2 production
  2. Decreased minute ventilation (V_E)
  3. Increased dead space ventilation (V_d)
- Arterial PCO_2 is described by the equation:
  - $PCO_2 = k \times VCO_2/\{V_E \times [1 - (V_d/V_t)]\}$, (where k is a constant, VCO_2 is metabolic CO_2 production in mL/min, V_E is total minute ventilation in L/min, V_d is dead space volume, and V_t is tidal volume).
- In the ICU setting, increased metabolic CO_2 production is multifactorial, and can result from increased metabolic rate or overfeeding.
- Decreased V_E arises from the following situations:
  1. Increased respiratory load
  2. Decreased central nervous system (CNS) drive
  3. Insufficient respiratory muscle strength/inadequate neuromuscular (NMS) coupling
- Respiratory load = Pr + Pel; [(Pr = inspiratory flow × resistance), (Pel = volume × elastance)].
- The respiratory load of spontaneous breathing is roughly 10 cmH_2O. An average individual is capable of generating a maximum negative inspiratory force well above this load, at 100 cmH_2O. In the setting of airways obstruction (increased Pr) or increased lung, chest wall, or abdominal wall elastance (increased Pel), however, respiratory load increases significantly. The respiratory system may not have sufficient respiratory muscle strength or reserve to overcome the increased mechanical load, hence leading to insufficient ventilation and consequently increased PCO_2.
- Decreased CNS drive to breathe in the ICU can develop secondary to medications (e.g., narcotics and sedatives), toxins, and CNS injury or CNS metabolic impairment (e.g., hypothyroidism).
- Respiratory muscle weakness/NMS uncoupling in the ICU can occur due to primary disease (e.g., amyotrophic lateral sclerosis [ALS] and Guillain-Barré) or secondary disease (e.g., severe hypophosphatemia and drug-induced myopathy).

- Dead space ventilation (V_d) refers to the portion of lung that are ventilated, but not perfused. Increased V_d can occur in a number of settings including emphysema and pulmonary embolus.

TYPES OF RESPIRATORY FAILURE

TYPE I: ACUTE HYPOXEMIC RESPIRATORY FAILURE (AHRF)

- Severe hypoxemia, decreased PCO_2 (a secondary response, not always present when respiratory failure is severe), and intrapulmonary shunting characterize acute hypoxemic respiratory failure (AHRF).
- AHRF results from airspace flooding (e.g., edema fluid, blood, and pus) with preserved perfusion but severely compromised ventilation. Since no gas exchange occurs, the PO_2 and PCO_2 of pulmonary arterial blood supplying areas of shunt are equal to the PO_2 and PCO_2 of pulmonary venous blood draining these regions. This is termed an intrapulmonary *shunt* lesion because blood flow bypasses normal gas exchange at the alveolar-capillary interface.
- Due to the absence of gas exchange in flooded alveolar units, increasing inspired O_2 has little impact on the level of hypoxemia in type I ARF.
- Positive end-expiratory pressure (PEEP) recruits flooded alveoli for gas exchange, and is frequently utilized in the setting of type I ARF to improve oxygenation.

TYPE II: ALVEOLAR HYPOVENTILATION

- Type II or hypoventilatory ARF presents with severe hypercarbia resulting from decreased CO_2 clearance. In contrast to type I ARF, isolated hypoventilatory ARF is not accompanied by severe, oxygen-refractory hypoxemia. Rather, hypoxemia typically corrects with modest supplemental oxygen therapy (or with improved ventilation).
- Etiologies of type II ARF are: (1) increased V_d, (2) increased respiratory load, (3) NMS insufficiency/respiratory muscle weakness, (4) decreased CNS drive, and (5) increased metabolic production of CO_2.
- Evaluation includes: measurement of peak and pause pressures on the mechanical ventilator during constant flow, volume-preset ventilation, to evaluate for airways obstruction or increased lung elastance; excluding obvious metabolic derangements (e.g., electrolyte abnormalities and hypothyroidism); examination of caloric intake and requirements; assessment of mental status in nonintubated patients; evaluation of medications administered (for toxicity); and vigilance in searching for additional sources of hypoventilation when obvious etiologies have been excluded, such as unrecognized sleep disordered breathing.
- Supplemental oxygen therapy and treatment of the primary etiology of alveolar hypoventilation dictate therapeutic management of type II ARF.

TYPE III: PERIOPERATIVE ACUTE RESPIRATORY FAILURE

- Postoperative atelectasis, due to supine positioning, splinting due to incisional pain and inadequate analgesia, impaired cough and overhydration (on some occasions), and tobacco use within 6 weeks of surgery, is the primary etiology of type III ARF.
- The aforementioned factors work synergistically to decrease functional residual capacity (FRC) below increased closing volumes. The result is collapse of dependent alveolar units.
- Surgery is not required to precipitate "perioperative" respiratory failure, which can also be seen in medical patients with severe obesity or ascites.
- Early institution of upright positioning, adequate analgesia, chest physiotherapy and PEEP in intubated patients (or mask continuous positive airway pressure [CPAP] in those not intubated), and avoidance of overhydration minimize the risk of developing significant postoperative atelectasis.
- If type III ARF does develop, the above factors should be enacted immediately and, on some occasions bronchoscopy can be attempted to clear endobronchial secretions.

TYPE IV: HYPOPERFUSION/SHOCK

- Type IV ARF is associated with severe hypoperfusion and an inability for Q (cardiac output) to meet the metabolic demands of the respiratory muscles.
- Endotracheal intubation is indicated in type IV ARF to minimize work of breathing and redirect Q from the lungs to other organ systems. Patients can be extubated on stabilization of shock/hypoperfusion, as long as some additional cause for respiratory failure has not developed.

CONCLUSIONS

- Acute respiratory failure in the ICU is often multifactorial. Identifying the primary cause(s) of ARF is critical to appropriate management of these patients.
- Assuring adequate oxygen transport and minimizing work of breathing are essential components in the treatment of patients with ARF.

- Expediency in liberation from mechanical ventilation should be instituted once the type of ARF has been identified and treated.

BIBLIOGRAPHY

Wood LDH. The pathophysiology of acute respiratory failure. In: Hall JB, Schmidt GA, Wood LH, eds., *Principles of Critical Care*, 2nd ed. New York, NY: McGraw-Hill; 1992/1998: 499–508.

Marino PL. Hypoxemia and hypercapnea. In: *The ICU Book*, 2nd ed. Baltimore, MD: Williams & Wilkins; 1990/1998: 339–354.

Waldman M. Overview of respiratory failure. In: Hall JB, Schmidt GA, Wood LH, eds., *Principles of Critical Care: Companion Handbook*, 2nd ed. New York, NY: McGraw-Hill; 1993/1999: 113–123.

West JB. Gas transport to the periphery. In: *Respiratory Physiology: The Essentials*, 5th ed. Baltimore, MD: Williams & Wilkins; 1995: 71–88.

28 NONINVASIVE POSITIVE PRESSURE VENTILATION

Nathan Sandbo

KEY POINTS

- During noninvasive ventilation, a nasal mask, oronasal mask, full facial mask, nasal pillows, or helmet is used to couple the ventilator to the patient.
- Many patients can be ventilated effectively with noninvasive means, especially those with exacerbations of COPD.
- In appropriately selected patients, noninvasive ventilation reduces the need for intubation, lowers the incidence of complications, shortens ICU stay, and improves survival.
- Improvement is generally evident within 1 hour in patients who will respond to noninvasive ventilation.

EPIDEMIOLOGY

- Noninvasive positive pressure ventilation (NIPPV) provides a less invasive alternative to endotracheal intubation (ETI) for the treatment of respiratory failure. Due to the less invasive nature of this intervention, complications normally associated with ETI can be minimized, while preserving the benefits of positive pressure ventilation.
- Use of NIPPV has dramatically increased over the past 15 years, as well as the indications for its use. Benefits in selected patients include a decrease in the need for ETI, shorter length of stay, decreased rates of complications (such as nosocomial pneumonia), and lower mortality rates.

TECHNICAL CONSIDERATIONS

- Positive pressure is delivered via a fitted mask in NIPPV, rather than an endotracheal tube. Adequate seal is required at the interface of the face and the mask to appropriately deliver positive pressure to the alveolar space. An oronasal mask is the primary interface used, and is superior to nasal mask or cushions in achieving adequate patient tolerance in the setting of acute respiratory failure.
- Both traditional ventilators and newer turbine ventilators specifically designed for NIPPV can be used. Ventilators specifically designed for NIPPV are used for reliable triggering despite air leaks, and are currently the preferred delivery system.
- A primary key to success is appropriate patient selection and achieving patient tolerance. An awake, spontaneously breathing patient who can protect the airway is the best candidate, although chronic obstructive pulmonary disease (COPD) patients obtunded due to ventilatory failure also often respond. Patient discomfort from claustrophobia, a tight fitting mask, and the sensation of positive pressure breathing are all common challenges which require experienced personnel to address and correct.
- The most common ventilator setting is characterized by the selection of both an inspiratory pressure level (IPAP) and an expiratory pressure level (EPAP). This correlates with a pressure support ventilator mode with a set level of positive end-expiratory pressure (PEEP). The two most studied strategies are continuous positive airway pressure (CPAP, where IPAP = EPAP), and bilevel positive airway pressure (BiPAP, where IPAP > EPAP).

INDICATIONS

- Acute-on-chronic respiratory failure:
  - COPD
    - Sine qua non is ventilatory failure characterized by rapid, shallow breathing. Patients experience increased work of breathing and respiratory

muscle fatigue due to disadvantageous respiratory system mechanics.
  - NIPPV can decrease work of breathing and improve respiratory mechanics. This is evidenced by improvement in tidal volumes, decreased respiratory rate, improved serum pH, and lowered PCO_2 within the first hour.
  - Clinical evidence for use includes several prospective randomized trials showing decreased need for ETI (from 67 to 9% in one study), shortened length of stay, lower rate of complications, and improved survival in patients with COPD. Most studies used BiPAP settings.
- Uncomplicated hypoxemic respiratory failure:
  - Both CPAP and BiPAP have been used successfully to treat respiratory failure due to cardiogenic pulmonary edema. Data suggest that rates of ETI, physiologic parameters, and 48 hours survival are all improved, but hospital survival was not changed. The subgroup which has shown the most benefit is patients with congestive heart failure (CHF) and coexistent hypercapnia.
  - In carefully selected patients, BiPAP, but not CPAP, is of benefit for other causes of hypoxemic respiratory failure. Uncomplicated respiratory failure without hemodynamic instability is an appropriate use of NIPPV and confers a benefit with regard to rates of ETI, duration of ventilation, ICU stay, and complication rate.
- Exclusions:
  - Severe or complicated hypoxemic respiratory failure, shock, need for airway protection, respiratory arrest, or coexistent organ failure.
- There is conflicting evidence regarding the role of NIPPV for postextubation respiratory distress.
- Evolving indications include respiratory failure due to asthma exacerbations, patients undergoing fiberoptic bronchoscopy with marginal oxygenation, and persistent weaning failure from invasive ETI.

RESPONSE

- Evaluation of clinical response to the initiation of NIPPV is critical to the successful implementation of this therapy. The presence of trained personnel familiar with the successful strategies in initiating NIPPV facilitates patient tolerance.
- Clinical response should be assessed in a timely fashion. Improvement in symptoms and physiologic parameters (respiratory rate, tidal volume, gas exchange) is usually apparent within 1 hour, with patients failing to demonstrate improvement unlikely to benefit from a longer trial.

BIBLIOGRAPHY

Brochard L. Noninvasive ventilation. In: Hall JB, Schmidt GA, Wood LDH, eds., *Principles of Critical Care*, 3rd ed. New York, NY: McGraw-Hill; 2005: 445–454.

Lightowler JV, Wedzicha JA, Elliott MW, et al. Non-invasive positive pressure ventilation to treat respiratory failure resulting from exacerbations of chronic obstructive pulmonary disease: Cochrane systematic review and meta-analysis. *BMJ* 2003;326:185–190.

Kramer N, Meyer TJ, Meharg J, et al. Randomized, prospective trial of noninvasive positive pressure ventilation in acute respiratory failure. *Am J Respir Crit Care Med* 1995;151: 1799–1806.

Evans TW. International Consensus Conferences in Intensive Care Medicine: non-invasive positive pressure ventilation in acute respiratory failure. Organised jointly by the American Thoracic Society, the European Respiratory Society, the European Society of Intensive Care Medicine, and the Societe de Reanimation de Langue Francaise, and approved by the ATS Board of Directors, December 2000. *Intensive Care Med* 2001;27:166–178.

Keenan SP, Powers C, McCormack DG, et al. Noninvasive positive-pressure ventilation for postextubation respiratory distress: a randomized controlled trial. *JAMA* 2002;287: 3238–3244.

Esteban A, Frutos-Vivar F, Ferguson ND, et al. Noninvasive positive-pressure ventilation for respiratory failure after extubation. *N Engl J Med* 2004;350:2452–2460.

Nava S, Ambrosino N, Clini E, et al. Noninvasive mechanical ventilation in the weaning of patients with respiratory failure due to chronic obstructive pulmonary disease. A randomized, controlled trial. *Ann Intern Med* 1998;128:721–728.

Ferrer M, Esquinas A, Arancibia F, et al. Noninvasive ventilation during persistent weaning failure: a randomized controlled trial. *Am J Respir Crit Care Med* 2003;168: 70–76.

29 COMMON MODES OF MECHANICAL VENTILATION

William Schweickert

KEY POINTS

- Consider NIV in appropriate patients before intubating.
- Ventilator modes are divided into those in which pressure is set by the clinician (pressure-preset modes) and those in which tidal volume is set (volume-preset modes).

- Advantages for pressure-preset modes are that variable and responsive inspiratory flow rates may be more comfortable for some patients.
- Advantages for volume-preset modes are that a lung-protective strategy using volume assist-control has been demonstrated in patients with acute lung injury and ARDS, and that respiratory system mechanics can be most easily measured and followed.

INTRODUCTION

- Advances in technology and critical care research have created a wide range of approaches to supporting the patient in respiratory failure. The most basic question to be asked prior to any intubation should be the following—Can the patient be supported with NIV?

NONINVASIVE VENTILATION (NIV)

- The role of noninvasive positive pressure ventilation (NIPPV) is rapidly increasing in clinical practice, and should be considered as an option before intubation and ventilation.
- Clinical scenarios that clearly warrant consideration of such include patients with respiratory failure in the absence of hemodynamic and neurologic compromise, or more specifically, acute exacerbations of chronic obstructive pulmonary disease, acute cardiogenic pulmonary edema, and postoperative ventilatory failure.

CONVENTIONAL MODES OF MECHANICAL VENTILATION

- Once intubation and mechanical ventilation are an established necessity, the next clinical question is: Does the clinical scenario and physician experience dictate a choice of volume-preset or pressure-preset mode of mechanical ventilation? Categorizing mechanical ventilation based on these headings can assist in defining the four most common ("conventional") modes of mechanical ventilation used in clinical practice. Either approach can provide full ventilatory support or allow for substantial patient exercise.
- All of the modes rely on a clinician-determined inspired fraction of oxygen (FiO_2) and positive end-expiratory pressure (PEEP), used primarily to modulate oxygenation. These variables are discussed in detail at the end of the chapter.

VOLUME-PRESET MODES

ASSIST-CONTROL (A/C) OR CONTROLLED MANDATORY VENTILATION (CMV)

- The clinician sets the tidal volume (Vt), minimum respiratory rate (f), and inspiratory flow rate ($\dot{V}$).
- The ventilator delivers the set tidal volume *every* time a breath is triggered by the patient. The inspiratory time (Ti), expiratory time (Te), and their ratio (I:E) are dictated by the Vt and $\dot{V}$.
- Passive patient: If the patient's spontaneous rate is less than the ventilator's set rate or if the patient is paralyzed, the ventilator delivers tidal volumes at the set rate.
- Active patient: Increases in the patient's spontaneous respiratory rate increase the minute ventilation delivered by the ventilator (i.e., the full tidal volume set is delivered for every breath).

COMMON CLINICAL USE

- This mode is frequently applied in patients with acute respiratory distress syndrome (ARDS), given evidence that ventilation with low tidal volumes ($\leq$ 6 cc/kg ideal body weight) improves overall mortality. In general, it is commonly used when the goal of care is to minimize the work of breathing.

ADVANTAGES

- Permits the measurement of respiratory mechanics.
- Ensures adherence to low tidal volume ventilation, even in the presence of changes in compliance of the respiratory system.

DISADVANTAGES

- Significant elevations in ventilator pressures may ensue in the setting of decreased respiratory compliance or increased airways resistance.
- In the presence of high inspiratory effort, the patient may trigger a second, superimposed breath, precluding rigid control of the tidal volume delivered.
- Obstructed patients can increase minute ventilation to jeopardize exhalation time and risk-resultant PEEPi (intrinsic PEEP).

SYNCHRONIZED INTERMITTENT MANDATORY VENTILATION (SIMV)

- The clinician sets Vt, f, and $\dot{V}$.
- The ventilator delivers exactly that number (f) of tidal volumes every minute, synchronizing those mandatory breaths with the patients' triggering efforts.
- Passive patient: identical to A/C ventilation.

- Active patient: Spontaneous efforts between ventilator-delivered breaths are unassisted. The resultant (additional) breath's Vt, $\dot{V}$, and inspiratory and expiratory duration are determined by patient effort and respiratory system mechanics. Often they are quite variable, frequently short duration and small in volume.

Common Clinical Use

- Often used to permit gradual increases in patient work of breathing via lowering of the mandatory f and/or Vt. However, this modality of weaning has been demonstrated to prolong ventilator dependence.
- Often used to limit minute ventilation in deeply sedated patients with severe airflow obstruction and dynamic hyperinflation.
- Patients without lung disease requiring intubation, in whom a concern for central drive cessation is possible.

Advantages

- Respiratory mechanics can be measured on mandated, ventilator-assisted breaths (only).

Disadvantages

- Studies document inferiority as a weaning mode.

PRESSURE-PRESET MODES

PRESSURE CONTROL VENTILATION (PCV)

- The clinician sets the inspiratory pressure (Pinsp), PEEP, f, and I:E ratio or Ti.
- The ventilator then delivers whatever flow rate and volume are required to maintain the Pinsp for the set Ti.
- Passive patient: Vt depends on a complex interplay of respiratory mechanics, pressure, Ti, and dynamic hyperinflation.
- Active patient: May demonstrate distress, unless adequately sedated. Otherwise, respiratory effort can change Vt (in either direction, depending on magnitude and timing of effort).

Common Clinical Use

- In ARDS patients, Palv should not exceed 30 cmH_2O in an attempt to avoid overdistention. The clinician can rigidly adhere to that limit by setting Pinsp to a value equaling ideal Pplat (usually ≤30); however, this approach has not been demonstrated to protect the lung adequately from ventilator-induced injury.
- Permits the utilization of salvage therapies for ARDS, such as inverse ratio ventilation (IRV), in which Ti exceeds Te.

Advantages

- May be the most comfortable mode for the patient with high drive, since the flow rate and profile are not limited.

Disadvantages

- Increased airway resistance or decreased compliance can result in marked hypoventilation (as resultant volume per pressure supplied falls).
- Most physicians and respiratory therapists are not familiar with this mode of ventilation. This becomes a clinical setting where errors may increase.

PRESSURE SUPPORT VENTILATION (PSV)

- The clinician sets ONLY Pinsp and PEEP.
- The ventilator then delivers Pinsp whenever the patient triggers a breath, at whatever flow is necessary to maintain Pinsp. Inspiration is terminated when the inspiratory flow rate falls to a threshold or fraction of initial flow (either via cessation of patient effort or increasing elastic recoil of the respiratory system as Vt increases).
- Passive patient: PSV requires a central ventilatory drive and neuromuscular coupling so this mode is not applicable in fully passive patients.
- Active patient: The minute ventilation is determined by the Pinsp and respiratory mechanics combined with the patient's respiratory rate and effort.

Common Clinical Use

- Utilized for titration of patient effort during liberation from mechanical ventilation.
- Patients with unimpaired respiratory drive and stable compliance of the respiratory system. Example: patients intubated for angioedema alone.
- Deeply sedated patients with severely obstructive airways (this requires vigilant monitoring for apnea).

Advantages

- Improved patient comfort (compared with volume-preset modes) and subsequent ventilator synchrony.

Disadvantages

- Lack of a backup respiratory rate (f) in the event of apnea.
- Potential decreases in minute ventilation in the event of changes in respiratory system compliance or resistance.
- Similar to A/C, high respiratory rates can lead to the development of PEEPi.
- No direct measurement of respiratory system mechanics.

CONTINUOUS POSITIVE AIRWAY PRESSURE (CPAP)

- Not a unique mode of mechanical ventilation since the ventilator pressure is constant (i.e., there is no inspiratory assistance).
- This is used for spontaneous breathing trials, in which the ventilatory support is minimized, while still permitting accurate evaluation of respiratory rate and tidal volume (see Chap. 33).

MIXED MODES OF VENTILATION

- Ventilators will often allow for the combination of the above modes, most commonly the usage of SIMV plus PSV.
- The clinician programs the SIMV as outlined above. In addition, a Pinsp is programmed into the ventilator.
- The ventilator delivers the exact number (f) of tidal volumes (Tv) every minute, synchronizing the mandatory breaths with the patient's triggering efforts. Spontaneous efforts between the ventilator-delivered breaths are then augmented with the Pinsp.
- The clinical utility of this mode is unclear, but has been applied in the following settings:
    - The addition of sighs (via the SIMV—volume-controlled breaths) to traditional PSV.
    - The patient in whom central respiratory drive is not guaranteed (e.g., central nervous system [CNS] injury or deep sedation) and PSV is the desired mode. The SIMV contribution will guarantee a minimum minute ventilation.

MODULATING OXYGENATION

FRACTION OF INSPIRED OXYGEN (FiO_2)

- It is only in the intubated setting that one can truly achieve 100% tracheal oxygen concentration.
- One of the first goals is to reduce the FiO_2 to <0.6 to minimize further lung injury (levels higher than 0.6 are generally viewed as toxic).

POSITIVE END-EXPIRATORY PRESSURE

- Positive end-expiratory pressure is best viewed as a continuous supply of positive pressure into the respiratory circuit, used to recruit alveoli (expanding collapsed units and translocating fluid from flooded units into the interstitial space) and to prevent alveolar derecruitment at end-expiration. These mechanisms serve to diminish intrapulmonary shunt and facilitate a decrease in FiO_2.
- An additional role of PEEP is to assist in the management of patients with obstructive lung disease, in whom PEEP can lower the inspiratory threshold load associated with PEEPi.
- Administration of PEEP may result in hypotension secondary to a rise in pleural (and therefore, right atrial) pressure and to increased resistance to venous return. Significant hypotension can be treated by reducing the PEEP temporarily and then infusing fluids or vasoactive drugs to restore cardiac output.

BIBLIOGRAPHY

Schmidt GA, Hall JB. Management of the ventilated patient. In: Hall JB, Schmidt GA, Wood LDH, eds., *Principles of Critical Care*, 3rd ed. New York, NY: McGraw-Hill; 2005:481–498.

30 MANAGING THE VENTILATED PATIENT

William Schweickert

KEY POINTS

- Choice of ventilator settings depends on what is wrong with the patient.
- PEEP should be set generally no lower than 5 cmH_2O and higher in patients who require it for oxygenation or who are obese and prone to alveolar collapse at low values.
- When the respiratory system is normal (no intrinsic lung or chest wall disease), nearly any mode is acceptable as long as the patient is comfortable.
- Patients with acute lung injury (ALI) or ARDS should be ventilated with volume assist-control with tidal volume set at 6 cc/kg ideal body weight. Patients at risk for ALI may also benefit from these "lung-protective" tidal volumes.
- Patients with severe airflow obstruction should be ventilated with modest minute ventilation (generally <8 L/min) to reduce the risk of dangerous dynamic hyperinflation. PEEP assists the patient with triggering.
- Patients with restrictive lung or chest wall disease should be ventilated with small tidal volume and rapid rates.

OVERVIEW

- Ventilator settings vary depending on the goals of ventilation (i.e., full rest vs. exercise), the etiology of respiratory failure, minute ventilation needs, and the comfort and familiarity of the physician with various modes.
- This chapter defines the five most commonly encountered types of patients with respiratory failure and supplies ventilatory strategies, including overall goals and specific ventilator modes and settings.

PATIENTS WITH NORMAL RESPIRATORY MECHANICS AND GAS EXCHANGE

- Patients with normal respiratory mechanics and gas exchange requiring mechanical ventilation are not uncommon. Examples of such situations include: (1) absence of central drive to breathe (narcotic overdose); (2) neuromuscular weakness (amyotrophic lateral sclerosis [ALS]); (3) upper airway obstruction (angioedema); and (4) hyperventilation therapy (elevated intracranial pressure).
- Initial volume-preset ventilator settings include an FiO_2 of 0.5–1.0, tidal volumes of 8–12 cc/kg, respiratory rate of 8–12 breaths/min, and an inspiratory flow rate of 60 L/min.
- Initial pressure-preset ventilator settings—if the patient has an intact central respiratory drive and is not excessively weak—include pressure support of roughly 10 cmH_2O above positive end-expiratory pressure (PEEP), which commonly generates tidal volumes of 1 L and spontaneous respiratory rates around 10 breaths/min.
- Regardless of the choice of mode, the administration of small amounts of PEEP (5 cmH_2O) is often necessary to prevent atelectasis.

PATIENTS WITH ACUTE HYPOXEMIC RESPIRATORY FAILURE

- Acute hypoxemic respiratory failure (AHRF) or type I respiratory failure is the result of alveolar filling (with blood, pus, or edema) or alveolar collapse. The resultant intrapulmonary shunt is characterized by hypoxemia that is minimally responsive to oxygen therapy.
- AHRF can be subdivided into diffuse and focal lung lesions. Diffuse lesions may be high-pressure (hydrostatic, cardiogenic) or low-pressure (acute respiratory distress syndrome [ARDS]) pulmonary edema. Focal lesions are often caused by lobar pneumonia or lung contusion.
- The goals of ventilation are to reduce intrapulmonary shunt, to avoid toxic concentrations of oxygen, and to select a ventilation strategy that does not propagate further lung injury.
- Initial therapy includes supplemental oxygen therapy in the highest concentration available—the initial FiO_2 should be 1.0 in view of the typically extreme hypoxemia (but this can be lowered promptly in most patients, guided by pulse oximetry).
- In *diffuse* lung lesions, the primary modality for reducing intrapulmonary shunt is the administration of PEEP, which recruits collapsed alveoli and translocates fluid from flooded units, and prevents derecruitment at end-expiration. PEEP may not be helpful in focal disease such as labor pneumonia.

EXAMPLE: LOW-PRESSURE EDEMA (ACUTE RESPIRATORY DISTRESS SYNDROME)

- Positive end-expiratory pressure should be instituted immediately, beginning with 10 cmH_2O then rapidly adjusted to either:
  - The least PEEP necessary to produce an arterial saturation of 88% on an FiO_2 no higher than 0.6 (the "least PEEP" approach).
  - A value of 2 cmH_2O higher than the lower inflection point of the inflation pressure-volume curve ("open-lung approach"). This more complex method has not been shown to be superior to the simpler "least PEEP" method.
- The tidal volume should be 4–6 cc/kg (ideal body weight) on volume assist-control as larger tidal volumes may overdistend the lung leading to ventilator-induced lung injury.
- Alternatively, pressure-controlled ventilation may be used, with an inspiratory pressure adjusted (and monitored) to drive tidal volumes of 6 cc/kg ideal body weight.
- In either mode, the respiratory rate should be set at 24–36 breaths/min as long as there is little intrinsic PEEP (PEEPi; see below).
- An occasional consequence of this ventilation strategy is hypercapnia, which is considered preferential to alveolar overdistention.

EXAMPLE: HIGH-PRESSURE EDEMA (CARDIOGENIC)

- Positive end-expiratory pressure should be titrated similarly to low-pressure edema (i.e., "least PEEP"). PEEP almost never depresses circulatory function in these patients since the pressure driving venous return to the heart is so high.
- Low tidal volume strategies have not been proven to reduce mortality in this setting, but it seems reasonable to use this approach for high-pressure pulmonary edema.

PATIENTS WITH SEVERE AIRFLOW OBSTRUCTION

- The primary goal of ventilation is to minimize alveolar overdistention and limit dynamic hyperinflation in an attempt to avoid barotrauma and impairment of cardiac output.
- The overall result of such ventilation strategy is diminution of the minute ventilation and subsequent elevation of $PaCO_2$ (levels > 40 mmHg).
- The hypercapnia, combined with preexisting anxiety or distress, prompt routine administration of (deep) sedation. Therapeutic paralysis should be reserved only for salvage therapy in extreme circumstances.
- An initial FiO_2 of 0.5 generally suffices, as the gas exchange limitations are generally limited to V/Q mismatch. If requirements are determined to be higher, re-evaluation for alveolar filling or collapse should be initiated.
- Ventilation should be initiated utilizing A/C mode. The tidal volume should be small (5–7 cc/kg), and the respiratory rate should be (relatively) lower (10–12 breaths/min).
- A peak flow of 60 L/min with a square inspiratory waveform is recommended. Higher flow rates do little to increase expiratory time, and lower flow rates or decelerating inspiratory waveforms can result in prolonging inspiration and limiting exhalation time. This can exacerbate auto-PEEP.
- Dynamic hyperinflation and auto-PEEP (PEEPi) occur when insufficient time has elapsed between inflation cycles to allow for complete expiration of tidal volume. It may occur in any situation in which there is a high demand for ventilation, but occurs most commonly in cases of airflow obstruction.
- In the event of PEEPi, the respiratory rate reduction is the most powerful means by which to increase exhalation time. This can usually be achieved with deep sedation with opioid medications.
- If the patient is triggering the ventilator, incremental PEEP should be added to reduce the work of triggering. PEEP levels should not exceed 85% of the PEEPi to avoid the risk of further hyperinflation.

PATIENTS WITH ACUTE-ON-CHRONIC RESPIRATORY FAILURE (ACRF)

- Most patients are intubated after days to weeks of progressive deterioration; as a result, most patients will appear exhausted and sleep with minimal sedation.
- The primary goals of ventilation include full respiratory muscle rest (usually for 36–72 hours).
- In stable health, these patients usually have a resting minute ventilation of 10 L/min or less with a resultant compensated respiratory acidosis. This should be recreated; more aggressive mechanical ventilation risks severe respiratory alkalosis and bicarbonate wasting by the kidney.
- Ventilation should be initiated utilizing A/C mode with lower tidal volumes (5–7 cc/kg) and moderate respiratory rates (20–24 breaths/min).
- Ventilation rules regarding oxygen supplementation and inspiratory flows and waveforms are similar to status asthmaticus.
- Patients still experiencing increased work of breathing or progressive hypotension should be evaluated for PEEPi, which may require administration of PEEP, akin to status asthmaticus.

PATIENTS WITH RESTRICTION OF THE LUNGS OR CHEST WALLS

- Restrictive diseases of the lungs (pulmonary fibrosis), chest wall (kyphoscoliosis), or abdomen (morbid obesity, tense ascites) can progress to overt respiratory failure, either individually or in conjunction with (even a small) ventilatory challenge.
- Goals of ventilation include small tidal volumes and rapid rates to minimize the hemodynamic consequences of positive pressure ventilation and to reduce the likelihood of barotrauma.
- Any reversible causes of restriction should be immediately addressed (e.g., paracentesis for ascites). Sitting the patient up can reduce abdominal pressure on the diaphragm, easing the work of breathing.
- Ventilatory approaches to achieve eucapnia may culminate in excessive intrathoracic pressures, which can compromise the circulation and subsequently evolve into hypoxemia. The clinician must recognize this scenario, as administration of further PEEP may augment the problem, not solve it.

BIBLIOGRAPHY

Schmidt GA, Hall JB. Management of the ventilated patient. In: Hall JB, Schmidt GA, Wood LDH, eds., *Principles of Critical Care*, 3rd ed. New York, NY: McGraw-Hill; 2005: 481–498.

31 RESPONDING TO CRISES IN THE VENTILATED PATIENT

William Schweickert

KEY POINTS

- Unplanned extubations occur commonly and may precipitate an urgent crisis.
- The distressed patient or alarming ventilator is best assessed at the bedside with attention to lung examination, tracheal position, ETT position, ability to pass a suction catheter through the ETT, and the shape of ventilator waveforms. A chest radiograph and arterial blood gas should generally be obtained unless the basis for the crisis is readily apparent.
- Endotracheal and tracheostomy tubes that appear to be in good position may not be.
- Hypotension may signal dynamic hyperinflation, sedative effect, tension pneumothorax, or one of the many causes applicable to critically ill patients.
- Pressure alarming (during volume-preset ventilation) is often caused by ETT obstruction, patient distress, or a change in the mechanical properties of the respiratory system (e.g., worse edema or obstruction).
- Low-pressure alarms often point to leaks, a failed ETT cuff, or ventilator disconnection.

OVERVIEW

- Ventilated patients are prone to a number of medical crises. The problem may be easy to discern (unplanned extubation); however, a ventilator alarm may be the only signal of the impending crisis.
- The physician's prompt recognition of the problem is necessitated, and this chapter should provide a systematic approach for responding to such warning signals.

THE OBVIOUS CRISIS: UNPLANNED EXTUBATION

- Unplanned extubation is common in the ICU, with reported frequency ranging from 3 to 12%. Endotracheal tube (ETT) or tracheostomy tube securement is paramount. Despite attention to this detail, the loss of artificial airway may occur in the agitated or delirious patient, or in association with patient manipulation (routine nursing care or during diagnostic studies).
- Evaluate the patient immediately, but don't just act. Stop and review the patient—do they truly need to be reintubated? Evaluate the work of breathing, oxygenation status, and the ability to protect the airway.
- Noninvasive ventilation may be a reasonable alternative if airway protection is not an issue. However, recognize its limitations—it should only be continued if a clear improvement is experienced within 1–2 hours of its initiation.
- Auscultation may reveal upper airway obstruction (stridor), which may be palliated with noninvasive ventilation or helium-oxygen mixtures (heliox).
- In the event of tracheostomy tube dislodgement, recognize the risk of the immature tract (<2 weeks old) which can be lost, and replacement of the trac tube may not be feasible or safe. When in doubt, reintubate through the nose or mouth.
- If airway protection is compromised, avoid a secondary aspiration injury by applying cricoid pressure until the reintubation is complete.

THE REMAINING CRISES: RESPONSE ALGORITHM

THE PRIMARY EVALUATION—GO TO THE BEDSIDE!

- Inspect vital signs, the patient, and ventilator waveforms.
  - Clues to patient distress may be as subtle as diaphoresis to the obvious wide-eyed patient with limbs akimbo.
  - The trachea should be midline with symmetrical rise of the chest. Listen for bilateral equal breath sounds (entertaining pneumothorax or collapse).
  - Abdominal paradox should be evaluated with a hand on the abdomen feeling for patient synchrony with inspiration or forced expiration.
  - The ETT should be properly secured at a proven-safe distance at the lip.

THE PRIMARY MANEUVER

- Whenever the quality of the artificial airway or ventilator function is in question, the patient should be removed from the ventilator and hand-bagged with 100% oxygen. The clinician should note the ease of bagging the patient and the resultant rise and fall of the chest.

HYPOXEMIA

- First, rescue the patient. Immediately apply increasing oxygen to return the saturation to ≥88% and begin the search for the cause of the deterioration.

- Review the possible mechanisms of hypoxemia: hypoventilation, ventilation/perfusion inequality, shunt, decrease in the mixed venous oxygenation, insufficient inspired oxygen, and diffusion block (rarely clinically present).
- Hypoventilation is usually obvious, signaled by concomitant hypercapnia.
- Ventilation/perfusion mismatch typically causes mild hypoxemia that is easily corrected with supplemental oxygen. Common culprits include airway secretions and mucous plugging, both remedied by aggressive suctioning. Bronchoconstriction, another common mediator, can be recognized by a high peak to plateau airway gradient during volume-preset ventilation.
- Shunt, recognized by its relative refractoriness to increased FiO_2, may be explained by progression of the primary cause of respiratory failure, or may implicate a new process. Atelectasis, ventilator-associated pneumonia, or pulmonary edema should be evident when combining the physical examination and chest x-ray. In general, diffuse lesions respond to positive end-expiratory pressure (PEEP), while focal lesions may require patient repositioning or maneuvers to maximize blood flow to the nondiseased lung.
- Mixed venous desaturation is detected by analyzing a venous blood sample, and invokes nonpulmonary causes of hypoxemia. Reductions in cardiac output (e.g., myocardial infarction) or hemoglobin concentration (e.g., gastrointestinal bleed) or increased systemic oxygen consumption (e.g., fever) may be culprits.

Hypotension (Soon After Initiation of Mechanical Ventilation)

- Shock is common in the ICU, and the clinician should have a focused approach to its diagnosis. However, abrupt hypotension following initiation of mechanical ventilation has several key etiologies which should be considered early.
- The introduction of positive intrathoracic pressure effectively reduces venous return. In addition, anesthetic induction agents and sedatives frequently cause venodilation. Both of these changes may uncover relative hypovolemia or right ventricular dysfunction. Both respond well to fluids; however, right heart dysfunction may require additive vasoactive drug administration. One approach is to infuse norepinephrine in the abruptly deteriorating patient (works to increase inotropy, venoconstrict, and improve coronary blood flow to the failing right heart), while dobutamine may be considered in the volume replete, relatively hypotensive patient.
- The physical examination provides clues to the two most common other causes: dynamic hyperinflation and tension pneumothorax.
- Dynamic hyperinflation usually responds to the primary maneuver—by disconnecting the patient from the ventilator, the lungs are able to decompress. Premorbid recognition of this condition is possible through evaluation of flow waveforms (inability to return to baseline) or through measurement of intrinsic PEEP. Its treatment necessitates changing ventilator settings to produce longer exhalation time or treatment of the underlying disease.
- Tension pneumothorax is usually signaled by unilateral decreased breath sounds, asymmetric rise of the chest, tracheal deviation, hypoxemia, hypotension, and increased pressure measurements on volume-preset ventilation. It requires immediate recognition and needle decompression, followed by tube thoracotomy.

VENTILATOR ALARM: "HIGH PRESSURE"

- This alarm signals the presence of obstruction of the ETT, airway, or reduced lung, chest wall, or abdominal compliance.
- Primary risks: (1) may signal worsening clinical status, and (2) may result in hypoventilation of the patient (ventilator potentially cycles prematurely to expiration as the upper pressure alarm is reached).
- First, perform the "primary maneuver"—manual bagging will remove the ventilator from the equation.
- Difficult bag ventilation should prompt passage of a suction catheter through the ETT. Inability to pass the catheter confirms artificial airway obstruction.
  - Proximal obstruction may be caused by the patient biting the ETT—evident on close physical examination—which can be remediated by bite block, sedative, or in extremes, a short-acting neuromuscular blocker.
  - In the absence of biting, the ETT may be kinked or occluded by desiccated secretions. Attempt repositioning the head; if there is no improvement, reintubation is necessitated.
- Difficult bag ventilation with an easily passed catheter should direct attention to patient effort. This should be apparent on examination (usually thoracoabdominal asynchrony), and should be treated with increasing sedative or adjustment to ventilator parameters.
  - Always review the possible reasons for the respiratory distress (e.g., pain, withdrawal, and progressive shock).
- Finally, if bagging remains difficult despite adequate sedation and relief of patient effort, the resistance may be caused by worsening compliance of the patient's respiratory system. Systematically evaluate for narrowing of the lower airway (bronchoconstriction), collapse or consolidation of the lung, pleural or chest

wall (pneumothorax) process, or abdominal (tense ascites) pathology.
- Combining the examination with chest x-ray should help to identify the cause. Additionally, placing the patient back on the ventilator and measuring peak and plateau pressures as well as auto-PEEP will further delineate the problem.
- Ventilator dysfunction—review appropriate settings (tidal volume, flow, inspiratory time, alarm limit), search for fluid pooling in circuit, or any other kinking.

VENTILATOR ALARM: "LOW INSPIRATORY PRESSURE/LOW EXHALED TIDAL VOLUME"

- Low-pressure alarms signal inspiratory effort by the patient, a leak, or ventilator malfunction.
- Effort, as described above, should be recognizable immediately by the examination.
- Large persistent leaks can occur within the ventilator, at any point of connection, including around the ETT, or through a bronchopleural fistula.
- Bag ventilation can isolate the problem to the ventilator and its tubing versus the ETT and the patient.
- If hand-bagging reveals minimal resistance, an ETT cuff leak is likely. This can be confirmed by listening over the neck or placing a hand over the mouth.
- Chest tube and pleural drainage systems should be interrogated for air leak, confirming bronchopleural fistula.

PROGRESSIVE RESPIRATORY ACIDOSIS

- An increasing $PaCO_2$ may be first recognized only as a result of increased patient agitation. The assessment of the arterial blood gas proves its presence. It can result from one of three processes: (1) decreased minute ventilation (clearance), (2) increased carbon dioxide production, or (3) increasing dead space.
- A fall in minute ventilation can be recognized by comparing rate and tidal volume values with those recorded by the therapist or saved in the ventilator's trend monitor.
- Increased carbon dioxide production may be mediated by such processes as fever, shivering, and agitation. Once recognized, each one has a distinct solution.
- Increasing dead space is the most challenging. Its presentation can be elusive, and may represent such diverse etiologies as pulmonary embolism, excessive PEEP, and hypovolemia. This recognition is vital, as instinctual increases in minute ventilation may exacerbate the underlying problem (e.g., auto-PEEP).

BIBLIOGRAPHY

Schmidt GA, Hall JB. Management of the ventilated patient. In: Hall JB, Schmidt GA, Wood LDH, eds., *Principles of Critical Care*, 3rd ed. New York, NY: McGraw-Hill; 2005: 481–498.

32 USING RESPIRATORY WAVEFORMS TO ADJUST VENTILATOR SETTINGS

Steve Mathai

KEY POINTS

- Waveform displays of flow convey rapidly important issues of ventilator mode and patient-ventilator interaction.
- From the pressures during volume-preset, constant flow ventilation, one can assess the respiratory mechanical properties.
- Patients must be passive in order to determine mechanical properties. It is essential to be able to recognize patient effort.

INTRODUCTION

- In the mechanically ventilated patient, bedside respiratory graphics ("waveforms") are a useful method for assessing ventilatory status and determining response to certain interventions.

BASIC WAVEFORMS

- Because patient effort can affect the waveforms, a passive patient is a prerequisite for determining accurate mechanical information.
- Effort can be recognized by transient drop in pressure before a breath (signaling triggering), scooping of the inspiratory pressure during constant flow, and variability in pressure waveforms.

PRESSURE-TIME WAVEFORMS

- Used for ventilator mode recognition, synchrony between patient and ventilator, assessment of adequacy of paralytic dose, among others (Fig. 32-1).

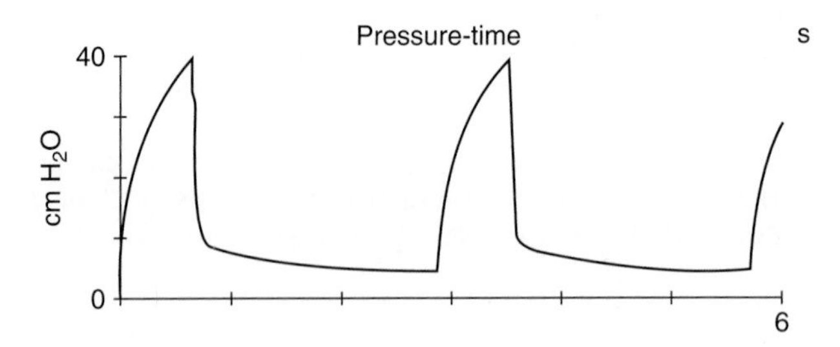

FIG. 32-1 Pressure waveform of volume breath. In the passive patient, the pressure rises smoothly and is convex upward.

- By setting a brief end-inspiratory pause (e.g., 0.4 seconds), the components of the airway opening pressure can be subdivided into resistive and elastic components (Fig. 32-2):
  - The resistive pressure is related to flow and resistance. This value is normally only 4–8 cmH2O when flow is roughly 1 L/min.
  - The elastic component is comprised of volume, compliance, and positive end-expiratory pressure (PEEP) or auto-PEEP. The elastic pressure is normally about 5 cmH2O when the tidal volume is 500 mL.
- These components can signal how the respiratory system is deranged, serve to direct therapy, and reveal changes related to treatment or time.
- Pressure on vertical axis, time on horizontal axis, positive pressure-upward deflection, negative pressure-downward deflection.

Ventilator Mode Recognition

- Volume-preset modes: assist-control (A/C), synchronized intermittent mandatory ventilation (SIMV):

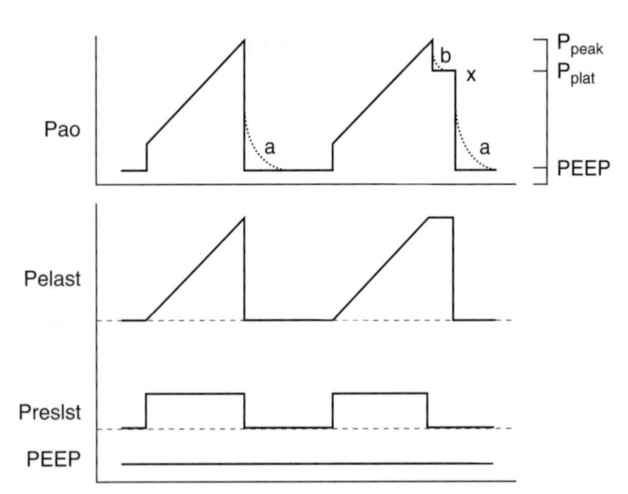

FIG. 32-2 Components of the pressure waveform. The top figure shows the pressure waveform, while the three tracings below reveal its components. The resistive pressure is found by noting the difference between peak airway pressure and the plateau pressure (at "x") during a brief end-inspiratory pause.

  - Volume is selected by clinician, pressure determined by respiratory system compliance and airway resistance.
  - A/C: volume, rate, inspiratory time, and sensitivity (pressure that must be overcome during patient initiated breath to trigger delivery of breath by ventilator; usually set at -2 cmH_2O) selected:
    - When patient initiates breath, ventilator delivers a breath of set volume to patient.
  - SIMV: volume, rate, inspiratory time, and sensitivity selected for mandatory breaths:
    - When patient initiates spontaneous breath between mandatory breaths, he or she receives only the self-generated volume (Fig. 32-3).
- Pressure-preset modes: pressure control (PC), pressure support ventilation (PSV):
  - Pressure is selected by clinician and is constant throughout inspiration.
  - PC: inspiratory pressure, rate, inspiratory time, and sensitivity selected by clinician:
    - When patient initiates breath, ventilator delivers set pressure; volume delivered varies.
  - PSV: inspiratory pressure and sensitivity selected by clinician:
    - Spontaneous breathing mode with constant pressure delivered during inspiration until flow rate decreases by some amount (Fig. 32-4).

Synchrony Between Patient and Ventilator

- Inspiration is normally shorter than expiration (normal ratio 1:2 or 1:3).
- During volume-preset modes, inspiratory time depends on inspiratory flow, set by clinician.
- When flow rate is too slow for the patient's demand, the inspiratory pressure waveform shows a "scooped" appearance (Fig. 32-5). This may be corrected by increasing the flow rate, raising the minute ventilation, or sedating the patient.
- When inspiratory flow rate is too fast, the patient may become uncomfortable and peak inspiratory pressures (PIP) rise.

Detection of Auto-PEEP

- Auto-PEEP: end-expiratory alveolar pressure exceeds pressure at the airway opening.
- Occurs secondary to insufficient expiratory time, high minute ventilation, and expiratory airflow limitation.
- If auto-PEEP is present, baseline pressure on waveform will rise to auto-PEEP level following an end-expiratory occlusion maneuver (Fig. 32-6).

Assessment of Adequacy of Paralytic Dose

- Monitoring of adequacy of paralysis by peripheral nerve stimulator may not be reliable in critically ill patients.

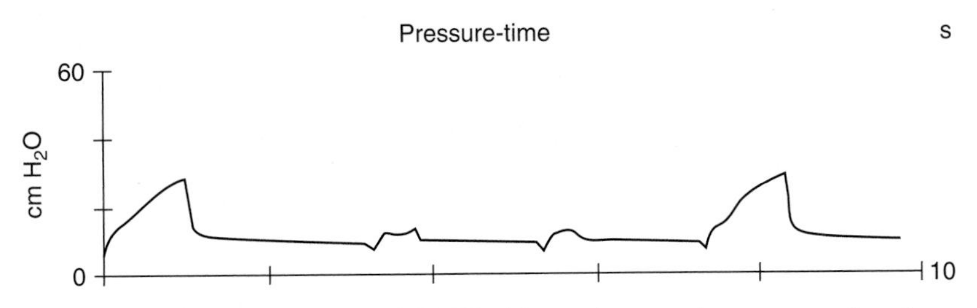

FIG. 32-3 Pressure waveform of SIMV with mandatory and spontaneous breaths.

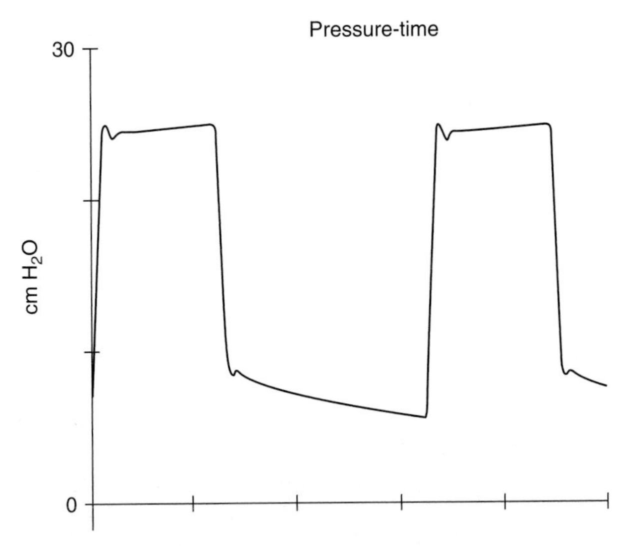

FIG. 32-4 Pressure waveform of pressure breath.

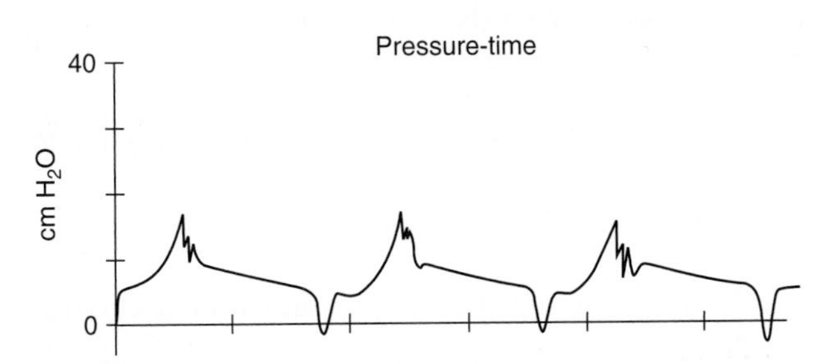

FIG. 32-5 Pressure waveform with inadequate flow and inspiratory scoop. Notice the signs of effort (drop in pressure before the breath, scooping of the pressure rise).

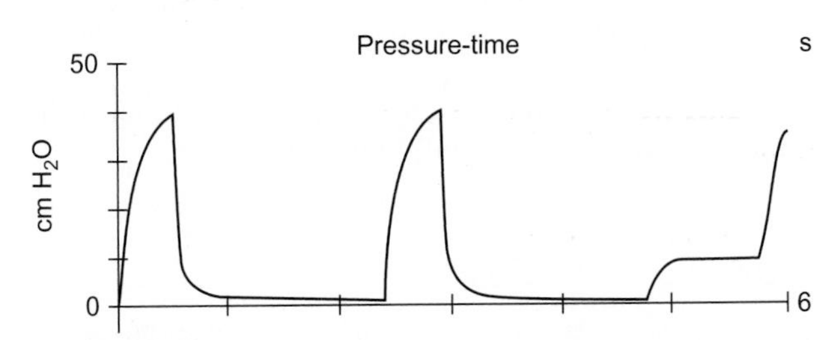

FIG. 32-6 Pressure waveform with auto-PEEP. Note the rise in pressure before the third breath, due to the end-expiratory pause maneuver.

- Detection of "breakthrough breathing" (trigger efforts, scooping of the inspiratory pressure) indicates incomplete paralysis.

FLOW-TIME WAVEFORMS

- Used to assess auto-PEEP and response to therapy.
- Flow on vertical axis, time on horizontal, inspiration-upward deflection, expiration-negative deflection.
- Different inspiratory waveforms for volume modes, pressure modes, and spontaneous breaths:
  - Volume modes: flow rate maintained throughout breath (square flow waveform; Fig. 32-7).
  - Pressure modes: flow at beginning of breath higher than end of breath (decelerating flow waveform; Fig. 32-7).
  - Spontaneous breathing: flow is variable and generally decreases throughout the breath.
  - Expiratory flow patterns are similar for all three.

DETECTION OF AUTO-PEEP

- Expiratory flow will not return to baseline (flow = 0) prior to inspiration if auto-PEEP present (Fig. 32-8).

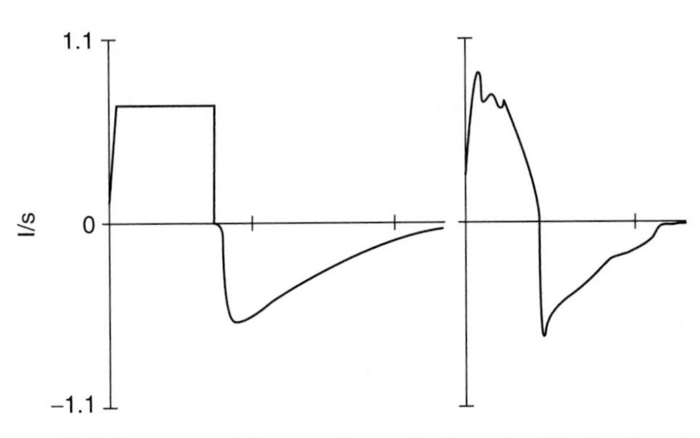

FIG. 32-7 Square flow waveform of volume breath, decelerating waveform of pressure breath, and sinusoidal waveform of spontaneous breath. Notice that volume-preset, constant-flow breaths (left panel) have a square profile, while pressure-preset breaths (right panel) typically show a decelerating flow profile.

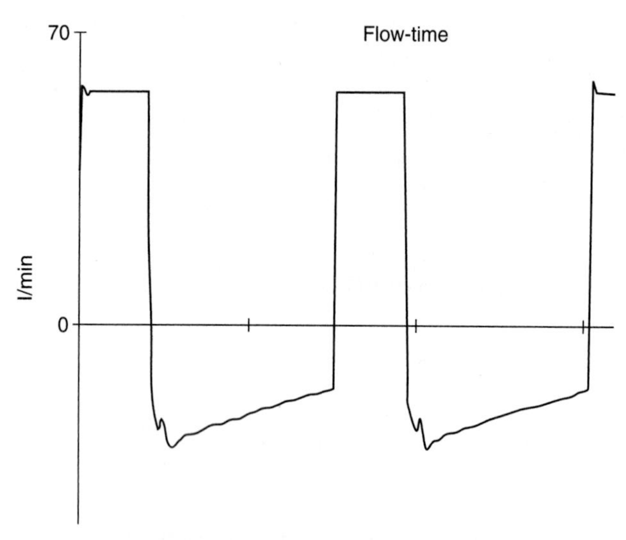

FIG. 32-8 Volume breaths with impaired expiratory flow secondary to auto-PEEP. Flow persists at end-expiration, revealing that the end-expiratory alveolar pressure is greater than the ventilator expiratory pressure (i.e., auto-PEEP is present).

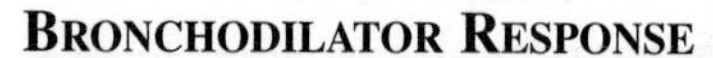

BRONCHODILATOR RESPONSE

- Expiratory flow is impeded in bronchospasm.
- If bronchodilator therapy is effective, expiratory flow may increase and return to baseline (flow = 0) more rapidly (Fig. 32-9), or the amount of auto-PEEP will fall.

PRESSURE-VOLUME LOOPS

- Used to assess changes in compliance and resistance.
- Orientation can vary, but most will have volume on vertical axis and pressure on horizontal axis.
- Varies based on type of breath:
  - Spontaneous breath: yields negative pressure as breath is initiated and continues as inspiration progresses along with an increase in volume; with expiration comes positive pressure and decrease in volume as expiration ends.
  - Mechanical ventilation breaths: yields positive pressure as breath is delivered by ventilator along with increase in volume; positive pressure diminishes during expiration.

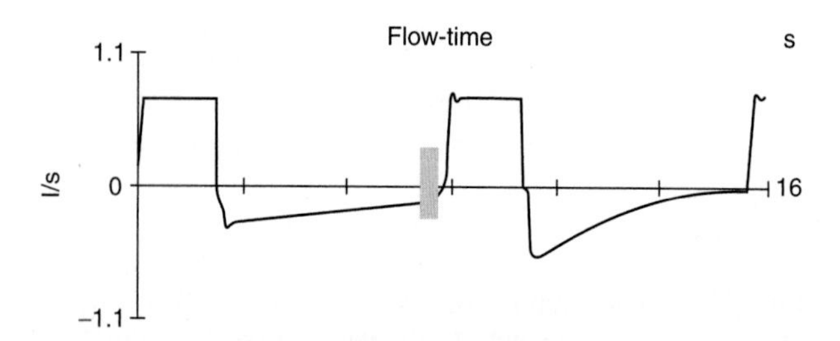

FIG. 32-9 Square flow waveform with expiratory waveform response to bronchodilator. Following successful bronchodilation, expiratory flow may increase, as shown.

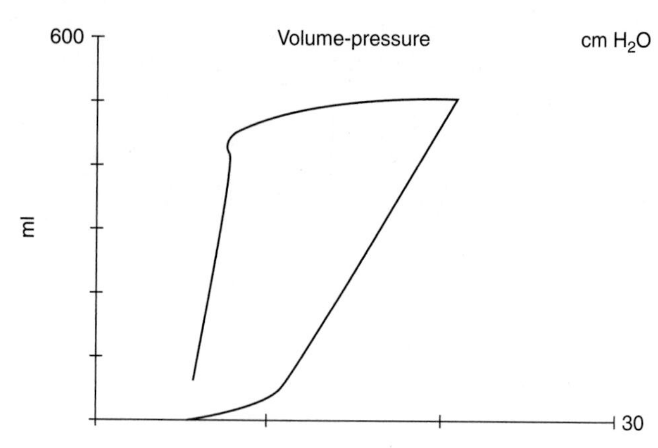

FIG. 32-10 Pressure-volume loop: mechanical breath.

  - Plotted counterclockwise (Fig. 32-10).
  - If patient initiates breath, there will be a negative pressure deflection that returns to positive deflection as breath is delivered by ventilator.

CHANGES IN COMPLIANCE

- Static compliance of the respiratory system can be expressed by the following equation:

$$\text{Static compliance} = \text{tidal volume}/(\text{plateau pressure} - \text{PEEP})$$

- Normal compliance: 80–100 mL/cmH_2O.
- Low compliance occurs with pulmonary edema, severe pneumonia, ARDS, tension pneumothorax, pulmonary fibrosis, kyphoscoliosis, and obesity.
- As compliance decreases, the pressure required to distend the lung increases.
  - Results in shift in slope of pressure-volume curve to the right.
- As compliance increases, the pressure required to distend the lung decreases.
  - Results in shift in slope of pressure-volume curve to the left.

CHANGES IN RESISTANCE

- Resistance in the pulmonary system results from frictional resistance of the gas passing through narrow tubes (airways, endotracheal tube), the secretions in airways.
- As resistance increases, the inspiratory portion of the pressure-volume loop will bow to the right.

FLOW-VOLUME LOOPS

- Used to detect response to therapy.
- Orientation can vary, but most will have flow on vertical axis and volume on horizontal axis.

RESPONSE TO BRONCHODILATORS

- Expiratory flow will improve with response to bronchodilator therapy.

BIBLIOGRAPHY

Schmidt GA. Waveforms: clinical interpretation. In: Hall JB, Schmidt GA, Wood LDH, eds., *Principles of Critical Care*, 3rd ed. New York, NY: McGraw-Hill; 2005: 427–443.

33 LIBERATION FROM MECHANICAL VENTILATION

Mark C. Pohlman

KEY POINTS

- Liberation from mechanical ventilation is the process by which patients are removed from the ventilator.
- This process has also been referred to as "weaning," but this implies a prolonged process of removal from a benevolent device.
- Patients' need for mechanical ventilation should be assessed daily; most patients considered for "weaning" don't need any and can be promptly extubated.
- The SBT and calculation of the RSBI guide most assessments about discontinuing mechanical ventilation.
- The following questions should be considered:
  - What is the cause of the respiratory failure, and has it been reversed?
  - Is the patient capable of performing an SBT?
  - How will the SBT be performed, and what is considered passing?
  - How will the patient be managed after failing an SBT?
  - What is the role of tracheostomy?

WHAT IS THE CAUSE OF RESPIRATORY FAILURE, AND HAS IT BEEN REVERSED?

- It is logical that unless the cause of respiratory failure has been thoroughly addressed and reversed, liberation of ventilation will not be possible. (Please see Chaps. 27 and 32 on respiratory failure and waveforms for more discussion.)
- Causes that can slow the process of liberation can be divided into two categories:
  - Strength/drive
    - Sedation
    - Encephalopathy
    - Malnutrition
    - Muscle weakness
    - Polyneuropathy of critical illness
    - Electrolyte disturbance
    - Circulatory adequacy
  - Load
    - Lung or chest wall compliance
    - Airways resistance
    - Minute ventilation requirements

WHICH PATIENTS ARE CAPABLE OF PERFORMING AN SBT?

- Prior to assessing liberation parameters and performing a spontaneous breathing trial (SBT), the patient should meet several requirements:
  - Oxygenation ($PaO_2 > 60$ on $FiO_2 \leq 50\%$, and positive end-expiratory pressure [PEEP] ≤ 8).
  - pH ≥ 7.25 (metabolic acidosis increases respiratory rate [RR] and places a "load" on the patient).
  - Hemodynamic stability (i.e., no active malignant arrhythmias, cardiac ischemia, or critical hypoperfusion).
  - Patient is initiating spontaneous breaths.
  - Presence of cough and gag reflexes (SBT/weaning parameters can be obtained without this).
- The most useful liberation parameter is the *rapid shallow breathing index (RSBI)*, also referred to as *rate volume ratio (RVR)*.
- The RSBI aims to quantitate the clinical observation that, when removed from the ventilator, patients who still have ventilatory failure will breath rapidly and shallowly, whereas those who have recovered will breath more slowly and deeply. Multiple trials have shown this index to have better sensitivity, specificity, positive predictive value, and negative predictive value than other means of assessing ventilatory readiness.
- RSBI sensitivity in multiple trials is about 70–90% in predicting successful liberation.
  - Threshold value < 105 bpm is "positive" and indicates a likelihood of weaning success.
  - However, false positives are the concern and the positive predictive value is about 80%, and specificity of 11–64% (i.e., those who pass but require reintubation or fail their SBT).
- PI_{max}/negative inspiratory force (NIF)/maximum inspiratory pressure (MIP):

- Measures pressure generated by patient from functional residual capacity (FRC), and requires patient effort.
- Poor indicator of success or failure of extubation.

- Minute ventilation (V_E):
  - Values <10 L/min thought to be an indicator of liberation success; however, several large trials found this to be a poor predictor of outcome.
  - Values >15–20 L/min helped identify those likely to fail.
- Too much importance is likely placed on obtaining weaning parameters: an SBT is always preferred.

HOW IS AN SBT PERFORMED? WHAT IS CONSIDERED "PASSING"?

- A typical SBT involves one of four methods: setting the ventilator to continuous positive airway pressure (CPAP; generally at 5 cmH_2O); pressure support (PS) of 5 cmH_2O over PEEP; PS of 7 cmH_2O over PEEP; or removing the ventilator and using a T-piece.
- Disadvantage of the T-piece method is the lack of respiratory monitoring (ventilator waveforms, V_T, alarms, and so forth).
- Monitoring is most important during the initial few minutes, as this is when most patients fail.
- If the patient does not fail (see below) within the first few minutes, then a trial of 30–120 minutes is attempted.
- If the patient passes an SBT, extubation is successful ≥80–90% of the time (assuming that the endotracheal tube [ETT] is no longer needed for other problems).
- Objective criteria used to indicate "success" during the SBT include:
  - Oxygenation/ventilation
    - $SpO_2 \geq 85$–90% or $PaO_2 \geq 50$–60
    - pH ≥ 7.32, increase in $PaCO_2 \leq 10$
  - Hemodynamic stability
    - Not requiring significant vasopressors
    - Heart rate (HR) < 120–140 bpm, change < 20%
    - SBP < 180–200, but > 90, and no change > 20%
  - Breathing pattern
    - RR ≤ 30–35
    - Not increased by >50%
- Subjective criteria used to indicate "success" during the SBT include:
  - No mental status changes (agitation, anxiety, lethargy, or somnolence)
  - No visible discomfort
  - No diaphoresis
  - No signs of dramatically increased work of breathing (accessory muscles, abdominal paradox, respiratory alternans)

HOW ARE PATIENTS MANAGED AFTER FAILING AN SBT?

- Two large randomized trials have evaluated the weaning process. In both, the majority of patients considered for weaning are already sufficiently recovered so as to be ready for extubation. For the minority of patients who fail an SBT, alternate modes for weaning were compared (T-piece vs. PS vs. synchronized intermittent mandatory ventilation [SIMV]).
  - In one, T-piece was found to be best, while in the other, PS was superior. Both trials found SIMV to delay weaning.
- Another trial found that identifying patients capable of breathing spontaneously leads to a reduction in duration of mechanical ventilation of 1.5 days, and therefore appropriate patients should be screened and SBTs should be conducted each day.
  - This trial also found that weaning protocols (nurse- or respiratory therapist-driven) lead to shorter duration of mechanical ventilation.
- Between SBTs, a stable, nonfatiguing mode of ventilation should be used (e.g., volume assist-control or sufficient PS). There is no role for SIMV.

WHAT IS THE ROLE OF TRACHEOSTOMY?

- Many possible benefits of tracheostomy are theoretical and have not been demonstrated conclusively in good clinical trials. Possible benefits include:
  - Improved patient comfort
  - Effective airway suctioning
  - Decreased airway resistance
  - More secure airway
  - Ability for speech, eating
  - Mobility
  - Decreased incidence of ventilator-associated pneumonia
  - More rapid weaning from ventilator
- No data clearly support that tracheostomy reduces risk of ventilator-associated pneumonia.
- It is not clear that early versus late tracheostomy reduces duration of prolonged mechanical ventilation.
- Tracheostomy should be considered after the patient has been stabilized on the ventilator and it appears prolonged (>2 weeks) ventilator support may be necessary.

BIBLIOGRAPHY

Ely EW, Baker AM, Dunagan DP, et al. Effect on the duration of mechanical ventilation of identifying patients capable of breathing spontaneously. *N Engl J Med* 1996;335: 1864–1869.

Esteban A, Frutos F, Tobin MJ, et al. A comparison of four methods of weaning patients from mechanical ventilation. *N Engl J Med* 1995;332:345–350.

Hall JB, Wood LD. Liberation of the patient from mechanical ventilation. *JAMA* 1987;257:1621–1628.

MacIntyre NR, Cook DJ, Ely EW Jr, et al. American College of Chest Physicians. American Association for Respiratory Care. American College of Critical Care Medicine. Evidence-based guidelines for weaning and discontinuing ventilatory support: a collective task force facilitated by the American College of Chest Physicians; the American Association for Respiratory Care; and the American College of Critical Care Medicine. *Chest* 2001;120:375S–395S.

Manthous CA, Schmidt GA, Hall JB. Liberation from mechanical ventilation. In: Hall JB, Schmidt GA, Wood LDH, eds., *Principles of Critical Care*, 3rd ed. New York, NY: McGraw-Hill; 2005: 625–637.

Yang KL, Tobin MJ. A prospective study of indexes predicting the outcome of trials of weaning from mechanical ventilation. *N Engl J Med* 1991;324:1445–1450.

34 VENTILATOR-INDUCED LUNG INJURY

Shashi Kiran Bellam

KEY POINTS

- Positive pressure ventilation can lead to functional and structural changes in the lungs, especially in the setting of underlying lung injury, and these changes can be termed VILI.
- VILI encompasses macroscopic air leakage (barotrauma), microscopic changes in lung function and structure, and the production of inflammatory mediators which may drive systemic inflammation and organ-system dysfunction.
- VILI has been shown to be related to excessive pressures as well as tidal volumes (volutrauma).
- VILI has been shown to be more common in younger and smaller animals.
- The most impressive clinical study related to minimizing VILI was the ARDS-NET "ARMA" trial which demonstrated that using tidal volumes of 12 mL/kg ideal body weight during mechanical ventilation of patients with acute lung injury or ARDS leads to greater mortality than using tidal volumes of 6 mL/kg ideal body weight.
- Ventilator management of patients with exudative-phase ARDS should begin with a FiO_2 of 1.0, tidal volume of 6 mL/kg ideal body weight, and respiratory rate 24–36 breaths/min. During initial stabilization on the ventilator, heavy sedation is advisable to minimize oxygen consumption.
- Goals of supportive therapy include achieving 88% saturation of an adequate hemoglobin on a nontoxic FiO_2 (<60%).

VENTILATOR-INDUCED LUNG INJURY (VILI)

- Barotrauma—a macroscopic injury to the airways leading to pneumothorax, pneumomediastinum, pneumoperitoneum, and subcutaneous emphysema.
  - Early studies correlated barotrauma to peak airway pressures, level of positive end-expiratory pressure (PEEP), tidal volume, and minute ventilation, but these correlations appear poor, at best.
  - Other studies have only demonstrated a correlation or worsening barotrauma in the setting of acute respiratory distress syndrome (ARDS).
  - Gas-trapping (or auto-PEEP) has been shown to relate to the development of barotrauma.
  - Underlying lung diseases (such as asthma, chronic obstructive pulmonary disease, and pneumonia) are risk factors for the development of barotrauma.
  - Barotrauma may often be occult with plain chest x-rays unrevealing.
  - Significant barotrauma may lead to hemodynamic consequences (e.g., a tension pneumothorax).
- Microscopic lung injury—abnormalities of the alveolar walls, surfactant dysfunction, and lung damage (consistent histologically with ARDS) that signify functional and anatomic changes that occur with mechanical ventilation.
  - Early animal studies have demonstrated microscopic lung injury that correlated to the peak airway pressures.
  - Clinical human studies have failed to confirm the importance of peak airway pressures as a predictor of the development of microscopic lung injury; more likely, plateau airway pressure (which more closely represents lung stretch) predicts the development of microscopic lung injury.
  - Lung injury related to tidal volumes (volutrauma) has been shown to correlate with some markers of microscopic lung injury—even with negative pressure ventilation, confirming that lung stretch, not pressures per se, are responsible for injury.
  - Heterogeneity of lung disease and injury may lead to regional differences in volume and pressure which may lead to regional microscopic lung injury without obvious whole lung overdistention (volutrauma) or elevated airway pressures.

- Low PEEP levels have been shown to lead to microscopic lung injury in experimental animals, presumably due to cyclic opening and closing of alveoli (atelectrauma), which can be ameliorated by higher levels of PEEP.
- Biotrauma—inflammatory mediators induced by cyclic stress or shear.
  - Various cells (epithelial, endothelial, fibroblasts, and white blood cells) can be induced to produce inflammatory mediators from lung stretching.
  - Increased inflammatory mediators are not limited to the lung and may drive systemic inflammation and systemic organ-system dysfunction.

ACUTE RESPIRATORY DISTRESS SYNDROME

- Definition:
  - Diffuse pulmonary infiltrates in all four quadrants of the lungs of acute onset.
  - Hypoxemia with a ratio of partial pressure of arterial oxygen (PaO_2) to fraction of inspired oxygen (FiO_2) of <200.
  - No evidence of elevated left atrial pressure.
- Greater than 50 causes have been identified, but the primary causes include: sepsis, aspiration of gastric contents, pneumonia, trauma and burns, massive blood transfusion, and drug reactions.
- Pathologic changes occur due to inflammatory injury to alveoli leading to the histology of diffuse alveolar damage.
- Clinical features include severe hypoxemia, decreased respiratory system compliance, and elevated pulmonary artery pressures.
- Common complications include barotrauma, commonly manifested as pneumothorax.
- Mortality is estimated at 40%. Long-term survivors may show relatively normal lung function and be symptom-free.
- Treatment: ventilator strategies:
  - Tidal volumes of 12 mL/kg ideal body weight are clearly associated with higher mortality than lower tidal volumes in the range of 6 mL/kg ideal body weight. Since most patients weigh more than predicted based on height and gender, lung protective tidal volumes may be closer to 4 mL/kg measured weight, on average.
  - Plateau pressures were maintained <30 cmH_2O in the low tidal volume group in the ARMA trial, but the average for the group was only 26 cmH_2O.
  - Limiting tidal volumes may lead to hypercapnia, so contraindications (such as increased intracranial pressure) should be considered.
  - In patients (as opposed to experimental animals) levels of PEEP higher than necessary for oxygenation have not been shown beneficial.

BIBLIOGRAPHY

Granton JT, Slutsky AS. Ventilator-induced lung injury. In: Hall JB, Schmidt GA, Wood LDH, eds., *Principles of Critical Care*, 3rd ed. New York, NY: McGraw-Hill; 2005: 499–515.

35 ACUTE RESPIRATORY DISTRESS SYNDROME

Nuala J. Meyer

KEY POINTS

- Patients with ALI or its most severe form, ARDS, present with hypoxemic respiratory failure which is characteristically resistant to oxygen therapy.
- Many primary insults can lead to ALI/ARDS, with sepsis, pneumonia, and aspiration being the most common.
- The clinician should seek to exclude other causes of diffuse alveolar flooding and hypoxemia, including pulmonary hemorrhage, atypical infection, or cardiogenic pulmonary edema.
- Management of ALI/ARDS hinges on providing adequate oxygenation, typically by intubation and mechanical ventilation using PEEP.
- A ventilation strategy employing lung-protective ventilation—tidal volumes of 6 mL/kg of ideal body weight (IBW) and the maintenance of plateau airway pressures below 30 cmH_2O—reduces mortality in ALI/ARDS.

DEFINITION

- The acute respiratory distress syndrome (ARDS) is a clinical syndrome of severe lung injury which results in damage to the alveolar-capillary membrane. Numerous initial insults, either directly injurious to the lung or indirectly injurious via systemic inflammation, can result in a final pattern of lung inflammation, which in turn causes protein-rich fluid to leak into the alveolar space. ARDS is commonly referred to as "low-pressure" or noncardiogenic edema.

- Acute lung injury (ALI) is defined as the acute onset of respiratory distress with hypoxemia, bilateral pulmonary infiltrates on frontal chest x-ray, and the absence of any clinical evidence of left atrial hypertension. The ratio of arterial partial pressure of oxygen to the fraction of inspired oxygen (PaO_2/FiO_2 ratio) in ALI is <300.
- ARDS describes those patients with the most severe form of ALI. Like ALI, patients with ARDS have an acute onset of respiratory distress, bilateral pulmonary infiltrates on chest radiograph, and the absence of evidence of left atrial hypertension, but hypoxemia is more severe and characterized by a PaO_2/FiO_2 ratio of <200.
- While historical definitions of ARDS often include "pulmonary capillary wedge pressure (PCWP) < 18 mmHg" as a criterion, pulmonary artery catheterization (PAC) is not necessary to define ARDS.

EPIDEMIOLOGY

- Obtaining an accurate incidence for ARDS has been notoriously difficult, but recent studies in the United States and Australia cite an incidence of between 22 and 38 cases per 100,000 persons per year.
- Of patients entering European ICUs, approximately 7% met criteria for ARDS. ARDS accounted for 16% of mechanically ventilated patients and 32% of hypoxemic mechanically ventilated patients in the same study.
- Mortality for ARDS remains high, at approximately 30% in the most recent trials. Mortality is as likely to be from sepsis or multisystem organ failure as from respiratory failure.
- As more patients survive, long-term outcomes such as neuromuscular weakness, psychological difficulties, and persistent dyspnea despite nearly normal pulmonary function are becoming increasingly recognized.

ETIOLOGY

- Acute respiratory distress syndrome is a clinical syndrome incited by numerous initial events, both pulmonary and extrapulmonary.
- Common pulmonary injuries include pneumonia, aspiration, or pulmonary contusion.
- Sepsis, an extrapulmonary insult, is the most common risk factor for ARDS. Other extrapulmonary etiologies include major trauma with multiple long bone or pelvic fractures, hypertransfusion of blood products (>10 units over a 12-hour period), disseminated intravascular coagulopathy, or acute pancreatitis.
- The likelihood of developing ARDS increases with the number of risk factors present.
- Several potentially treatable conditions can mimic ARDS and should be actively considered and excluded depending on patient history. They include:
  - Acute eosinophilic pneumonia (AEP), characterized by >20% eosinophils in bronchoalveolar lavage fluid.
  - Acute hypersensitivity pneumonititis (HP), typically with respiratory distress beginning within 6 hours of organic exposure to birds or hay.
  - Acute cryptogenic organizing pneumonia (COP), best diagnosed by biopsy.
  - Diffuse alveolar hemorrhage (DAH), which may be present even when hemoptysis is absent. Unless clinically obvious, the source of alveolar hemorrhage should always be sought with bronchoscopy. Occasionally, angiography with embolization or surgery is necessary for life-threatening hemorrhage.
  - Pneumocystis pneumonia, or PCP, is pulmonary infection with the fungus *Pneumocystis jirovecii* (formerly *Pneumocystis carinii*) which is most often encountered in patients with human immunodeficiency virus or chronic corticosteroid therapy. Diagnosis is made by staining sputum or bronchoalveolar lavage fluid for *P. jerovecii*.

PATHOGENESIS

- Acute lung injury results from damage to the alveolar-capillary membrane which allows proteinaceous fluid to flood the alveolar space. Damage likely results from damage to both the pulmonary capillary endothelium, and to the alveolar epithelium.
- Type II respiratory epithelial cells, which typically comprise only 10% of normal respiratory epithelium, proliferate in response to injury, yet become deficient in their usual roles of fluid transport and surfactant production.
- The cascade of events causing such endothelial and epithelial damage is not fully elucidated, but may involve free radical damage from oxygen metabolites, cytokine or leukotriene elaboration, complement fixation, or vasoactive substances.
- Both oxygen therapy, especially at FiO_2 > 60%, and ventilator stretch of the alveoli may also contribute to lung injury.

CLINICAL FEATURES

- Acute respiratory distress syndrome is classically described as passing through several distinct clinical, radiographic, and pathologic stages.

- The initial or exudative phase involves an acute respiratory decompensation, where the patient is often extremely hypoxemic and relatively refractory to high levels of inspired oxygen. As alveoli are flooded, the patient's alveolar dead space fraction rises, forcing the patient to have a high minute ventilation to maintain near-normal levels of arterial carbon dioxide.
  - Patients are hypoxemic, extremely tachypneic, and have a very low lung compliance ("stiff lungs"), manifested by very high plateau airway pressures on the ventilator when excessive tidal volumes are given.
  - Chest radiographs at this phase show a rapid development of bilateral infiltrates, often resembling cardiogenic pulmonary edema.
  - The pathologic description of this exudative phase is "diffuse alveolar damage," characterized by thickening and edema of the alveolar septae and spaces, with hyaline membranes layering the alveolar epithelium.
- The subacute phase, often from days 5 to 7 onwards, occurs in a subset of patients who fail to rapidly resolve. These patients may have ongoing, oxygen-refractory hypoxemia, low lung compliance, and persistent radiographic infiltrates.
  - Pathologically, the subacute phase is defined by fibrosing alveolitis, whereby the alveolar ducts begin to lay down collagen and fibroblasts in their septae.
- In a small proportion of patients, ARDS persists for 10 days or more, and pathologically enters a proliferative or fibrotic stage.
  - Clinically, patients have persistent hypoxemia and low lung compliance.
  - Pathologically, extensive fibrosis is present, to the extent that this stage may be difficult to distinguish from any other form of pulmonary fibrosis.
  - Radiographic studies, especially computed tomography (CT), at this stage will often show cystic or bullous formations in the lungs, predisposing the patients to complications such as pneumothorax or pneumomediastinum.

DIAGNOSTIC EVALUATION

- Bilateral pulmonary infiltrates on frontal chest x-ray are necessary to meet criteria for ARDS (Fig. 35-1). When patients with ARDS undergo CT, it often highlights striking inhomogeneity between areas of the lung which are well ventilated and those which are completely consolidated (Fig. 35-2). CT is not necessary for the diagnosis.
- While ARDS may coexist with left ventricular failure, ARDS is considered a low-pressure or noncardiogenic form of edema. Appropriate approaches to distinguish cardiogenic from noncardiogenic edema can be difficult.
  - Echocardiogram to evaluate left ventricular function, combined with central venous catheterization

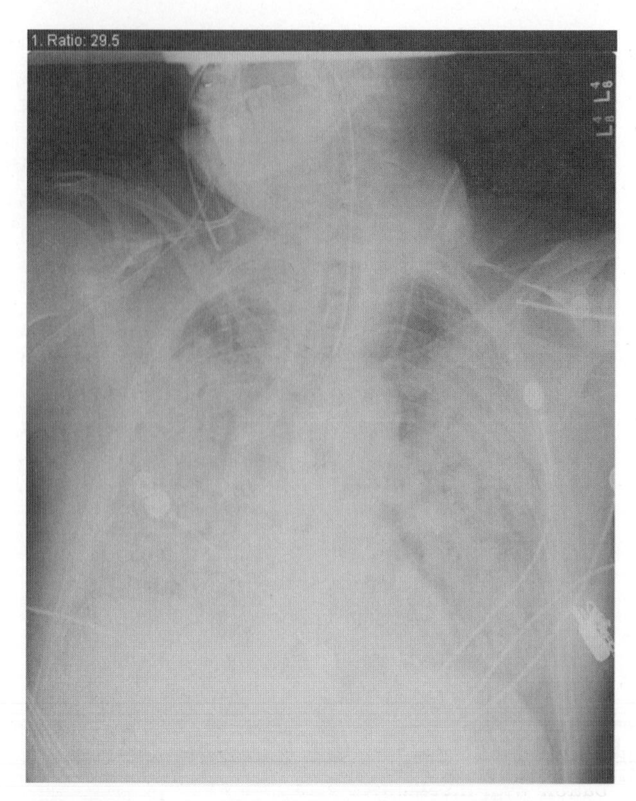

FIG. 35-1 Chest radiograph of a patient with ARDS.
SOURCE: Adapted from Meyer NJ and Schmidt GA. Chapter 10C: ARDS. In: Fein A, Kamholz S, Ost D, ed. Respiratory Emergencies. London, England: Hodder Arnold, 2006;179–199.

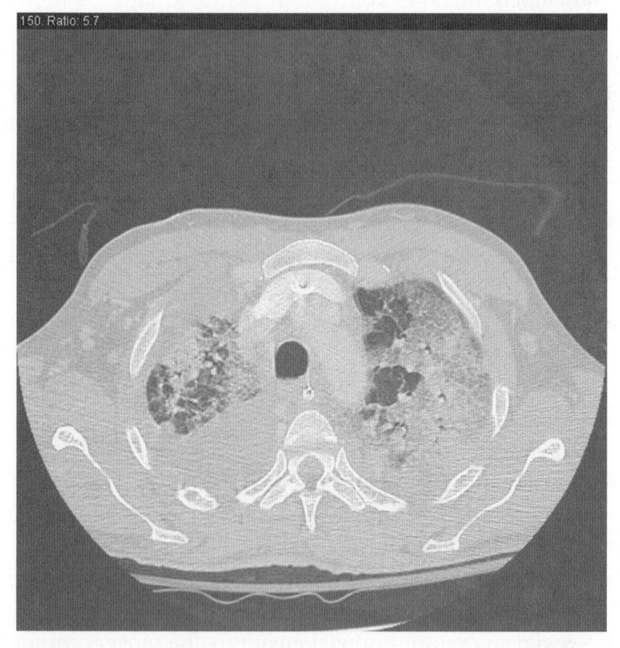

FIG. 35-2 Chest CT image of the same patient with ARDS, demonstrating heterogenous airspace flooding and consolidation.
SOURCE: Adapted from Meyer NJ and Schmidt GA. Chapter 10C: ARDS. In: Fein A, Kamholz S, Ost D, ed. Respiratory Emergencies. London, England: Hodder Arnold, 2006;179–199.

to assess the right atrial filling pressure, can be helpful in confirming normal systolic function.
- PAC, with direct measurement of the PCWP, is also possible, and historically a limit of 18 mmHg is considered the threshold below which ARDS is more likely than left ventricular failure. However, PAC is not necessary for the diagnosis of ARDS, and as PAC can incur risk such as pulmonary embolism or arrhythmia, we do not routinely advocate its use. A large multicenter trial comparing PAC to central venous catheter in this setting showed that the PAC conferred no benefit, but was associated with more complications.
- Bronchoscopy with bronchoalveolar lavage can be helpful to exclude treatable disease, such as AEP, DAH, or an infectious agent. Lung biopsy can also be helpful to exclude treatable conditions such as COP or HP.
- Edema fluid protein analysis, while not frequently performed, can suggest low-pressure edema when the initial edema-to-serum protein ratio is >0.6.

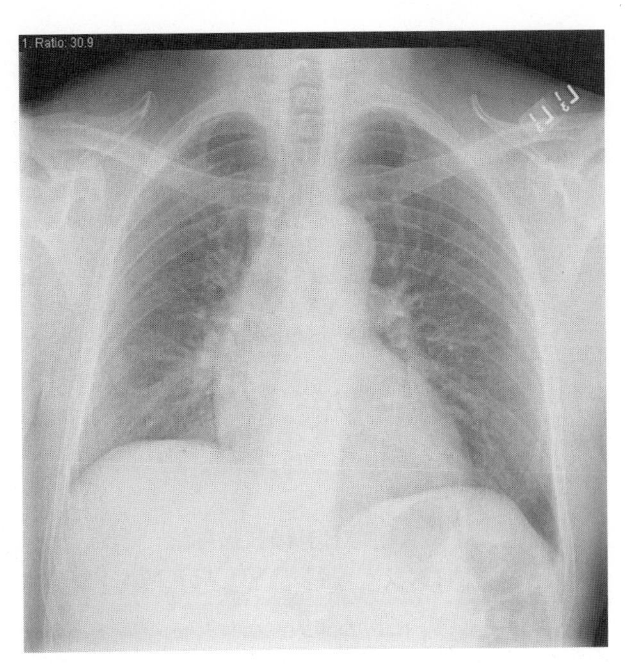

FIG. 35-3 Chest radiograph of the same patient 3 months later, with near-total resolution of his lung disease.
SOURCE: Adapted from Meyer NJ and Schmidt GA. Chapter 10C: ARDS. In: Fein A, Kamholz S, Ost D, ed. Respiratory Emergencies. London, England: Hodder Arnold, 2006;179–199.

INTENSIVE CARE UNIT MANAGEMENT

- Most patients with ALI and ARDS will require intubation with mechanical ventilation. All patients with hemodynamic compromise in addition to ALI should be intubated.
- Early use of noninvasive positive pressure ventilation (NIPPV) can be considered, and has been proven to decrease the rate of intubation and infection in immunosuppressed patients when compared to oxygen administered by face mask. ARDS and sepsis are risk factors for failure of NIPPV.
- Mechanical ventilation should achieve specific goals, which have been validated in large multicenter trials:
  - A lung-protective strategy, defined by tidal volumes (Vt) ≤ 6 mL/kg of IBW, where IBW is calculated as = 50 + 0.91 (height in cm - 152.4) for males, and IBW = 45.5 + 0.91 (height in cm - 152.4) for females. For an average male of 5'10", IBW = 73 kg, and initial Vt should be 438 mL. Similarly, an average woman of 5'4" has an IBW = 55 kg, making the initial Vt 330 mL.
  - Plateau pressure (P_{PLAT}) should be ≤ 30 cm of water. If P_{PLAT} is >30 cm of water with a tidal volume of 6 mL/kg, tidal volume should be reduced further, to as low as 4 mL/kg IBW.
  - Permissive hypercapnia, whereby the PCO_2 is allowed to rise as tidal volumes are deliberately kept low for lung protection, is generally a safe and effective strategy without the use of sodium bicarbonate to offset the respiratory acidosis. In specific patients—those with elevated intracranial pressure or recently postmyocardial infarction—the PCO_2 should not be allowed to rise dramatically.
  - PEEP—positive end-expiratory pressure—should be employed in order to keep the fraction of inspired oxygen (FiO_2) in the presumed nontoxic range, below 0.6. PEEP is felt to decrease ventilator-induced lung injury by lessening mechanical shear forces caused by repetitive opening and closing of alveoli in atelectatic regions of the lung, and reducing stretch between aerated and collapsed lung regions. PEEP may also recruit alveoli by preventing their collapse at end-expiration.
  - Reducing the circulating volume of the patient with diuresis or by withholding extra hydration may help to decrease edemagenesis. A large clinical trial showed that an aggressive diuretic regimen reduced time on the ventilator for ALI/ARDS patients.
- Aside from diuresis, no pharmacologic therapy—including corticosteroids, ketoconazole, inhaled nitric oxide, surfactant, or prostaglandin therapy—has been proven effective in reducing mortality or otherwise changing outcomes in ARDS.
- With proper management, patients can survive to discharge with resolution of symptoms and chest x-ray findings (Fig. 35-3).

BIBLIOGRAPHY

Bernard GB, Artigas A, Brigham KL, et al. The American-European Consensus Conference on ARDS: definitions, mechanisms, relevant outcomes, and clinical trial coordination. *Am J Respir Crit Care Med* 1994;149:818–824.

The Acute Respiratory Distress Syndrome Network. Ventilation with lower tidal volumes as compared with traditional tidal volumes for acute lung injury and the acute respiratory distress syndrome. *N Engl J Med* 2000;248:1301–1308.

The National Heart, Lung, and Blood Institute ARDS Clinical Trials Network. Higher versus lower positive end-expiratory pressures inpatients with the acute respiratory distress syndrome. *N Engl J Med* 2004;351:327–336.

Rubenfeld GD, Caldwell E, Peabody E, et al. Incidence and outcomes of acute lung injury. *N Engl J Med* 2005;353:1685–1693.

Ware LB, Matthay MA. The acute respiratory distress syndrome. *N Engl J Med* 2000;342:1334–1349.

36 EXTRACORPOREAL MEMBRANE OXYGENATION

Anna N. Kamp

KEY POINTS

- Extracorporeal membrane oxygenation (ECMO) improves outcome in neonates with severe respiratory failure.
- Several trials in adults have failed to demonstrate any advantage.
- ECMO should be considered a salvage strategy for adults to buy time in the setting of potentially reversible respiratory disease.
- Complications of ECMO include clotting, hemorrhage, accidental decannulation, air embolism, problems maintaining flow.

HISTORY

- Extracorporeal membrane oxygenation (ECMO) has been used routinely since 1975; however, collection of systemic data was not begun until 1985. Since 1989, all neonatal, pediatric, and adult patients from participating ECMO centers have been registered with the Extracorporeal Life Support Organization (ELSO).
- The first successful use of ECMO support was in 1971. An adult with acute posttraumatic respiratory failure was maintained on ECMO for 3 days and survived.
- After this first adult survivor, about 150 additional adults received ECMO for severe respiratory failure with a survival rate of about 10–15%.
- A National Institutes of Health (NIH) sponsored multicenter prospective, randomized-controlled trial in the late 70s of the use of ECMO for adults with acute respiratory failure showed such a high mortality rate that it was stopped early and for years, little research was pursued in adults.
- It was not until 1974 that ECMO was first used in a neonate. This sentinel case occurred at the Orange County Medical Center in a neonate with severe meconium aspiration whose PaO_2 went as low as 12 mmHg when a decision was made to try ECMO. After 3 days on ECMO, the newborn recovered completely.
  - After the initial success with a newborn, the physicians involved continued to treat neonates with severe respiratory failure with ECMO. While these infants had an estimated 90% mortality rate, the infants supported on ECMO were found to have a 75% survival rate. However, this was not a randomized-controlled trial.
  - The physicians reporting this success in neonates in the late 1970s and early 1980s were met with much skepticism because there was no randomized-controlled trial.
- Because of the initial success with ECMO in neonatal severe respiratory failure, several initial studies at the University of Michigan and Boston Children's Hospital were organized using an adaptive design. This adaptive design allowed for initial randomization; however, the design was then adjusted so that more patients would be randomized to the treatment that seemed to be superior. These adaptive randomized studies showed a survival rate of 97% for ECMO patients compared with a 60% survival rate for conventional ventilator patients. However, there was still much criticism of the adaptive design.
- In 1996, a true multicenter, randomized study was conducted in the United Kingdom. This trial was halted prematurely when early analysis showed a statistically significant survival rate of 70% for ECMO infants compared with a 41% survival for the conventional ventilator infants.
- There are about 120 centers worldwide that participate in the ELSO registry. The ELSO originates from the University of Michigan ECMO program. The registry data are presented annually at the meeting of the American Society of Artificial Internal Organs.
- Currently, there is an ongoing randomized trial in the United Kingdom for ECMO in adults with severe respiratory failure.

INDICATIONS/CONTRAINDICATIONS

- It has been recommended, but not proven for all instances, that ECMO be considered in acute severe reversible respiratory or cardiac failure when the risk of dying from the primary disease despite optimal conventional treatment is 50–100%.

TABLE 36-1 Contraindications for the Use of ECMO

Relative
Ventilator 6–10 days
Immunosuppression
Systemic sepsis
Active bleeding
Absolute
Terminal disease
Brain injury
Ventilator >10 days
Septic shock
Cardiac arrest

- Because ECMO is a supportive measure, the main requirement in considering ECMO is that the patient has reversible disease.
- It is important to note that institutional experience plays a large role in patient selection.
- Contraindications for the use of ECMO are based predominantly on the reversibility of the patient's condition. ECMO is not a treatment; rather, it is a means by which to sustain a patient while other treatments are employed. Therefore, terminal disease, brain injury, and cardiac arrest are some absolute contraindications. Table 36-1 lists relative and absolute contraindications to the use of ECMO.
- The oxygen index (OI) is a measurement that compares the amount of ventilator support with the patient's oxygenation. In neonates, ECMO is considered as the OI increases toward 40.

$$OI = \frac{MAP \times FiO_2 \times 100}{PaO_2}$$

where MAP is mean airway pressure in cmH_2O and FiO_2 is expressed as a fraction of 1.

- In neonates, gestational age and birth weight are significant factors when considering a patient for ECMO. Patients <34 weeks gestational age are at higher risk for intracranial hemorrhage. Additionally, weight <2.0 kg limits the use of ECMO due to the size of the catheters.

PHYSIOLOGY OF EXTRACORPOREAL MEMBRANE OXYGENATION

- Extracorporeal membrane oxygenation may be delivered via venovenous (VV) or venoarterial (VA) cannulation. VA cannulation is used commonly in pediatric cardiac patients.
- VV cannulation drains the right atrium, usually through the right internal jugular vein. Venous blood drains from the right atrium by both venous flow and aspiration by a siphon. Blood passes through a self-regulating pump where it is pumped through a membrane lung (referred to as the "oxygenator"); this is where oxygen, water vapor, and carbon dioxide are transferred. The oxygenated blood is then returned to the patient.
  - If the ECMO application is purely for respiratory support, the oxygenated blood is returned to the venous circulation, via cannulation of the femoral vein or with a second catheter in the right internal jugular vein. This is called VV cannulation.
  - However, if cardiac support is required, the oxygenated blood is returned to the arterial circulation, usually through a catheter in the right common carotid. This is called VA cannulation (Fig. 36-1).
- Once the ECMO circuit is attached and functioning, circulation and gas exchange are supported mechanically, and the native heart and lungs are "rested." That is, ventilator settings and inotropic support are decreased to low, safe levels. ECMO support is continued until heart or lung function improves.
- The amount of blood flow through the circuit depends on the degree of support required.
- While VA ECMO may seem to be conceptually identical to operating room cardiopulmonary bypass, it is actually quite different in that it is partial bypass. The patient is maintained at normothermia with normal blood flow and normal hematocrit to maintain normal systemic oxygen delivery (Table 36-2).
- An ECMO circuit has a semipermeable membrane of silicone rubber between the blood and the gas, avoiding a direct blood-gas interface, which is a significant difference from an operating room (O.R.) cardiopulmonary bypass machine.
- VA ECMO is run at about 80% of normal resting cardiac output.

GAS EXCHANGE IN EXTRACORPOREAL MEMBRANE OXYGENATION

- Oxygen delivery during ECMO is a combination of blood oxygenation in the membrane, flow through the circuit, cardiac output, and gas exchange through the native lung.
  - However, in planning the size of the ECMO circuit, it is assumed there will be no gas exchange across the native lung.
- Oxygenation in the membrane is described as the "rated flow." Rated flow is the amount of venous blood that can be raised from a hemoglobin saturation

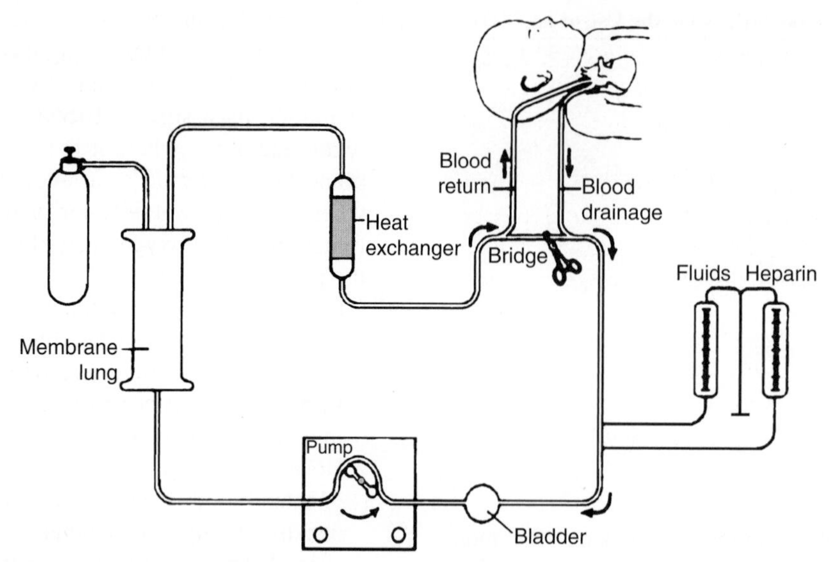

FIG. 36-1 A schematic of the venoarterial ECMO circuit.
SOURCE: Adapted from Wolfson PJ. The development and use of extracorporeal membrane oxygenation in neonates. *Ann Thorac Surg* 2003;76:S2224–S2229.

of 75–95% in a specific time. The rated flow is used to determine which type of membrane will be used for ECMO and to evaluate how the membrane is functioning during ECMO.

- If the extracorporeal blood flow is less than the rated flow of the membrane, the blood leaving the membrane will be fully saturated. Therefore, the oxygen delivery is controlled by the blood flow of the circuit and the oxygen uptake capacity of the patient.
- If the hemoglobin concentration is low, the amount of oxygen that can be bound in the oxygenator is decreased.
- If the venous blood saturation is high, the amount of oxygen that can be bound in the oxygenator is also decreased.
- One can compensate for decreased oxygen uptake in the oxygenator by increasing the flow of the circuit.

TABLE 36-2 Venoarterial Mechanical Circulation

	O.R. CARDIOPULMONARY BYPASS	ICU ECMO
Venous reservoir	Yes	No
Heparin (ACT)	Large dose (>600)	Titrated (120–180)
Autotransfusion	Yes	No
Hypothermia	Yes	No
Hemolysis	Yes	No
Anemia	Yes	No
Arterial filter	Yes	No

SOURCE: Adapted from Zwischenberger JB, Bartlett RH, eds., *ECMO: Extracorporeal Cardiopulmonary Support in Critical Care.* 3rd ed. Ann Arbor, MI: Extracorporeal Life Support Organization; 2005:6.

- In VV bypass, the arterial PO_2 will be identical to the mixed right atrial blood. The hemoglobin saturation will usually be close to 80% with a PO_2 of 40, and as long as there is an increase in cardiac output to compensate, oxygen delivery will be adequate.
    - Improvement in native lung function will be identified as a step up from venous to arterial saturation.
- In VA bypass, however, the arterial blood gases may be interpreted several ways, depending on the amount of venous return going through the ECMO circuit and the flow of the membrane. An increasing PO_2 may be read as:
    - Improving lung function at constant flows.
    - Decreasing native cardiac output at constant extracorporeal flows.
    - Increasing ECMO flow at constant native cardiac output.
- The carbon dioxide removal in ECMO is determined by the membrane lung surface area, the blood PCO_2, and membrane lung gas flow (called the sweep flow).
- The ventilating gas usually contains no CO_2, so the gradient for transfer of CO_2 is the difference between the blood CO_2 and zero.
- As blood passes through the membrane lung, the PCO_2 drops; thus the gradient decreases and less CO_2 is removed near the blood outlet end of the membrane lung compared to the blood inlet end.
- Carbon dioxide transfer can be increased by increasing both the sweep flow and the surface area of the membrane lung.
- The ECMO circuit is extremely efficient at removing CO_2. For this reason, if the circuit is set to supply total

oxygen requirements, it will remove excessive CO_2, resulting in a respiratory alkalosis. Adding CO_2 to the sweep gas will decrease the gradient between the blood PCO_2 and the membrane lung, thus decreasing the removal of CO_2.

- If CO_2 removal is the primary goal and the native lung can supply oxygen absorption, CO_2 removal can be achieved with VV access and low blood flow. This is termed extracorporeal carbon dioxide removal ($ECCO_2R$).

HEMODYNAMICS DURING EXTRACORPOREAL MEMBRANE OXYGENATION

- At initiation of ECMO, the exposure of blood products to artificial surfaces of the circuit and oxygenator triggers an inflammatory response, leading to an increase in capillary permeability. This capillary leak lasts about 2–3 days as long as there is no associated sepsis. The capillary leak itself resolves spontaneously; however, the associated increase in total body water may linger.
- Normal blood flow through the circuit to maintain systemic perfusion is about 100 cc/kg/min.
- Blood flow through the extracorporeal circuit is limited by the size of the venous drainage catheter. The shortest and largest diameter catheter that can be placed in the right atrium will allow the highest rate of blood flow.
- A catheter in the right internal jugular vein will usually allow venous drainage that approximates the normal resting cardiac output of patients of all ages and sizes.
- If total blood flow through the circuit is too low, the result is inadequate oxygen delivery, shock, and acidosis; this typically occurs at a flow <40 cc/kg/min.
- Resistance through the membrane lung and reinfusion catheter causes the pressure on the oxygenated side of the circuit to increase with increasing blood flow. These postoxygenator pressures must be monitored because higher pressures increase the chances of blood leaks or circuit disruption.
- The redistribution of blood flow is significantly different between VV and VA ECMO.
  - During VA ECMO, the blood is withdrawn from the venous circulation and pumped through the circuit; as a larger percentage of venous blood is directed through the circuit, left ventricular preload decreases. This results in normal mean arterial pressure but with a reduced pulse pressure (since only the flow contributed by the native circulation is pulsatile) and dampened arterial waveform.
  - During VV ECMO, blood is withdrawn and returned to the venous circulation at exactly the same rate. Therefore, there is no net effect on left ventricular preload. The cardiac output is all native left ventricular ejection.
- Hypertension on ECMO is a common complication.
  - One etiology that has been investigated is the stimulation of the renin-angiotensin-aldosterone axis by the nonpulsatile flow to the kidney from the circuit. This usually responds to vasodilator therapy with angiotensin-converting enzyme (ACE) inhibitors, nitroglycerine, and hydralazine.
  - Other causes of hypertension include hypervolemia, exogenous inotropes and pressors, and inadequate sedation.
- The ECMO circuit is set up with a self-regulatory system to avoid excessive negative pressure on the venous circulation. There is a small collapsible bladder in the venous line; when this bladder collapses, the pump shuts off automatically. When the bladder refills, the pump restarts.
  - As ECMO is initiated and the circuit flow is increased, the collapse of the bladder will identify the physical limitations of the venous drainage. If this maximal flow is not adequate to support the patient, additional venous drainage may be necessary to increase flow.
  - If the pump shuts off once ECMO has been ongoing, it may signal other problems such as pneumothorax or hypovolemia.
- The regulation of negative pressure on the venous circulation is important to avoid serious problems with the circuit.
  - Negative pressure over 200 mm can cause hemolysis.
  - The right atrium and superior vena cava can become sucked into the catheter at high pressures and cause endothelial damage.
  - Negative pressure within the circuit can increase the risk of air embolus.
- The University of Michigan group described a standard system for explaining the pressure flow in the catheters called the "M number." Using the M number of a catheter, the pressure and flow of that catheter can be determined using a nomogram.
- If ECMO is being used for cardiac support and the left ventricle is not ejecting adequately, the left side of the circulation can become overdistended. This can lead to pulmonary edema or cardiac damage, and left-sided decompression may be necessary.
  - In neonatal VA ECMO, this is not a problem because the left side can decompress via the patent ductus arteriosus.
  - In children and adults, however, just a few minutes of left-sided overdistention can cause significant pulmonary edema or cardiac damage.

- If cardiac failure is severe and the left ventricle is not able to eject against the pressure of VA ECMO, arterial resistance should be decreased by vasodilatory agents. If vasodilation is unsuccessful, left-sided venting may be necessary. This can be achieved by direct cannulation of the left atrium via thoracotomy or by creating an atrial septal defect in the catheterization laboratory.

MANAGEMENT OF THE PATIENT ON EXTRACORPOREAL MEMBRANE OXYGENATION

- Several monitors, in addition to patient vital signs, blood gases, and ventilator settings, are used to maintain a patient on ECMO.
- Blood flow through the circuit is monitored continuously. Blood flow is set at a level that will provide appropriate oxygenation and CO_2 exchange.
- Pressure is measured before and after the membrane lung; an increasing pressure gradient across the membrane lung may be a sign that thrombosis has occurred.
- Mixed venous saturation is monitored continuously.
- Patient arterial blood gases are used to calibrate the continuous monitors of the extracorporeal circuit.
- Systemic blood pressure is maintained by adjusting the blood volume.
- Hemoglobin is maintained between 14 and 15 g/dL.
- Systemic anticoagulation is standard practice with an extracorporeal circuit. Continuous heparin is given to maintain the whole blood activated clotting time (ACT) at about 180–200 seconds or less if the circuit has a nonthrombogenic coating.
- Platelet transfusions are usually required to maintain the platelet count >80,000 during ECMO.
- Ventilator settings while the patient is maintained on ECMO are directed at recruiting alveoli while avoiding ventilator-induced lung injury. Typically, the FiO_2 is 20–30% and peak airway pressures are <40 cmH_2O.
  - Other methods of managing severe lung injury are continued in an ECMO patient: lung-protective tidal volumes; prone positioning (in neonates); postural drainage; maintenance at dry weight; adequate nutrition.
- Backup ventilator settings to provide full support are posted near the patient in the event that ECMO is abruptly discontinued.
- Measuring end-tidal CO_2 in the airway is helpful in assessing native lung recovery.
- Following the pulmonary and systemic mean blood pressures during ECMO is a good indicator of the likelihood of lung recovery.

COMPLICATIONS

PUMP COMPLICATIONS

- Clots in the circuit are the most common mechanical complication. Major clots can lead to a consumptive coagulopathy or oxygenator failure, as well as systemic or pulmonary emboli.
- Cannulas can be a significant source of complications while on ECMO.
  - If the venous cannula is advanced too little or too much, it can become obstructed, causing the pump to shut down.
  - The arterial cannula can be inserted too far into the ascending aorta, causing increased afterload or aortic insufficiency, or too far into the descending aorta, compromising coronary and cerebral blood flow.
  - Cannula placement should be confirmed using echocardiography.
- Inadequate venous drainage can cause the pump to "cut out" or quit pumping blood, and one must consider all causes of decreased venous return in managing this problem. Figure 36-2 outlines the management of low venous drainage.
  - If hypovolemia is the cause of low venous return, correct it with fluid resuscitation or decrease the flow rate of the pump.
  - Any kinks in the tubing of the circuit can obstruct venous return and should be assessed.

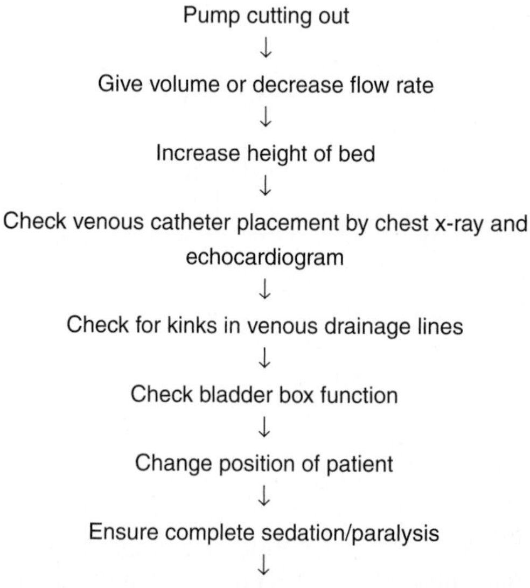

FIG. 36-2 Management of low venous drainage.
SOURCE: Adapted from Zwischenbeger JB, Bartlett RH, eds., *ECMO: Extracorporeal Cardiopulmonary Support in Critical Care.* 3rd ed. Ann Arbor, MI: Extracorporeal Life Support Organization; 2005:138.

  - An echocardiogram may be necessary to ensure that cardiac tamponade is not the etiology of obstruction.
- If the circuit is squirting blood or pumping air, the patient must be emergently removed from ECMO. To emergently remove the patient from ECMO, the technician immediately clamps the **V**enous line, opens the **B**ridge, and clamps the **A**rterial line (VBA)—a common reminder for this management is that the patient has had a Very Bad Accident. The patient must then be hand-bagged or the ventilator settings adjusted to pre-ECMO settings in an attempt to maintain respiratory support.
- Massive air embolism, such as that which may develop if a tear develops in the membrane lung, is the one exception to the VBA rule. In this situation, the arterial line is clamped first.

PATIENT COMPLICATIONS

- Bleeding complications are common because of systemic heparinization.
- The neck cannulation site is most frequently the source of moderate bleeding. Surgeons may vary in their treatments to achieve hemostasis; however, if the neck incision bleeds more than 10 cc/h for 2 hours regardless of treatment strategies used, the neck wound should be explored.
- Hemorrhages in the intrathoracic, abdominal, or retroperitoneal cavities will need to be drained, as allowing bleeding to tamponade in these sites is not usually successful.
- A new intracranial hemorrhage is an indication to discontinue ECMO support. Most ECMO centers have routine transfusion orders to maintain hemoglobin levels, so routine pupil examination may be the only indication of an intracranial hemorrhage.
- While a patient is on ECMO, it is unusual to have severe hemodynamic instability. If this occurs, one should immediately consider the venous catheter placement, volume status, and circuit failure.
- A pericardial tamponade, tension pneumothorax, or hemothorax may all present as decreased venous return causing the pump to cut out. The ECMO circuit does not affect the appearance of pneumothorax or hemothorax on chest x-ray.
- Accidental decannulation is an emergent reason to come off ECMO and is best avoided by adequate sedation and paralytics.
- Hemolysis is a commonly recognized complication and can often be attributed to the ECMO circuit, as clots in the membrane can promote a coagulopathy. However, disseminated intravascular coagulopathy must be considered by checking ACT, platelet count, fibrinogen, fibrin degradation products, prothrombin time (PT), and partial thromboplastin time (PTT). Then the circuit must be checked for clots, kinks, an arterial catheter occlusion, and high temperatures and pressures.

WEANING OFF EXTRACORPOREAL MEMBRANE OXYGENATION

- Extracorporeal membrane oxygenation may be necessary for anywhere from 1 day to 14 days or longer, depending on the patient's clinical situation.
- If the patient's initial insult was severe respiratory failure, one must look for evidence of native lung recovery before attempting to wean off ECMO. This includes: better breath sounds on physical examination and improved chest x-ray, higher venous saturation levels, increasing PaO_2 or decreasing $PaCO_2$ without changing ventilator or ECMO settings, and improving lung mechanics.
- For a patient with cardiogenic shock on VA ECMO, evidence of cardiac recovery includes: increasing arterial pulse contour, improving contractility by echocardiography, increasing mixed venous oxygenation with no change in other parameters.
- As a patient improves and is approaching a weaning trial, it is important to evaluate total body fluid and maximize diuresis if possible, as most patients on ECMO have a significant amount of third-spacing.
- Before beginning to wean, ensure the patient is properly sedated or paralyzed, as inadequate sedation contributes to higher oxygen consumption and may result in failure to wean from ECMO.
- Ventilator settings should be gradually increased to recruit collapsed lung tissue prior to weaning off EMCO.

OUTCOMES EVIDENCE IN ADULTS

- The National Heart, Lung, and Blood Institute of the NIH conducted a randomized-controlled trial at nine medical centers of severe acute respiratory failure in 1975–1979. Patients were randomized to either conventional mechanical ventilation or mechanical ventilation with VA ECMO. The study was discontinued after 90 patients because the mortality rate in each group was about 90%. Once this study was published, clinical research in adult ECMO was significantly slowed.
- The University of Michigan has published the largest series of extracorporeal life support to date. Between 1980 and 1998, 1000 patients were managed with

ECMO at U of M. ECMO use was initially limited to neonates with respiratory failure; however, it was expanded to the pediatric population in 1982 and to adults in 1990.
  - Of these patients, the survival to hospital discharge in patients with respiratory failure was 88% in 586 neonates, 70% in 132 children, and 56% in 146 adults.
  - Survival to hospital discharge in patients with cardiac failure was 48% in 105 children and 33% in 31 adults.
- In a retrospective review of 36 adult patients with severe respiratory failure managed with ECMO at the University of Michigan, mortality was found to be directly related to the duration of mechanical ventilation prior to the initiation of ECMO. These 36 patients were initially treated with conventional ventilation and had a predicted mortality of 90% based on previously established NIH criteria published in 1974.
  - 18 of the 36 patients survived to hospital discharge.
  - Of the 18 patients who died, ECMO was discontinued in 11 patients due to irreversible lung disease.
  - Patients who received conventional ventilation for 1–2 days and 3–4 days prior to management on ECMO had a survival rate of 72% and 75%, respectively.
  - Patients receiving conventional ventilation for 5–6 days and ≥7 days had a survival rate of 25% and 20%, respectively.
- A retrospective analysis of 219 adult patients in Germany managed with ECMO for refractory postoperative cardiogenic shock (after aortic valve replacement, coronary artery bypass grafting, or both) found that 52 of the 219 ECMO patients survived to hospital discharge.
- The CESAR Trial, a randomized-controlled trial comparing **C**onventional ventilation or **E**CMO for **S**evere **A**dult **R**espiratory failure in adults is currently ongoing in the United Kingdom.

BIBLIOGRAPHY

Anderson HL, Edmunds LH, Coagulation, anticoagulation, and the interaction of blood and artificial surfaces. In: Zwischenberger JB, Bartlett RH, eds., *ECMO: Extracorporeal Cardiopulmonary Support in Critical Care.* 3rd ed. Ann Arbor, MI: Extracorporeal Life Support Organization; 2005:29–58.

Bartlett RH, Roloff DW, Custer JR, et al. Extracorporeal life support: the University of Michigan experience. *JAMA* 2000;283:904–908.

Bartlett RH. Physiology of extracorporeal life support. In: Zwischenberger JB, Bartlett RH, eds., *ECMO: Extracorporeal Cardiopulmonary Support in Critical Care*. 3rd ed. Ann Arbor, MI: Extracorporeal Life Support Organization; 2005:5–28.

Chapman RA, Bartlett RH. *Extracorporeal Life Support Manual for Adult and Pediatric Patients.* Ann Arbor, MI: The University of Michigan Medical Center; 1991.

Doll N, Kiaii B, Borger M, et al. Five-year results of 219 consecutive patients treated with extracorporeal membrane oxygenation for refractory postoperative cardiogenic shock. *Ann Thorac Surg* 2004;77:151–157.

Kanto WP, Shapiro MB. The development of prolonged extracorporeal circulation. In: Zwischenberger JB, Bartlett RH, eds., *ECMO: Extracorporeal Cardiopulmonary Support in Critical Care*. Ann Arbor, MI: Extracorporeal Life Support Organization; 1995:15–27.

Pranikoff T, Hirschl RB, Steimle CN, et al. Mortality is directly related to the duration of mechanical ventilation before the initiation of extracorporeal life support for severe respiratory failure. *Crit Care Med* 1997;25:28–32.

Wolfson PJ. The development and use of extracorporeal membrane oxygenation in neonates. *Ann Thorac Surg* 2003;76: S2224–S2229.

Zapol WM, Snider MT, Hill JD, et al. Extracorporeal membrane oxygenation in severe acute respiratory failure. A randomized prospective study. *JAMA* 1979;242:2193–2196.

Zwischenberger JB, Upp JR. Emergencies during extracorporeal membrane oxygenation and their management. In: Zwischenberger JB, Bartlett RH, eds., *ECMO: Extracorporeal Cardiopulmonary Support in Critical Care*. 3rd ed. Ann Arbor, MI: Extracorporeal Life Support Organization; 2005:133–156.

37 ACUTE-ON-CHRONIC RESPIRATORY FAILURE

Timothy K. Baker, Steven Q. Davis

KEY POINTS

- Acute-on-chronic respiratory failure represents acute decompensation of a chronically diseased respiratory system.
- ACRF is most often caused by new respiratory system loading, deterioration in neuromuscular competence, or depressed drive.
- Auto-PEEP is a major contributor to the elastic load during ACRF.
- Oxygen, bronchodilators, and corticosteroids are the mainstays of treatment.
- Noninvasive positive pressure ventilation improves outcomes in selected patients.

OVERVIEW

- Chronic respiratory failure (CRF) is a significant and growing cause of morbidity and mortality in the United States and across the world. The majority of the clinical manifestations of CRF are related to the

spectrum of diseases related most significantly to cigarette smoking—that of emphysema and chronic bronchitis, known as chronic obstructive pulmonary disease (COPD).
- Acute-on-chronic respiratory failure (ACRF) occurs when the chronically compromised respiratory system suffers an incremental insult and becomes incapable of adequately excreting carbon dioxide or maintaining oxygenation.

PATHOPHYSIOLOGY

- Three components, respiratory drive, neuromuscular competence, and respiratory load are essential to the physiology and proper functioning of the respiratory system.
- Respiratory drive is mediated by the central nervous system (CNS), specifically in the medulla by the dorsal and ventral respiratory groups and in the pons by the pneumotaxic center. Given this, insults to the CNS can lead to a depressed respiratory drive and ACRF.
- Possible etiologies include cerebrovascular events such as hemorrhage or embolic phenomena. Additionally, spinal cord compromise, especially in the upper cervical area, can lead to loss of respiratory drive. Beyond primary neurologic events, other and often iatrogenic causes also exist. These are most commonly due to pharmacologic complications. Drugs, both illicit and prescribed, such as sedatives and narcotics are often implicated in the pathogenesis of ACRF. Additionally, other metabolic causes such as hypothyroidism should be excluded.
- The second component of the respiratory system is neuromuscular function, primarily involving the muscles of respiration, including the diaphragm and intercostal muscles and their innervation. The increased load of the chronically disease respiratory system puts at risk the neuromuscular component, such that only modest loss of function may precipitate failure. As the respiratory muscles are forced to work harder against an increasing load, they may fail as force generators, a condition called "fatigue."
- Fatigue is related to a muscle's work and its duration, in concert with the amount of energy that is supplied to the muscle by the circulation in the form of oxygen and nutrients. Fatigue may also hinge on the concentration of electrolytes such as phosphate.
- Several of the medicines that are commonly used to treat ACRF can further contribute to metabolic derangements, especially hypophosphatemia. Malnutrition and other muscle disease play a role in some patients.
- To accomplish the work of the respiratory system, the respiratory muscles must consistently sustain the ventilatory load. In health the balance of neuromuscular function and respiratory load is tipped greatly in favor of function, clinically apparent as the "pulmonary reserve." Patients without preexisting chronic lung disease can suffer a significant insult to their systems, resulting in a large increase in respiratory load, without developing respiratory failure.
- This is not the case for those with chronic lung disease; these patients have a very low pulmonary reserve and even slight insults, such as a mild viral respiratory illness, can tip the balance toward ventilatory failure. The load on the respiratory system can be divided into resistive and elastic components.
- Factors that contribute to the resistive load include bronchoconstriction, compression of airways by pulmonary edema (cardiac asthma), airway secretions, and obstructive sleep apnea.
- The elastic load can be raised by pulmonary edema, infiltrative processes such as pneumonia and tumors, as well as inflammation, interstitial fibrosis, and atelectasis. Chest wall elastic loads include obesity, rib fracture with splinted breathing, pneumothorax, pleural effusion, structural abnormalities, and abdominal distention from factors such as ascites and ileus.
- In most patients with ACRF, one of the most important elastic loads is the inspiratory threshold load presented by auto-PEEP.
- Finally, all of these loads are amplified when minute ventilation demands rise, such as during exercise, acidemia, or elevated dead space.

CLINICAL MANIFESTATIONS

- Patients with ACRF can present with acute worsening of pulmonary status over a very short period of time, or with a more prolonged course that ultimately leads them to seek medical attention. Patients typically present with worsening of their baseline dyspnea, with an increased and productive cough. Sputum may be reported as becoming thicker and more purulent in nature.
- As the patient's pulmonary function continues to worsen, the signs and symptoms become more ominous and include those of acute respiratory distress such as tachypnea, nostril flaring, accessory muscle use, and pursed lip breathing. Examination usually reveals prolonged expiration and wheezing that persists to end-expiration.
- Other signs include rhonchi from worsened mucous production and crackles from pulmonary edema, consolidation, or atelectasis.
- Pulse oximetry is an important bedside tool in assessing the patient in ACRF and guiding oxygen therapy.

- Blood tests should include arterial blood gas analysis; a complete blood count; and tests to exclude common and treatable precipitants, such as hypophosphatemia and hypothyroidism.

TREATMENT

- Initial choice of treatment for ACRF depends largely on the severity of the symptoms, clinical signs, and laboratory and radiographic data. In mild cases in which the patient has not yet progressed to severe respiratory distress and failure, bronchodilators, systemic corticosteroids, antibiotics, and supplemental oxygen may be enough to avert a more severe exacerbation. However, in some cases, patients have already progressed to overt respiratory failure and require more intensive therapy.

OXYGEN

- There is a long-standing myth that administration of oxygen to patients with COPD is contraindicated. This is due to the belief that drive is depressed during ACRF and that oxygen might undercut hypoxemic respiratory drive, leading to worse ventilatory failure and the need for intubation. While ACRF patients do have a component of hypoxic drive, their overall drive is supranormal. Raising PaO_2 lowers drive modestly, but leaves it supranormal. While patients with sleep disordered breathing may critically hypoventilate following oxygen, in the majority of ACRF patients we believe the benefit of assuring adequate tissue oxygenation far exceeds any risk of suppressing drive.
- Oxygen therapy can be guided with pulse oximetry, seeking a saturation in excess of 88%; this can often be accomplished with 3–5 L/min by nasal cannula or by a face mask delivering an FiO_2 of 30–35%.

BRONCHODILATORS

- Bronchodilators, such as beta$_2$-agonists and anticholinergic agents, are the mainstays of treatment of ACRF, as they act on the reversible component of airflow obstruction, which is a significant contributor to the load on the respiratory system.
- Beta$_2$-agonists (albuterol, metaproterenol) act to relax the smooth muscle of the airway. The most common beta$_2$-agonist in use is albuterol, which can be delivered by a metered-dose inhaler (MDI), 90 μg per puff, or as a nebulized solution of 2.5 mg per treatment. The two dosage forms appear to be equally efficacious when equivalent doses are used, but the clinical situation may necessitate the use of a nebulizer as patients with severe respiratory distress may become less able to tolerate administration via MDI.
- Anticholinergic agents such as ipratropium are also used to provide bronchodilation in patients experiencing ACRF. Like albuterol, ipratropium can also be administered in either an MDI or in a nebulized form. The MDI delivers 18 μg per puff while the nebulized form delivers 500 μg per treatment. Combined use of ipratropium and albuterol in stable COPD has been shown to be of benefit and is therefore often used in this way during ACRF. The role for tiotropium during acute exacerbations is uncertain.

CORTICOSTEROIDS

- There is often a significant amount of airway inflammation associated with an exacerbation of COPD and subsequent development of ACRF. Therefore, administration of systemic corticosteroids is a useful component of the treatment regimen. The agent chosen and the dose administered are based on the severity of the exacerbation.
    - In mild exacerbations, it is often appropriate to start with oral prednisone at a dose of 60 mg/day. This can either be dosed as a rapid pulse of 60 mg daily for 3 days, or tapered slowly over the course of 10–14 days.
    - In more severe cases, the use of intravenous methylprednisolone sodium succinate at a dose of 0.5–1.0 mg/kg every 6 hours is preferred. This is then transitioned to an oral formulation, often prednisone, as the patient's clinical status improves.

ANTIBIOTICS

- This is an area of considerable debate in the treatment of ACRF. In the situation where acute pulmonary infection such as community acquired or nosocomial pneumonia has lead to the development of ACRF, appropriate antibiotic therapy is prudent.
- Less clear is what to do in the situation of a relatively normal chest radiograph and the absence of fever or leukocytosis, as is often seen in an acute exacerbation of chronic bronchitis. The presence of purulent sputum may aid in the decision to initiate antibiotic therapy. Often, inexpensive, oral, broad-spectrum antibiotics such as azithromycin, doxycycline, or trimethoprim-sulfamethoxazole are given empirically for a course of 5–10 days.

NONINVASIVE POSITIVE PRESSURE VENTILATION

- For patients with severe ACRF, it is appropriate to consider noninvasive positive pressure ventilation (NIPPV). This technique has been shown to ameliorate symptoms, avert invasive mechanical ventilation in many instances, and improve outcomes such as complications, length of stay, and mortality.
- Patients must be carefully selected with regard to their appropriateness for NIPPV. Criteria for selection include the ability to maintain the airway, cardiovascular stability, spontaneous respiration, and tolerance of the facial appliance. Recommended initial settings are an inspiratory positive airway pressure (IPAP) of 10 cmH_2O and an expiratory positive airway pressure (EPAP) of 2–4 cmH_2O. Both of these can be adjusted in the first few minutes with a goal of IPAP 14–20 and EPAP 3–6.
- EPAP counterbalances auto-PEEP, in part, reducing the inspiratory threshold load, and substantially reducing the work of breathing. Even a CPAP mask (without a ventilator) can improve symptoms, blood gases, and the measured work of breathing.
- The key to the successful use of NIPPV is for the clinician to be prepared to act early in instituting therapy but also to recognize when it is failing.
- NIPPV generally improves subjective and blood gas measures within 1 hour. Failure to improve should lead to steps to adjust the ventilator settings, address sources of patient-ventilator dyssynchrony, and seek and correct leaks.

INVASIVE MECHANICAL VENTILATION

- While NIPPV is an appropriate initial therapy, it fails approximately 25% of the time, at which time endotracheal intubation and standard mechanical ventilation are indicated. A key for successful transition to traditional ventilation is recognize the need for intubation at a time when it can be performed in a controlled, elective setting rather than in an emergency. Clinical signs that may be useful are respiratory rate, mentation, pattern of breathing, and the patient's own assessment of their respiratory status.
- Initial ventilator settings should employ low tidal volume (5–7 cc/kg) and a respiratory rate of 20–24 breaths/min. Modest amounts of PEEP (5–10 cmH_2O) should be set to aid triggering. Any mode of ventilation will work, as long as the work of ventilation is done by the ventilator, allowing the patient to rest. We rest the patient for at least 24–48 hours, during which time attention is paid to treating the underlying condition that led to ACRF.
- Following an initial period of rest and treatment, we perform daily spontaneous breathing trials to identify the earliest opportunity for extubation. Some studies in subjects failing a spontaneous breathing trial have shown that extubation to NIPPV (despite failing the SBT) improves outcomes, but whether this is prudent requires experienced bedside judgment.

BIBLIOGRAPHY

Douglas IS, Schmidt GA, Hall JB. Acute-on-chronic respiratory failure. In: Hall JB, Schmidt GA, Wood LDH, eds., *Principles of Critical Care*, 3rd ed. New York, NY: McGraw-Hill; 2005: 549–566.

Kress JP, Hall JB. Principles of critical care medicine. In: Braunwald E, Fauci A, Kasper DL, eds., *Harrison's Principles of Internal Medicine*, 16th ed. New York, NY: McGraw-Hill; 2004.

Stoller JK. Clinical practice: acute exacerbations of chronic obstructive pulmonary disease. *N Engl J Med* 202;346:988–994.

38 STATUS ASTHMATICUS

Maria Dowell

KEY POINTS

- Status asthmaticus is a life-threatening exacerbation of asthma.
- Ventilatory failure is precipitated by excessive respiratory mechanical load due largely to increased airways resistance and auto-PEEP; oxygenation is only modestly impaired.
- The mainstays of therapy include oxygen, beta-agonists, ipratropium, and early intravenous corticosteroids.
- Parenteral magnesium, heliox, and noninvasive positive pressure ventilation may be useful in severe exacerbations.
- Circulatory depression due to pneumothorax or auto-PEEP must be recognized.
- Minute ventilation should be limited in intubated patients to prevent dangerous hyperinflation (DHI); hypercapnia is well-tolerated in adequately sedated patients.

EPIDEMIOLOGY AND DEFINITION

- Asthma is characterized by wheezing, dyspnea, cough, airway hyperreactivity, and reversible airflow

obstruction. Status asthmaticus is a life-threatening episode of asthma that is refractory to usual therapy.
- Severe attacks and death can occur regardless of the asthma severity classification.
- More than 5000 people die from asthma each year in the United States and this has increased significantly during the last two decades.

PATHOPHYSIOLOGY

- One consequence of airway inflammation in asthma is plugging of the large and small airways with tenacious mucus that can be striking on postmortem analysis. Less commonly, "sudden-onset asthma" results from a more pure form of smooth muscle-mediated bronchospasm.
- Triggers of sudden attacks include nonsteroidal anti-inflammatory agents, beta-blockers in susceptible patients, allergen/irritant exposure, exercise, stress, sulfites, and crack cocaine or heroine inhalation, and medical noncompliance.
- Airway obstruction causes V/Q mismatch. Intrapulmonary shunt is trivial so modest amounts (1–3 L/min) of supplemental oxygen generally correct hypoxemia. Supplemental oxygen reverses hypoxic vasoconstriction and bronchodilates the airways. Refractory hypoxemia is rare and suggests additional pathology.
- Respiratory alkalosis is a feature of acute asthma and may result in compensatory renal bicarbonate wasting (nongap metabolic acidosis). As airflow obstruction increases, $PaCO_2$ rises due to poor alveolar ventilation and a rise in CO_2 production from increased work of breathing.
- Lung mechanical abnormalities: hallmarks of expiratory airflow obstruction include incomplete alveolar gas emptying and elevated positive end-expiratory alveolar pressure. In the ventilated patients, the amount of intrinsic or auto-PEEP can be measured by the end-expiratory port occlusion technique as long as the patient is relaxed at end-expiration.
- Circulatory abnormalities reflect a state of cardiac tamponade resulting from dynamic hyperinflation (DHI) and pleural pressure changes. During expiration, high intrathoracic pressure decreases right-side preload. Vigorous inspiration augments right ventricular (RV) filling and shifts the interventricular septum to cause incomplete left ventricular (LV) filling. Lung hyperinflation increases RV afterload and may cause transient pulmonary hypertension. The net effect is to accentuate the normal inspiratory reduction in stroke volume, a phenomenon termed as *pulsus paradoxus*.
- Ventilatory failure is the result of several mechanisms including increased airway resistance, the inspiratory threshold load presented by auto-PEEP, respiratory muscle fatigue, systemic academia, and hypoperfusion from circulatory abnormalities.

CLINICAL FEATURES

- No single clinical measurements reliably predicts outcome.
- Characteristic of prior exacerbations that predict a fatal or near-fatal outcome include intubation, hypercapnia, barotrauma, hospitalization despite corticosteroids, psychiatric illness, substance abuse, and medical nonadherence.
- Severe exacerbations include several, but not necessarily all, of the following features: dyspnea at rest, upright positioning, inability to speak entire phrases, respiratory rate (RR) > 30/min, use of accessory muscle of respiration, heart rate (HR) > 120/min, pulsus paradoxus > 25 mmHg, peak expiratory flow rate < 50% predicted or personal best, hypoxemia and eucapnia or hypercapnia.
- Imminent respiratory arrest is characterized by altered mental status, paradoxical respirations, bradycardia, quiet chest from insufficient airflow, and absence of *pulsus paradoxus*. Bradycardia is an ominous sign as the usual rhythm is sinus tachycardia. Presence of subcutaneous emphysema suggests pneumomediastinum or pneumothorax.
- A peak expiratory flow rate or forced expiratory volume in one second (FEV_1) < 50% of predicted or personal best is an objective measure suggesting severe exacerbation and may be used to assess progress in the less critically ill patient.
- Hypercapnia on arterial blood gas suggests severe disease but is not always present. Patients who deteriorate clinically with impending respiratory failure should be intubated regardless of $PaCO_2$. Conversely, improving patients should not be intubated despite hypercapnia.
- Chest radiography is indicated when it is unclear if asthma is the cause of respiratory distress; when there are localizing signs or suspected barotraumas; and to check endotracheal tube position in mechanically ventilated patients.

THERAPY PRIOR TO INTUBATION

- Pharmacotherapy should start with inhaled albuterol and data support the addition of ipratropium to albuterol in any patient who is extremely ill on presentation or not responding quickly to albuterol alone.

- Systemic corticosteroids should be given early to treat the inflammatory component of acute asthma and there is evidence that this reduces the number of relapses in the first week and the risk of death. There is little benefit to the addition of inhaled corticosteroids.
- There is no benefit to adding aminophylline to inhaled beta-agonist, however, it is recommended to continue its use in those already taking it if attention is paid to serum levels.
- Several trials have failed to justify the routine use of IV magnesium sulfate but it is safe, inexpensive, and may be beneficial in severe exacerbations. Administration by inhalation is also being studied.
- Heliox (20% oxygen:80% helium) is less dense than air and allows more laminar flow and possibly increased distal delivery of albuterol. Concentrations of helium < 60% are ineffective, precluding its use in patients with significant hypoxemia.
- Noninvasive positive pressure ventilation is an option for patients with hypercapneic respiratory failure who do not require intubation as it helps overcome the adverse effects of auto-PEEP and unloads the inspiratory muscles.

MANAGEMENT OF THE INTUBATED ASTHMATIC

- The decision to intubate rests on the patient's ability to maintain spontaneous respiration.
- Goals of intubation/mechanical ventilation are to maintain oxygenation and prevent respiratory arrest.
- Hypotension is reported in 25–35% following intubation due to loss of vascular tone from sedation and loss of sympathetic activity. Hypovolemia and DHI may also contribute to the hypotension.
- DHI may be present if breaths sounds diminish, blood pressure (BP) falls, and HR rises. A trial of hypopnea (2–3 breaths/min) or apnea is both diagnostic and therapeutic for DHI.
- To avoid dangerous levels of DHI, minute ventilation should not exceed 115 mL/kg/min. RR is recommended at 12–14 breaths/min and tidal volume (TV) between 6 and 8 mL/kg. High inspiratory flow rates (above 60 L/min) do not prolong expiratory time meaningfully. Supplemental PEEP (at least 5 cmH_2O) should always be given, since auto-PEEP is universally present and will frustrate the patient's effort to trigger the ventilator. In some patients, higher levels of PEEP are useful to reduce the work of breathing. Externally applied PEEP generally does not raise the end-expiratory alveolar pressure, so there is little risk of worsening the hyperinflation or depressing the circulation.
- There is no consensus as to which ventilator mode to use. Both pressure-preset and volume-preset modes can be used successfully.
- Measurement of plateau pressure (Pplat) and auto-PEEP requires patient-ventilator synchrony and patient relaxation; however, neither measurement has been validated as a predictor of complications. Despite this, Pplat < 30 cmH_2O is generally safe and auto-PEEP < 15 cmH_2O is acceptable.
- Sedation is indicated to improve comfort, safety, and patient-ventilator synchrony. A continuous infusion of narcotic in combination with propofol or benzodiazepine is recommended. Short-term muscle paralysis is indicated if effective ventilation cannot be achieved by sedation alone; however, these agents should be minimized whenever possible to avoid the risk of postparalytic myopathy.
- Often 24–48 hours of treatment is needed before patients are ready for extubation. Readiness for extubation can generally be judged based on improving mechanical parameters. Prior to extubation, only a brief spontaneous breathing trial is recommended since a longer trial may provoke bronchospasm.

BIBLIOGRAPHY

Corbridge T, Hall JB. Status asthmaticus. In: Hall JB, Schmidt GA, Wood LDH, eds., *Principles of Critical Care*, 3rd ed. New York, NY: McGraw-Hill; 2005:567–582.

39 HEMOPTYSIS AND PULMONARY HEMORRHAGE

Maria Dowell

KEY POINTS

- Massive hemoptysis is defined as more than 300–600 mL in 12–24 hours.
- Massive lung hemorrhage can cause asphyxiation or severe hypoxemia.
- Causes of lung hemorrhage may be anatomic or diffuse and related to disordered coagulation or vascular integrity.
- Some patients with life-threatening DAH will have no hemoptysis.

- The plain chest radiograph usually discloses the side of bleeding.
- Any coagulopathy should generally be corrected aggressively, even when it is not the primary basis for the lung hemorrhage.
- Specialized airway, bronchoscopic, and angiographic techniques may be called for in protecting the lung, diagnosing the source of bleeding, or achieving control.
- Multidisciplinary involvement of a pulmonary specialist, interventional radiologist, rheumatologist, and thoracic surgeon is often helpful.

HEMOPTYSIS

- Most patients with hemoptysis do not require intensive care unless they have such large rates of bleeding that result in hemodynamic instability or they have life-threatening hypoxemia from parenchymal hemorrhage or extensive aspiration of blood.
- Massive hemoptysis is defined as >300–600 mL of blood in 12–24 hours although it is often clinically difficult for the patient to estimate. Also, some patients may have life-threatening hypoxemia due to alveolar hemorrhage, along with diffuse parenchymal infiltrates that satisfy criteria for acute respiratory distress syndrome (ARDS), yet have no hemoptysis.
- Many conditions may cause hemoptysis outlined in Table 39-1. The more common causes include bronchiectasis, mycetoma, tuberculosis, bronchogenic carcinoma, lung abscess, and vascular-bronchial fistulas.
- The most common cause of death in patients with hemoptysis is asphyxia from aspirated blood. If the site of bleeding is known, lateral decubitus positioning (bleeding lung down) may serve to protect the opposite lung. Small doses of codeine or morphine may be helpful to blunt the cough reflex and slow the rate of bleeding but at the risk of depressing the sensorium. Some patients, especially those with diffuse parenchymal hemorrhage, require intubation. In extreme circumstances, mainstem bronchus intubation of the nonbleeding side may protect the uninvolved lung.

TABLE 39-1 Causes of Hemoptysis

LOCALIZED BLEEDING	DIFFUSE BLEEDING
Infection • Bronchiectasis • Bronchitis • Bacterial pneumonia • Fungal infections • Tuberculosis (especially cavitary disease) • Lung abscess • Leprospirosis	Drug-induced • Anticoagulants • D-Penicillamine • Trimellitic anhydride (plastic, paint, epoxy manufacturing) • Cocaine • Propylthiouracil • Amiodarone • Dilantin
Tumors • Bronchogenic carcinoma (squamous cell) • Necrotizing parenchymal cancer (usually adenocarcinoma) • Bronchial adenoma	Blood dyscrasias • Thrombotic thrombocytopenic purpura • Hemophilia • Leukemia • Thrombocytopenia • Uremia • Antiphospholipid antibody syndrome
Cardiovascular problems • Mitral stenosis	Pulmonary-renal syndromes • Goodpasture syndrome • Wegener granulomatosis • Pauci-immune vasculitis
Pulmonary vascular problems • Pulmonary arteriovenous malformations • Pulmonary embolism with infarction • Bechet syndrome • Pulmonary artery catheterization with rupture	Vasculitis • Pulmonary capillaritis • Polyarteritis • Churg-Strauss syndrome • Henoch-Schönlein purpura • Necrotizing vasculitis • Connective tissue diseases • Pulmonary veno-occlusive disease
Others • Broncholithiasis • Sarcoidosis • Ankylosing spondylitis	Others • Hemosiderosis

INITIAL EVALUATION

- Initial evaluation includes careful inspection of the nose and mouth to exclude an upper airway source. Coagulation screening should include platelet count, prothrombin time (PT), partial thromboplastin time (PTT), fibrinogen level, and, in appropriate patients, antiphospholipid antibody assays. Blood should also be sent for blood urea nitrogen (BUN), creatinine, urinalysis, and serology screen (antinuclear antibodies [ANA], Rheumatoid factor [RF], complement levels, cryoglobulins, antineutrophil cytoplasmic antibodies [ANCA], antiglomerular basement membrane antibody) when excluding connective tissue disease and vasculitis.
- Chest x-ray will reveal the region of bleeding in 60% of cases. Fiberoptic bronchoscopy can locate endobronchial lesions or may at least locate the lobe or segment form which the bleeding is coming. If bleeding is brisk, visualization may be suboptimal and rigid bronchoscopy may be more useful. Chest computed tomography (CT) is similarly effective at determining the site of bleeding and may be very useful in detecting the source of bleeding as well. CT angiography is the gold standard and has an 80% sensitivity, 84% specificity, and 84% positive predictive value.

TREATMENT

- General treatment measures include maintaining platelet count >50,000 in an actively bleeding patient.

Platelet transfusion is common and intravenous immunoglobulin (IVIG) may be used if there is platelet destruction from immune-mediated causes. Dialysis, cryoprecipitate, or desmopressin (DDAVP) may be used for platelet dysfunction due to uremia. PT and PTT should be corrected to near normal with fresh frozen plasma or vitamin K.
- Bronchial arterial embolization is the treatment of choice for life-threatening hemoptysis from localized parenchymal lesions. Endobronchial ablation is reserved for palliative therapy in unresectable tumors affecting the larger airway. External beam irradiation has been used for mycetomas and occasionally for unresectable tumors.
- In the setting of diffuse disease, surgery is precluded. Indications for surgery include recurrence of bleeding after embolization, inability to embolize due to anatomic problems, or multiple bleeding vessels on angiography.

DIFFUSE ALVEOLAR HEMORRHAGE

- Up to 30% of patients with diffuse alveolar hemorrhage (DAH) will not have hemoptysis. Chest x-rays often show diffuse disease but localized disease may also be seen. DAH occurs in up to 33% of patients with microscopic polyangiitis, 10% of patients with Wegener granulomatosis, 10% of patients with Goodpasture syndrome, and 5% of patients with systemic lupus.
- Diagnosis is easily established when patients present with hemoptysis, diffuse infiltrates, falling hematocrit, and other manifestations of systemic disease. In those without hemoptysis or infiltrates, the diagnosis is more difficult. Increasingly bloody serial aspirations on bronchoalveolar lavage may be diagnostic. A renal biopsy or thoracoscopic lung biopsy is frequently recommended when DAH is diagnosed in order to differentiate the various types of vasculitis and to definitively diagnose or exclude Goodpasture disease since its treatment differs markedly from that of vasculitis.
- Despite treatment, >50% of patients with DAH from vasculitis or collagen vascular disease require mechanical ventilation. The mortality is 25% in patients with Wegener granulomatosus and 50% in patients with lupus.

BIBLIOGRAPHY

Albert RK. Massive hemoptysis. In: Hall JB, Schmidt GA, Wood LDH, eds., *Principles of Critical Care*, 3rd ed. New York, NY: McGraw-Hill; 2005:583–586.

40 RESTRICTIVE DISEASES OF THE RESPIRATORY SYSTEM

Maria Dowell

KEY POINTS

- Disorders of the chest wall that most profoundly impact ventilatory function include kyphoscoliosis (KS) and restrictive disease resulting from previous thoracoplasty.
- Respiratory mechanics and gas exchange are also significantly altered by the restrictive physiology of pulmonary fibrosis.
- Diseases of the respiratory muscles can depress ventilatory function.
- During mechanical ventilation, tidal volume should generally be limited to prevent lung injury and circulatory depression.

KYPHOSCOLIOSIS

- KS is the prototypical severe thoracic deformity seen in as many as 1 in 10,000 people in the United States.
- KS consists of anteroposterior angulation (kyphosis), lateral displacement (scoliosis), and often some rotation of the spine around its long axis.
- The most common form of KS is idiopathic (80%) although secondary KS may be seen (polio, muscular dystrophy).
- Clinical symptoms correlate with the degree of curvature. Less than 70° rarely results in cardiopulmonary sequelae. Angles >70° put patients at risk of developing respiratory failure, >100° are associated with dyspnea, and >120° may result in alveolar hypoventilation and cor pulmonale. On examination, patients exhibit a rapid shallow breathing pattern due to the reduction in lung and chest wall compliance. Often crackles or coarse wheezing are detected and reflect the atelectatic and deformed lung.
- Pulmonary function alterations typically include severe reduction in total lung capacity (TLC) and vital capacity (VC) due to reduced IC (inspiratory capacity; IC = TLC − FRC). Functional residual capacity (FRC) is reduced, expiratory reserve volume (ERV) is also low (ERV = FRC − RV), and residual volume (RV) is relatively spared. In advanced KS and neuromuscular disease associated with secondary KS, inspiratory muscle function is severely reduced and contributes to respiratory dysfunction.
- Gas exchange abnormalities include nocturnal hypercapnia and hypoxemia during rapid eye movement

(REM) sleep that may contribute to cardiovascular complications. Significant arterial hypoxemia often occurs late in the development of hypercapnia. A-a gradients are usually no more than 25 mmHg and result primarily from V/Q mismatch. Patients may have normal or reduced ventilatory response to inspired CO_2.

- As the spinal curvature increases, pulmonary hypertension may occur. This is a consequence of increased pulmonary vascular resistance from hypoxic vasoconstriction or anatomic abnormalities and not from elevated left atrial (LA) pressure. An increased gradient between the pulmonary artery diastolic pressure and the pulmonary wedge pressure usually exists. Early use of O_2 as well as correcting reversible causes of hypercapnia and sleep disordered breathing helps delay the onset of right ventricular (RV) failure.
- Acute cardiopulmonary failure: Often precipitated by pneumonia, upper respiratory tract infection, congestive heart failure (CHF), and occasionally pulmonary embolism (PE). Conservative management without invasive mechanical ventilation is effective in the majority of cases. One needs to look for potentially reversible causes (reversible airflow obstruction, aspiration). Arterial hypoxemia is aggravated by low venous saturation; therefore, raising the cardiac output or hemoglobin concentration or decreasing O_2 consumption will help. If shock occurs, mechanical ventilation is necessary. Patients in shock from sepsis may not mount the usual hyperdynamic response and if unresponsive to volume challenge, right heart catheterization may be helpful. Shock from right heart failure requires adequate circulating volume and correction of hypoxemia to reduce pulmonary vasoconstriction.
- Acute hypercapnic respiratory failure: Acute exacerbations are characterized by a dramatic decrease of respiratory system compliance and increase in work of breathing. Noninvasive positive-pressure ventilation (NIPPV) is considered first-line therapy and has the advantage of decreased incidence of nosocomial pneumonia/otitis/sinusitis, need for sedation, as well as improved patient comfort. Increased risk of aspiration, facial pressure necrosis, and less control of patient's ventilation compared with invasive ventilation are the disadvantages. Invasive ventilation is required for cardiopulmonary arrest, refractory hypoxemia, progressive ventilatory failure, and shock. Use small tidal volumes (6–7 mL/kg) and high respiratory rates (RR, 20–36/min) since large tidal volumes will raise the pleural pressure far more than usual, risking hemodynamic compromise. The addition of 5 cmH_2O positive end-expiratory pressure (PEEP) helps avoid collapse of alveoli at low lung volumes. Hypercapnia is generally well tolerated.

THORACOPLASTY

- A common surgical procedure used in the past to treat tuberculous empyema and cavitary pulmonary tuberculosis. It is second to KS in producing severe restrictive physiology as a result of distortion of the chest wall, pleural thickening, and secondary scoliosis.
- Other factors contributing to restriction in thoracoplasty include reduced respiratory system compliance, inspiratory muscle weakness, fibrothorax, lung resection, and phrenic nerve injury.
- Pulmonary function abnormalities are similar to those in KS. Unlike other restrictive diseases, however, coincident airflow obstruction is common.

PULMONARY FIBROSIS

- With extensive fibrosis, gas exchange units are deformed and dysfunctional and the lungs become small and stiff. Traction bronchiectasis may result in excess mucus production.
- As the fibrosis progresses, dyspnea occurs both at rest and with exercise, leading to a sedentary lifestyle and deconditioning. Dyspnea is often associated with a persistent, nonproductive cough.
- Rapid shallow breathing with higher than normal minute ventilation is common. Dry "Velcro" crackles may be heard on auscultation. Loud P_2, RV heave, jugular venous distention, and right-sided S_3 suggest pulmonary hypertension.
- Respiratory mechanics typically reveal reduced TLC, VC, and IC. Less of a reduction is seen in FRC and RV. Forced expired volume in one second (FEV_1) and forced vital capacity (FVC) are often reduced. Lung stiffness requires large negative pleural pressures to adequately breathe.
- Exercised-induced hypoxemia and low diffusing capacity (DLCO) are hallmarks of early disease. Later, resting hypoxemia and mild respiratory alkalosis are common. Sleep-related desaturation is due to exaggerated effects of normal nocturnal hypoventilation and V/Q variations or to respiratory muscle dysfunction and obstructive sleep apnea.
- Pulmonary hypertension and cor pulmonale are common in end-stage fibrosis (DLCO $< 45\%$ and VC $< 50\%$ of predicted).
- Acute cardiopulmonary failure: Common causes include pneumonia, bronchospasm, pulmonary embolus, aspiration, heart failure, and pneumothorax. If deterioration is seen over weeks to months, suspect progressive fibrosis, bronchogenic carcinoma, steroid myopathy, drug toxicity, cor pulmonale, or left ventricular (LV) failure. First-line therapy is targeted at

correcting hypoxemia with supplemental O_2, NIPPV or intubation, and mechanical ventilation if necessary to minimize the adverse effects of hypoxic pulmonary vasoconstriction. If intubated, the approach to mechanical ventilation is similar to acute respiratory distress syndrome (ARDS; tidal volume 6 mL/kg, RR 20–36/min, plateau pressure < 30 cmH_2O, PEEP 5 cmH_2O) to help reduce ventilator-induced lung injury. Unfortunately, there are several studies reporting the outcome of patients referred to the ICU for acute respiratory failure without a clearly identified reversible cause as very poor and not improved by mechanical ventilation.

RESPIRATORY MUSCLE WEAKNESS

- Reduced inspiratory muscle function (diaphragm, internal intercostals, and accessory muscles) produces restrictive respiratory mechanics and results in hypercapnia and respiratory failure. Impaired clearance of airway secretions is a common and potentially life-threatening problem in these patients.
- Causes include but are not limited to myasthenia gravis, postpoliomyelitis syndrome, amyotrophic lateral sclerosis, Guillain-Barré syndrome, Eaton-Lambert syndrome, muscular dystrophies, botulism, and critical illness polyneuropathy.
- Severe hypoxemia, hypercapnia, and acidemia are indications for respiratory support.
- Physical examination may reveal rapid, shallow breathing and paradoxical abdominal movements. Patients should be observed during sleep for nocturnal hypoventilation and obstructive sleep apnea.
- PI_{max} and PE_{max} are the most sensitive ways to quantify respiratory muscle weakness.
- Hypoxemic respiratory failure can often be treated adequately with supplemental O_2.
- With significant decline in lung volume and muscle strength, NIPPV or intubation and mechanical ventilation are needed. No particular mode of mechanical ventilation is superior; however, PEEP should be used to prevent atelectasis.

BIBLIOGRAPHY

Conti G, Rocco M, Antonelli M, et al. Respiratory system mechanics in the early phase of acute respiratory failure due to severe kyphoscoliosis. *Intensive Care Med* 1997;23:539–544.

Corbridge T, Wood LDH. Restrictive disease of the respiratory system and the abdominal compartment syndrome. In: Hall JB, Schmidt GA, Wood LDH, eds., *Principles of Critical Care*, 3rd ed. New York, NY: McGraw-Hill; 2005:587–598.

Fumeaux T, Rothmeier C, Jolliet P. Outcome of mechanical ventilation for acute respiratory failure in patients with pulmonary fibrosis. *Intensive Care Med* 2001;27:1868–1874.

Mason RJ, Murray JF, Broaddus VC, et al. *Textbook of Respiratory Medicine*, 4th ed. Philadelphia, PA: Elsevier; 2005.

Perrin C, Unterborn JN, D'Ambrosia C, et al. Pulmonary complications of chronic neuromuscular diseases and their management. *Muscle Nerve* 2004;29:5–27.

41 SLEEP-DISORDERED BREATHING

D. Kyle Hogarth

KEY POINTS

- The incidence of sleep-disordered breathing (SDB) is rising. Currently, SDB affects 2–4% of adults in the United States. In patients with COPD, the incidence can be as high as 20%.
- Untreated SDB leads to neurocognitive and cardiovascular end-organ effects.
- Untreated SDB can result in periods of profound hypoxemia and hypercapnia.
- OHS can be an end-stage manifestation of SDB, usually requiring admission to the ICU. These patients will usually require tracheostomy for definitive management of their disease.

SLEEP APNEA

- Sleep apnea is a disease state characterized by periods of absent breathing (apnea) or reduced tidal volumes (hypopneas). The apnea-hypopnea index (AHI) is the total number of apnea/hypopnea events per hour of sleep.
- Sleep apnea is divided into two categories: obstructive or central apnea. Obstructive apnea represents the majority of patients, though mixed obstructive/central apnea is not uncommon.
- Obstructive sleep apnea (OSA) is characterized by limitation of airflow in the upper airways due to a variety of factors, including anatomy, pharyngeal muscle tone, and obesity.
- Central sleep apnea (CSA) is characterized by disordered regulation of breathing and lack of appropriate neural output for control of respiratory function.

RISK FACTORS FOR OBSTRUCTIVE SLEEP APNEA

- Obesity
- Increased neck circumference
- Craniofacial abnormalities
- Hypothyroidism
- Acromegaly

FACTORS THAT CAN WORSEN/AGGRAVATE OBSTRUCTIVE SLEEP APNEA

- Upper airway injury
- Upper airway edema
- Alcohol or sedative use
- Hypothyroidism
- Hypoxia

RISK FACTORS FOR CENTRAL SLEEP APNEA

- Long-standing untreated OSA
- Poliomyelitis
- Encephalitis
- Brainstem neoplasm or infarction
- Spinal cord injury

DIAGNOSIS OF SLEEP APNEA

- Many patients with ICU admissions attributed to congestive heart failure or chronic obstructive pulmonary disease (COPD) actually suffer from profound OSA. It is important to maintain a high index of suspicion in patients with the risk factors mentioned above.
- Polysomnography remains the gold-standard study to accurately diagnose OSA.
- Portable systems for home use are available, but are not as proven as full polysomnography.
- Clinical scoring systems are useful, but are not reliable enough yet to accurately predict OSA.

COMPLICATIONS OF SLEEP APNEA

- Complications of sleep apnea are due to hypoventilation and hypoxemia. These complications can include:
  - Increased diurnal hypertension
  - Pulmonary hypertension
  - Left and right heart failure
  - Increased somnolence
  - Myocardial infarction
  - Stroke
- Complications of OSA that can lead to needs for critical care management include:
  - Postoperative respiratory failure:
    - General anesthesia decreases upper airway pharyngeal tone.
    - Upper airway edema may increase the resistance of the upper airway.
    - Central drive may be reduced from anesthetics.
    - Hypoxemia can be present from atelectasis and splinting.
  - Acute-on-chronic respiratory failure:
    - Can be difficult to discern whether respiratory failure is directly from an underlying illness such as COPD or directly from poorly treated OSA.
    - However, patients with both COPD and OSA have a higher risk for acute respiratory failure and have higher daytime $PaCO_2$ and lower daytime PaO_2.
- Long-term untreated OSA can progress to the obesity hypoventilation syndrome (OHS), a disease state characterized by:
  - Hypercapnia while awake
  - Hypersomnolence
  - Stupor
  - Right heart failure
  - Left heart failure
- OHS can be the principal cause of admission for respiratory failure to the ICU and should be considered in all patients with chronic hypercapnia.
- OHS can also aggravate other underlying conditions, such as ischemic cardiomyopathy and COPD.

MANAGEMENT OF SLEEP APNEA

- Positive pressure ventilation (PPV) is the management of choice for OSA. The application of external positive pressure maintains potency of the narrowed upper airway.
- Noninvasive ventilation may be helpful but, before this is relied on solely, the likelihood of compliance and follow-up, along with the potential for response must be considered along with the life-threatening nature of the patient critically ill from OSA.
- Oral appliances that move the mandible forward are also available, and may help some patients.
- Surgical options to reduce upper airway obstruction include uvulopalatopharyngoplasty, tonsillectomy, tongue ablation, and tracheostomy.
- Adequate treatment in the ICU is generally signaled by spontaneous diuresis, improved alertness, and (more gradually) lower $PaCO_2$.

BIBLIOGRAPHY

Flemmons WW. Obstructive sleep apnea. *N Engl J Med* 2002; 347:498–504.

Hall JB, Schmidt GA, Wood LA. An approach to critical care. In: Hall JB, Schmidt GA, Wood LA, eds., *Principles of Critical Care*, 3rd ed. New York, NY: McGraw-Hill; 2005:3–10.

Strollo PJ, Rogers RM. Obstructive sleep apnea. *N Engl J Med* 1996;334:99–104.

42 INHALATION INJURIES

Rekha Vij, Shashi Kiran Bellam

KEY POINTS

- Inhalation injury refers to the inhalation of toxic products of combustion.
- Early management focuses on maintaining airway patency and determining the need for intubation. Although obstruction is rarely present initially, serial assessments are required as inflammation and edema progress.
- Symptoms of bronchospasm and bronchorrhea may be minimal initially, and peak after 24–48 hours. These lead to increased work of breathing and decreased lung compliance.
- Late airway complications are primarily infectious.
- Treatment is primarily supportive, involving intubation, removal of secretions, and the use of PEEP.

PATHOPHYSIOLOGY/MECHANISMS OF INJURY

- *Thermal injuries*: These injuries tend to be limited to the upper airways, where mucosal damage results in erythema and ulceration. Edema may take up to 24 hours to develop, and typically resolves within 5 days.
- *Hypoxic gas inhalation*: As fire burns, it utilizes oxygen, decreasing the FiO_2 of ambient air. Inhaling hypoxic air not only decreases oxygen supply to vital organs, but also increases the toxic effects of other inhaled compounds, such as carbon monoxide.
- *Bronchospasm*: Several compounds found in smoke are irritants to the bronchial mucosa and alveoli, which trigger bronchospasm (Table 42-1).

TABLE 42-1 Common Components of Housefire Smoke

GAS	PROPERTY	SOURCE
Ammonia	Irritant	Nylon
Hydrogen chloride	Irritant	Polyvinyl chloride, insulation
Nitrogen oxides	Irritant	Wall paper, acetylene torches, jet engine fuel, diesel fumes
Phosgene	Irritant	Chlorinated hydrocarbons (paint stripping, welding)
Acrolein	Irritant	Wood, cotton, paper, acrylic, polyethylene, polypropylene
Benzene	Irritant	Petroleum plastics
Carbon monoxide	Asphyxiant	Incomplete combustion of any organic matter
Hydrogen cyanide	Asphyxiant	Wood, silk, nylon, polyurethane

SOURCE: Adapted from <<utdol.com>>—Smoke Inhalation.

- *Mucosal edema*: Inhaled toxins can damage tight junctions between epithelial cells, increasing vascular permeability, and causing mucosal edema. If severe, this may lead to airway obstruction.
- *Intrapulmonary shunting*: The combination of pulmonary edema and endobronchial debris contribute to V/Q mismatch and shunting.
- *Diminished compliance*: Persistent bronchospasm, bronchorrhea, and airway edema lead to decreased lung compliance and increased airway resistance.

DIAGNOSIS

- Early diagnosis relies on high clinical suspicion and a history of closed space exposure or aspiration of hot liquid or steam.
- Physical examination may reveal facial burns, singed nasal hairs, carbonaceous sputum, soot in the oropharynx, wheezing, cough, or altered mental status.
- Laboratory data should include arterial blood gas, carboxyhemoglobin and cyanide levels, and plasma lactate concentration.
- Initial chest radiographs are often normal. Serial studies are nonspecific, but may show bronchial wall thickening, air trapping, or diffuse interstitial, alveolar, or mixed infiltrates.
- Bronchoscopy is considered the gold standard for diagnosis. Direct visualization of the airways reveals endobronchial erythema and ulceration, providing information about the extent and severity of injury (Fig. 42-1).
- Radionuclide imaging using xenon-133 or technicium-99 can support the diagnosis, but are not widely used due to expense and logistic difficulty.

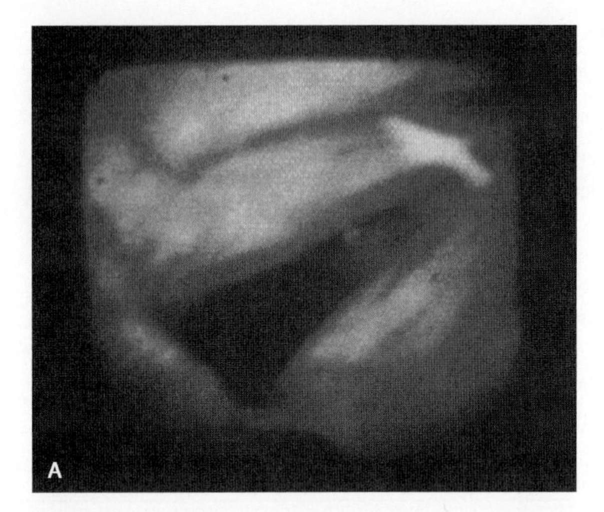

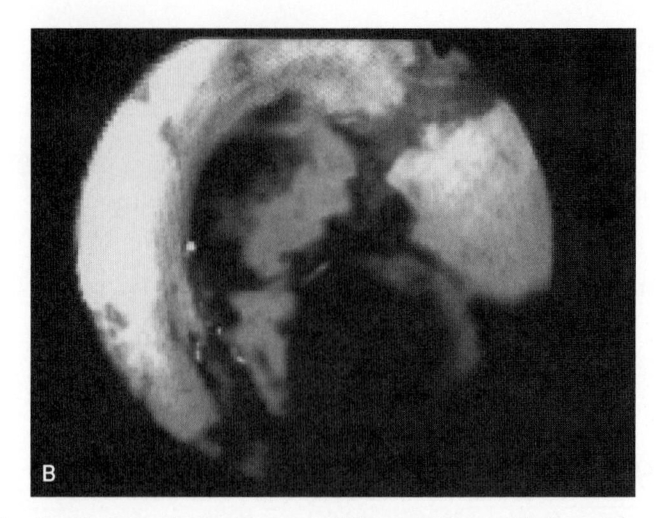

FIG. 42-1 Upper airway damage from smoke inhalation. (A) Vocal cord edema; (B) carbonaceous debris, erythema, and ulceration.
SOURCE: *Adapted from www.burnsurgery.com/Modules/initial_mgmt/sec_3.htm; pedsccm.wustl.edu/FILE-CABINET/Pulmonary/smoke_inhalation.html.*

RISK OF INFECTION

- In the setting of severe airway injury, there are several factors that contribute to an increased likelihood of tracheobronchitis or pneumonia:
  - Necrotic epithelium sloughs off, leading to obstruction of distal airways and atelectasis.
  - Neutrophils and alveolar macrophages function abnormally.
  - Mucociliary clearance is decreased.
- Classic radiographic findings of pneumonia may not be present because of the diffuse nature of the infection and its location in central airways.
- Corticosteroids and prophylactic antibiotics have not been shown to be effective.

MANAGEMENT

- Treatment is largely supportive, focusing on airway protection/intubation, oxygen supplementation, and antibiotics for documented infection.
- Pulse oximetry is affected by carboxyhemoglobin and methemoglobin; arterial oxygen saturation should be measured with co-oximetry instead.
- Criteria for intubation include: stridor, respiratory distress, deep burns to the face or neck, significant oropharyngeal edema.
- Aerosolized bronchodilators can be helpful in the initial treatment of bronchospasm. However, after the first 24 hours, airway resistance is more likely to be due to airway edema, and bronchodilators may no longer be effective.
- Intubation should be performed with a large endotracheal tube (7.0 mm in internal diameter or larger) to facilitate the clearance of secretions. The use of humidified oxygen can also help mobilize secretions.
- Positive end-expiratory pressure (PEEP) should be used to maintain small airway patency, recruit atelectatic alveoli, and improve oxygenation.
- Extubation is appropriate after upper airway edema has resolved. Although no test accurately predicts airway patency, serial laryngoscopy and cuff-leak tests may be helpful.
- Long-term sequelae of inhalation injury include bronchiectasis, tracheal stenosis, interstitial fibrosis, and bronchiolitis obliterans.

FUTURE THERAPIES

- Several studies in animal models may help shape future treatment recommendations for inhalation injury.
  - Exogenous surfactant has been shown to improve lung compliance and oxygenation in a dog model.
  - Leukotriene inhibitors decreased the severity of pulmonary edema in a sheep model.
  - Intravenous lisofylline decreases inflammatory mediators and inhibits neutrophil recruitment. When used with nebulized heparin, this reduces intrapulmonary shunting and improves ventilation.

BIBLIOGRAPHY

American Burn Association. Inhalation injury: diagnosis. *J Am Coll Surg* 2003;196:308–312.

Hales CA, Musto S, Hutchinson WG, et al. BW-755C diminishes smoke-induced pulmonary edema. *J Appl Physiol* 1995;78: 64–69.

Hall JB, Schmidt GA, Wood LDH, eds. *Principles of Critical Care*, 3rd ed. New York, NY: McGraw-Hill; 2005.

Haponik E, Munster A. *Respiratory Injury: Smoke Inhalation and Burns*. New York, NY: McGraw-Hill; 1990.

Miller K, Chang A. Acute inhalation injury. *Emerg Med Clin North Am* 2003;21:533–557.

Monafo W. Initial management of burns. *N Engl J Med* 1996;335: 1581–1583.

Nieman GF, Paskanik AM, Fluck RR,et al. Comparison of exogenous surfactant in the treatment of wood smoke inhalation. *Am J Respir Crit Care Med* 1995;152:597–602.

Rabinowitz PM, Siegel MD. Acute inhalation injury. *Clin Chest Med* 2002;23:707–715.

Tasaki O, Mozingo DW, Ishihara S, et al. Effect of Sulfo Lewis C on smoke inhalation injury in an ovine model. *Crit Care Med* 1998;26:1238–1243.

Section 4
INFECTIOUS DISORDERS

43 SEPSIS, SEVERE SEPSIS, AND SEPTIC SHOCK

Michael Moore

KEY POINTS

- Sepsis is defined as the combination of infection and systemic inflammation.
- Mortality and morbidity is particularly high in the subset of patients with sepsis and at least one organ failure, termed "severe sepsis."
- Complications of sepsis may involve the circulation, lung, kidney, liver, hematologic system, gastrointestinal tract, CNS, peripheral nerves, and the metabolic milieu.
- Treatment begins with source control, antimicrobial therapy, and supportive measures.
- Most patients require large volumes of intravenous fluids. If these fail to restore blood pressure, vasoactive drugs (such as norepinephrine) should be infused and adrenal insufficiency excluded.
- Initial antibiotics should cover any organism of greater than trivial probability but the spectrum of coverage should be narrowed as additional diagnostic information is gained.
- For patients with severe sepsis and septic shock, urgent resuscitation to a central venous oxyhemoglobin saturation ($ScvO_2$) >70% and infusion of drotrecogin alpha may improve outcome.
- Patients requiring mechanical ventilation should generally be ventilated using a lung-protective strategy including volume assist-control mode with 6 mL/kg predicted body weight.
- The roles of intensive insulin therapy and low-dose corticosteroids remain subject to study.

INTRODUCTION

- Sepsis is a complex syndrome that results from severe infection that leads to systemic inflammation and widespread tissue damage, often remote from the initial site of injury.
- It can produce a range of clinical conditions that can rapidly result in hypotension, perfusion abnormalities, global tissue hypoxia with single or multiple organ dysfunction, and ultimately death.
- Rapid and timely intervention is critical to successful treatment.
- Only recently have clinical trials suggested that specific strategies and new therapies may improve survival in severe sepsis.
- Effective interventions require rapid diagnosis and prompt and appropriate treatment including cardiopulmonary support, antibiotics, source control, general supportive care, and, for those with severe sepsis at high risk of death, drotrecogin alpha.
- Because sepsis and the clinical consequences of sepsis have been historically difficult to define, diagnose, and treat, the American College of Chest Physicians (ACCP) and the Society of Critical Care Medicine (SCCM) sponsored a consensus conference to improve definitions and set up a framework for research and patient care.

AMERICAN COLLEGE OF CHEST PHYSICIANS/SOCIETY OF CRITICAL CARE MEDICINE DEFINITION OF SEPSIS AND RELATED DISORDERS

- *Infection*: Microbial phenomenon characterized by an inflammatory response to the presence of microorganisms or the invasion of normally sterile host tissue by those organisms.

- *Bacteremia*: The presence of viable bacteria in the blood.
- *Systemic inflammatory response syndrome (SIRS)*: Generalized inflammatory response to a variety of clinical insults. The syndrome is characterized by two or more of the following:
  - Temperature >38°C or <36°C
  - Heart rate >90 beats/min
  - Respiratory rate >20 breaths/min or $PaCO_2$ <32 mmHg
  - WBC >12,000 cells/mm^3, <4000 cells/mm^3, or >10% immature (band) forms
- *Sepsis*: The systemic response to infection manifested by two or more SIRS criteria resulting from an infection.
- *Severe sepsis*: Sepsis is defined as severe when it is associated with hypotension, hypoperfusion, or organ dysfunction.
- *Septic shock*: Sepsis associated with hypotension that persists despite adequate fluid resuscitation and resulting in one or more organ failures. This includes oliguria, lactic acidosis, acute mental status changes, respiratory failure, or the need for vasopressor support.

EPIDEMIOLOGY

- The incidence of sepsis is increasing and is expected to increase approximately 1.5% per year until at least 2050 (Angus et al., 2001).
- The incidence of sepsis has increased 8.7% per year from 1979 through 2000, now with almost 660,000 cases per year.
- The incidence is higher among men versus women and among nonwhite persons versus white persons (Martin et al., 2003).
- Angus et al. evaluated over 6.5 million discharge records from seven large states in 1995:
  - Estimated 750,000 cases of sepsis per year.
  - Mortality rate was 28.6% with a national estimate of 215,000 deaths.
  - Average cost per case was $22,100.
- Most common causative organisms in 2000 (Martin et al., 2003):
  - Gram-positive bacteria 52.1%
  - Gram-negative bacteria 37.6%
  - Polymicrobial infections 4.7%
  - Fungi 4.6%
  - Anaerobic bacteria 1.0%
  - No specific organism is cultured in approximately 50% of cases (Martin et al., 2003)
- Most common sites of infection (Angus et al., 2001):
  - Respiratory tract (44%)
  - Bacteremia (17.3%)
  - Genitourinary (9.1%)
  - Abdominal (8.6%)
  - Wound/soft tissue (6.6%)
  - Device-related (2.2%)
  - Central nervous system (CNS) (0.8%)
  - Endocarditis (0.6%)
- Mortality:
  - About 30% of patients die within the first month of diagnosis and 50% die within 6 months.
  - Up to 135,000 European and 215,000 American deaths each year.
  - Kills approximately 1400 people worldwide every day.
  - Severe sepsis is the leading cause of death in the noncoronary intensive care unit (ICU).
- Sepsis is increasingly recognized as a disease of the elderly with an age-specific incidence of severe sepsis of 26.2/1000 in persons >85 years old.

PATHOGENESIS

- The sepsis syndrome results from the host's immune response to infection: concepts related to its pathogenesis are evolving.
- The normal host response to infection is the activation of local and circulating phagocytic cells and generation of proinflammatory and anti-inflammatory mediators designed to limit and control bacterial invasion of host tissues.
- The prevailing theory has been that sepsis is the result of an uncontrolled or hyperimmune response to infection.
- The balance of proinflammatory and anti-inflammatory elements serves to facilitate tissue repair and healing.
- Remote tissue injury may ensue if the equilibrium between these opposing forces is lost and new data suggest that death may result from a prolonged systemic hypoimmune response.
- Host factors that confer an increased risk of sepsis:
  - Break in membrane integrity (surgery, toxic injury to epithelium)
  - Age (very young, elderly)
  - Gender (men > women)
  - Race (nonwhite > white)
  - Genetic polymorphisms (e.g., tumor necrosis factor [TNF] promoter gene and toll-like receptors)
  - Comorbidities (e.g., diabetes mellitus and immunosuppression)
- Pathogenic microbial factors:
  - Properties of capsule or envelope:
    - Pili of *Escherichia coli* enable colonization of urinary epithelium.
    - Capsular polysaccharides of *Streptococcus pneumoniae* prevent phagocytosis.
  - Cell wall components:
    - Lipopolysaccharide of Gram-negative organisms is known to trigger the septic response.

- Exotoxins:
  - Gram-positive organisms can secret exotoxins that act as superantigens bypassing normal antigenic specificity and costimulatory signals required for T-cell activation.
  - Hyaluronidase can promote bacterial spread along tissue planes.

EXPANDED DEFINITIONS OF ACUTE ORGAN DYSFUNCTION IN SEVERE SEPSIS OR SEPTIC SHOCK

CARDIOVASCULAR SYSTEM

- Arterial systolic blood pressure ≤90 mmHg or the mean arterial pressure (MAP) ≤70 mmHg for at least 1 hour despite adequate fluid resuscitation or the use of vasopressors in an attempt to maintain a systolic blood pressure of ≥90 mmHg or a MAP of ≥65 mmHg (Levy et al., 2003)
- Tachycardia
- Arrhythmias
- Cardiac arrest

RESPIRATORY SYSTEM

- The ratio of PaO_2 to FiO_2 ≤250 in the presence of other dysfunctional organs or systems or ≤200 if the lung is the only dysfunctional organ
- PaO_2 <70 mmHg
- SaO_2 <90%
- Tachypnea
- Mechanical ventilator dependence with or without positive end-expiratory pressure (PEEP)

RENAL

- Urine output <0.5 mL/kg of body weight/h for 1 hour, despite adequate fluid resuscitation
- Acute elevation of serum creatinine
- Oliguria
- Anuria
- Requirement for renal replacement therapy

HEMATOLOGIC

- Platelet count <80,000/mm^3 or having decreased by 50% in the preceding 3 days
- Leukocytosis/leukopenia
- Increased prothrombin time
- Elevated partial thromboplastin time
- Decreased protein C
- Increased D-dimer
- Impaired leukocyte function

GASTROINTESTINAL

- Elevated pancreatic enzymes (amylase, lipase)
- Decreased gastric pHi
- Ileus
- GI bleeding or perforation
- Intestinal ischemia
- Acalculous cholecystitis
- Acute pancreatitis
- Intolerance of enteral nutrition

HEPATIC

- Hyperbilirubinemia
- Elevated aminotransferases
- Increased lactate dehydrogenase (LDH)
- Elevated alkaline phosphatase
- Hypoalbuminemia
- Elevated prothrombin time
- Jaundice
- Asterixis

NEUROLOGIC

- Delirium
- Altered consciousness
- Impaired mentation
- Confusion
- Psychosis
- Abnormal electroencephalogram (EEG)

METABOLIC/ENDOCRINE

- pH <7.30 or a base deficit ≥5.0 mmol/L in association with a plasma lactate level >1.5 times the upper limit of the normal value
- Hyperglycemia
- Hypertriglyceridemia
- Hypoalbuminemia

PROGNOSIS

- Prognosis in severe infections has multiple determinants including host defense mechanisms, the environment, and the specific microorganisms involved.

- Specific risk factors for death include comorbid conditions, severity of acute illness and acute organ dysfunction, shock, nosocomial infection, and infection caused by aerobic gram-negative bacilli, enterobacteria, *Staphylococcus aureus*, and infection from a gastrointestinal or unknown source.
- The number and severity of organ failures are significantly associated with outcome.
  - Risk factors for hospital mortality were evaluated in 3608 ICU patients included in the European Sepsis Study.
  - Mortality was similar for patients with infection and sepsis but increased in patients with sepsis and organ dysfunction (i.e., severe sepsis or septic shock).

MANAGEMENT

INITIAL EVALUATION

- Severe sepsis is a medical emergency and immediate attention to the "ABCs" or airway, breathing, and circulation is appropriate.
- After initial stabilization, the source of infection should be established, controlled, and broad-spectrum antibiotics should be administered.
- Source control of infection includes identifying all potential foci of infection and directly examining material from these sites by Gram's stain, culture, and immunologic studies (where appropriate).
- After these initial steps, consider additional support for dysfunctional or failing organs, disease-specific interventions, and other general supportive care measures.
- Consider early hemodynamic monitoring including arterial line and central venous catheter for measurement of central venous pressure (CVP) and the $ScvO_2$.
- Eleven international organizations have published Surviving Sepsis Campaign (SSC) guidelines for managing severe sepsis and septic shock (Table 43-1).

INITIAL RESUSCITATION

- Initial intervention is administration of large amount of intravenous fluids to reverse organ hypoperfusion in the setting of relative hypovolemia.
- Fluid deficits may be in the range of 6–10 L of crystalloids.
- Fluid choice has been controversial in the past but the recent SAFE (Saline vs. Albumin Fluid Evaluation) study has shown that there is no therapeutic advantage to colloids versus crystalloids.
- Early (first 6 hours), goal-orientated resuscitation, aimed at raising the $ScvO_2$ to at least 70% in severe sepsis or septic shock, improved outcome in a single study. Those

TABLE 43-1 Synopsis of Major SSC Practice Guidelines

INTERVENTION	GUIDELINES RECOMMENDATION
Initial resuscitation	1. Resuscitate within 60 min to achieve a MAP ≥ 65 mmHg, urine output ≥ 0.5 mL/kg/h, and a CVP of 8–12 mmHg (12–15 mmHg in mechanically ventilated patients) 2. Packed red blood cells or dobutamine to achieve an $ScvO_2$ of ≥70%
Fluids	1. Crystalloids or colloids 2. Packed red blood cells to achieve a target Hb of 7–9 g/dL
Source control and antibiotics	1. The site of infection should be rapidly identified and appropriate source control measures instituted 2. When the specific infecting organism is unknown, empiric antibiotics should be administered within the first hour of treatment
Mechanical ventilation	1. 6 mL/kg tidal volume (IBW) for patients with ALI/ARDS 2. Avoid increased V_T plus increased plateau pressure (PP)—maintain end-expiratory PP <30 cmH_2O 3. PEEP should be employed to avoid oxygen toxicity in patients treated with high FiO_2 4. Consider prone positioning in patients with dangerous FiO_2 levels
Drotrecogin alfa (activated)	1. Indicated for all patients at high risk of death 2. No absolute contraindication 3. Administer as soon as possible after "high-risk of death" identified
Steroids	1. Indicated for patients with vasodepressor-dependent shock despite fluids 2. Administer 200–300 mg/day × 7 days by either continuous intravenous infusion or in divided doses at 6-h intervals. 3. The following steroid-related issues remain unresolved: adrenocorticotropic hormone (ACTH) stimulation test, weaning, mineralocorticoid, need to discontinue after resolution of shock
Glycemia control	1. Maintain blood glucose <150 mg/dL with insulin and glucose* 2. Monitor glucose concentrations at the bedside
Sedation	1. Intermittent as required, or; 2. Continuous with daily interruption

*The SSC group expressed concerns that an initial recommendation for strict glycemic management (80–110 mg/dL) might be so stringent that it might not be adopted.

randomized to goal-directed resuscitation received more fluid, blood, and dobutamine in the early hours.

HEMODYNAMIC SUPPORT

- Vasopressor and inotropes are added if fluid resuscitation fails to restore adequate arterial pressure and organ perfusion.
- Invasive monitoring of blood pressure is recommended.
- A number of different agents are available and the choice of agents requires knowledge of the pharmacodynamic properties as well as appropriate application to the clinical situation.
- There have been no large scale, randomized, controlled trials to determine which vasoactive drug strategy is best, but norepinephrine is the most commonly used initial vasoconstrictor.
- Vasopressin may be useful as a catecholamine-sparing agent.
- Monitor for restoration of perfusion to vital organs and peripheral tissues.
- Typical goals include MAP >65 mmHg, warm extremities, normal capillary refill, increased urinary output, and improved mentation.
- Careful monitoring for complications of vasoactive drugs including impaired splanchnic blood flow and oxygenation, impaired distal extremity perfusion, and worsening acidemia.

RESPIRATORY SUPPORT

- Sepsis is a significant stressor on the respiratory system.
- Up to 85% of patients with severe sepsis require ventilatory support.
- Supplemental oxygen should be given to maintain SaO_2 >87%.
- Recognition of the signs of impending respiratory failure is critical.
- Endotracheal intubation and mechanical ventilation may stabilize the septic patient and redirect cardiac output from the respiratory muscles to vital organs.
- A lung-protective strategy (V_T 6 mL/kg ideal body weight [IBW]) for patients with evidence of acute lung injury (ALI) or acute respiratory distress syndrome (ARDS) should be considered the standard of care (see Chaps. 34 and 35).

IMPORTANCE OF EARLY GOAL-DIRECTED THERAPY

- Rivers et al. (2001) recently showed that the early provision of therapy to maintain specific hemodynamic goals significantly reduced in-hospital mortality in severe sepsis and septic shock patients compared to standard hemodynamic therapy (30.5% vs. 46.5%; $P = .009$).
- 28-day (33.3% vs. 49.2%; $P = .01$) and 60-day (44.3% vs. 56.9%; $P = .03$) mortality rates significantly decreased.
- This study indicates the importance of the early identification and resuscitation of patients with severe sepsis to restore the balance between oxygen supply and demand to avoid cardiovascular collapse and death.

INFECTION MANAGEMENT

- Includes source control and prompt administration of anti-infective agents that cover the microbial organisms suspected in the context of the patient's presentation.
- Source control can be divided into three broad categories (Jimenez and Marshall, 2001):
  - Drainage of an abscess
  - Debridement of devitalized or infected tissue
  - Removal of foreign bodies colonized by pathogens and diversion, repair, or excision of an infected focus in a hollow viscus
- The presentation of infected foci can be subtle and requires a thoughtful search.
- Principles of anti-infective therapy in severe sepsis are:
  - Obtain cultures of suspected sources of infection
  - Promptly administer parenteral antibiotics
  - Antibiotic choice is based on many factors:
    - Most probable diagnosis and suspected pathogens
    - Site of acquisition (i.e., community or nosocomial)
    - Results of Gram's stain
    - History of prior antimicrobial treatment
    - Known resistance patterns in the community or institution
    - The drug's tissue penetration
    - Comorbidities
    - The patient's hepatic and renal function
    - History of allergy to antibiotics
    - Potential toxicity
    - Risk of influencing resistance
  - Initial therapy should be broad spectrum and progressively narrowed as microbiologic data become available
  - Patients should be monitored closely:
    - Evidence of a response
    - Development of drug toxicity
    - Selection of antibiotic-resistant strains
    - Appearance of a superinfection
- Specific antibiotics are discussed elsewhere.

SEPSIS-SPECIFIC INTERVENTIONS

- Early goal-directed therapy aimed at raising the $ScvO_2$ to at least 70%.

- Drotrecogin alfa (activated):
  - Drotrecogin alfa (activated) is a recombinant human version of activated protein C that represents the first therapy against sepsis to show efficacy in a phase III clinical trial.
  - The PROWESS (Recombinant Human Activated Protein C Worldwide Evaluation in Severe Sepsis) trial is discussed in detail in Chap. 45.
  - In general, patients with severe sepsis and a high risk of death without contraindications are candidates for therapy.
- Replacement dose corticosteroids:
  - Despite earlier negative trials, recent studies have indicated that low-dose corticosteroids may reduce morbidity and mortality in septic shock patients.
  - Stress dose steroids are indicated in patients with known adrenal insufficiency.
  - A French multicenter placebo-controlled, randomized, double-blind, parallel group trial (n = 300) demonstrated improved survival in patients with septic shock treated with low-dose hydrocortisone and fludrocortisone:
    - 28-day survival benefit was limited to patients with relative adrenal insufficiency (change in cortisol level <9 mg/dL after cosyntropin stimulation).
    - No increase of adverse events in the treatment group was found.
    - A larger European trial to confirm these results is underway.

GENERAL SUPPORTIVE MEASURES

- Adequate nutritional support is necessary as in any other critically ill patient.
- Glycemic control:
  - Critically ill patient commonly have hyperglycemia associated with insulin resistance which can contribute to severe infections, polyneuropathy, multiple organ failure, and death.
  - Intensive insulin therapy in a group of surgical ICU patients reduced in-hospital mortality by 34%.
  - A similar protocol in medical critical illness failed to show any benefit to strict glycemic control.
  - Other benefits in the surgical trial:
    - Decreased incidence of acute renal failure
    - Decreased incidence of episodes of septicemia
    - Decreased incidence of bloodstream infections
    - Reduced levels of inflammatory markers
    - Less prolonged use of antibiotics
    - Fewer red cell transfusions required
    - Less risk of polyneuropathy
    - Shorter length of stay in the ICU (16.8% of patients in the intensive treatment group stayed for over 5 days vs. 26.3% of control patients)
- Dialysis:
  - The risk of mortality in sepsis patients with acute renal failure is >50%.
  - Renal replacement therapies in critically ill patients are primarily limited to intermittent renal replacement therapy (IRRT) and continuous renal replacement therapy (CRRT).
  - A recent meta-analysis suggested that CRRT was associated with a significant mortality reduction ($P < .01$) when adjustments were made for study quality and severity of illness.
- Stress ulcer prophylaxis.
- Thromboembolism prophylaxis.

BIBLIOGRAPHY

American College of Chest Physicians/Society of Critical Care Medicine. Consensus Conference: definitions for sepsis and organ failure and guidelines for the use of innovative therapies in sepsis. *Crit Care Med* 1992;20:864–874.

Angus DC, Linde-Zwirble WT, Lidicker J, et al. Epidemiology of severe sepsis in the United States: analysis of incidence, outcome, and associated costs of care. *Crit Care Med* 2001;29:1303–1310.

Annane D, Bellissant E, Bollaert PE, et al. Corticosteroids for severe sepsis and septic shock: a systematic review and meta-analysis. *BMJ* 2004;329:480–488.

Balk RA. Pathogenesis and management of multiple organ dysfunction or failure in severe sepsis and septic shock. *Crit Care Clin* 2000;16;337–352.

Bernard GR, Vincent J-L, Laterre P-F, et al. Efficacy and safety of recombinant human activated protein C for severe sepsis. *N Engl J Med* 2001;344:699–709.

Bollaert PE, Chapentier C, Levy B, et al. Reversal of late septic shock with supraphysiologic doses of hydrocortisone. *Crit Care Med* 1998;26:645–650.

Briegel J, Forst H, Haller M, et al. Stress doses of hydrocortisone reverse hyperdynamic septic shock: a prospective, randomized, double-blind, single center study. *Crit Care Med* 1999;27:723–732.

Hall JB, Schmidt, GA, Wood LDH. *Principles of Critical Care*, 3rd ed. New York, NY: McGraw-Hill; 2005:1123–1136.

Hollenberg SM, Ahrens TS, Annane D, et al. Practice parameters for hemodynamic support of sepsis in adult patients: 2006 update. *Crit Care Med* 2004;32:1928–1948.

Hotchkiss SR, Karl IE. The pathophysiology and treatment of sepsis. *N Engl J Med* 2003;348:138–150.

Jimenez MF, Marshall JC. Source control in the management of sepsis. *Intensive Care Med* 2001;27(Suppl):S49–S62.

Kellum JA, Angus DC, Johnson JP, et al. Continuous versus intermittent renal replacement therapy: a meta-analysis. *Intensive Care Med* 2002;28:29–37.

Levy MM, Fink MP, Marshall JC, et al. 2001 SCCM/ESICM/ACCP/ATS/SIS International Sepsis Definitions Conference. *Crit Care Med* 2003;31:1250–1256.

Martin GS, Mannino DM, Eaton S, et al. The epidemiology of sepsis in the United States from 1979 through 2000. *N Engl J Med* 2003;348:1546–1554.

Natanson C, Esposito CJ, Banks SM. The sirens' songs of confirmatory sepsis trials: selection bias and sampling error. *Crit Care Med* 1998;26:1927–1931.

Patel BM, Chittock DR, Russell JA, et al. Beneficial effects of short-term vasopressin infusion during severe septic shock. *Anesthesiology* 2002;96:576–582.

Surviving Sepsis Campaign guidelines for management of severe sepsis and septic shock. *Crit Care Med* 2004;32: 858–873.

van den Berghe G, Wouters P, Weekers F, et al. Intensive insulin therapy in the surgical intensive care unit. *N Engl J Med* 2001;345:1359–1367.

44 EARLY GOAL-DIRECTED THERAPY FOR SEPSIS

Jonathan D. Paul

KEY POINTS

- Severe sepsis and septic shock are associated with severe morbidity and mortality, and rapid intervention is critical.
- Patient-specific end points, as opposed to global end points not accounting for the body's metabolic status, are necessary for successful resuscitation.
- For patients with severe sepsis and septic shock, central venous oxyhemoglobin saturation should be monitored and resuscitation in the first 6 hours should be aimed at raising its value to at least 70%.

PRINCIPLES

- A landmark study of sepsis resuscitation was performed to determine whether early goal-directed therapy (EGDT) in the emergency department improves outcomes in patients with severe sepsis and septic shock.
- Resuscitation of septic patients to restore a normal central venous oxyhemoglobin saturation was hypothesized to ensure a balance between systemic oxygen delivery and oxygen demand.
- Simple hemodynamic monitoring of the patient, as assessed by vital signs, physical examination, central venous pressure determination, and measurement of urinary output are useful screening tools to identify severe sepsis and septic shock.
- Resuscitation to mean arterial pressure (MAP) >65 mmHg, central venous pressure (CVP) 8–12 cmH_2O, and urine output (UO) of 0.5 mL/kg/h did not resuscitate effectively many subjects with sepsis. In contrast, titration in the first 6 hours to raise the central venous oxyhemoglobin saturation from a starting average value of 49% to a value exceeding 70% significantly reduced mortality.

METHODS

- The study was prospective, randomized, blinded, and controlled.
- Inclusion criteria included fulfillment of two out of four criteria for the systemic inflammatory response syndrome (SIRS) and a systolic blood pressure <90 mmHg (after a small fluid challenge) or a serum lactate concentration of at least 4 mmol/L.
- Criteria for SIRS are temperature ≥38°C or <36°C, heart rate >90, respiratory rate >20 or partial pressure of arterial CO_2 <32 mmHg, and WBC count >12,000/mm^3 or <4000/mm^3 or the presence of more than 10% immature band forms.
- Exclusion criteria included age <18, pregnancy, or the presence of an acute cerebral vascular event, acute coronary syndrome, acute pulmonary edema, status asthmaticus, cardiac dysrhythmias (as a primary diagnosis), contraindication to central venous catheterization, active gastrointestinal hemorrhage, seizure, drug overdose, burn injury, trauma, a requirement for immediate surgery, uncured cancer, immunosuppression, do-not-resuscitate status, or advance directives preventing implementation of the protocol.
- Standard therapy consisted of treatment at the clinicians' discretion according to a protocol for hemodynamic support (CVP ≥8–12 mmHg, MAP ≥65 mmHg, and UO ≥0.5 mL/kg/h).
- EGDT patients were monitored in the emergency department for at least 6 hours according to the same end points, but additionally to a central venous oxygen saturation ($ScvO_2$) ≥70% (Fig. 44-1).
- $ScvO_2$ ≥70% was raised by additional fluid infusion, transfusion of RBCs until the hematocrit was ≥30%, administration of inotropic agents, or intubation and mechanical ventilation.

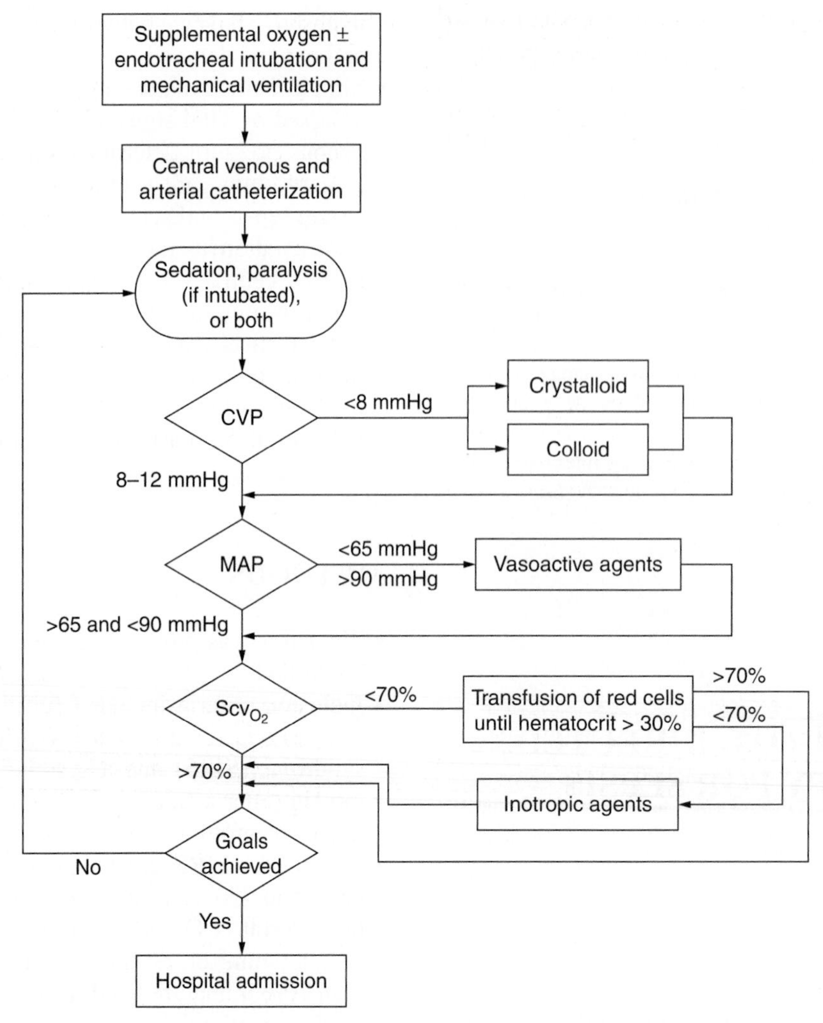

FIG. 44-1 Protocol for EGDT.
SOURCE: Rivers E, Nguyen B, Havstad S, et al. Early goal-directed therapy in the treatment of severe sepsis and septic shock. *N Engl J Med* 2001;345:1368–1377.

- Patients in both groups were subsequently transferred to intensive care units (ICU) under the care of critical care clinicians, and these physicians were blinded to which protocol each patient was assigned.

RESULTS

- During the initial 6 hours in the emergency department, the goal of $ScvO_2$ ≥70% was met by 60.2% of patients in the standard therapy group and 94.9% of patients in the EGDT group. The goals for CVP, MAP, and UO were achieved in 86.1% of patients in the standard therapy group and 99.2% of patients in the EGDT group.
- In the ICU, during 7–72 hours, patients in the standard therapy group had significantly higher heart rates and lower MAPs than patients in the EGDT group. Also, patients in the EGDT group had significantly higher $ScvO_2$ values than those in the standard therapy group. The two groups had similar CVP values.
- Common indices of organ dysfunction in the ICU (acute physiologic and chronic health evaluation [APACHE II] score, simplified acute physiology score [SAPS II], and multiple organ dysfunction score [MODS]) were significantly more deranged in patients in the standard therapy group.
- Overall in-hospital mortality rates were significantly higher in the standard therapy group than in the EGDT group. Mortality at 28 and 60 days was also higher in the standard therapy group (Table 44-1).
- Of the patients surviving until hospital discharge, those in the standard therapy group had significantly longer hospital stays.

TABLE 44-1 Kaplan-Meier Estimates of Mortality and Causes of In-Hospital Death*

VARIABLE	STANDARD THERAPY (N = 133) NO. (%)	EARLY GOAL-DIRECTED THERAPY (N = 130)	RELATIVE RISK (95% CI)	P VALUE
In-hospital mortality†				
All patients	99 (46.5)	38 (30.5)	0.58 (0.38–0.87)	.009
Patients with severe sepsis	19 (30.0)	9 (14.9)	0.46 (0.21–1.03)	.06
Patients with septic shock	40 (56.8)	29 (42.3)	0.60 (0.36–0.98)	.04
28-Day mortality†	61 (49.2)	40 (33.3)	0.58 (0.39–0.87)	.01
60-Day mortality†	70 (56.9)	50 (44.3)	0.67 (0.46–0.96)	.03
Causes of in-hospital death‡				
Sudden cardiovascular collapse	25/119 (21.0)	12/117 (10.3)	—	.02
Multiorgan failure	26/119 (21.8)	19/117 (16.2)	—	.27

*CI denotes confidence interval. Dashes indicate that the relative risk is not applicable.
†Percentages were calculated by the Kaplan-Meier product limit method.
‡The denominators indicate the number of patients in each group who completed the initial in-hour study period.
SOURCE: Rivers E, Nguyen B, Havstad S, et al. Early goal-directed therapy in the treatment of severe sepsis and septic shock. *N Engl J Med* 2001;345:1368–1377.

TABLE 44-2 Recommended Goals of Initial Resuscitation of Sepsis-Induced Hypoperfusion Within 6 H of Presentation to the Emergency Department

CVP	8–12 mmHg
MAP	≥65 mmHg
UO	≥0.5 mg/kg/h
$ScvO_2$	≥70%

CONCLUSIONS

- Early trials studying resuscitation aimed at normalizing the venous oxyhemoglobin saturation may have failed to show benefit because patient-specific therapy was delayed until later in the clinical course (after the first 6 hours).
- Rivers et al. demonstrated that EGDT, designed to achieve specific hemodynamic end points (Table 44-2) in the emergency department, leads to increased survival in patients with severe sepsis and septic shock.

BIBLIOGRAPHY

Rhodes A, Bennet D. Early goal-directed therapy: an evidence-based review. *Crit Care Med* 2004;32(11):S448–S450.

Rivers E, Nguyen B, Havstad S, et al. Early goal-directed therapy in the treatment of severe sepsis and septic shock. *N Engl J Med* 2001;345:1368–1377.

45 DROTRECOGIN ALFA (ACTIVATED)

Michael Moore

KEY POINTS

- Drotrecogin alpha (activated) is recombinant, human, activated protein C.
- Drotrecogin possesses antithrombotic, profibrinolytic, and anti-inflammatory properties that may explain its benefit in sepsis.
- Drotrecogin lessens the duration of organ failures and reduces mortality in patients with severe sepsis at high risk of death. It is not effective in pediatric sepsis or in patients with low risk of death. Because of its anticoagulant properties, drotrecogin is contraindicated when there is active bleeding or a high risk of bleeding.
- Drotrecogin is infused intravenously at a constant dose (24 μg/kg/h) for 96 hours.

BACKGROUND

- Drotrecogin alfa (activated) was approved by the Food and Drug Administration (FDA) in November 2001 for the reduction of mortality in severe sepsis in adults at high risk of death.
- Observational data collected during studies of sepsis and septic shock point to an association between

coagulopathy (subclinical or clinical) or low protein C levels and mortality.
- A phase II prospective, randomized, placebo-controlled study of drotrecogin alfa (activated) in 131 patients with severe sepsis was conducted to determine its safety and effect on the coagulopathy of severe sepsis. This study showed an acceptable safety profile with a dose/dose-duration effect on the reduction of D-dimer levels.
- Subsequently, the PROWESS trial was designed to detect a difference in mortality in patients with severe sepsis treated with drotrecogin alpha (activated).

MECHANISM OF ACTION

- The exact mechanism of action in terms of the reduction of mortality as seen in the PROWESS (Recombinant Human Activated Protein C Worldwide Evaluation in Severe Sepsis) trial is not certain. However, the biologic activity of activated protein C is well described.
- Protein C is a vitamin-K-dependent protein factor synthesized by the liver. Protein C is converted to its active state by complexing thrombin and thrombomodulin in the presence of endothelial cell protein C receptor. After conversion, it has antithrombotic, profibrinolytic, and anti-inflammatory effects mediated through inactivation of factor Va and VIIIa, inactivation of plasminogen activator inhibitor, and effects on tumor necrosis actor (TNF), macrophage migration, thrombin-induced inflammation, and nuclear factor kB (NF-kB).
- Experimental and animal data suggest multiple potential mechanisms, and it has been suggested that synergy among drotrecogin alpha's antithrombotic, profibrinolytic, and anti-inflammatory effects may be responsible for its clinical effects.
- Finally, it is postulated that the restoration and preservation of microcirculatory blood flow prevents ischemia-reperfusion injury while the anti-inflammatory effects prevent organ dysfunction and failure.

PROWESS TRIAL

STUDY DESIGN

- Phase III randomized, double-blind, placebo-controlled, multicenter trial.
- Primary end point was 28-day all-cause mortality including prospectively defined stratification by age, acute physiologic and chronic health evaluation [APACHE II] score, and plasma protein C activity; changes in baseline level of plasma D-dimer level and serum interleukin (IL)-6 levels were also analyzed.
- Patients received drotrecogin alfa (activated) 24 μg/kg/h continuous infusion for 96 hours or placebo.
- Analysis was by intention-to-treat.

INCLUSION/EXCLUSION CRITERIA

- Patients with severe sepsis defined as having a known or suspected source of infection with evidence of SIRS (systemic inflammatory response syndrome) and at lease one organ dysfunction
- Excluded patients (Table 45-1)

RESULTS

- 1728 patients were randomized and 1690 received the study drug or placebo.
- Baseline characteristics were similar in the study groups including demographics, severity of illness, appropriateness of initial antibiotic therapy, and baseline indicators of coagulopathy and inflammation.
- There was a statistically significant reduction in 28-day all-cause mortality rate (24.7% vs. 30.8%; *P* = .005):
  - The study was terminated after second planned interim analysis
  - Absolute risk reduction 6.1%
  - Relative risk reduction 19.4%
- Thrombosis as determined by plasma D-dimer levels was significantly lower in the drotrecogin group on days 1–7 after the start of the infusion versus placebo.
- Inflammation measured by IL-6 levels was also significantly decreased for the majority of days after start of infusion of drotrecogin during the first 7 days.
- Serious bleeding was higher in the drotrecogin group:
  - 3.5% vs. 2.0% (*P* = .06) over 28 days
  - 2.4% vs. 1.0% (*P* = .044) during infusion period
  - Rate of intracranial hemorrhage was 0.2% versus 0.1% in the drotrecogin and placebo groups, respectively
  - Number needed to harm = 66

CONCLUSIONS

- PROWESS demonstrated the safe and effective use of drotrecogin alfa (activated) for the reduction of mortality in patients with severe sepsis.
- An antithrombotic effect was demonstrated by a significant reduction of D-dimer levels.
- An anti-inflammatory effect was demonstrated by a significant reduction in IL-6 levels.
- An increase in serious bleeding events was seen in the drotrecogin alfa (activated) group versus controls. The

TABLE 45-1 Trial Inclusion and Exclusion Criteria

Inclusion criteria

Known or suspected infection

Three of four SIRS criteria:

- Temperature ≥38.0°C or ≤36.0°C
- Heart rate ≥90 beats/min
- Respiratory rate ≥20 breaths/min or $PaCO_2$ of ≤32 mmHg
- White cell count ≥12,000/mm³ or ≤4000/mm³

At least one dysfunctional organ or system:

- Systolic BP ≤90 mmHg or MAP ≤70 mmHg despite adequate fluid resuscitation, adequate volume status, or use of vasopressors
- Urine output, 0.5 mL/kg/h despite adequate volume status
- PaO_2/FiO_2 ratio ≤250 or ≤200 if lung was only dysfunctional organ
- Platelet count <80,000/mm³ or 50% decrease during last 3 days
- pH ≤7.30 or base deficit ≥5.0 mmol/L with plasma lactate >1.5 times upper limit of normal

Exclusion criteria

Pregnancy or breast-feeding

Age >18 years or weight >135 kg

Conditions that increased risk of bleeding: surgery or anticipation of need for surgery with general or spinal anesthesia, postoperative bleeding; severe head trauma, intracranial surgery, or stroke within 3 months or any history of intracerebral AVM, cerebral aneurysm, or CNS mass lesion; history of congenital bleeding diathesis; gastrointestinal bleeding within 6 weeks without corrective surgery; trauma considered to increase risk of bleeding

Known hypercoagulable condition or recently documented (within 3 months) or highly suspected DVT or PE

Advance directive to withhold life-sustaining treatment; physician, or family, or both not in favor of aggressive treatment

Moribund state or patients not expected to survive 28 days because of uncorrectable medical condition

HIV with CD4 <50/mm³

History of bone marrow, lung, liver, pancreas, or small-bowel transplantation

Chronic renal failure requiring renal replacement therapy

Known or suspected portosystemic hypertension, chronic jaundice, cirrhosis, or chronic ascites

Acute pancreatitis with no known source of infection

Use of banned medication including therapeutic anticoagulation, ASA >650 mg/day within 3 days, systemic thrombolytic therapy within 3 days, glycoprotein IIb/IIIa antagonists within 7 days, antithrombin III, or protein C

ABBREVIATIONS: BP, blood pressure; MAP, mean arterial pressure; AVM, arteriovenous malformation; CNS, central nervous system; DVT, deep vein thrombosis; PE, pulmonary embolism; ASA, aspirin.

difference was primarily seen during drug infusion and in patients with identifiable risk factors for bleeding.

CONTROVERSIES

- The PROWESS trial has generated a number of controversies. These primarily relate to changes made to the protocol midway through the trial, risk of serious bleeding, FDA labeling restricting use based on APACHE II scores, and cost-effectiveness.

PROTOCOL CHANGES

- Two main changes were made:
  - The trial was amended to more effectively exclude patients with a high risk of death from preexisting illness.
  - The master cell line used to manufacture drotrecogin was changed.
- The observed reduction in mortality was improved after these changes were made.
- However, a subsequent analysis showed that the mortality benefit was greater in the subgroup of patient who would have been excluded after the protocol changes. The protocol changes made drotrecogin alpha (activated) less effective than if the protocol were not amended.
- The manufacturer conducted extensive testing of the new master cell line prior to its use in PROWESS. No significant differences were seen. While it is not possible to rule out all potential changes in a complex protein drug product, the new master cell line would then be more effective, not less.

RISK OF SERIOUS BLEEDING

- More serious bleeding events were observed in the drotrecogin alpha (activated) group: this was both predicted based on the known actions of drotrecogin, and has been confirmed in studies subsequent to PROWESS.
- Bleeding was seen primarily during the infusion period and in patients with known risk factors for bleeding (e.g., platelet count <30,000/mm³).
- Some authors have noted increased rates of fatal intracranial hemorrhage in patients treated with drotrecogin alpha (activated) in open-label use. In published data to date, the rate of intracranial hemorrhage is 0.5% (open-label use).

USE OF APACHE II SCORES

- The APACHE II score was developed and validated as a measure to predict mortality in critically ill ICU patients.
- The FDA approved drotrecogin alpha (activated) in patients who are at high risk of death, such as those who have an APACHE II score greater than the mean value in PROWESS (APACHE II score = 25).
- Subsequent analysis has showed that the APACHE II score can identify patients more likely to benefit from drotrecogin alpha (activated).

TABLE 45-2 Contraindications/Warnings/Precautions

Contraindications
Hypersensitivity to drotrecogin alpha (activated)
Active internal bleeding
Recent hemorrhagic stroke (within 3 months)
Sever head trauma (within 2 months)
Recent intracranial or intraspinal surgery (within 2 months)
Intracranial neoplasm or mass
Evidence of cerebral herniation
Presence of epidural catheter
Trauma with increased risk of life-threatening bleeding
Warnings/Precautions
Increased bleeding risk in patients with:
Concurrent therapeutic heparin
Oral anticoagulants
Glycoprotein IIb/IIIa antagonists
Platelet aggregation inhibitors
High dose aspirin (>650 mg/day within 7 days)
International normalized ratio (INR) >3.0
GI bleeding (within 6 weeks)
Platelet <30,000/mm^3
Thrombolytic therapy (within 3 days)
Recent ischemic stroke (within 3 months)
Intracranial AVM or aneurysm
Known bleeding diathesis
Chronic severe liver disease

COST-EFFECTIVENESS

- Manns et al. used data from PROWESS and FDA analyses to compare the cost-effectiveness of drotrecogin alpha (activated) and standard therapy for severe sepsis:
  - Cost per life-year gained was $27,936 for all patients
  - Cost per life-year gained stratified by APACHE II scores (FDA analysis)
    - $24,484 for APACHE II scores >25
    - $575,054 for APACHE II scores ≤24
  - Cost per life-year gained increased with increasing age and was higher in patients with lower expected survival based on comorbid conditions
- Angus et al. conducted a prospective cost-effectiveness analysis based on the PROWESS cohort:
  - Drotrecogin alpha (activated) cost $160,000 per life saved
  - $48,000 per quality-adjusted life-year with an 82% probability that the ratio is <$100,000 per quality-adjusted life-year
  - $27,000 per quality-adjusted life-year in patients with APACHE II >25
  - Drotrecogin alpha (activated) was cost-ineffective in patient with APACHE II ≤24
  - The cost-effectiveness profile was comparable to other well-accepted therapeutic interventions

RECOMMENDED USE

- Drotrecogin alpha (activated) should be considered for adult patients with recent onset of severe sepsis or septic shock who are at a high risk of death, such as those with APACHE II score >25 or with at least two organ failures.
- Careful evaluation of patients including assessment of potential benefits and risks of adverse event is essential especially with regard to patients who were not studied in the PROWESS trial (Table 45-2).
- APACHE II scores most effectively discriminated among patients likely to benefit from therapy in the PROWESS trial, but this single measure should not replace clinical judgment regarding high risk of death.

BIBLIOGRAPHY

Bernard GR, Vincent JL, Laterre PF, et al. Efficacy and safety of recombinant human activated protein C for severe sepsis. *N Engl J Med* 2001;344:699–709.

Hall JB, Schmidt, GA, Wood LDH. *Principles of Critical Care*, 3rd ed. New York, NY: McGraw-Hill; 2005:1123–1136.

Manns BJ, Lee H, Doig CJ, et al. An economic evaluation of activated protein C treatment for severe sepsis. *N Engl J Med* 2002;347:993–1000.

Package insert/prescribing information. Drotrecogin alfa (activated): Drotrecogin alfa (activated), Lilly Inc. Available at: http://www.Xigris.com. Accessed March 30, 2004.

Siegel JP. Assessing the use of activated protein C in the treatment of severe sepsis. *N Engl J Med* 2002;347:1030–1034.

Vincent JL, Angus DC, Artigas A, et al. Effects of drotrecogin alfa (activated) on organ dysfunction in the PROWESS trial. *Crit Care Med* 2003;31:834–840.

Warren HS, Suffredini AF, Eichacker PQ, et al. Risks and benefits of activated protein C treatment for severe sepsis. *N Engl J Med* 2002;347:1027–1030.

Wheeler AP, Bernard GR. Treating patients with severe sepsis. *N Engl J Med* 1999;340:207–214.

46 AN APPROACH TO SEPSIS OF UNKNOWN ETIOLOGY

Nina M. Patel

KEY POINTS

- A thorough history and physical examination, repeated at frequent intervals, are essential in primary bacterial or nonbacterial sepsis to guide diagnostic workup and empiric antimicrobial therapy.

- The detection of secondary sepsis in the ICU requires extreme vigilance, a high clinical index of suspicion on a daily basis, and focused attention to local and systemic risk factors for infection.
- Broad-spectrum antibiotic therapy should be initiated promptly in all septic patients, even amidst investigation for the primary source of infection. If a causative infectious agent is identified, the spectrum of antibiotic therapy should be narrowed to offer coverage specific to that pathogen.
- Immunosuppressed patients require more extensive empiric antimicrobial therapy than the normal host.
- Sepsis has a high mortality rate, but vigilance toward detecting infection early and instituting appropriate therapy expediently improve morbidity and mortality.

EPIDEMIOLOGY

- 750,000 people per year acquire sepsis in the US.
- The mortality rate associated with sepsis is 35–45%.

DEFINITION

- Sepsis is defined as infection-provoked systemic inflammatory response syndrome (SIRS; see Chap. 43).
- If acute organ dysfunction or hypotension accompanies SIRS, severe sepsis is present.
- Septic shock is severe sepsis accompanied by refractory hypotension.
- Primary sepsis is the sepsis syndrome or septic shock in the absence of a clear source of infection.
- Secondary sepsis is the development of hemodynamic instability and recurrent sepsis syndrome despite adequate antimicrobial therapy for a known initial source of infection.

DIFFERENTIAL DIAGNOSIS

- Primary and secondary sepsis may be bacterial or nonbacterial in nature. In addition, a number of noninfectious syndromes can mimic the clinical picture observed in sepsis.

PRIMARY SEPSIS

- A thorough history and physical examination, with attention to timing of onset of symptoms, localization of symptoms and signs, travel and past medical history (in particular, risk factors for immunosuppression), are essential to guiding the diagnostic evaluation of sepsis.
- Diagnostic evaluation begins with basic laboratory tests: complete blood count (CBC) with differential, comprehensive metabolic panel, blood cultures, urine culture, and a chest radiograph.
- Fever, hypotension, tachycardia, tachypnea, decreased urine output, and decreased mental status are seen frequently in septic patients. Laboratory perturbations suggestive of sepsis include leukocytosis or leukopenia; thrombocytopenia; hyper- or hypoglycemia; anion gap metabolic acidosis (lactic acidosis, in particular); elevated transaminases or bilirubin (direct); respiratory alkalosis; and hypoxemia.
- Clinical history and examination should guide further testing:
    - If mental obtundation or nuchal rigidity is present or there is concern for central nervous system (CNS) pathology, head computed tomography (CT) and lumbar puncture should be performed to evaluate for meningitis.
    - If productive cough, shortness of breath, or other respiratory symptoms are present, sputum should be sent for Gram's stain, culture, and susceptibility. Thoracentesis should be performed to rule out an empyema if there is a pleural effusion. If purulent nasal drainage is present, CT of the sinuses should be performed with a plan to aspirate the sinuses if there is an air-fluid level.
    - If indwelling vascular devices are present, one set of blood cultures should be drawn through the device. If the site looks infected or in the setting of bacteremia, the catheter should be removed and sent for culture. Also, transesophageal echocardiography should be considered to evaluate for endocarditis.
    - If ascites or indwelling drains are present, the peritoneal or drain fluid should be sampled and sent for Gram's stain and culture. Also, abdominal imaging with CT or ultrasound should be considered.
    - If there is a history of nephrolithiasis, pyelonephritis, or other renal pathology, renal ultrasound should be ordered to assess for a perinephric abscess and to exclude urinary obstruction.
    - If swollen, hot, tender joints are present, septic arthritis should be ruled out with aspiration of the affected joint. If persistent bacteremia and focal bony pain are identified, plain films or bone scan should be ordered to evaluate for osteomyelitis.
- If no obvious source of infection is present following a detailed history and physical examination, one should reconsider common sources of infection that

may be presenting in an uncommon fashion. A chest radiograph should be repeated after hydration to reassess for pneumonia if there are respiratory symptoms. Abdominal films and serial abdominal examinations should be performed if there is even a mildly abnormal abdominal examination.

- If no source is identified, sepsis is presumed due to bacteremia or endocarditis. *Staphylococcus aureus* is the most common cause of in-hospital bacteremia.
- Nonbacterial causes of sepsis include malaria (*Plasmodium falciparum*), dengue fever, or other parasitic infections in the returned traveler, rickettsial infection (Rocky Mountain spotted fever, ehrlichiosis), and viral hepatitis.
- Noninfectious sources of sepsis syndrome are drug intoxication or withdrawal, anaphylaxis, vasculitis, acute pancreatitis, massive tissue injury (e.g., rhabdomyolysis), and heat stroke.
- Patients with diabetes mellitus, chronic renal disease, chronic liver disease, asplenia, and immunodeficiency or on immunosuppressive medical therapy should be evaluated meticulously due to increased risk for infection with encapsulated organisms, fungus, gram-negative bacteria, *S. aureus*, or opportunistic pathogens.

NOSOCOMIAL INFECTION

- Patients who redevelop fever or hemodynamic instability and sepsis syndrome despite what is deemed adequate antibiotic therapy should be evaluated for four major possibilities: (1) initial antibiotic coverage was not adequate, (2) secondary antimicrobial resistance to the antibiotic has emerged, (3) the antibiotic was unable to penetrate the site of infection (e.g., abscess), (4) a new primary infection has developed.
- These patients should undergo resampling of the initial site of infection. They also should have inspection of all indwelling devices (e.g., lines) to assess for access device-related infection. Workup for fungal and viral infection should be completed in an immunosuppressed host with no other source of infection.
- Other occult or subtle infectious sources in the ICU patient are ventilator-associated pneumonia, acalculous cholecystitis, multidrug-resistant urinary tract infection, frontal or maxillary sinusitis, suppurative parotitis, wound or decubitus ulcer infection, secondary peritonitis, and pseudomembranous colitis.
- Several antibiotics, antiarrhythmics, and other medications used in the ICU can lead to drug fever. The possibility that drugs may be responsible for fever should be considered in all ICU patients, particularly if there is no obvious source of infection.

TREATMENT AND PREVENTION

- Appropriate antibiotic therapy decreases the mortality rate of sepsis by 11%. However, delay in initiating adequate therapy can lead to increased mortality and morbidity from sepsis.
- Broad-spectrum antibiotic coverage with reasonable gram-positive and gram-negative coverage is recommended for initial therapy for primary sepsis if no causative organism is identified. Particular attention should be directed toward evaluating for the possibility of anaerobic infection, meningitis, methicillin-resistant S. aureus (MRSA) infection, or pseudomonal infection. These bacteria are not always covered by standard broad-spectrum antibiotic coverage.
- Empiric broad-spectrum antibiotic therapy for secondary sepsis should always include coverage for MRSA and *Pseudomonas aeruginosa*. Additional factors in antibiotic selection are local bacterial susceptibility and resistance patterns as well as impaired host immunity (e.g., neutropenia).
- Empiric antifungal therapy should be considered in patients with neutropenia or severe immunosuppression who have not responded clinically to antibiotic therapy.
- At 48–72 hours, all microbiologic data should be reviewed and the antibiotic regimen tailored if possible. If a clear source of infection is identified, antibiotic coverage should be narrowed to prevent the development of resistant organisms or bacterial superinfection.
- An adequate response to therapy is marked by a normalization of vital signs, resolution of leukocytosis or leukopenia, and resolution of acidosis and other lab abnormalities.
- Source control signifies: (a) drainage of abscesses or fluid collections, (b) debridement of devitalized or necrotic tissue, (c) removal of infected devices (e.g., catheter) or excision of an infected viscus. Aggressive source control prevents extension of infection and worsening of clinical status.

BIBLIOGRAPHY

Ely EW, Goyette RE. Sepsis with acute organ dysfunction. In: Hall JB, Schmidt GA, Wood LDH, eds., *Principles of Critical Care*, 3rd ed. New York, NY: McGraw-Hill; 2005:699–734.

Pittet D, Thievent B, Wenzel RP, et al. Bedside prediction of mortality from bacteremic sepsis. A dynamic analysis of ICU patients. *Am J Respir Crit Care Med* 1996;153:684–693.

Wheeler AP, Bernard GR. Treating patients with severe sepsis. *N Engl J Med* 1999;340:207–214.

47 EMPIRIC ANTIBIOTIC SELECTION FOR SEVERE INFECTIONS

Kevin Gregg

KEY POINTS

- Incorrect empiric antibiotic selection has been shown to lead to increased mortality and longer hospital stays in critically ill patients.
- Initial antibiotic coverage in a critically ill patient should be broad, covering likely community-acquired and nosocomial infectious organisms.
- Appropriate cultures should be drawn *prior to* the administration of antibiotics whenever possible. These should include samples from urine, peripheral blood from multiple sites (including indwelling catheters and arterial lines), and sputum.
- When selecting initial antibiotic coverage in the ICU, the risk factors for infection should be carefully assessed in each patient.
  - Is the patient immunocompromised?
  - Do they have instrumentation that could be a source for infection?
  - Are they mechanically ventilated?
  - Have they been hospitalized or institutionalized recently?
  - Have they recently been on antibiotics?
- Antimicrobial resistance patterns vary in different hospitals and communities. These patterns may help determine appropriate empiric therapy.

SEPSIS AND SEPTIC SHOCK IN THE IMMUNOCOMPETENT PATIENT

- The most frequent sites of infection leading to sepsis are the lungs, the blood, the abdomen, the urinary tract, and the skin.
- Gram-positive organisms are most often responsible for sepsis, followed by gram-negative organisms.
- Fungal infections account for only 5% of all cases of sepsis.
- Initial antibiotic therapy should broadly cover gram-positive, gram-negative, and anaerobic organisms if the infecting organism is unknown.
- Ureidopenicillins + β-lactamase inhibitors, carbapenems, and third- or fourth-generation cephalosporins have very similar, broad antimicrobial spectra.
- Evidence shows that empiric monotherapy with a carbapenem or a third- or fourth-generation cephalosporin is as efficacious as combination therapy with a β-lactam and an aminoglycoside.
- Ureidopenicillins with β-lactamase inhibitors have also been as effective as combination antibiotic therapy in several small studies.
- If there is concern for methicillin-resistant *Staphylococcus aureus* (MRSA), vancomycin or linezolid should be included in the initial regimen.
- If there is concern for vancomycin-resistant *Enterococcus* spp. (VRE), linezolid should be included in the initial regimen.
- Combination antimicrobial therapy ("double coverage") for *Pseudomonas aeruginosa* remains controversial. The results of a meta-analysis suggest that routine combination therapy in gram-negative bacteremia does not decrease mortality. However, if *P. aeruginosa* or multidrug-resistant (MDR) gram-negative bacilli are suspected, combination therapy may still be warranted. In that setting, increasing the likelihood of adequate coverage by utilizing a second agent aids in alleviating the increased morbidity and mortality associated with inadequate coverage at the onset of sepsis.
- An algorithm for empiric selection of antibiotic therapy is presented in Fig. 47-1.

SEPSIS AND SEPTIC SHOCK IN THE IMMUNOCOMPROMISED PATIENT

- An infectious disease specialist should be consulted as soon as possible; these patients are at risk for significant morbidity and mortality if not managed appropriately.
- Immunocompromised patients are at risk for the same infections that most often cause sepsis in immunocompetent patients, but are at higher risk for systemic fungal and viral infections than an immunocompetent patient.
- Initial antimicrobial coverage should be the same as in an immunocompetent host (carbapenem, third- or fourth-generation cephalosporin, ureidopenicillin + β-lactamase inhibitor) *and* should include vancomycin or linezolid.
- In a neutropenic patient, combination therapy to treat *P. aeruginosa* infection is recommended, although to date there are not data to support improved patient outcomes with this practice.
- If the immunocompromised patient is at high risk for fungal infection, antifungal therapy with amphotericin B, caspofungin, or voriconazole should be initiated.
- Empiric therapy with antiviral agents is generally not warranted.

INTRAVENOUS CATHETER-RELATED INFECTIONS

- There are little or no data to support the use of one particular empiric antibiotic regimen for catheter-related infections.

Carbapenem[1]	OR	Third/fourth generation-Cephalosporin[2]	OR	Ureidopenicillin/β-lactamase inhibitor[3]
-Imipenem -Meropenem		-Cefotaxime -Ceftriaxone -Cefotaxime -Ceftizoxime -Cefepime		-Piperacillin/tazobactam -Ticarcillin/clavulanate

[1] Carbapenems do not cover *Bacteroides* spp., *L. pneumophila* or atypical organisms
[2] Cephalosporins do not cover *L. monocytogenes, L. pneumophila*, spp. or *C. difficile*
[3] Ureidopenicillins do not cover *L. pneumophila* or atypical organisms.

If Pseudomonas aeruginosa is a likely pathogen, add:

Aminoglycoside	OR	Anti-pseudomonal fluoroquinolone*
-Gentamicin -Amikacin -Tobramycin		-Ciprofloxacin -Levofloxacin

* Other fluoroquinolones (gatifloxacin, moxifloxacin) have some activity against Pseudomonas spp.

If MRSA is a likely pathogen, add:

Vancomycin	OR	Linezolid

FIG. 47-1 Empiric antibiotic therapy in sepsis and septic shock in the immunocompetent patient.

- In hospitals or communities with significant MRSA prevalence, the recommended empiric therapy is vancomycin.
- In immunocompromised or severely ill patients, additional coverage with an antipseudomonal agent is recommended.
- If fungemia is suspected, amphotericin B or intravenous fluconazole may be initiated.

VENTILATOR-ASSOCIATED PNEUMONIA, HOSPITAL-ACQUIRED PNEUMONIA, AND HEALTH CARE-ASSOCIATED PNEUMONIA

- Nosocomial pneumonia and ventilator-associated pneumonia (VAP) cause significant morbidity and mortality in critically ill patients including increased organ dysfunction, length of stay, cost, and death.
- Patient risk factors requiring broad-spectrum antibiotics in suspected VAP, hospital-acquired pneumonia (HAP), and health care-associated pneumonia (HCAP) (American Thoracic Society [ATS] guidelines):
    - Recent antibiotic therapy (within 3 months)
    - Hospitalization for 2 or more days in the last 3 months
    - Immunosuppression
    - Chronic dialysis within the past 30 days
    - Residence in a nursing home or other health care institution
    - Home infusion therapy
    - Home wound care
    - Family member with MDR organism
    - High level of antibiotic resistance in hospital or community
- If none of the risk factors requiring broad-spectrum antibiotics are present, patients may be covered for typical pneumonia pathogens (*Streptococcus pneumoniae, Haemophilus influenzae, MSSA*) and enteric gram-negative bacilli (*Escherichia coli, Klebsiella pneumoniae, Serratia marcesans*). Coverage can often be a single antibiotic covering these organisms: most fluoroquinolones, ampicillin/sulbactam, or ceftriaxone.
- Empiric broad-spectrum antibiotics should cover gram-positive and gram-negative organisms, atypical organisms (including *Legionella pneumophila*), MRSA, *P. aeruginosa, K. pneumoniae*, and *Acinetobacter* spp.
- If *P. aeruginosa* is suspected, two antipseudomonal antibiotics should be used (β-lactam + fluoroquinolone or aminoglycoside).
- A treatment selection algorithm is presented in Fig. 47-2.

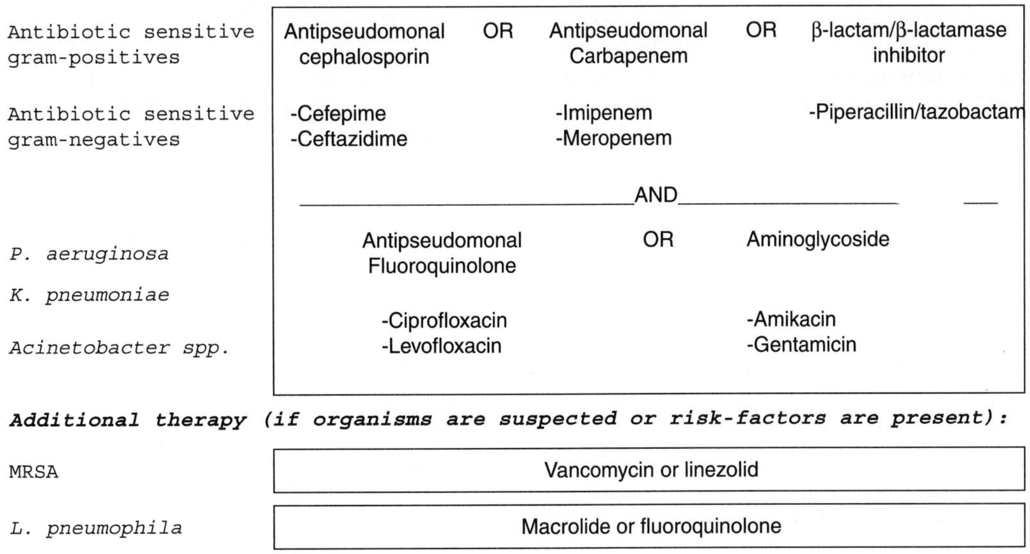

Antibiotic sensitive gram-positives	Antipseudomonal cephalosporin	OR	Antipseudomonal Carbapenem	OR	β-lactam/β-lactamase inhibitor
Antibiotic sensitive gram-negatives	-Cefepime -Ceftazidime		-Imipenem -Meropenem		-Piperacillin/tazobactam
			AND		
P. aeruginosa *K. pneumoniae* *Acinetobacter spp.*	Antipseudomonal Fluoroquinolone -Ciprofloxacin -Levofloxacin		OR		Aminoglycoside -Amikacin -Gentamicin

Additional therapy (if organisms are suspected or risk-factors are present):

MRSA	Vancomycin or linezolid
L. pneumophila	Macrolide or fluoroquinolone

FIG. 47-2 Empiric antibiotic therapy for VAP, HAP, and HCAP in patients at risk for MDR pathogens. SOURCE: Adapted from ATS guidelines.

SEVERE COMMUNITY-ACQUIRED PNEUMONIA

- Community-acquired pneumonia (CAP) necessitating admission to the ICU should broadly cover typical organisms (*S. pneumoniae, H. influenzae, S. aureus*), atypical organisms (*Mycoplasma pneumoniae, Clamydia pneumoniae*), and *L. pneumophila.*
- Empiric antibiotic selection for patients without risk factors for *P. aeruginosa* infection should include an intravenous third-generation cephalosporin and an intravenous macrolide or nonpseudomonal fluoroquinolone.
- For patients with risk factors for *P. aeruginosa* infection, empiric antibiotic selection should include: (1) carbapenem *or* ureidopenicillin + β-lactamase inhibitor *or* antipseudomonal cephalosporin *and* intravenous antipseudomonal fluoroquinolone OR (2) carbapenem *or* ureidopenicillin + β-lactamase inhibitor *or* antipseudomonal cephalosporin *and* aminoglycoside *and* fluoroquinolone.

FUNGAL INFECTIONS

- Fungal infections cause approximately 5% of all cases of sepsis; therefore, the empiric use of antifungal therapies should be based on patient risk factors.
- Patients at higher risk for fungal sepsis include: patients on broad-spectrum antibiotics, patients who are immunocompromised, and patients known to be colonized with *Candida* spp.

TABLE 47-1 Dosages of Antibiotics Commonly Used as Empiric Therapy in the Critical Care Setting*

Ureidopenicillins + β-lactamase inhibitor	
Piperacillin/tazobactam	3.375 g IV q 6 h†
Ticarcillin/clavulanate	3.1 g IV q 4–6 h†
Carbapenems	
Meropenem	0.5–1.0 g IV q 8 h†
Imipenem/cilastatin	500 mg IV q 6 h†
Third-generation cephalosporins	
Ceftriaxone	2.0 g IV q 24 h‡
Ceftizoxime	1.0–4.0 g IV q 8 h†
Cefotaxime	1.0–2.0 g IV q 4-12 h†
Ceftazidime	1.0–2.0 g IV q 8-12 h†
Fourth-generation cephalosporins	
Cefepime	1.0–2.0 g IV q 12 h†
Aminoglycosides	
Gentamicin	5.1 mg/kg IV q 24 h†,§
Amikacin	15 mg/kg IV q 24 h†,§
Tobramycin	5.1 mg/kg IV q 24 h†,§
Fluoroquinolones	
Ciprofloxacin	200–400 mg IV q 24 h†
Gatifloxacin	200–400 mg IV q 24 h†
Moxifloxacin	400 mg IV q 24 h
Levofloxacin	250–750 mg IV q 24 h†
Glycopeptides	
Vancomycin	15 mg/kg IV q 24 h†
Oxazolidinones	
Linezolid	600 mg IV q 12 h†

*This list does not include all antibiotic options available.
†Antibiotic dose must be altered if renal function is impaired.
‡Dose for persons <65 years old. Dose 1.0 g IV q 24 h if >65 years old.
§Multiple daily dosing regimens available.

- Caspofungin is as effective as liposomal amphotericin B and is associated with fewer side effects in neutropenic patients with persistent fever.
- Amphotericin B, liposomal amphotericin B, caspofungin, itraconazole, and voriconazole have different antifungal spectra and associated toxicities which should be considered on a patient-by-patient basis when administering these drugs as empiric therapy.

DOSING REGIMENS

- Recommended dosing regimens by antibiotic option are listed in Table 47-1.

BIBLIOGRAPHY

American Thoracic Society. Guidelines for the management of adults with hospital-acquired, ventilator-associated, and healthcare-associated pneumonia. *Am J Respir Crit Care Med* 2005;171:388–416.

Bochud P, Bonten M, Marchetti O, et al. Antimicrobial therapy for patients with severe sepsis and septic shock: an evidence-based review. *Crit Care Med* 2004;32(Suppl):S495–S512.

Gea-Banacloche JC, Opal SM, Jorgensen J, et al. Sepsis associated with immunosuppressive medications: an evidence-based review. *Crit Care Med* 2004;32(Suppl):S578–S590.

Gilbert DN, Moellering RC, Eiopoulos GM, eds., *The Sanford Guide to Antimicrobial Therapy*, 34th ed. Antimicrobial Therapy, Inc.; 2004.

Mermel LA, Farr BM, Sherertz RJ, et al. Guidelines for the management of intravascular catheter-related infections. *Clin Infect Dis* 2001:32:1249–1269.

Niederman MS, Mandell LA, Anzueto A, et al. Guidelines for the management of adults with community-acquired pneumonia. *Am J Respir Crit Care Med* 2001;163:1730–1754.

Safdar N, Handelsman J, Maki DG. Does combination antimicrobial therapy reduce mortality in gram-negative bacteraemia? A meta-analysis. *Lancet* 2004;4:519–527.

Walsh TJ, Teppler H, Donowitz GR, et al. Caspofungin versus liposomal amphotericin B for empirical antifungal therapy in patients with persistent fever and neutropenia. *N Engl J Med* 2004;351:1391–1402.

48 NEUTROPENIC PATIENTS

Nathan Sandbo

KEY POINTS

- The risk of infection rises when the ANC falls below 500/mm^3 and is highest once the count is below 100/mm^3.
- Fever is defined as an oral temperature of >38°C sustained over 1 hour, or a single measurement of >38.3°C in neutropenic patients.
- Evaluation of the febrile, neutropenic patient should include a meticulous physical examination, seeking even subtle evidence of infection, involving sites not often involved in infection (periodontal, perianal), and assessing any hardware, especially semipermanent intravenous catheters.
- High-risk patients can be treated with intravenous antibiotics either in combination (extended spectrum β-lactam combined with an aminoglycoside) or as monotherapy (third- or fourth-generation cephalosporin, such as ceftazidime or cefepime, or carbapenems, such as imipenem-cilastin). In selected patients at higher risk for β-lactam-resistant gram-positive organisms, vancomycin should be added.
- Fungal infections become more likely when fever fails to respond to 3–5 days of broad-spectrum antibiotic therapy.

BACKGROUND

- The use of chemotherapies to treat malignancy has evolved over the past two decades, and has resulted in increasing doses with resultant increases in systemic toxicity.
- Commonly used chemotherapeutic agents differentially affect rapidly dividing cells, and myelosuppression is a frequent result, usually occurring around days 10–14. Furthermore, there is a simultaneous impairment of both cell-mediated and humoral host immune responses, resulting in significant immunosuppression after treatment.
- Risk of opportunistic infections increases as the absolute neutrophil count (ANC) drops below 500/mm^3, with the highest risk occurring when ANC is <100/mm^3. Increased duration of neutropenia also is associated with increasing risk of morbidity and mortality.
- In addition, the basal epithelial cells lining the upper and lower gastrointestinal (GI) tract, upper and lower respiratory tract, and genitourinary tract are differentially sensitive to the effects of chemotherapeutic agents, resulting in disruption of the mucocutaneous barrier, and further predisposition to infection. Severe damage manifests clinically as mucositis and diffuse GI ulcerations.
- The presence of other integumentary defects from indwelling central venous lines, urinary catheters, or other devices further increases the risk of opportunistic infection.

APPROACH TO FEVER IN NEUTROPENIC PATIENTS

- Fever is most strictly defined in neutropenic patients as an oral temperature of >38°C sustained over 1 hour, or a single measurement of >38.3°C.
- The presence of fever in a neutropenic patient is assumed to represent infection unless a clear alternative etiology is present. As a result, the workup of a neutropenic patient is necessarily focused on the identification of a possible infectious focus, and subsequent risk stratification.
- History should focus on the timing and nature of recent cytotoxic therapy, the administration of new drugs or blood products, and the onset of new symptoms.
- Physical examination should be directed at identifying a potential focus of infection, with attention to disruptions in the integument. Physical findings may be extremely subtle or absent, especially with profound neutropenia.
  - *Eyes*: evidence of conjunctival abnormalities, scleral hemorrhage, icterus, or retinal exudates
  - *Skin*: appearance of new rashes, lesions, or purpura. The presence of swelling or fluctuance. Examination of indwelling lines and catheters for erythema, tenderness, or exudates
  - *Upper respiratory*: examination of tympanic membranes for erythema or pus; evidence of sinus tenderness or erythema
  - *Lower respiratory*: presence of tachypnea, focal crackles, or consolidation
  - *Upper GI*:– presence of mucosal ulcers, focal pain, or periodontal fluid collection
  - *Lower GI*: presence of focal abdominal pain, perianal tenderness, erythema, ulcerations, or fluid collections
- Initial diagnostics may include laboratory inquiry of cell counts, electrolytes, and hepatic enzymes. Chest radiography should be obtained looking for infiltrates. Relevant body fluid specimens (urine, cerebrospinal fluid [CSF], sputum, stool) should be sent for microbial cultures if clinical suspicion warrants. It is recommended for all febrile neutropenic patients that blood be sent from two independent sites for bacterial culture, with one from an indwelling central venous catheter if present (including catheters with port reservoirs).
- Empiric antimicrobial therapy should be initiated immediately, and should target aerobic gram-negative bacteria, as well as catheter-associated gram-positive bacteria. The type of empiric regimen should be determined by patient risk (low vs. high).
  - Low-risk patients (absence of pulmonary findings, abdominal findings, or other evidence of focal infection, and lack of systemic toxicity or circulatory compromise) can be treated with oral combination therapy (ciprofloxacin and amoxicillin/clavulanate).
  - High-risk patients can be treated with intravenous antibiotics either in combination or as monotherapy. Combination therapy usually consists of an extended spectrum β-lactam combined with an aminoglycoside. Monotherapy may consist of a third- or fourth-generation cephalosporin, such as ceftazidime or cefepime, or carbapenems, such as imipenem-cilastin.
  - The addition of coverage for β-lactam-resistant gram-positive organisms with agents such as vancomycin can be considered in selected patients at higher risk for these infections (evidence of line infection on examination, known colonization with resistant organisms, positive blood cultures, and evidence of circulatory compromise).
- Persistent fevers despite 3–5 days of broad-spectrum antimicrobials should lead to the entertainment of invasive fungal infections as possible etiologies, and a further search for a focus of infection. An antifungal agent is usually given at this time. Liposomal amphotericin B or voriconazole has been shown to be equally efficacious to standard formulations of amphotericin B, with less systemic toxicity.

COMMON INFECTIOUS SYNDROMES IN NEUTROPENIC PATIENTS

- *Mucositis*: This syndrome usually presents at days 10–14, and is often complicated by secondary superinfection with polymicrobial organisms, *Candida* species, or reactivation of herpes simplex virus. Management is targeted toward symptomatic relief with topical anesthetics, topical or oral antifungals for candida superinfection, and antiviral agents for herpes.
- *Clostridium difficile enterocolitis*: The risk of this opportunistic infection increases with broad-spectrum antimicrobial use, which frequently is present in neutropenic patients. Diagnosis is obtained through the identification of toxin in the stool, and therapy usually consists of oral metronidazole and adequate hydration.
- *Typhlitis*: The range of clinical presentation can be from mild mucosal inflammation to frank necrosis and perforation. Symptoms are characterized by abdominal pain (either diffuse or localized to the right lower quadrant) and fever. Computed tomography (CT) scan is usually needed to make the diagnosis, most often showing thickening and edema of the cecal wall, with or without inflammatory changes in the surrounding tissues. Management consists of bowel rest, nasogastric decompression, intravenous fluids,

and broad-spectrum antibiotics directed against enteric bacteria. Surgical consultation is required, but most patients can be managed medically. Mortality can be as high as 50%.

- *Perirectal infections*: Most patients who develop perirectal infections do not have a known predisposing condition such as anal fissures or hemorrhoids, so examination of the perirectal area for erythema, tenderness, or fluid collections is important in any neutropenic patient. Medical therapy with appropriate antibiotics is the most important therapeutic intervention, with surgical drainage recommended for obvious fluid collections.
- *Disseminated candidiasis*: The presence of indwelling catheters, interruption of mucosal barriers, and broad-spectrum antibiotics in neutropenic patients all predispose to the development of candidiasis, either focal or disseminated. Hematogenous spread is common, with consequent eye, skin, renal, hepatic, or splenic lesions. Diagnosis is established through the isolation of organisms from the blood or tissue biopsy. Treatment is initiated with amphotericin B, fluconazole, or caspofungin.
- *Aspergillosis*: Aspergillosis is a common etiology of persistent fever despite broad-spectrum antibiotics. The clinical syndrome consists of multiple sites of tissue infection, with a predilection for the lung. Diagnosis requires identification of branching septate hyphae on tissue biopsy, or growth in culture. Treatment is usually initiated with liposomal amphotericin or voriconazole. Complete resolution of infection usually requires reconstitution of the neutrophil count.
- *Catheter-related infections*: Risk for the development of catheter-related infection increases with degree of neutropenia, duration of neutropenia, type of indwelling line, and duration of use. Most etiologic organisms are gram positives such as *Staphylococcus aureus* or *S. epidermiditis*, and *Corynebacterium*. Severely neutropenic patients are also at risk for more unusual species, however, such as Enterobacteriaceae and *Acinetobacter anitratus*. Removal of the line is indicated when there is infection of the tunnel site, evidence of hematogenous spread of infection, persistent bacteremia, or infection with highly pathogenic organisms such as *S. aureus*, *Serratia* species, and fungus.

PROPHYLAXIS IN NEUTROPENIC PATIENTS

- Trimethoprim/sulfamethoxazole is recommended for prophylaxis for any neutropenic patient at higher risk for pneumocystis pneumonia.
- Currently, no consensus exists for general bacterial prophylaxis with oral quinolones, but they are widely used.
- Use of vancomycin for prophylaxis for gram-positive infections is discouraged.
- Oral fluconazole for prophylaxis of topical or systemic fungal infections is still controversial, and not currently recommended for all patients.
- Oral acyclovir for patients at high risk for herpes simplex virus reactivation may be appropriate in high-risk patients, but is not currently recommended for all patients.

GROWTH FACTORS IN NEUTROPENIC PATIENTS

- Granulocyte colony-stimulating factor (GCSF) can shorten the duration of neutropenia, but has not been shown to decrease infectious complications, length of stay, or mortality.

BIBLIOGRAPHY

Bow EJ. Approach to infection in patients receiving cytotoxic chemotherapy for malignancy. In: Hall JB, Schmidt GA, Wood LDH, eds., *Principles of Critical Care*, 3rd ed. New York, NY: McGraw-Hill; 2005:735–770.

Freifeld A, Marchigiani D, Walsh T, et al. A double-blind comparison of empirical oral and intravenous antibiotic therapy for low-risk febrile patients with neutropenia during cancer chemotherapy. *N Engl J Med* 1999;341:305–311.

Hughes WT, Armstrong D, Bodey GP, et al. 2002 Guidelines for the use of antimicrobial agents in neutropenic patients with cancer. *Clin Infect Dis* 2002;34:730–751.

Mora-Duarte J, Betts R, Rotstein C, et al. Comparison of caspofungin and amphotericin B for invasive candidiasis. *N Engl J Med* 2002;347:2020–2029.

Pizzo PA. Management of fever in patients with cancer and treatment-induced neutropenia. *N Engl J Med* 1993;328: 1323–1332.

Vento S, Cainelli F. Infections in patients with cancer undergoing chemotherapy: aetiology, prevention, and treatment. *Lancet Oncol* 2003;4:595–604.

Walsh TJ, Finberg RW, Arndt C, et al. Liposomal amphotericin B for empirical therapy in patients with persistent fever and neutropenia. National Institute of Allergy and Infectious Diseases Mycoses Study Group. *N Engl J Med* 1999;340: 764–771.

Walsh TJ, Pappas P, Winston DJ, et al. Voriconazole compared with liposomal amphotericin B for empirical antifungal therapy in patients with neutropenia and persistent fever. *N Engl J Med* 2002;346:225–234.

49 AIDS IN THE ICU

William Schweickert

KEY POINTS

- A large number of opportunistic infections may need to be considered: knowledge of the CD4 count helps limit the differential diagnosis.
- Some critical illness is a consequence not of infection, but of antiretroviral treatment [lactic acidosis, Immune-Reconstitution Syndrome (IRS), pancreatitis] or organ-specific complications of HIV infection, such as cardiomyopathy or renal failure.
- The antiretroviral regimen should generally be discontinued when a patient with AIDS is admitted to the ICU, both to remove a potential confounding cause of illness and to reduce the risk of provoking resistance.
- Infections should generally be diagnosed specifically, even when invasive procedures are necessary, rather than relying on empirical therapy.

OVERVIEW

- The acquired immunodeficiency syndrome (AIDS) is caused by chronic infection with the human immunodeficiency virus (HIV), which replicates to progressively deplete T-helper (CD4+) lymphocytes leading to severe cellular immunodeficiency. Without treatment, this immunodeficiency results in the development of otherwise unusual opportunistic infections and neoplasms characteristic of AIDS.
- The number of HIV-infected individuals continues to increase, as does the potential for prolonged survival. Therefore, critical care specialists can expect to care for more HIV-infected patients admitted to the ICU for complications related to their HIV infection or their treatment. When presented with a patient with AIDS or suspected to have HIV, a broad differential diagnosis, including opportunistic diseases, should be kept in mind to avoid delays in diagnosis.

KNOWN HIV PATIENT—UNDERSTAND THE SEVERITY OF DISEASE

- The severity of a patient's HIV disease burden will help to navigate the differential diagnosis. Important historical clues include most recent CD4+ count and viral load, known previous opportunistic infections or malignancy, current medications, including prescribed prophylactic medicines. Trimethoprim-sulfamethoxazole (TMP-SMX) prophylaxis implicates a (recent) historical nadir CD4+ <200 cells/μL, while azithromycin may implicate levels <100 cells/μL.
- Antiretroviral therapy may include nucleoside or nucleotide reverse transcriptase inhibitors (NRTIs, NtRTIs), nonnucleoside reverse transcriptase inhibitors (NNRTIs), protease inhibitors (PIs), and fusion inhibitors. Decisions to continue therapy must be carefully considered, but temporary interruption of the full regimen is commonly performed during hospitalizations for severe HIV-related complications.
- Adverse effects, toxicities, and possible drug interactions must be considered in respect to antiretroviral medicines. Severe reported toxicities include pancreatitis and lactic acidosis.

SUSPICION FOR HIV/AIDS

- The history of opportunistic infections, wasting, otherwise unexplained extensive herpes zoster, or persistent generalized lymphadenopathy combined with a history (or clinical evidence) of high-risk activities will necessitate consideration of HIV infection and related diseases.
- Common laboratory features found among HIV-infected individuals may provide the initial consideration, including: lymphopenia, anemia, thrombocytopenia, and hypergammaglobulinemia.
- HIV infection should not be diagnosed without specific serologic tests—enzyme-linked immunosorbent assay (ELISA) and Western blot.

NECESSARY DATA COLLECTION

- Lymphocyte subsets for CD4 count and viral load should be sent immediately. All microbiologic tests should include cultures for bacterial, fungal, viral, and mycobacterial pathogens (especially sputum and blood). Patients with respiratory distress should have a lactate dehydrogenase level (LDH) drawn to help stratify risk for *Pneumocystis jiroveci* infection (see "*Pneumocystis jiroveci* (formerly *P. carinii*) Pneumonia," below).

PULMONARY COMPLICATIONS

BACTERIAL PNEUMONIAS

- Pneumonias are the most common cause for hospitalization of the HIV-infected patient.
- Bacterial pneumonia should be suspected with acute onset of fever, cough, and lobar consolidate on chest x-ray (CXR).

- HIV engenders higher rates of usual bacterial infections (vs. the non-HIV population) including *Streptococcal pneumoniae* (150-fold), *Haemophilus influenzae* (100-fold), and *Legionella* (40-fold).
- *Pseudomonas aeruginosa* should be considered in late stages of disease (CD4 <100 cells/μL) and in the presence of cavitary disease or a history of broad-spectrum antibiotics.

PNEUMOCYSTIS JIROVECI (FORMERLY *P. CARINII*) PNEUMONIA

- Although classified as a fungus (with properties of a protozoan), this pathogen is given special attention as effective diagnostic testing and therapy mediate marked survival improvement.
- *Presentation*: dyspnea, nonproductive cough, and fever usually progressing over several days to weeks; physical examination usually demonstrates acute respiratory distress with scant findings on chest auscultation.
- *Studies implicating possible P. jiroveci*: (1) CXR—diffuse bilateral interstitial pattern (most commonly); although varying degrees of alveolar involvement can be seen, including multiple atypical presentations such as cystic changes, pneumothoraces, nodular disease, and even a normal radiograph (up to 30%); (2) elevated LDH levels—tends to correlate with disease severity and changes tend to parallel the clinical course (N.B. this is a nonspecific finding); and (3) CD4 count—*P. jiroveci* rarely occurs when the CD4 count is >200 cells/μL.
- *Diagnosis*: visualization of organism in pulmonary secretions or a lung biopsy. Most commonly, the modality of choice is bronchoscopy with bronchoalveolar lavage (BAL)—the sensitivity of BAL for *P. jiroveci* and other treatable pathogens commonly found in AIDS patients exceeds 95%. In the few patients with a nondiagnostic BAL, transbronchial or open lung biopsy should be considered. Empiric therapy is not recommended.
- TMP-SMX is first-line drug therapy, administered intravenously at a dose of 75 mg/kg daily in three divided doses. Adverse drug reactions are common, including rash, fever, liver, and renal dysfunction, thrombo- and leukocytopenia, anemia, and hyponatremia.
- Adjunctive systemic corticosteroid therapy (prednisone 40 mg twice daily) is recommended for moderate and severe infection recognized by impaired gas exchange, defined as PaO_2 <70 mmHg on room air.

MYCOBACTERIAL INFECTIONS

- *Mycobacterium tuberculosis (MTB)*. HIV infection is the most significant predisposing factor for reactivation of latent infection, and the radiographic presentation is often similar to primary TB; apical infiltrates or cavities are seen only in a minority. Extrapulmonary TB may present as lymphadenitis and disseminated disease. Purified protein derivative (PPD) testing is reasonable, but of limited use—nearly 30% of AIDS patients are anergic. Sputum, blood, or BAL stain and cultures are the mainstays of diagnosis.
- *Mycobacterium avium complex (MAC)* is usually disseminated (90%) and occurs later than MTB in the course of HIV, typically when the CD4 lymphocyte count is <50 cells/μL. Findings include fever, night sweats, diarrhea, weight loss, anemia, and elevated serum alkaline phosphatase levels. The diagnosis is established by isolating the organism from blood (mycobacterial blood culture) or less often from tissue biopsy or other normally sterile body fluids. Recovery of the organism from sputum, BAL, bowel, or stool specimens may represent colonization or localized or disseminated disease.

NEUROLOGIC COMPLICATIONS

BACTERIAL MENINGITIS

- The most common causes are *S. pneumoniae*, *H. influenzae*, and less commonly, *Listeria*, *M. tuberculosis*, and endemic fungi (coccidioidomycosis and histoplasmosis).

CRYPTOCOCCAL MENINGITIS

- The disease starts as a pulmonary infection and then disseminates to the brain and other organs. Presenting symptoms are often indolent and include headache, fever, nausea, vomiting, and occasionally, skin lesions or seizures.
- Serum cryptococcal antigen titer is a rapid and sensitive screening test, and diagnosis is confirmed with cerebrospinal fluid (CSF) analysis. Findings include lymphocytic-predominant pleocytosis, elevated protein, depressed glucose, and most importantly, *cryptococcal antigen testing*, smear, and culture. Alternatively, organism isolation from blood, urine, sputum, or other skin lesions is possible.
- Treatment of AIDS-related cryptococcal meningitis should be initiated with amphotericin B, 0.7 mg/kg/day plus flucytosine (100 mg/kg/day in four divided doses).

TOXOPLASMA ENCEPHALITIS

- The most common *focal* neurologic complication of HIV infection.

- Results from reactivation of latent infection and presents as a subacute headache with focal neurologic findings (majority), and seizures (30%).
- Risk of toxoplasma is most pronounced in those with CD4 counts <100 cells/μL without appropriate prophylaxis (TMP-SMX).
- Diagnosis is made empirically with visualization of multiple ring-enhancing lesions on contrast-enhanced brain imaging (magnetic resonance imaging [MRI] preferred over computed tomography [CT]) in a patient with positive serology. CSF analysis is often normal.
- Treatment is with pyrimethamine (100–200 mg loading does and then 50–100 mg/day) plus folinic acid (10 mg/day) plus sulfadiazine (4–8 g/day). Repeat brain imaging after 2–3 weeks of treatment; absence of improvement may require brain biopsy for definitive diagnosis.

OTHER CAUSES OF FOCAL NEUROLOGIC DISEASE

- Primary central nervous system lymphoma is the second most common cause of focal brain disease in this population. Brain imaging is necessary to implicate the diagnosis, but it is radiographically indistinguishable from toxoplasmosis. If toxoplasma therapy yields no improvement, lymphoma is quite possible, and a brain biopsy is required for a definitive diagnosis.
- Progressive multifocal leukoencephalopathy is mediated by the Jakob-Creutzfeldt virus, and can present with seizures or focal neurologic symptoms. MRI reveals single or multiple white matter lesions without surrounding edema, and definitive diagnosis requires brain biopsy.

IMMUNE RECONSTITUTION SYNDROME

- Immune reconstitution syndrome (IRS) is the augmentation of the immune response to preexisting clinical or subclinical infection, and can mediate clinical deterioration in almost any organ system.
- Most reports have been related to cytomegaloviral (CMV) retinitis, TB, MAC, *P. carinii* pneumonia (PCP), cryptococcosis, progressive multifocal leukoencephalopathy, and herpes zoster. Its frequency is increasing with the more pervasive use of highly active antiretroviral therapy.
- A diagnosis of IRS begins with a suspicion of clinical events occurring usually within weeks or months after initiating or revising an antiretroviral regimen. The differential diagnosis includes adverse drug effects and unrecognized infections. The diagnosis of IRS is one of exclusion, but requires convincing evidence of a response to the antiretroviral regimen (reduction in HIV RNA and usually a CD4 increase).
- The incidence of this complication may be reduced by delaying the initiation of antiretroviral therapy until after therapy directed at the opportunistic infection has been completed, and case reports suggest a possible benefit from systemic corticosteroids.

OTHER ORGAN SYSTEM DISEASE COMPLICATING AIDS

- *Cardiovascular*: Pericarditis (infectious and noninfectious), valvular heart disease (infectious or marantic endocarditis), and importantly, dilated cardiomyopathy (characterized by myocarditis pathologically).
- *Renal*: HIV-associated nephropathy (nephritic syndrome or renal insufficiency), renal toxicity from medications (either antibiotics or antiretrovirals). *Electrolytes*, especially hyponatremia (syndrome of inappropriate antidiuretic hormone [SIADH], hypovolemia, adrenal insufficiency), hypokalemia (GI losses), and hyperkalemia (medications, renal insufficiency).
- *Gastrointestinal*: Diarrhea from infectious colitis (bacterial, parasitic, viral) may lead to severe hypovolemia.
- *Endocrinology*: Adrenal insufficiency (infectious—TB, CMV, MAC).
- *Pulmonary*: Accelerated emphysema independent of inhalational toxins.
- *Hematology*: Cytopenias from the disease itself, marrow infiltration by infection or malignancy, or most commonly, from medication effect.

BIBLIOGRAPHY

Afessa B, Green B. Clinical course, prognostic factors, and outcome prediction for HIV patients in the ICU. The PIP (Pulmonary complications, ICU support, and prognostic factors in hospitalized patients with HIV) study. *Chest* 2000;118(1):138–145.

Morris A, Masur H, Huang L. Current issues in critical care of the human immunodeficiency virus-infected patient. *Crit Care Med* 2006;34(1):42–49.

Phillips P, Montaner JSG, Russell JA. AIDS in the intensive care unit. In: Hall JB, Schmidt GA, Wood LDH, eds., *Principles of Critical Care*, 3rd ed. New York, NY: McGraw-Hill; 2005: 1161–1199.

Vincent B, Timsit JF, Auburtin M, et al. Characteristics and outcomes of HIV-infected patients in the ICU: impact of the highly active antiretroviral treatment era. *Intensive Care Med* 2004;30(5):859–866.

50 ENDOCARDITIS

D. Kyle Hogarth

KEY POINTS

- The possibility of an endocardial (or intravascular) infection should be considered in all critically ill patients with the following:
  - Bacteremia or fungemia of uncertain origin
  - Fever of unknown origin
  - Hemodynamic instability of unclear etiology
- Blood cultures are the most important diagnostic test.
- Successful treatment requires prolonged duration of antimicrobial agents and removal of indwelling devices.
- Classic organisms causing endocarditis are staphylococci, enterococci, aerobic gram-negative bacilli, and yeasts.
- All patients with an indwelling intravascular device are at risk for the development of endocarditis.

PATHOGENESIS

- Microbial invasion into the bloodstream, even if transient, can lead to adherence to a heart valve. The organism replicates in a layer of fibrin and platelets, allowing it to escape the normal immune defenses.
- The likelihood of endocarditis developing will depend on the following factors: species of microbe, the inoculating concentration of microorganisms, presence of antimicrobials, and the characteristics of the endocardium.
- *Staphylococcus aureus*, enterococci, and other streptococci are the most adherent of organisms and are the most likely to cause endocarditis, even in undamaged valves. For example, *S. aureus* commonly causes skin infections and can result in transient bacteremia. Also, dental work on the teeth or gingiva may lead to transient bacteremia with viridans-type streptococci.

CLINICAL AND LABORATORY FEATURES

- Common symptoms include fever, malaise, myalgias and arthralgias, headache, and backache.

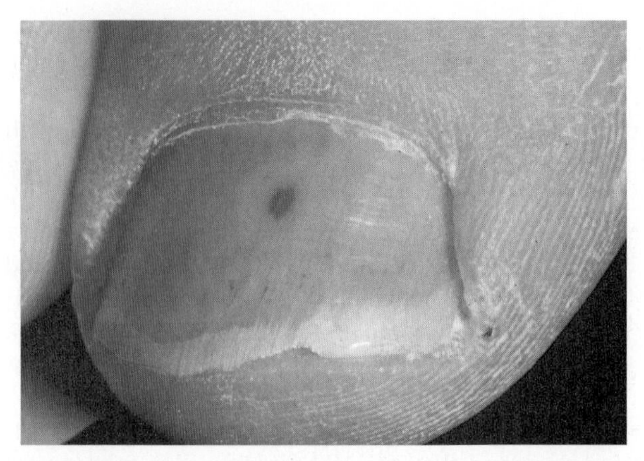

FIG. 50-1 Splinter hemorrhages in infective endocarditis.

- Common signs include fever, cardiac murmur, petechiae, Osler nodes, Janeway lesions, change in mental status, stroke.
  - Petechiae may be located on conjunctivae, the soft palate, and distal portions of the legs and arms.
  - Splinter hemorrhages may be located under the nail beds (Fig. 50-1).
  - Roth spots are hemorrhages in the fundus seen with an ophthalmologic examination.
  - Osler nodes are tender subcutaneous erythematous papules that occur on the finger pads, while Janeway lesions are nontender, larger, and occur on the palms and soles (Figs. 50-2 and 50-3).
- Common lab findings include: anemia, thrombocytopenia, increased white blood cells, elevated sedimentation rate, proteinuria, and hematuria.
- Systemic emboli from the endocarditis can lead to stroke, splenic infarctions, mesenteric ischemia, and

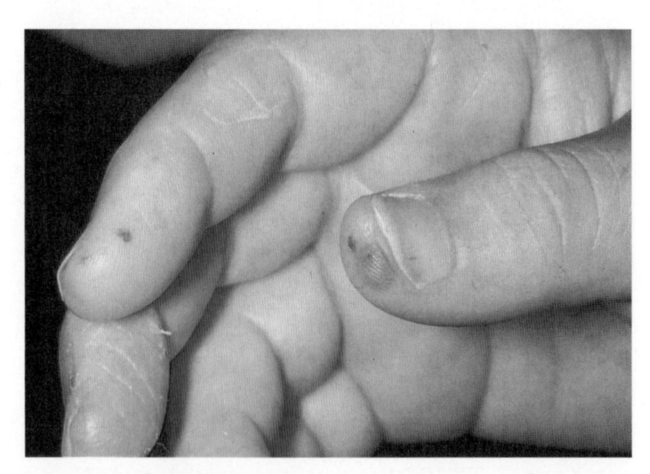

FIG. 50-2 Osler nodes in infective endocarditis. Osler nodes are tender, papulopustules located on the pulp of the finger in a patient with bacterial endocarditis caused by *S. aureus*.

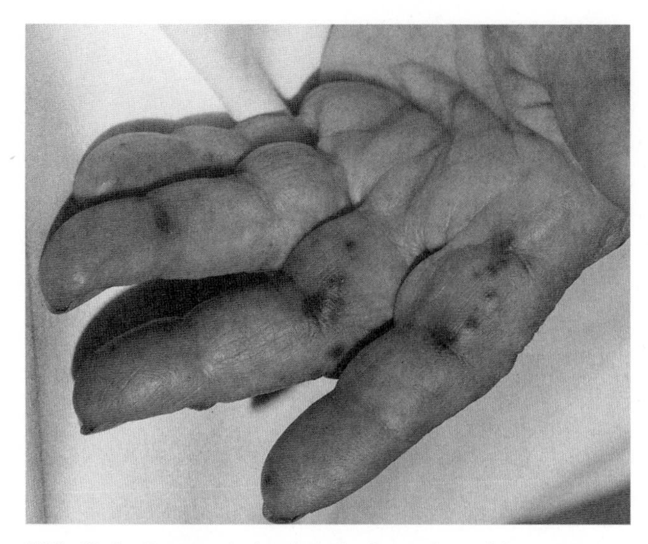

FIG. 50-3 Janeway lesion in infective endocarditis.

renal infarcts. Right-sided endocarditis can lead to septic pulmonary emboli.
- Many patients may have heart failure symptoms due to valvular dysfunction from the infection.

DIAGNOSIS

- The most important lab test is the blood culture, and it will be positive in 90% of cases of endocarditis.
- In approximately 5–10% of patients with presumed endocarditis, no etiologic organism is initially isolated.
- The causes of "culture-negative endocarditis" are the following:
  - Prior antibiotics given before blood cultures.
  - Endocarditis due to fastidious organisms, such as anaerobes, *Coxiella burnetii, Legionella pneumophila, Chlamydia psittaci, Chlamydia pneumoniae*, various fungi, and the HACEK organisms. (HACEK is an acronym for *Haemophilus* species, *Actinobacillus actinomycetemcomitans, Cardiobacterium hominis, Eikenella corrodens*, and *Kingella kingae*.)
  - Culture negative endocarditis can become "culture positive" using longer incubation times and special culture techniques to aid in isolation of fastidious microorganisms. Serologic studies for *Coxiella*, *Bartonella*, and *Chlamydia* can be used to help with the diagnosis.
- Echocardiography is useful for detecting vegetations.
- Transthoracic echocardiography (TTE) has 60% sensitivity for endocarditis.
- Transesophageal echocardiography (TEE) has a sensitivity of 90–99% with a specificity of 90%.

MANAGEMENT

- In hospitals with low rates of methicillin-resistant *S. aureus* (MRSA), initial therapy should be intravenous (IV) nafcillin, 2 g every 4 hours plus ampicillin 2 g IV every 4 hours and gentamicin, 1 mg/kg every 8 hours.
- Many centers have high rates of MRSA, and therefore empiric therapy with vancomycin or linezolid should be considered.
- Once the organism and its sensitivities are known, then therapy directed to the specific organism should be started.
- Parenteral antibiotics are always preferred over oral drugs.
- Bacteriocidal agents are superior to bacteriostatic drugs and are therefore preferred.
- Long-term antimicrobial therapy (6 weeks) is almost always required for cure of endocarditis.
- Indications for urgent valve replacement include:
  - Ineffective antimicrobial therapy
  - Severe heart failure
  - Valvular obstruction
  - Fungal endocarditis
  - The presence of an unstable prosthetic device (e.g., loose artificial mitral valve)

PROGNOSIS

- Outcomes are dependent on:
  - Pathogenicity of the organism
  - Location of infected valve (*S. aureus* is fatal in one-third of patients with aortic or mitral valve disease.)
  - Complications associated with the infection, especially congestive heart failure, shock, systemic emboli, and myocardial abscess
  - Size of the vegetation (>1 cm associated with an increased morbidity and mortality

BIBLIOGRAPHY

Alsip SG, Blackstone EH, Kirk JW, et al. Indications for cardiac surgery in patients with active infective endocarditis. *Am J Med* 1985;78:138–148.

Daniel WG, Mugge A. Transesophageal echocardiography. *N Engl J Med* 1995;332:1268–1278.

Moreillon P, Que YA. Infective endocarditis. *Lancet* 2004;363: 139–149.

Mylonakis E, Calderwood SB. Infective endocarditis in adults. *N Engl J Med* 2001;345:1318–1330.

Sizemore JM Jr, Cobbs CG, Carr MB. Endocarditis and other intravascular infections. In: Hall JB, Schmidt GA, Wood LDH, eds., *Principles of Critical Care*, 3rd ed. New York, NY: McGraw-Hill; 2005:801–814.

51 INFECTIOUS COMPLICATIONS OF INTRAVENOUS DEVICES

Ajeet Vinayak

KEY POINTS

- Catheter-related infections are common, costly, and associated with significant morbidity and mortality.
- CNS, *S. aureus*, enterococci, aerobic gram-negative bacteria, and *C. albicans* are most often responsible for catheter-related infection.
- The risk of catheter-related infection can be reduced by preferring the subclavian site, using a chlorhexidine-containing disinfectant, enforcing full barrier precautions, and removing catheters at the earliest opportunity. Antimicrobial impregnated catheters may be useful especially when the incidence of catheter-related infections is high despite other precautions.
- Infected catheters must be removed when patients are critically ill due to the catheter infection; the pocket or tunnel of a long-term catheter is involved; infection recurs following treatment; or certain resistant organisms are involved.
- Empirical treatment of catheter-related infection should cover *staphylococcal* species; vancomycin should be used where methicillin-resistant strains are prevalent. Antibiotics to cover gram-negative organisms and fungi should be added in patients who are critically ill or immunocompromised pending microbiologic confirmation of antimicrobial susceptibility.

EPIDEMIOLOGY

- It is estimated that 15 million patients days are spent with a central catheter and over 5 million central venous catheters (CVCs) are placed a year in the United States.
- The overwhelmingly largest complication associated with the use of CVCs is the development of serious catheter-related infections.
- The mortality rate associated with this complication is estimated to be as high as 25% with costs related to its treatment reaching half a billion dollars a year.
- CVCs account for over 90% of all cases of catheter-related infection.
- The following risk factors are associated with a higher risk of infection:
  - Inappropriate barrier protection
  - The internal jugular vein and femoral vein insertion sites
  - Distant site of infection
  - Concurrent bacteremia
  - Skin breakdown
  - The use of multilumen catheters
- Infections are much more likely to occur from transmission of skin flora to the tip of the catheter than from an intraluminal origin of infection related to tubing manipulation, or seeding from distant sources.
- Intraluminal (vs. extraluminal) infections are more likely with prolonged catheter duration (>2 weeks).

MICROBIOLOGY

- Common organisms include coagulase-negative staphylococci (CNS), *Staphylococcus aureus*, and *enterococcal* species. Other relatively common organisms include aerobic gram-negative bacteria and yeasts (e.g., *Candida albicans*).
- Cultures of *Corynebacterium* species, *Bacillus cereus*, *Trichophyton*, *Malassezia furfur*, and *Fusarium* all should raise suspicion for catheter-related infection.
- The majority of CNS, over 50% of *S. aureus*, and a quarter of enterococci have broad resistance patterns.

PREVENTION

- Site of CVC placement influences risk of infection: subclavian CVCs are superior to femorally placed CVCs, and may be slightly safer than those inserted in the internal jugular vein.
- The use of prophylactic vancomycin flushes has not been shown to reduce the incidence of infection and should be avoided given the risk of resistant organisms.
- Chlorhexidine-containing skin antiseptics appear to reduce the risk of infection over traditional povidone-iodine preparations.
- Full barrier protections (sterile gloves, gowns, mask, cap, and large drapes) during insertion of CVCs are clearly effective in prevention and should also be considered when central catheters are inserted peripherally.
- Gauze-based dressings have not been shown to be clearly superior to transparent dressings.
- Triple antibiotic ointments may increase the risk of candidal infections.
- Mupirocin may affect polyurethane catheter integrity and should be avoided.
- Povidone-iodine ointment has been shown to be beneficial with the insertion of hemodialysis catheters and should be considered for use in other immunocompromised patient groups.

- A variety of antibiotic-impregnated catheters are available. Benzalkonium chloride-coated pulmonary artery catheters may prevent infections. Combined chlorhexidine and silver sulfadiazine-coated catheters reduce infection and are cost-effective if these CVCs are used for 14 days or less. While the combination of minocycline and rifampin may be superior to the chlorhexidine and silver sulfadiazine-coated CVCs, the documentation of resistance to this combination has been reported over longer dwell times. Therefore, this catheter should also be employed for short-term use.
- The use of prophylactic doses of unfractionated and low-molecular weight heparin has been shown to reduce the incidence of catheter-related thrombosis. Lower infection rates with the use of heparin may be related to effects on thrombus formation or on packaged antimicrobial preservatives.
- Appropriate nurse-to-patient ratios should be in place in ICUs.
- Scheduled exchanges of catheters over a wire are not indicated.
- Daily assessment for the continued need of intravenous access is imperative to minimize preventable days with the catheter.

DIAGNOSIS

- No uniform consensus definition exists for intravenous catheter-related infections.
- Only 50% of line infections occur with local evidence of exudation or inflammation at the insertion site.
- Suspected cases should be investigated with two sets of blood cultures. Some experts recommend both samples be drawn from a peripheral site to avoid confusing skin/hub contamination with clinical device infection. Yet, the most recent consensus statement advises that at least one sample be from a peripheral site.
- Semiquantitative (roll plate method) and quantitative (sonification of flush) cultures are accepted as more diagnostically accurate than qualitative cultures.
    - While the former may be more accurate with recently placed (<1 weeks) catheters, the latter process may be superior to detect intraluminal infections associated with longer catheter placement.
    - Accepted positive results include >15 colony forming units (CFU) by the semiquantitative method and $>10^3$ CFU by quantitative procedures.
- Time to culture positivity data may make two simultaneous qualitative cultures more accurate for catheter-related infection if central samples are positive 2 or more hours earlier than peripheral samples.
- If metastatic seeding is considered possible, transesophageal echocardiography is indicated.

MANAGEMENT

- Catheters should be removed in the following situations:
    - Sepsis or septic shock with a clear diagnosis of catheter-related bloodstream infection or those cases without any other identifiable source of infection.
    - Tunnel or pocket infection of long-term devices.
    - Recurrent disease following treatment course completion.
    - Bacteremia with Corynebacteria, *Bacillus* sp., gram negatives, or fungi.
    - Subsequent tip positivity following replacement of a catheter via changing the original catheter over a wire. In this situation a new site should be used if intravenous access is still needed.
- Initial parenteral antibiotic therapy should be directed at treating *staphylococcal* species. The upfront choice of vancomycin should be reserved in areas where methicillin-resistant *S. aureus* is prevalent. Fungemia or gram-negative organisms should be empirically treated if patients are severely ill or immunocompromised.
- Once sensitivities are known and with clinical stability, therapy can be tailored to less broad-coverage agents and eventually to oral therapy including quinolones, linezolid, or trimethoprim-sulfamethoxazole. Cases of corynebacterium and bacillus infections should be treated with vancomycin.
- Antibiotic lock therapy consists of a mixture of antibiotic agent and heparin that is allowed to dwell within the volume of the catheter between periods of catheter use.
- CVC infections should be treated for 5–7 days following CVC removal. If the CVC is not removed, coagulase-negative staphylococcal infections should be treated for 10–14 days with systemic antibiotics and concomitant antibiotic lock therapy. Retained, tunneled devices with coagulase-negative staphylococcal bloodstream infection should be treated with 7 days of systemic therapy and a total of 14 days of antibiotic lock therapy.
- Given the metastatic potential of *S. aureus* bacteremia, treatment should likely be no less than 2 weeks for uncomplicated, quickly resolving cases, 4–6 weeks for cases with endocarditis, and even longer when there is osteomyelitis.
- Therapy directed at gram-negative organisms should be adjusted from 10–14 days up to 4–6 weeks based on suspicion of seeding, prolonged bacteremia, or the presence of risk factors such as valvular heart disease.
- Amphotericin B should be preferred initially over intravenous fluconazole in cases of candidemia associated with organ dysfunction, prolonged prior exposure to fluconazole, or prior known azole-resistant candidal infection. Caspofungin may also be a useful alternative drug in these situations, while reducing drug complications associated with amphotericin.

BIBLIOGRAPHY

McGee DC, Gould MK. Preventing complications of central venous catheterization. *N Engl J Med* 2003;342:1123–1133.

Mermel LA, Farr BM, Sherertz RJ, et al. Guidelines for the management of intravascular catheter-related infections. *Clin Infect Dis* 2001;32:1249–1272.

Mermel LA. Prevention of intravascular catheter-related infections. *Ann Intern Med* 2000;132:391–402.

Nucci M, Anaissie E. Should vascular catheters be removed from all patients with candidemia? An evidence-based review. *Clin Infect Dis* 2002;34:591–599.

O'Grady NP, Alexander M, Dellinger EP, et al. Guidelines for the prevention of intravascular catheter-related infections. Centers for Disease Control and Prevention. *MMWR Recomm Rep* 2002;51:1–29.

52 SEVERE COMMUNITY-ACQUIRED PNEUMONIA

Shashi Kiran Bellam

KEY POINTS

- Community-acquired pneumonia is a common cause of respiratory failure and ICU admission.
- CAP requiring ICU admission has a mortality rate near or >50%.
- Prompt identification, assessment of sputum for culture, and empiric antibiotics are the principles of specific therapy.
- Most critically ill patients with CAP should be treated with a third-generation cephalosporin plus either azithromycin or a fluoroquinolone. As an increasing incidence of MRSA is seen, VANCOMYCIN or LINEZOLID may be needed as well.
- For those at risk of *Pseudomonas*, use an intravenous antipseudomonal β-lactam plus an intravenous antipseudomonal fluoroquinolone.
- General therapy primarily involves supportive care to maintain hemodynamic stability and adequate oxygenation.

GENERAL CLINICAL FEATURES

- Definition: "Community-acquired" is defined as patients who present with pneumonia from outside the hospital. Common reasons for ICU admission include respiratory failure (both hypoxemic or hypercarbic) and circulatory failure (ranging from volume-responsive hypotension to septic shock).
- Pneumonias developing within 2 days of admission to a hospital are still considered community-acquired, since the infecting organism is likely to have been acquired before the hospitalization.
- Community-acquired pneumonia (CAP) needs to be distinguished from hospital-acquired pneumonia, as well as the newly described entity "health care"-associated pneumonia. The latter two are commonly caused by organisms different from the community pneumonia microbes (see Chap. 53).
- Microbiologic features: Common causes for CAP in general include *Streptococcus pneumoniae, Staphylococcus aureus*, and *Haemophilus influenzae*. Patients with severe CAP requiring ICU care may be more prone to have been infected with less common pathogens than those listed above, such as *Legionella pneumophila*.

ROUTES OF ENTRY

ASPIRATION

- Small amounts of oral or gastric bacteria are aspirated commonly and those organisms are cleared routinely by the bronchial mucociliary clearance mechanisms as well as normal immunologic responses in the alveoli. If the aspirate contains potentially virulent organisms or the normal pulmonary clearance mechanisms are dysfunctional, the organisms can proliferate and lead to pneumonia.
- Aspiration of potentially virulent bacteria occurs with large volumes of aspirated material (such as with seizures, alcoholics with altered mental status, or with oral disease) or if the normal clearance mechanisms are ineffective (such as cases of foreign body aspiration or malignancy with bronchial obstruction, or muscular dysfunction in the oropharynx, or after a viral respiratory infection which impairs ciliary function).
- Pneumonia can occur with small amounts of aspiration and no dysfunction of normal clearance if a virulent organism is involved (including *S. pneumonia, S. aureus*, and enteric gram-negative rods).

INHALATION

- As the number of organisms inhaled is usually small, only highly virulent organisms lead to pneumonia by this route, including respiratory viruses, *Legionella* spp., *Mycoplasma pneumoniae*, *Chlamydia* spp., *Coxiella burnetii, Mycobacterium tuberculosis*, and fungi.

HEMATOGENOUS

- Organisms within the venous circulation can lodge in the pulmonary vasculature and proliferate.

- Infections by this route are more often diffuse or multinodular and bilateral, and commonly include *S. aureus* and *Pseudomonas aeruginosa*. Skin entry and hematogenous dissemination can be seen in tularemia, brucellosis, and melioidosis.

TYPICAL CLINICAL FEATURES

- Common symptoms include cough with sputum (often purulent or bloody), shortness of breath, pleuritic chest pain, all of an acute onset. Common signs include fever, elevation in the white blood cell count with a neutrophil predominance, arterial hypoxemia, and possibly hypocarbia or hypercarbia (in respiratory failure). Chest x-rays often disclose an infiltrate.
- Less common causes of pneumonia with specific clinical features are:
  - *Legionnaire disease*: Transmitted via infected water, Legionnaire disease may be indistinguishable clinically from pneumococcal pneumonia, but often includes symptoms of dry cough, diarrhea or other gastrointestinal upset, or encephalopathy not explained by hypoxemia or shock.
  - *M. pneumoniae infection*: Often in younger patients (20s–30s) and frequently with an initial upper respiratory tract infection followed by a dry cough with low grade fevers and occasionally with symptoms such as diarrhea, myalgia, arthralgia, skin rash, and bullous myringitis. In severely ill patients, infiltrates may be bilateral and accompanied by myocarditis or encephalomyelitis.
  - *Chlamydia psittaci*: Transmitted from birds, clinically characterized by high fever and persistent dry cough and occasionally with myalgia, headache, gastrointestinal symptoms, or a macular rash. Frequently, hepatomegaly, splenomegaly, and pleural or pericardial friction rubs are found on physical examination. Severely ill patients can present with dyspnea, hypoxemia, and encephalopathy (including coma).
  - *Viral pneumonia*: Viral causes of critical illness usually are due to influenza viruses, predominantly in winter or early spring, and predominantly in nonimmunized patients, more so in the elderly or in patients with other comorbid conditions. Influenza is often complicated by a bacterial pneumonia (often *S. aureus*).

MANAGEMENT

- Laboratory studies: White blood cell count, Gram's stain and culture of lower respiratory tract secretions (defined as <10 epithelial cells per high-powered field), and blood cultures should be obtained.
- *L. pneumophila* is not detectable on routine Gram's stain or cultures and requires specific cultures; direct fluorescent antibody testing of sputum (neither highly sensitive nor specific) and urinary antigen testing (highly specific but not highly sensitive for pneumonia) are also available.
- Antibiotics should be started within 4–8 hours of the patient presenting for evaluation. Ideally, cultures will be obtained prior to antibiotics being administered, but antibiotics should not be delayed while waiting for lab testing or cultures.
- An understanding of local resistance rates, as well as characteristics of the patient, can help to guide initial empiric antibiotic selection. Guidelines published by the American Thoracic Society (ATS) and the Infectious Disease Society of America provide management guidelines for CAP.
- Empiric therapy with an appropriate regimen should be provided until culture data dictate more specific therapy. For patients sufficiently ill from CAP to require ICU admission, the ATS guidelines recommend:
  - Third-generation cephalosporin (cefotaxime, ceftriaxone) combined with either azithromycin or an intravenous fluoroquinolone.
  - If the patient is at risk for *Pseudomonas* infection (structural lung disease, such as bronchiectasis; on corticosteroids equivalent to >10 mg/day prednisone; on broad-spectrum antibiotics more than 7 days of the past month; or significantly malnourished), use an intravenous antipseudomonal β-lactam (cefepime, imipenem, meropenem, piperacillin/tazobactam) plus an intravenous antipseudomonal fluoroquinolone (or intravenous aminoglycoside plus azithromycin).
  - Chlamydia infection should be treated with a tetracycline (e.g., doxycycline 100 mg intravenously q 12 h).
  - *Legionella* infection should be treated with macrolides and rifampin.
- Pleural effusions: If an effusion is present, then thoracentesis to assess pH, Gram's stain and culture is indicated. If empyema is present, then a chest tube should be inserted.
- Supportive therapy:
  - Mechanical ventilation as needed for respiratory failure (via an endotracheal tube; current literature does not support routine use of noninvasive mechanical ventilation for severe CAP).
  - Intravenous volume infusion will be required by most patients with severe CAP to meet the criteria for goal-directed management of early shock (see Chap. 44).
  - Intravenous medications to maintain systemic blood pressure may be required, but should be instituted once the intravascular volume has been resuscitated.
  - Drotrecogin (as a therapy for sepsis) has been suggested to be particularly useful in cases of severe CAP from post hoc analysis of primary study data.

BIBLIOGRAPHY

Bartlett JG, Breiman RF, Mandell LA. Community-acquired pneumonia in adults: guidelines for management. *Clin Infect Dis* 1998;26:811–838.

Light RB. Pneumonia. In: Hall JB, Schmidt GA, Wood LDH, eds., *Principles of Critical Care*, 3rd ed. New York, NY: McGraw-Hill; 2005: 823–844.

Mandell LA, Bartlett JG, Dowell SF, et al. Update of practice guidelines for the management of community-acquired pneumonia in immunocompetent adults. *Clin Infect Dis* 2003;37: 1405–1433.

Niederman MS, Mandell LA, Anzueto A, et al. Guidelines for the management of adults with community-acquired pneumonia. Diagnosis, assessment of severity, antimicrobial therapy, and prevention. *Am J Respir Crit Care Med* 2001;163:1730–1754.

53 VENTILATOR-ASSOCIATED PNEUMONIA

D. Kyle Hogarth

KEY POINTS

- Ventilator-associated pneumonia is common in mechanically ventilated patients and associated with increased cost, duration of ventilation, and mortality.
- Prevention includes limiting time on the ventilator by performing daily spontaneous breathing trials, elevating the head of the bed, and keeping ETT cuff pressures >20 cmH_2O.
- Organisms causing VAP differ from those causing CAP (e.g., *S. aureus and Pseudomonas aeruginosa*) and are often drug-resistant.
- Treatment should take into account the local microbiologic susceptibility patterns, along with patient risk factors, but should cover both gram-negative and gram-positive organisms frequently identified to cause VAP.

DEFINITION

- Ventilator-associated pneumonia (VAP) is pneumonia developing in mechanically ventilated patients 48 hours or more after intubation and mechanical ventilation.
- This definition is important to distinguish from community-acquired pneumonia (CAP) requiring mechanical ventilation at initial presentation. Severe CAP has a different microbiologic epidemiology than VAP.
- The new entity of Health Care Associated Pneumonia (HCAP) has been developed to distinguish the patient type that is never truly "in the community" but not in the hospital (e.g., dialysis patients and nursing home residents).

EPIDEMIOLOGY

- Ventilator-associated pneumonia is the most common nosocomial infection in mechanically ventilated patients.
- VAP is associated with increased length of stay, time on ventilator, cost, morbidity (acute renal failure [ARF], shock, liver dysfunction), and mortality.
- Risks for drug-resistant organisms causing VAP include:
  - Antimicrobial therapy in preceding 90 days
  - Current hospitalization of 5 days or more
  - High frequency of antibiotic resistance in the community or in the specific hospital unit. This risk factor stresses the importance of knowing the "local flora" of your ICU or hospital
  - Presence of risk factors for HCAP:
    - Hospitalization for 2 days or more in the preceding 90 days
    - Residence in a nursing home or extended care facility
    - Home infusion therapy (including antibiotics)
    - Chronic dialysis within 30 days
    - Home wound care
    - Family member with multidrug-resistant pathogen
    - Immunosuppressive disease or therapy

RISKS FOR VENTILATOR-ASSOCIATED PNEUMONIA

- Mechanical ventilation (consider noninvasive ventilation for your patients)
- Length of time on ventilator
- Reintubation following unsuccessful extubation
- Aspiration of gastric contents
- Acid suppression
- Supine positioning of patient

INDEPENDENT RISKS FOR MORTALITY FROM VENTILATOR-ASSOCIATED PNEUMONIA

- Inadequate antibiotics
- Cancer

- Immunosuppression
- Poor premorbid lifestyle score
- Advanced age

TYPICAL FLORA CAUSING VENTILATOR-ASSOCIATED PNEUMONIA

- *Serratia* species, *Pseudomonas* species, *Staphylococcus aureus*, and *Enterococcus* species.
- A majority of these organisms will be resistant to various antibiotic agents available.

PREVENTION OF VENTILATOR-ASSOCIATED PNEUMONIA

- Minimizing time on the ventilator. This involves good strategies of sedation, pain control, and daily spontaneous breathing trials (see Chaps. 5, 6, and 33)
- Semirecumbent positioning (30–45°)
- Oral, rather than nasal, intubation for endotracheal tubes (ETT) and gastric tubes
- Aspiration of subglottic secretions with new ETT that have a side port for subglottic aspiration
- Maintaining endotracheal cuff pressures at least 20 cmH_2O
- Rotational bed therapy (for surgery patients only)
- Prevention of condensation collection in the tubing from the ventilator to the ETT
- Antiseptic hand solution and strict infection control
- Maintaining adequate staffing in the ICU
- Postpyloric feeding

DIAGNOSIS OF VENTILATOR-ASSOCIATED PNEUMONIA

- Tracheal colonization and ETT colonization occur within 24 hours of intubation. This can make the interpretation of sputum Gram's stains and cultures very difficult.
- Mechanically ventilated patients should be examined daily with an eye toward detecting VAP. Fevers, increased sputum, increasing oxygen requirement, or new infiltrates on chest radiograph should raise the concern for VAP.
- If a patient develops a new or worsening infiltrate plus two of the following three criteria, then the probability of a VAP is high and empiric antibiotics should be begun:
  - Fever >38°C
  - Leukocytosis or leukopenia
  - Purulent secretions
- The Clinical Pulmonary Infection Score (CPIS) can be used to aid in diagnosis:
  - CPIS is a score derived from the patient's temperature, blood leukocytes, quantity of tracheal secretions, cultures of tracheal aspirates, level of oxygenation (PaO_2/FiO_2 ratio), and evaluation of the radiograph for new infiltrates.
  - The CPIS has been demonstrated to have 93% sensitivity for VAP confirmed by bronchoscopy.
  - Follow-up studies indicate that patients initially suspected of having VAP who have low CPIS by day 3 of empiric therapy can have antibiotics discontinued with improved outcomes.
- Some experts advocate the use of an "invasive" strategy of deep pulmonary cultures using bronchoscopy with lavage and protected brush specimen.
- Not all patients can have a bronchoscopy safely performed in the ICU.
- While there is debate as to the best way to make the diagnosis of VAP, what is agreed on is that initial empiric antibiotic selection is very important. Equally important is a policy of "de-escalation" when further evidence shows that the patient does not have VAP and then empiric antibiotics can be stopped. (See Fig. 53-1 for a treatment algorithm from the American Thoracic Society (ATS)/Infectious Diseases Society of America (IDSA) 2005 guidelines for VAP.)

VENTILATOR-ASSOCIATED PNEUMONIA THERAPY

- Empiric therapy must begin by covering both gram negatives and gram positives.
- Resistance is a major concern and knowing the resistance patterns of the local flora of the ICU is extremely important.
- Results of Gram's stains of tracheal isolates or bronchoscopy cultures can allow the therapy to be appropriately narrowed.
- Empiric broad-spectrum therapy should be narrowed as soon as possible.

THE GRAM-NEGATIVE ORGANISMS

- Therapy for VAP must begin by empirically covering for *Pseudomonas* and *Serratia* species. Thus, one of the following agents should be employed.
- β-Lactams
  - Piperacillin/tazobactam 3.375 g IV every 4–6 hours
  - Imipenem/cilastatin 500 mg to 1 g IV every 6–8 hours
  - Meropenem 1 g IV every 8 hours

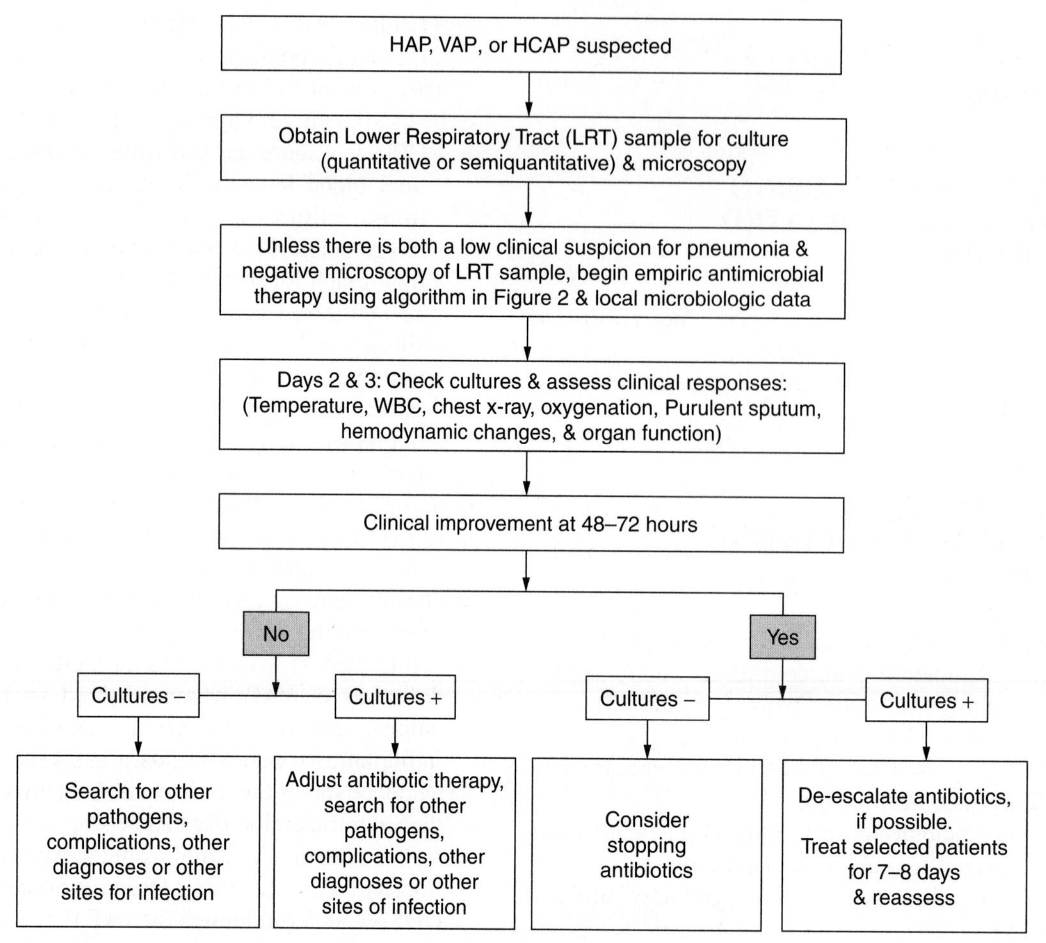

FIG. 53-1 Treatment algorithm from the ATS/IDSA 2005 guidelines for VAP.

- Cefepime 1 g IV every 8 hours or 2 g IV every 12 hours
- Ceftazidime 2 g IV every 8 hours
- Aztreonam 2 g IV every 6–8 hours (*Note*: not to be used as monotherapy)

• Fluoroquinolones
- Ciprofloxacin 400 mg IV every 8–12 hours

• Aminoglycosides (*Note*: not to be used as monotherapy)
- Amikacin 5–7.5 mg/kg IV every 8–12 hours
- Gentamicin 1.5–2.5 mg/kg IV every 8–24 hours or 5–7 mg/kg IV every 24 hours
- Tobramycin 1.5–2.5 mg/kg IV every 8–24 hours or 5–7 mg/kg IV every 24 hours

THE GRAM-POSITIVE ORGANISMS

• At least 50% of all isolates of *S. aureus* are methicillin resistant (MRSA) in the United States. There are two options for gram-positive coverage:
- Vancomycin 10–15 mg/kg IV every 8–24 hours
- Linezolid 600 mg IV every 12 hours

BIBLIOGRAPHY

American Thoracic Society, Infectious Diseases Society of America. Guidelines for the management of adults with hospital-acquired, ventilator-associated, and healthcare-associated pneumonia. *Am J Respir Crit Care Med* 2005;171:388–416.

Celis R, Torres A, Gatell JM, et al. Nosocomial pneumonia: a multivariate analysis of risks and prognosis. *Chest* 1988;93:378–324.

Koleff MH, Sherman G, Ward S, et al. Inadequate antimicrobial treatment of infections: a risk factor for hospital mortality among critically ill patients. *Chest* 1999;115:462–474.

Light RB. Pneumonia. In: Hall JB, Schmidt GA, Wood LDH, eds., *Principles of Critical Care*, 3rd ed. New York, NY: McGraw-Hill; 2005:823–844.

Richards M, Edwards JR, Culver DH, et al. Nosocomial infections in medical intensive care units in the United States. *Crit Care Med* 1999;27:887–892.

54 FUNGAL INFECTIONS IN THE INTENSIVE CARE UNIT

Ben Freed, Steve Davis

KEY POINTS

- Fungal infections most frequently affect immunocompromised patients. However, even patients with an intact immune system are susceptible if they are either severely ill or have a breach in their skin or mucous membranes.
- Clinical presentation varies depending on the type of fungus and severity of illness. In general, patients present with fever, chills, and myalgias. Rash, meningitis, and cough are symptoms that characterize certain kinds of fungi. In progressive cases, disseminated disease involving infection of multiple organs is possible.
- Culturing sources of infection including blood, CSF, and urine can sometimes make the diagnosis. Biopsies of skin lesions, pulmonary nodules, or bone marrow can also be helpful. In some cases, antigens can be detected easily.
- Treatment usually involves antifungal medications and, in certain cases, removal of the infected hardware. In recent years, many species of fungi have emerged that are resistant to what was considered standard treatment. Fortunately, new antifungals are showing promise for even the most resistant types of fungi.

OVERVIEW AND EPIDEMIOLOGY

- Although rare in the general population, fungal infections are increasingly becoming the cause for unexplained fevers in the intensive care unit (ICU).
- Fungi account for about 9% of all sepsis, severe sepsis, and septic shock cases and the mortality rate for fungemia is still extremely high at about 50%.
- There has been a threefold increase in fungemia between 1979 and 2000.
- Fungal infections can be difficult to diagnose in many cases. Empirical antifungal treatment is not appropriate in all cases of severe sepsis or septic shock. Clinical judgment is used in many instances in determining whether or not the patient should be treated.

THE HOST

- Identifying which patients are at high risk for fungal infections helps in determining whether or not that patient should be treated with antifungal medications.
- Patients with HIV/AIDS are very susceptible to fungal infections. In one prospective study, 84% of patients with AIDS were infected with *Candida*. The CD4 count of these patients helps in determining the type of fungus causing the infection. The most common types are *Candida albicans*, *Pneumocystis jiroveci*, and *Cryptococcus neoformans*. Dimorphic fungi such as *Histoplasma capsulatum* and *Coccidioides immitis* are found less frequently but occur most often in this patient population. Molds such as *Aspergillus fumigatus* and *Fusarium* spp. are rarely, if ever, the cause for infection.
- Patients with neutropenia secondary to chemotherapy or bone marrow transplant are also likely to be infected with fungi. Almost any kind of fungus can infect neutropenic patients. *C. albicans* and *A. fumigatus* are the most common but mold such as *Fusarium* spp. is occasionally the culprit.
- Any patient taking chronic corticosteroids or immune modulators for solid organ transplants or rheumatologic conditions is subject to a wide variety of fungal infections. Like with neutropenic patients, *A. fumigatus* and *C. albicans* are frequent causes of infection. Aspergillosis is found mostly in lung and heart transplant recipients and candidiasis in liver, kidney, and pancreas transplants.
- Patients with a relatively intact immune system can also fall victim to fungal infections if their first-line of defense against these diseases (i.e., skin or mucus membranes) is somehow breached. Patients with extensive burns often develop infections involving highly resistant fungi such as *Fusarium* spp. In addition, patients with indwelling catheters such as central lines, Foley catheters, peritoneal dialysis catheters, and feeding tubes are also subject to fungal infections. In fact, in one study, 95% of all patients with Foley catheters were found to have candiduria.
- Severely ill patients such as those with uncontrolled diabetes and frequent episodes of diabetic ketoacidosis are sometimes infected with rhinocerebral zygomycosis.
- Broad-spectrum antibiotics cause changes in normal bacterial flora such that fungal infections can thrive.

TREATMENT

- Current recommendations for treating severe sepsis or septic shock in the ICU state that empirical antifungal therapy should not be used on a routine basis but may be justified in selected subsets at high risk.
- Amphotericin B deoxycholate, one of the oldest antifungal therapies, is a polyene antifungal medication that is fungistatic in standard doses and fungicidal at

higher doses. It works by increasing membrane permeability, which leads to cell death. Used only in intravenous form, amphotericin B successfully treats a variety of fungal species. It is not used alone for fungal meningitis because it does not cross the blood-brain barrier. Side effects include chills, acute febrile reactions, anemia, and nephrotoxicity. Anaphylaxis occurs in 1% of all patients.

- Lipid-associated formulations of amphotericin B include amphotericin B lipid complex (ABLC) (Abelcet®; Enzon), amphotericin B colloidal dispersion (ABCD) (Amphotec®; InterMune), and liposomal amphotericin B (AmBisome®; Vestar). These antifungals are less toxic and are used as second-line agents for fungal diseases that are refractory to amphotericin B and for patients with underlying renal dysfunction. They are more expensive than amphotericin B.
- Flucytosine works by inhibiting fungal protein synthesis. It can be given enterally or intravenously. It is not recommended as monotherapy but can be used in association with other antifungals especially for meningitis, endocarditis, and endophthalmitis. Side effects include nausea, vomiting, diarrhea, and myelosuppression.
- Itraconazole is a triazole derivative that selectively inhibits the fungal cytochrome P450 resulting in decreased ergosterol synthesis and increased membrane permeability. It is available in either enteral or intravenous preparations. It works well against most mucosal forms of candidiasis but has fallen out of favor with the advent of newer triazoles. Its side effects include nausea, vomiting, headache, and rash.
- Fluconazole is also a triazole derivative but has different pharmacologic properties than itraconazole. This antifungal is used as first-line treatment for many types of fungal infections because, while it has similar efficacy to amphotericin B, it is far less toxic. Recently, certain strains of *Candida* and other types of fungi have developed resistance to this drug.
- Voriconazole is one of the newest triazoles that is similar to fluconazole but has a higher potency and has been effective against many fluconazole-resistant fungi, invasive *Aspergillus*, and emerging fungi such as *Blastomyces dermatitidis*, *Fusarium* spp., and *Penicillium marneffei*. It is available in both oral and parenteral formulations. Rare side effects include visual disturbances, transaminitis, and rash but it is relatively nontoxic.
- Caspofungin is in a new class of antifungal medications called echinocandins, which increases cell wall permeability by inhibiting a certain component of its synthesis. Caspofungin is only used in intravenous form. It has shown to be successful against fluconazole-resistant species of *Candida* but it appears not to have significant activity against *C. neoformans* or filamentous fungi other than *Aspergillus* (i.e., *Fusarium* spp. and *P. boydii*).
- For most fungal infections caused by an indwelling catheter, it is recommended that the hardware be removed and, if possible, the tip cultured.

PREVENTION

- Certain fungi such as *Candida* can be spread by the hands of health care workers. Basic infection-control measures such as hand-washing between patient contact and sterile technique prior to insertion of any device reduce risk of fungal infections.
- Antifungal prophylaxis has been successfully used for patients with neutropenia and for patients with advanced HIV or AIDS in decreasing the incidence of invasive fungal infections.
- Preemptive therapy for nonneutropenic but critically ill patients is controversial. Many physicians will treat this patient population without a definitive diagnosis if they are highly colonized with fungi or if they continue to remain febrile despite the use of broad-spectrum antibiotics.

SPECIFIC FUNGAL INFECTIONS

CANDIDA ALBICANS

- No matter the patient, the most common type of fungal infection in the ICU is *Candida*. In fact, 60% of all fungal infections are caused by this yeast. *C. albicans* is still the most frequent culprit but, in recent years, a growing number of nonalbicans species such as *C. parapsilosis*, *C. glabrata*, and *C. krusei* have been implicated.
- *Candida* spp. is now the fourth most common cause of nosocomial bloodstream infections in the United States.
- *Candida* spp. are yeasts that can form pseudohyphae. They are a normal part of the gut flora and can also be found on the skin. They can cause infection by either being translocated from the gut into the bloodstream, or by translocation from the skin or urine into the bloodstream.
- In the ICU, colonization with this yeast is frequent and does not always lead to infection. However, *Candida* found in the blood is never normal.
- The clinical manifestations vary since *Candida* spp. can affect a multitude of organs. In the general population, skin, nail, and vulvovaginal candidal infections are common.

- In the intensive care setting, oropharyngeal and esophageal candidiasis are commonly seen especially in patients with HIV/AIDS. This can present as a sore throat, dysphagia, or as thrush (patches of thick, white, creamy exudate on the tongue that is difficult to remove).
- *Candida* spp. can also infect the bloodstream causing fevers, chills, and possibly septic shock. Once in the bloodstream, *Candida* spp. can spread hematogenously to many organs including the lungs, liver, spleen, gallbladder, pancreas, peritoneum, heart, meninges, skin, and eyes.
- *Candida* spp. are found in the urine in 20–30% of critically ill patients with Foley catheters. Candiduria can potentially cause urosepsis but it is rare. Most patients with candiduria are asymptomatic.
- Diagnosis is made by detecting pseudohyphae in the blood. Only one positive culture is needed, but the sensitivity of this test is so low, many patients with disseminated candidiasis will have negative blood cultures. The lysis-centrifugation method is best for detecting this fungus in blood but it still takes 2–4 days for a blood culture to turn positive.
- If a blood culture is positive, an ophthalmologic examination should be performed in order to identify white cotton wool exudates consistent with endophthalmitis or chorioretinitis.
- A punch biopsy of skin lesions which consist of clusters of painless pustules or macules on any part of the body might be helpful in making the diagnosis.
- Culturing the tips of invasive catheters after removal might be beneficial.
- Other tests such as antigen/antibody assays or polymerase chain reaction (PCR) have proved disappointing.
- For most cases of candidiasis, therapy consists of fluconazole instead of amphotericin B. The combination of these two drugs has also been recommended for the first 5–6 days of treatment.
- In cases of fluconazole-resistant *Candida* such as *C. glabrata*, patients who are unstable with multiple organs involved, and patients who received prophylaxis with fluconazole, amphotericin B is used instead of fluconazole.
- Both voriconazole and caspofungin are quickly becoming first-line agents for candidal disease. Both antifungal drugs have excellent activity against all *Candida* strains including triazole-resistant *Candida* and they have less toxicity than amphotericin B.
- Although removal of the Foley catheter is recommended for all, the use of antifungal treatment for candiduria is usually reserved for the critically ill and immunocompromised.
- In cases of candidal meningitis, endophthalmitis, and endocarditis, flucytosine has been recommended in combination with amphotericin B.
- For cases of candidemia, treatment should continue for 2 weeks after the last negative blood culture. A longer course of treatment might be required depending on which organs are involved.

CRYPTOCOCCUS NEOFORMANS

- *C. neoformans* is a polysaccharide-encapsulated yeast which grew in prevalence during the 1980s with the rapid growth of HIV.
- Almost 10% of all patients with HIV/AIDS have *C. neoformans* but it can affect other immunocompromised patients as well.
- The species exists in several varieties: the *gatti* variety (serotype B) which has been associated with eucalyptus trees, and *neoformans* (serotype D) and *grubii* (serotype A) which have been associated with fruits, trees, and bird excreta.
- *C. neoformans* is inhaled and usually causes an asymptomatic pulmonary infection. It then travels hematogenously to the cerebrospinal fluid (CSF) where it can cause signs and symptoms of meningitis including fever, headache, mental status changes, and photophobia.
- Cryptococcosis can be detected in the CSF or blood using the cryptococcal latex antigen test. India ink stains are no longer used.
- The treatment is usually a combination of amphotericin B and flucytosine followed by fluconazole. Patients with HIV/AIDS should be treated for life since recurrence is common.
- Although voriconazole shows good activity, caspofungin has not been shown to be effective against cryptococcosis.

ASPERGILLUS FUMIGATUS

- *Aspergillus* is a mold which produces hyaline or colorless, septate hyphae.
- The species *A. fumigatus* is the most common type and is responsible for over 90% of invasive fungal infections. Although uncommon in the United States, *A. flavus* produces toxins called aflatoxins which can cause liver cancer.
- A population-based study for San Francisco shows an incidence of 1–2 cases per 100,000 a year.
- *A. fumigatus* is commonly found in patients with lung and heart transplants but has also been described in burn patients and those with alcoholic liver disease and is increasing in patients with HIV/AIDS.

- Patients with lung cavitations from tuberculosis or sarcoidosis can grow *Aspergillus* 'fungal balls' (aspergillomas).
- *A. fumigatus* is diagnosed by detecting the acute angle branching septae in bronchoalveolar lavage or biopsy.
- Amphotericin B was used as the primary weapon against *A. fumigatus* but, since the advent of amphotericin B-resistant species such as *A. terreus*, voriconazole and caspofungin have been used with much greater success.

HISTOPLASMA CAPSULATUM, COCCIDIOIDES IMMITIS, BLASTOMYCES DERMATITIDIS

- All three fungi are dimorphic in that they grow as mycelial forms, with spores, at 25°C on Sabouraud agar and as yeast at 37°C on blood agar.
- These fungi commonly affect patients with HIV/AIDS but have been found in other immunocompromised patients.
- *H. capsulatum* is the most common of the three overall and *B. dermatitidis,* the least common but the incidence for each fungus, is dependent on geographic regions.
- *H. capsulatum* is found primarily in the Ohio and Mississippi River valley states. It is isolated in the soil where avian and bat excreta exist.
- *C. immitis* is endemic in the desert areas of the Southwest United States and Northern Mexico. It, too, is found in soil.
- *B. dermatitidis* is most commonly seen in the Ohio and Mississippi River Valley states as well. It is isolated from soil and rotten wood.
- All three fungi are transmitted by inhalation of spores which can result in pneumonia and, possibly, dissemination into the bloodstream.
- *C. immitis* commonly causes pneumonia with calcified granulomas in HIV/AIDS patients. The clinical presentation is typically fevers, chills, and cough. Disseminated disease is rare but is seen more commonly in critically ill patients without HIV/AIDS.
- Unlike *Coccidioides*, *H. capsulatum* and *B. dermatitidis* more commonly cause disseminated disease in patients with HIV/AIDS. In one study, 10–25% of patients with AIDS developed disseminated histoplasmosis. Meningitis, bone lytic granulomas, skin granulomas, and other organ lesions have been reported.
- Diagnostic tests for *H. capsulatum* include blood and bone marrow cultures but detecting the polysaccharide antigen in the serum or urine is faster and just as sensitive. The specificity for the antigen assay is not as good because false positive results are seen in patients with blastomycosis, paracoccidioidomycosis, and *P. marneffei* infection.
- *C. immitis* is commonly seen on the chest radiograph as a diffuse reticulonodular pattern that is often confused with *Pneumocystis*. Complement-fixation serologic tests are also useful.
- *B. dermatitidis* can be detected by antigen assay.
- Amphotericin B followed by fluconazole has been the recommended therapy for each fungus but voriconazole is gaining favor as first-line treatment.

PNEUMOCYSTIS JIROVECI (FORMERLY CARINII)

- *P. jiroveci* (still referred to as *PCP*) is an atypical fungus that is neither yeast nor mold. In fact, it was classified as a protozoan for many years but is more recently considered a fungus.
- This fungus is considered the most common opportunistic infection in patients with HIV/AIDS. About 80% of patients with AIDS will be infected with *PCP* at least once in their lifetime unless prophylactic antibiotics are taken.
- *PCP* infects its host through respiratory transmission and will commonly cause a clinical picture consisting of dyspnea, hypoxemia, cough, and sometimes fever.
- The chest radiograph will typically show a diffuse interstitial pattern: an elevated serum lactate dehydrogenase (LDH) is a fairly sensitive, yet not specific, marker.
- Diagnosis is made by direct fluorescent antibody (DFA) of induced sputum or bronchoalveolar lavage. Silver stains are no longer used.
- Unlike other fungi, *PCP* has been successfully treated with trimethoprim/sulfamethoxazole and steroids (prednisone, 40 mg twice daily, for 5 days, followed by a tapering dose, to be used when the PaO_2 is <70 mmHg). Many patients with HIV/AIDS are placed on prophylaxis.

PENICILLIUM MARNEFFEI

- Once rare in the Unites States, the incidence of the dimorphic fungus, *P. marneffei*, is rising especially in the HIV/AIDS population.
- This fungus is endemic in Southeast Asia, Hong Kong, and Taiwan where penicilliosis is considered the third most common opportunistic infection (following cryptococcus and tuberculosis) among HIV-infected patients.

- The transmission for this infection is thought to be both from inhaled spores from the soil and direct inoculation of skin wounds.
- Patients with this infection present with fever, cough, lymphadenopathy, and weight loss. Skin lesions are characterized by umbilicated papules or nodules with necrotic centers located mostly on the trunk and upper extremities.
- The chest radiograph might show interstitial infiltrates and anemia is commonly reported.
- Diagnosis of this fungus is currently made by culture of blood, stool, urine, CSF, and bone marrow. *P. marneffei* produces a red soluble pigment on Sabouraud agar. Biopsies of skin lesions or lymph nodes are also helpful. PCR and antigen assays have been used with some success but are not yet in clinical use.
- Treatment consists of amphotericin B, itraconazole, or voriconazole. The fungus is resistant to fluconazole. The activity of caspofungin against this fungus has yet to be studied. Lifelong secondary prophylaxis with itraconazole or voriconazole has been recommended.

FUSARIUM SPP.

- Like *Aspergillus*, *Fusarium* is a saprophytic filamentous mold that produces septate hyphae.
- *F. solani* is the most common type to produce infection but *F. oxysporum*, *F. moniliforme*, and *F. proliferatum* have also been recovered from humans.
- Fusarial infections were epidemic in Russia in the early 1900s secondary to the ingestion of contaminated grains and is now becoming more common especially among patients with hematologic malignancies, bone marrow transplants, and those with severe burns.
- *Fusarium* spp. usually cause disseminated disease by direct inoculation or the ingestion of *Fusarium* toxins.
- Clinically, patients present with severe myalgias, fevers, and skin lesions that are characterized as initially macular with central pallor and progress to necrotic lesions with a surrounding rim of erythema. These lesions can be seen on all extremities.
- Definitive diagnosis can be made by culturing blood and skin biopsies. The fungus produces downy, cotton colonies that are lavender to purple-red on Sabouraud agar. Microscopically, they appear as sickle-shaped and multicellular. The histopathology can be indistinguishable from *Aspergillus*.
- *Fusarium* is extremely resistant to many antifungal medications. Only high-dose amphotericin B and voriconazole have been effective in eradicating this fungus.

BIBLIOGRAPHY

Ampel NM. Emerging disease issues and fungal pathogens associated with HIV infection. *Emerg Infect Dis* 1996;2:109–116.

Avecillas JF, Mazzone P, Arroliga AC. A rational approach to evaluation and therapy of the infected patient in the intensive care unit. *Clin Chest Med* 2003;24:645–669.

Bochud PY, Bonten M, Marchetti O, et al. Antimicrobial therapy for patients with severe sepsis and septic shock: an evidence-based review. *Crit Care Med* 2004;32:S495–S512.

Eggimann P, Garbino J, Pittet D. Epidemiology of *Candida* species infections in critically ill non-immunosuppressed patients. *Lancet Infect Dis* 2003;3:685–702.

Eggimann P, Garbino J, Pittet D. Management of *Candida* species infections in critically ill patients. *Lancet Infect Dis* 2003;3:772–785.

Flanagan PG, Barnes RA. Fungal infection in the intensive care unit. *J Hosp Infect* 1998;38:163–177.

Garnacho-Montero J, Garcia-Garmendia JL, Barrero-Almodovar A, et al. Impact of adequate empirical antibiotic therapy on the outcome of patients admitted to intensive care unit with sepsis. *Crit Care Med* 2003;31:2742–2751.

Gea-Banacloche JC, Opal SM, Jorgensen J, et al. Sepsis associated with immunosuppressive medications: an evidence-based review. *Crit Care Med* 2004;32:S578–S590.

Hadley S, Lee WW, Ruthazer R, et al. Candidemia as a cause of septic shock and multiple organ failure in nonimmunocompromised patients. *Crit Care Med* 2002;30:1808–1814.

Jain P, Sandur S, Meli Y, et al. Role of flexible bronchoscopy in immunocompromised patients with lung infiltrates. *Chest* 2004;125:712–722.

Richards MJ, Edwards JR, Culver DH, et al. Nosocomial infections in combined medical-surgical intensive care units in the United States. *Infect Control Hosp Epidemiol* 2000;8:510–515.

55 CENTRAL NERVOUS SYSTEM INFECTIONS

John A. Schneider

KEY POINTS

- Imaging plays little role in the diagnosis of acute bacterial meningitis but CT should be performed before lumbar puncture when an intracranial mass lesion is suspected (antibiotics should not be delayed).
- Dexamethasone has been shown to reduce morbidity in children with acute *H. influenzae* type B meningitis and, when given before antibiotics, in adults with pneumococcal meningitis.

- Rapid surgical decompression is indicated in patients with spinal epidural abscess with worsening deficit.
- Herpes simplex encephalitis benefits from prompt diagnosis and treatment with acyclovir.

EPIDEMIOLOGY AND ETIOLOGY

- Viruses are the major cause of *aseptic meningitis*—a general term to describe a meningitis that is infectious or noninfectious with a lymphocytic pleocytosis, for which a cause is not apparent after initial evaluation and routine stains and cultures of cerebrospinal fluid (CSF).
- A specific viral etiology is established in only up to 70% of aseptic meningitides. Enteroviruses are the most likely causative pathogen in 85–95% where a diagnosis is made. Arboviruses and herpes viruses are also pathogens that cause aseptic meningitis, however, they much more commonly cause *encephalitis*—distinguished by the presence of decreased mentation (i.e., confusion or stupor).
- *Bacterial meningitis* causes significant morbidity and mortality with rates that remain unacceptably high despite the availability of effective antimicrobial therapy.
- *Subdural empyema* refers to a collection of pus in the space between the dura and arachnoid. It accounts for up to 20% of all localized intracranial infections.
- *Epidural abscess* refers to a localized collection of pus between the dura mater and the overlying skull or vertebral column. Because cranial epidural abscess can cross the cranial dura, an accompanying subdural empyema can be present. Spinal epidural abscess usually occurs secondary to hematogenous dissemination from foci elsewhere in the body to the epidural space, or by extension from vertebral osteomyelitis.
- *Suppurative intracranial thrombophlebitis* includes both venous thrombosis and suppuration which usually begins in the paranasal sinuses, middle ear, mastoid, face, or oropharynx. Its development depends on the close proximity of various structures to the dural venous sinuses.
- The three most common meningeal pathogens (accounting for 80% of cases) have remained the top three for the last 25 years, however, their relative order has reversed completely from *Haemophilus influenzae, Neisseria meningitidis, Streptococcus pneumoniae* in 1978 to *Streptococcus pneumoniae, Neisseria meningitidis, Haemophilus influenzae* by 2005. Other causative organisms include *Streptococcus agalactiae* and *Listeria monocytogenes*.
- In infants (0–3 months), *S. agalactiae* and *L. monocytogenes* are more prominent than in adults (18–50 years) where *S. pneumoniae* and *N. meningitidis* are dominant. *L. monocytogenes* returns as an important pathogen in those >50 years.
- Certain predisposing factors should raise awareness of other pathogens: immunocompromised state—gram-negative bacilli (*Pseudomonas*); basilar skull fracture—group A β-hemolytic streptococci; head trauma/postneurosurgery/CSF shunt—*Staphylococcus* species, gram-negative bacilli (*Pseudomonas*).
- The organisms responsible for a brain abscess (case fatality 30–60%) are highly variable and depend on the predisposing condition: otitis media or mastoiditis—streptococci, anaerobes, Enterobacteriaceae; sinusitis—streptococci, anaerobes, *S. aureus*, *Haemophilus* spp.; dental sepsis—*Fusobacterium*, other anaerobes, and streptococci; penetrating trauma or postneurosurgical—*S. aureus*, streptococci, Enterobacteriaceae, *Clostridium* spp.; lung abscess, empyema, bronchiectasis—*Fusobacterium*, *Actinomyces*, other anaerobes, streptococci, *Nocardia* spp.; bacterial endocarditis—*S. aureus*, streptococci; neutropenia—aerobic gram-negative bacilli, *Aspergillus* spp., Mucorales, *Candida* spp.; transplantation—*Aspergillus* spp., *Candida* spp., Mucorales, Enterobacteriaceae, *Nocardia* spp., *Toxoplasma gondii*; HIV infection—*T. gondii*, *Nocardia* spp., *Mycobacterium* spp., *L. monocytogenes*, *Cryptococcus neoformans*.

PATHOGENESIS

- For bacterial meningitis, colonization is followed by local invasion, bacteremia, meningeal invasion, and finally bacterial replication in the subarachnoid space.
- Microorganisms can reach the brain and cause abscess by three mechanisms in decreasing frequency: spread from contiguous focus, hematogenous spread, and traumatic spread.
- Specific virulence factors overcome host defense mechanisms to cause meningitis. The new arrival of an organism which colonizes the nasopharynx is the first step in this process. Fimbria, polysaccharide capsule, and IgA protease production are a few of the bacterial factors that allow for colonization and subsequent invasion.
- Intravascular survival is facilitated as the most common meningeal pathogens are encapsulated. The mechanism for meningeal invasion is unknown. Once meningeal pathogens enter the subarachnoid space, host defense mechanisms are inadequate to control the replication and infection that occurs.
- Marked inflammation occurs in the subarachnoid space which manifests in the clinical symptoms and signs of meningitis. Alterations in the blood-brain barrier occur, which allows for increased permeability of both pathogen and antimicrobials.

- Vasogenic, cytotoxic, and interstitial mechanisms contribute to cerebral edema which creates increased intracranial pressure which may lead to subsequent herniation. A vasculitis can occur which can lead to narrowing or thrombosis of cerebral blood vessels and subsequent ischemia and infarction. Direct neuronal injury can also occur.

CLINICAL FEATURES

- Viral meningitis almost always has fever as one of its presenting signs. Accompanying symptoms of vomiting, anorexia, headache, and rash are common. Other neurologic symptoms and signs are often reported.
- Bacterial meningitis classically presents with four components: headache, fever, meningismus, and altered mental status. At least one of these components is present in all patients with acute bacterial meningitis. Kernig or Brudzinski sign is present in over 50% of patients. Emesis (35%), seizures (30%), focal neurologic signs (10–20%), and papilledema (<1%) may also be present.
- Rash present on the extremities occurs in 50% of patients with meningococcemia. Rash is erythematous and macular, and matures rapidly into petechial and subsequent purpuric phases. This rash is more commonly seen in younger patients with meningococcal meningitis.
- Neonates may not have meningismus and may present with temperature instability (hypo/hyperthermia), listlessness, irritability, refusal to eat, vomiting, diarrhea, or respiratory distress. Likewise, elderly and neutropenic patients may present with lethargy and obtundation.
- CSF shunt infections may not present with meningeal signs. Frequent symptoms are headache, nausea, lethargy, and change in mental status. Fever is variable, and pain is often related to infection at the peritoneal or pleural endings of the shunt or may be absent altogether.
- Brain abscess may be indolent or fulminant with some clinical manifestations mimicking those for meningitis. However, the clinical symptoms and signs may be more due to the size and location of a space-occupying lesion and the virulence of the infecting organism.
- Subdural empyema may be rapidly progressive, with symptoms and signs secondary to the presence of increased intracranial pressure, meningeal irritation, or focal cortical inflammation. This acute presentation of subdural empyema is seen most often in patients with contiguous spread of infection. Headache, which may be localized to the infected sinus or ear, is a prominent complaint and becomes generalized as the infection progresses.
- Spinal epidural abscess may develop within hours to days, or the course may be more chronic, over weeks to months. The presentation in most patients demonstrates four clinical stages: (1) backache and focal vertebral pain, with tenderness on examination; (2) nerve root pain, manifested by radiculopathy or paresthesias, or both; (3) spinal cord dysfunction, characterized by defects of motor, sensory, or sphincter function; and (4) complete paralysis. Pain is the most consistent symptom and is usually accompanied by local tenderness at the affected level.
- Suppurative intracranial thrombophlebitis may damage the nerves that traverse the cavernous sinuses. The most common complaints in patients with septic cavernous sinus thrombosis are periorbital swelling and headache. Other symptoms include drowsiness, diplopia, eye tearing, photophobia, and ptosis.

DIAGNOSIS

- For viral meningitis, CSF pleocytosis is almost always present with the cell count ranging from 100 to 1000 mm^3. Early in infection neutrophils may dominate the CSF profile; however, a lymphocytic predominance occurs over the first 6–48 hours of infection. Protein and glucose perturbations are minimal. A specific virologic diagnosis depends on the isolation of virus from the CSF in tissue culture. PCR for herpes simplex virus or for varicella-zoster virus may also be diagnostic.
- Bacterial meningitis usually has the following typical findings: opening pressure > 180 mmHg; WBC count 1000–5000/mm^3; ≥80% neutrophils; protein 100–500 mg/dL; glucose ≤40 mg/dL. The Gram stain is positive in 60–90% and the culture 70–85% of cases. A rapid streptococcal urinary antigen may help with the diagnosis.
- Cranial computed tomography (CT) or magnetic resonance imaging (MRI) does not aid in the diagnosis of acute meningitis. If the symptoms are prolonged or there are neurologic deficits, it may be warranted. Cranial imaging should be obtained prior to lumbar puncture when there is evidence of papilledema or focal neurologic deficits, however, it should not delay the initiation of antibiotics and corticosteroids.
- Cranial CT or MRI is key to the diagnosis of brain abscess or subdural empyema and MRI for spinal epidural abscess and suppurative intracranial thrombophlebitis. For brain abscesses, CT characteristically demonstrates a hypodense center with a peripheral uniform ring enhancement following the injection of contrast material; this is surrounded by a variable hypodense area of brain edema. MRI is more sensitive than CT and assists in early detection of cerebritis, cerebral

edema, inflammation into ventricles and subarachnoid space, and earlier detection of satellite lesions.

- A lumbar puncture is contraindicated for the diagnosis of subdural empyema due to risk of herniation.
- Blood cultures should be obtained for all patients presenting with stigmata of meningitis or brain abscess.

MANAGEMENT AND TREATMENT

- Imaging should be performed to verify the suspicion of brain abscess. If single or multiple ring-enhancing lesions are found, the patient should be taken urgently to surgery and all lesions >2.5 cm in diameter should be excised or stereotactically aspirated and sent to microbiology and pathology.
- Subdural empyema and epidural abscesses are medical emergencies. Prompt surgical decompression through a drainage procedure is necessary as antimicrobial agents alone do not reliably sterilize the empyema. Antibiotics for 3–6 weeks are recommended (longer if bone is involved).
- Suppurative thrombophlebitis can usually be managed with antibiotics. Ligation of the internal jugular vein along with thrombectomy via a surgical procedure may be needed with severe disease of cavernous sinus thrombosis with sphenoid involvement. Anticoagulation can be used in conjunction with antibiotics for severe disease; however, risk of intracranial hemorrhage or venous hemorrhagic infarcts does exist.
- For acute meningitis, the institution of antimicrobial therapy should be based on the results of Gram stain of the CSF. If a positive Gram stain is not obtained from the CSF or the lumbar puncture is delayed longer than 90–120 minutes, empirical antibiotic therapy should be initiated after blood cultures are obtained.
- Dexamethasone (10 mg q6h × 2 days) should be initiated 30 minutes prior to or concomitantly with antibiotics when a diagnosis of meningitis is made or if empiric treatment is to begin.
- Specific antiviral chemotherapy is not available for the enteroviruses.
- Early recognition and treatment improves outcome in herpes simplex encephalitis. The treatment is acyclovir at a dose of 10 mg/kg every 8 hours for 10–14 days.
- Empirical therapy for purulent meningitis depends on the predisposing factors as outlined above. For infants (0–3 months) ampicillin plus a third-generation cephalosporin (ceftriaxone) should be administered. For children and adults (3 months–50 years) a third-generation cephalosporin should be administered and for adults >50, ampicillin should be added to this regimen. Vancomycin should be added to all the above regimens in areas where there is *S. pneumoniae* resistance to penicillin (PCN; United States). With penicillin allergy, trimethoprim/sulfamethoxazole (TMP/SMX) should replace ampicillin for treatment of *L. monocytogenes* and vancomycin + rifampin for treatment of *S. pneumoniae*.
- For specific targets of antimicrobial therapy, the following should be administered: *S. pneumoniae* (ceftriaxone or cefotaxime + vancomycin + dexamethasone); *N. meningitidis* (Pen G); *L. monocytogenes* (ampicillin + gentamycin 2); *H. influenzae*, coliforms, and *Pseudomonas aeruginosa* (ceftazidime 2 + gentamycin).
- Duration of therapy is for 10–14 days.
- Empirical antimicrobial therapy for bacterial brain abscess includes a third-generation cephalosporin (ceftriaxone) and metronidazole.

BIBLIOGRAPHY

Gilbert DN, Moellering RC, Eliopoulos JM, et al., eds. *The Sanford Guide to Antimicrobial Therapy*, 35th ed. New Rochelle, NY: Antimicrobial Therapy, Inc; 2005.

Tunkel L AR, Scheld M, Bacterial infection of the central nervous system. In, Hall JB et al., *Principles of Critical Care,* 3rd ed. New York, NY: McGraw-Hill.

Mandell GL, Bennett JE, Dolin R. *Mandell, Douglas, and Bennett's Principles and Practices of Infectious Diseases*, 6th ed. Edinburgh: Churchill Livingstone; 2004.

56 VIRAL ENCEPHALITIS

D. Kyle Hogarth

KEY POINTS

- A diagnosis of encephalitis should be considered in any patient with unexplained headaches, fevers, change in mental status, or seizures.
- The most common cause of fatal viral encephalitis is HSV. Outcomes in patients with HSV encephalitis are significantly improved by early recognition and prompt institution of acyclovir therapy.
- 90% of cases of HSV encephalitis will have focal neurologic abnormalities.

- Early LP should be performed in all cases of suspected encephalitis, but CT or MRI imaging should first be performed in patients with focal neurologic findings.
- The CSF is generally abnormal in encephalomyelitis: usual findings include increased leukocytes, normal glucose, mildly elevated or normal protein.
- PCR detection of HSV in CSF is the gold standard for the diagnosis of HSV encephalitis. However, a negative PCR result cannot always exclude HSV encephalitis and acyclovir therapy should continue until culture results are definitive or an alternative diagnosis is made.
- Worldwide, the arboviruses are the most common cause of encephalitis. In North America, West Nile virus has become an increasingly common cause of encephalitis.
- Viral encephalitis patients should receive full intensive care support, as many can regain full neurologic function, even after prolonged alteration of their mental status.

APPROACH TO THE ENCEPHALITIS PATIENT

- There are no specific clinical signs or symptoms that can easily distinguish between causes of encephalitis. Patients must be approached with a wide differential diagnosis of etiologies.
- Patients will typically present with fever, headache, and behavioral changes or altered mental status.
- The setting of the disease may provide helpful clues as to the etiology. The likelihood of arbovirus encephalitis depends on the season, location, degree of insect exposure the patient has experienced, and current prevalence of disease in a given community.
- Often, there are clues in the community as to the current risk of viral encephalitis. For example, West Nile virus infections are typically preceded by outbreaks and deaths among birds.
- The rate of progression of the encephalitis may offer suggestions as to the cause of disease. For example, disease developing 1–2 weeks after a viral syndrome or recent immunization is likely postinfectious, whereas an acute fulminant course suggests herpes simplex virus (HSV).
- Physical examination is usually only helpful if a characteristic rash is present, such as the exanthems of varicella, measles, Lyme disease, or Rocky Mountain spotted fever.
- Urgent diagnostic imaging by CT or MRI should be obtained. These tests are limited in diagnosing viral encephalitis, but are useful in ruling out other causes of the patient's symptoms.
- Early lumbar puncture (LP) should be performed, especially to rule out bacterial meningitis as the cause of symptoms.
- Cerebrospinal fluid (CSF) should be sent for cell count, chemistry, viral studies and cultures, and stains and culture for fungi, bacteria, and mycobacteria.
- Completely normal findings on LP significantly reduce the likelihood of encephalitis and raise the possibility of toxic or metabolic encephalopathy.

HERPES SIMPLEX VIRUS ENCEPHALITIS

- Herpes simplex virus encephalitis is the most common fatal encephalitis.
- It is seen in all age groups, in both sexes, immunocompetent and immunocompromised, in all seasons, and accounts for 5% and 10% of all reported cases of encephalitis.
- The early use of acyclovir therapy at a dose of 10 mg/kg every 8 hours for 10–14 days significantly improves morbidity and mortality. The dosage of acyclovir should be adjusted in patients with renal failure.
- A temporal lobe syndrome in the setting of nonspecific constitutional symptoms is the most common clinical presentation for HSV, but parietal or frontal lobes involvement is occasionally seen.
- Adult HSV encephalitis does not require mucocutaneous HSV lesions to be present.
- Examination of the CSF reveals an abnormality in 90–97% of cases. The white blood cell count is elevated with a lymphocyte predominance, but early in the course polymorphonuclear leukocytes will predominate. Red blood cells are present in 75–80% of samples. Glucose is normal, and the protein content is only moderately elevated.
- Viral cultures for HSV are almost always negative. Polymerase chain reaction (PCR) analysis to detect HSV DNA in CSF is the gold standard for the diagnosis of HSV, especially in the early phase of the disease. PCR has a demonstrated sensitivity of 96% and a specificity of 99%.
- In 80–90% of cases, the initial electroencephalogram (EEG) is abnormal, with predominantly spiked and slow wave patterns localized to the area of the brain involved.
- Long-term consequences include residual dysphasias, paresis, paresthesias, behavioral changes, and amnesia. The mortality rate is 28% for HSV encephalitis, even with acyclovir therapy. Only 38% of patients recover with little residual deficit.

ARBOVIRUS ENCEPHALITIS

- Arboviruses are insect-transmitted viruses and are the most common cause of encephalitis worldwide.
- The risk of arboviruses infection depends on many factors that determine the predominance of the virus in the environment. These include geography, season, and local weather conditions.
- West Nile virus is an arboviral infection with increasing frequency in the United States, causing significant mortality and morbidity, including a polio-like illness and seizures.
- Human beings are incidental hosts and most infections are asymptomatic and mild.
- Encephalitis from an arbovirus is typically an acute fever with headaches, followed by neck pain and then alteration in mental status.
- Examination of the CSF usually shows fewer than 500 leukocytes per microliter, with a lymphocyte predominance, though polymorphonuclear leukocytes may predominate early. The glucose is normal. The protein content is normal or may be slightly elevated. Virus isolation is rare, and enzyme immunoassays for IgM antibodies in blood or CSF remain the best way to detect West Nile or Japanese B viruses.
- There is no proven antiviral therapy that helps with arboviral infections.

BIBLIOGRAPHY

Galbraith JC, Verity R, Tyrell DL. Encephalomyelitis. In: Hall JB, Schmidt GA, Wood LDH, eds., *Principles of Critical Care*, 3rd ed. New York, NY: McGraw-Hill; 2005:863–880.

Griffin DE. Encephalitis, myelitis and neuritis. In: Mandell GL, Bennett JE, Dolin R, eds., *Mandell, Douglas, and Bennett's Principles and Practice of Infectious Diseases*, 5th ed. Philadelphia, PA: Churchill Livingstone; 2000:1009–1016.

Koskiniemi M, Vaheri A, Taskinen E. Cerebrospinal fluid alterations in herpes simplex virus encephalitis. *Rev Infect Dis* 1984;6:608–618.

Lakeman FD, Whitley RJ. Diagnosis of herpes encephalitis: application of polymerase chain reaction to cerebral spinal fluid from brain-biopsied patients and correlation with disease. *J Infect Dis* 1995;171:857–863.

McGrath N, Anderson NE, Croxson MC, et al. Herpes simplex encephalitis treated with acyclovir: diagnosis and long term outcome. *J Neurol Neurosurg Psychiatry* 1997;63: 321–326.

Solomon T. Flavivirus encephalitis. *N Engl J Med* 2004;351: 370–378.

Whitley RJ, Soong S-J, Linneman C Jr, et al. Herpes simplex encephalitis. *JAMA* 1982;247:317–320.

57 LIFE-THREATENING INFECTIONS OF THE HEAD AND NECK

Nuala J. Meyer

KEY POINTS

- Serious infections of the head and neck can pose life-threatening situations due to their potential for encroachment on either the airway or CNS.
- As deep neck or facial infections tend to spread along fascial planes, a thorough understanding of the anatomic spaces in the neck is essential to proper management of such infections.
- Deep infections of the head and neck are classically polymicrobial, reflecting the normal mouth flora. Anaerobes tend to greatly outnumber aerobic bacteria. Accordingly, empiric antibiotic therapy should consist of broad gram-positive and anaerobic coverage.
  - Penicillin with clindamycin or metronidazole remains an excellent choice in immunocompetent patients.
  - Clindamycin alone may be considered in penicillin-allergic patients.
- Immunocompromised patients may lack the classic manifestations of life-threatening infections—such as edema, fluctuance, or systemic toxicity—and are at much greater risk for unusual organisms causing virulent disease. Antimicrobial coverage in such patients is by necessity broad-spectrum, and frequently requires consideration of mold-fighting antifungal agents.

SUBMANDIBULAR SPACE INFECTIONS

- Classically described "Ludwig angina," this pyodermic induration of the tissue of the neck extends into the muscles between the larynx and over the floor of the mouth.
- Aggressive, rapidly spreading cellulitis of the submandibular space, often described as "woody."
- Etiology is typically infection of the 2nd or 3rd molar teeth.
- Clinically, patient is febrile with mouth pain, drooling, and dysphagia, often sitting up and leaning forward to maximize the airway size.
  - Respiratory distress is common.
  - Stridor and cyanosis are ominous signs.
  - Potential for direct extension of infection into the lateral pharyngeal space, retropharyngeal space, or mediastinum. Any asymmetry of the submandibular

area should be viewed with great concern for lateral extension.

- Treatment: First priority is the maintenance of an adequate airway.
  - Urgent tracheostomy may be necessary, and should be performed *before* the development of stridor or cyanosis.
  - If intubation is attempted, it should be done fiberoptically with a flexible scope and with a surgeon present to perform immediate tracheostomy should the intubation fail.
  - Infected teeth should be extracted.
  - If cellulitis fails to respond to antibiotics alone or if fluctuance is present, needle aspiration or surgical incision and drainage is indicated.
- Prognosis: Mortality has declined dramatically with aggressive management, but may still be as high as 4%.

LATERAL PHARYNGEAL SPACE INFECTIONS

- Anatomically, this space is defined as an inverted cone with its base at the skull, its apex at the hyoid bone, bounded medially by the carotid sheath, and laterally by the parotid. The space is divided into anterior and posterior compartments.
  - The posterior compartment of the lateral pharyngeal space contains the 9th through 12th cranial nerves, the carotid sheath, and the cervical sympathetic trunk.
  - Symptoms from infection in this space often relate to the structures located within this posterior compartment.
    - Postanginal sepsis involves lymphatic spread of infection into the carotid sheath, often 1–3 weeks following clinical pharyngitis. The carotid artery itself can be involved, leading to arteritis and even rupture. This rare but potentially fatal complication is often signaled by several minor bleeds prior to major hemorrhage, and must be treated with urgent surgical intervention.
    - Lemierre syndrome, or suppurative jugular thrombophlebitis, is the most common vascular complication of lateral pharyngeal space infections.
    - Vocal cord paralysis may result from suppurative compression of lower cranial nerves.
- Dental infections are the most common source of infection, followed by peritonsillar abscess. More rarely, parotitis, otitis, or mastoiditis can occur.
- Infection of the anterior compartment often causes trismus—inability to open the mouth—as well as induration below the mandible. Suppurative infections can lead to systemic toxicity with fever and rigors and medial bulging of the pharyngeal wall.
- Treatment of these infections depends on the presence of local suppuration; if pus is present—as determined by computed tomography (CT) or direct visualization—needle aspiration or surgical incision and drainage is indicated. With the absence of abscess formation, many such infections can be managed by a prolonged course of antibiotics, usually on the order of 3–6 weeks.
  - Penicillin plus clindamycin or metronidazole is often required, as mouth anaerobes such as *Fusobacterium* and *Bacteroides* species are frequently recognized as penicillin-resistant.
  - Surgical ligation is required for an infected carotid artery with potential for rupture, whereas involvement of the internal jugular vein can frequently be treated by antibiotics alone. The role of anticoagulation in vascular infections is unclear, and has not been proven to be helpful.
- Prognosis of lateral pharyngeal space infections depends on the extent of the infection, but both morbidity—often stroke—and mortality remain high (20–40%).

RETROPHARYNGEAL INFECTIONS

- Also known as the "danger" space, the retropharyngeal space extends between the fascia from the esophagus and pharynx back to the vertebral spine. Infections here can spread from the base of the skull through the entire posterior mediastinum down to the diaphragm.
- In children, these infections arise typically via lymphatic drainage following suppurative adenitis. In adults, infection may follow penetrating trauma—often trauma to the esophagus, or choking injuries—or may result from tooth or peritonsillar abscess.
- Symptoms include fever, drooling, trismus, and possible nuchal rigidity, with the neck held tilted to the unaffected side. On examination, there may be bulging of the posterior pharyngeal wall but occasionally direct examination is compromised by the patient's pain and trismus.
  - CT and x-ray of the lateral neck may show cervical lordosis with swelling.
  - Occasionally, gas collections are seen in the retropharyngeal space.
- The main dangers are laryngeal edema with airway obstruction, or abscess rupture with aspiration.
- Acute necrotizing mediastinitis can also follow infections in the danger space, with potential necrotic extension into the retroperitoneum, pleural space, pericardial space, or rupture into the airways. In adults, this diagnosis carries a 25% mortality rate despite prompt antibiotic therapy, and surgical debridement is the rule.

CLINICAL SYNDROMES

PERITONSILLAR ABSCESS

- Also known as quinsy, peritonsillar abscess is a complication of acute tonsillitis and typically strikes young adults.
- Classically, patients are febrile with unilateral sore throat, dysphagia, trismus, drooling, and muffled voice.
- Drainage may be attempted by experienced physicians, with the patient in the Trendelenburg position, and with recognition of potentially life-threatening hazards:
  - Airway obstruction
  - Aspiration of purulent material
  - Lateral extension to deep lateral pharyngeal space

DIPHTHERIA

- Pharyngeal infections caused by toxigenic strains of *Corynebacterium diphtheriae*, still sporadically occurs despite widespread immunization against the bacterium.
- Inflammation may occur at any site in the upper airway, with tonsillitis being the most common presentation.
- Diphtheria classically forms a tenacious membrane on the airway mucosa, which frequently discolors and becomes necrotic.
  - Airway obstruction may follow either membrane formation or mucosal swelling.
  - Membranes tend to bleed extensively, especially with attempts at removal.
  - Urgent tracheostomy may be required, as well as bronchoscopy to identify and remove any membrane in the lower airways.
  - Distant complications of diphtheria include myocarditis and peripheral neuropathy, usually within 2 weeks after the initial infection. These occur secondary to circulating toxin, and can progress to shock, heart failure, and dysrhythmia.
  - Treatment for all suspected cases of diphtheria should include administration of equine diphtheria antitoxin immediately—to reduce the risk of myocarditis—in addition to antibiotic therapy with penicillin or a macrolide.

EPIGLOTTITIS

- Involves typically nonsuppurative inflammation of the supraglottic structures and epiglottis (also called "supraglottitis").
- Can affect young children and adults.
- *Haemophilus influenzae* was once the most common bacterial cause of epiglottitis, but with vaccination efforts it has been replaced by other oral flora, such as *Streptococcus pneumoniae* and *Staphylococcus aureus*.
- Triad of fever, stridor, and drooling; adults may complain of sore throat and exquisite odynophagia. Patients are classically found sitting up, leaning forward, with noticeably slow inspirations. Inspiration draws the epiglottis down, which can further obstruct the airway, so slowing inspiration can minimize obstruction.
- Cyanosis, pallor, or bradycardia reflect severe airway obstruction and signal the need for urgent tracheostomy or intubation.
- Treatment involves ICU monitoring, antimicrobial therapy, and, not infrequently, an artificial airway.
  - Children require artificial airway management more often than adults.
  - Intubation, if indicated, should be done under direct visualization and in the operating room, with immediately available equipment and personnel for a surgical airway if necessary.

LARYNGOTRACHEOBRONCHITIS

- Also known as croup; primarily affects young children.
- Follows typically a viral upper respiratory infection.
- Causes swelling of the conus elasticus, which narrows the infraglottic structures and produces the classic "barking" or "brassy" cough.
- May involve inspiratory stridor, hoarseness, and respiratory distress.
- Lateral neck x-ray may show infraglottic narrowing, or "steeple sign."
- Treatment includes humidified oxygen, hydration, and antibiotics if a secondary bacterial infection is suspected.
  - Artificial airway—either surgical or via intubation—may be necessary and is fraught with potential complication and loss of airway.
  - Airway manipulation should be performed only by experienced personnel.

SINUSITIS AND OTITIS

- Although typically quite treatable with antibiotic therapy alone, can have devastating complications due to their vascularity and proximity to the central nervous system (CNS).
- Sinus infection is especially common in the ICU setting as a nosocomial infection, particularly in patients with nasotracheal, nasogastric, or (less commonly) orotracheal or orogastric tubes.

- Malignant otitis externa is a necrotizing infection of the ear caused by *Pseudomonas aeruginosa*, which tends to occur in diabetic or otherwise immunocompromised patients.
- Immunocompromised patients are also at risk for fungal disease of the sinus or ear, which can be invasive and aggressively necrotizing. Common molds implicated in disease derive from the Aspergillus, Rhizopus, and Mucor families.
- Both sinus and ear disease can extend directly or via the hematogenous route into the skull itself or to intracranial structures. The myriad CNS effects of such extension are beyond the scope of this chapter, but include:
  - Periorbital cellulitis
  - Cranial osteomyelitis
  - Septic intracranial thrombophlebitis involving the cavernous venous sinus or superior sagittal vein
  - Brain abscess
  - Cranial epidural abscess
  - Subdural empyema
- Early consultation with otolaryngologists, potential imaging either by direct endoscopy or by CT, and quick surgical intervention can be lifesaving in such cases.

BIBLIOGRAPHY

Bansal A, Miskoff J, Lis RJ. Otolaryngologic critical care. *Crit Care Clin* 2003;19:5–72.

Chow AW. Life-threatening infections of the head, neck, and upper respiratory tract. In: Hall JB, Schmidt GA, Wood LDH, eds., *Principles of Critical Care*, 3rd ed. New York, NY: McGraw-Hill; 2005:881–896.

Riordan T, Wilson M. Lemierre's syndrome: more than a historical curiosa. *Postgrad Med J* 2004;80:328–334.

58 SOFT-TISSUE INFECTIONS

Joseph Levitt

KEY POINTS

- Serious soft-tissue infections causing necrosis of subcutaneous tissue, fascia, and muscle are rare but can be rapidly fatal without prompt diagnosis and early definitive therapy.
- The characteristic presentation of extensive subcutaneous involvement and systemic toxicity in the absence of significant superficial signs can hamper diagnosis in early stages.
- Severe pain and loss of functionality (when involving an extremity) with signs of systemic toxicity should trigger urgent surgical exploration and debridement.
- Delaying definitive surgical therapy while obtaining confirmative radiographic testing may significantly increase morbidity and mortality.

MAJOR SOFT-TISSUE INFECTIONS

SUPERFICIAL PYODERMAS

- Characterized by superficial infections limited to the dermis, including erysipelas, impetigo, furunculosis, and carbunculosis.
- While they may require treatment, they rarely cause systemic involvement and are not life-threatening infections.

CELLULITIS

PATHOGENESIS

- Most cases occur with inoculation from minor trauma, underlying skin lesions, or surgical wounds, or spread from other soft tissue or bone. However, they can occur without predisposing event, particularly with group A streptococcus.
- Other risk factors include mild immunosuppression (e.g., diabetes or steroid use), impaired lymphatic drainage (e.g., saphenous vein harvest, mastectomy, heart failure, or previous infection in same lymphatic system), or specific recreational or occupational exposure (e.g., swimming, butcher, or fish handler).
- *Streptococcus pyogenes* and *Staphylococcus aureus* are the most common causative organisms. *S. pneumoniae* and other streptococci are less common. Gram-negative bacilli can be seen in immunosuppressed states and with chronic illness and nursing home exposure predisposing to colonization.
- Rare but fulminant forms of cellulitis are caused by *Aeromonas hydrophila* (fresh-) and vibrio species (salt-) water exposure.

PRESENTATION

- Pain, local tenderness, erythema, and edema with ill-defined borders are the hallmark signs. Fever may be absent or low-grade with limited infections.
- Lymphangitis and regional lymphadenopathy are ominous signs of progression to systemic involvement.

Management

- Cultures of wound drainage or skin biopsy are recommended, but the yield is low (25%). Aspiration after injection of 0.5 mL of nonbacteriostatic saline in the leading edge of erythema may also be attempted. Superficial swabs of uninterrupted skin are not useful and blood cultures are rarely positive but should be taken nevertheless in patients showing systemic signs.
- In the absence of specific culture data, antibiotic choices are empirically based on site and predisposing risk factors. Penicillinase-resistant penicillins (nafcillin, dicloxacillin) or first-generation cephalosporins are the most common first-line agents. Vancomycin may be appropriate in settings with a high prevalence of methicillin-resistant *S. aureus* (MRSA). Diabetic wounds also should prompt coverage for gram negatives and anaerobes. Infections related to bites need specific coverage based on the offending animal. Aminoglycosides (gentamicin, tobramycin) should be added if there is a history of water injury.
- Borders of erythema should be marked with a pen at the time of initial evaluation to aid subsequent judgment of progression. Areas of fluctuance, suppuration, or crepitus should be sought carefully.
- Analgesia is an important part of therapy.
- Failure to defervesce on appropriate antibiotics after 48–72 hours should prompt reinspection for an undrained source.

ANAEROBIC CELLULITIS

- Also referred to as gangrenous cellulitis, this subclass of cellulitis results from inoculation of nonviable tissue in inadequately debrided wounds or areas of disrupted vascular supply (e.g., diabetic ulcers).
- Presentation is characterized by suppurative drainage and gas formation in discolored tissue with little pain or systemic signs.
- Organisms most commonly include clostridial species or polymicrobial infections with gram-negative rods, gram-positive cocci, and facultative anaerobes.
- Once fluid or tissue is cultured, therapy consists of appropriate antibiotics and adequate surgical debridement. While its limitation to nonviable tissue and thus lack of symptoms distinguishes it from more serious soft-tissue infections, systemic spread is inevitable if inadequately treated.

NECROTIZING FASCIITIS

Pathogenesis

- While inciting events are similar to those of cellulitis, necrotizing fasciitis is characterized by inoculation of subcutaneous tissue and spread along deep fascial planes with relative sparing of the overlying skin.
- Any site may be involved but the perineum and extremities are seen most commonly. Most cases are related to minor trauma (80%), surgical wounds, and decubitus ulcers.
- Chronic illness (diabetes, renal disease, arteriosclerosis) or poor nutrition is usually present, but group A streptococcal infections can occur without precipitating event.
- Histology of deep tissues shows nonspecific inflammation with fibrinoid necrosis and thrombosis of vessels, highlighting the need for surgical intervention as antibiotics and host immunity are inadequate in the ischemic tissue where infection progresses.
- Group A streptococcus species, usually *S. pyogenes*, produce toxins with the ability to act as superantigens, inducing a nonspecific inflammatory cascade and a toxic shock syndrome (TSS).
- In polymicrobial infections, virulent organisms such as streptococci, gram-negative rods (*Escherichia coli, Klebsiella, Proteus*), or *S. aureus* create a necrotic milieu that supports growth of anaerobes.

Presentation

- Symptoms usually occur several hours to several days after a history of minor trauma, although with group A streptococcal infections, the onset may be sooner. Presentation is characterized by severe pain that is out of proportion to the superficial appearance of the involved area.
- Swelling and erythema can progress rapidly to pallor, bluish discoloration, appearance of superficial vesicles, and frank gangrene. Crepitus is a rare and late finding.
- Pain progressing to numbness is an ominous sign of compression and destruction of superficial nerves.
- Systemic toxicity, disorientation, and shock are not uncommon as the condition progresses.
- Computed tomography (CT) scan and magnetic resonance imaging (MRI) are useful in determining the extent of deep fascial involvement when clinical suspicion exists but signs and symptoms are lacking. However, time-consuming studies should never be used as confirmatory tests prior to definitive surgical exploration once signs and symptoms are present.

Management

- Early surgical exploration and wide debridement is the mainstay of effective therapy. Failure to adequately debride all involved tissue adversely affects survival.
- Blood and fluid drainage should be cultured immediately. Debrided tissue is especially likely to provide useful microbiologic information (more than intraoperative wound swabs).

- Aminoglycosides and clindamycin are considered first-line therapy in most cases. Clindamycin targets ribosomes and has the potential added benefit of reducing toxin-mediated inflammation out of proportion to bacterial killing. Alternatively, extended spectrum fourth-generation penicillins may be used as monotherapy. If a group A streptococcal infection is suspected, penicillin G with clindamycin is the treatment of choice.
- Drotrecogin may be indicated in many of these very sick patients, but a careful working relationship with the surgeon is important to time therapy appropriately and reduce the risk of wound hemorrhage.
- In streptococcal Toxic Shock Syndrome (TSS), intravenous immunoglobulin may reduce toxin-mediated inflammation and improve host immunity, however, clinical trials demonstrating its effectiveness are lacking.
- Mortality rates have been reported from 4 to 74%. Higher APACHE (Acute Physiology and Chronic Health Evaluation) scores at presentation, age >50, diabetes, truncal location, and inadequate initial debridement are associated with worse outcomes.

MYONECROSIS

PATHOGENESIS

- Myonecrosis, also known as gas gangrene, can be divided into clostridial and nonclostridial causes.
- Historically, clostridial myonecrosis was seen with penetrating war wounds but now more commonly results from penetrating trauma or open fractures (particularly motor vehicle or agricultural accidents), surgical or burn wounds, malignancy (particularly colorectal), arterial insufficiency, septic abortions, or intramuscular injections.
- Necrosis is exotoxin-mediated and can progress to shock, disseminated intravascular coagulation, and multisystem organ failure while bacteremia only occurs in 10–15% of cases.
- Nonclostridial organisms and pathogenesis are similar to that of necrotizing fasciitis.

PRESENTATION

- Symptoms usually present 2–3 days after initial injury. In clostridial etiologies, severe pain and tense edema are hallmark signs. With disease progression, woody edema spreads and the skin takes on a characteristic bronze appearance. Gas bubbles may be present in wound drainage. Muscle may herniate through open wounds.
- With nonclostridial organisms, pain is constant but erythema is more prominent than edema.

MANAGEMENT

- As in necrotizing fasciitis, early debridement and fasciotomy are critical. Surgical exploration reveals dusky "cooked" appearing muscle that is noncontractile.
- Penicillin G is therapy of choice for clostridial organisms with chloramphenicol or metronidazole first-line in penicillin-allergic patients. Polymicrobial infections are treated with aminoglycosides and clindamycin.
- Hyperbaric oxygen may be a useful adjuvant therapy in clostridial infections but clinical data are lacking and its use controversial. The main utility may be in limiting debridement of extensive infections when wide excisions may be life threatening or require sacrifice of a limb.

BIBLIOGRAPHY

Conly JM. Soft tissue infections. In: Hall JB, Schmidt GA, Wood LDH, eds., *Principles of Critical Care*, 3rd ed. New York, NY: McGraw-Hill; 2005:897–904.

Seal DV. Necrotizing fasciitis. *Curr Opin Infect Dis* 2001;14: 127–132.

Swartz MN. Clinical practice. Cellulitis. *N Engl J Med* 2004;350:904–912.

59 URINARY SYSTEM INFECTIONS

Michael Moore

KEY POINTS

- The urinary tract is the most common site of nosocomial infection.
- 80% of nosocomial genitourinary infections follow urinary catheterization.
- These infections prolong hospital stay and increase costs.
- Bacteremia complicates 1–3% with an attributable mortality of 13%.
- UTIs are a common cause of ICU admission and a common consequence of ICU care and urinary catheterization.
- Urinary catheters act as a reservoir of multidrug-resistant hospital pathogens.

DEFINITIONS

- Bacteriuria—presence of bacteria in the urine
- Significant bacteriuria—10^5 organisms/mL by quantitative method or 10^2 aerobic gram-negative organisms/mL in symptomatic patients with pyuria
- Pyuria—presence of ≥5 WBCs per high-powered field in urine
- Complicated urinary tract infections (UTIs)
  - A UTI in a healthy, young, nonpregnant woman is considered uncomplicated
  - All others are considered complicated
  - Complicated UTIs are associated with an underlying condition which increases the risk of treatment failure
    - Obstruction
    - Diverticulae
    - Fistulae
    - Surgical urinary diversions
    - Neurogenic bladder
    - Vesicoureteral reflux
    - Indwelling catheter
    - Ureteral stent
    - Nephrostomy tube
    - Pregnancy
    - Diabetes
    - Renal failure
    - Renal transplantation
    - Immunosuppression
    - Multidrug-resistant pathogens
    - Hospital-acquired infection

REVIEW OF SPECIFIC GENITOURINARY SYNDROMES

ACUTE PYELONEPHRITIS

Microbiology

- Nosocomial urinary tract pathogens:
  - *Escherichia coli* (47%)
  - *Enterococcus* spp. (13%)
  - *Klebsiella* (11.0%)
  - *Pseudomonas aeruginosa* (8%)
  - *Proteus mirabilis* (5.0%)
- ICU urinary tract pathogens:
  - *Enterococcus* spp. (24%)
  - *Candida albicans* (21%)
  - *E. coli* (15%)
- Resistant *Enterococcus* spp. are of increasing concern in nosocomial UTI and bacteremia in ICU patients.
- Vancomycin-resistant enterococci may serve as a reservoir of resistant genes for *Staphylococcus aureus.*
- Persistent or relapsing bacteriuria caused by *P. mirabilis* should prompt a search for a staghorn calculus.
- Chronic bacteriuria due to *Corynebacterium urealyticum* can be associated with alkaline urine and renal stones.

Pathogenesis

- Women with recurrent UTIs often have vaginal and periurethral cells to which *E. coli* adhere more readily compared to controls.
- Most *E. coli* implicated in UTIs have several virulence factors including adhesins, siderophores, toxins, polysaccharide coatings, and other properties that assist the bacteria in avoiding or subverting host defenses, injuring or invading host cells and tissues, and stimulating a noxious inflammatory response.
- These various factors allow adhesion to periurethral cells, multiplication in the bladder, ascent via the ureters, and invasion of renal tissue in patients with anatomically normal urinary tracts.
- Regular bladder voiding is the most important host defense.

Diagnosis and Assessment

- Acute pyelonephritis is a syndrome of fever with renal inflammation suggested by costovertebral angle tenderness or flank pain, often with signs of systemic toxicity and bacteremia.
- Silent pyelonephritis is present in up to a third of patients with cystitis.
- Spinal cord injury patients are prone to silent, complicated, life-threatening pyelonephritis which presents with fever and nonspecific abdominal discomfort, increased spasms, and autonomic dysreflexia.
- Pyelonephritis requiring ICU admission should prompt a search for urinary tract obstruction, renal abscess or perinephric abscess, and resistant pathogens.
- Features suggestive of obstruction: classic renal colic, severe costovertebral angle tenderness, and palpable kidney (hydronephrosis).
- At presentation, Gram's stain of a drop of unspun urine can provide rapid, specific information and can be valuable for distinguishing less common etiologies including *S. aureus*, *Enterococcus* spp., *Candida* spp., and polymicrobial-anaerobic organisms.
- Urine culture identifies the organism except in the case of prior antibiotic therapy, complete obstruction, or perinephric abscess.
- Obtain blood cultures to rule out concomitant bacteremia.

Antimicrobial Therapy

- Many antimicrobial regimens have been shown to be effective empiric therapy as most antibiotics are excreted through the kidney. Treatment includes a β-lactam plus aminoglycoside, cephalosporins, carbapenems, trimethoprim-sulfamethoxazole monobactams, and quinolones.

- An initial combination of two agents effective against aerobic gram-negative bacilli and *Enterococcus* spp. is appropriate in septic patients with UTI.
- For patients with a high risk of aminoglycoside toxicity consider a nonaminoglycoside regimen or limit to a single dose to cover the first 24 hours.
- Resistance:
  - β-Lactamase inhibitors usually eliminate ampicillin resistance in *E. coli* and other Enterobacteriaceae.
  - Resistance rates in uropathogens to trimethoprim-sulfamethoxazole are growing.
  - A quinolone plus aminoglycoside double covers aerobic gram-negative bacilli but will not reliably kill enterococci.
  - Piperacillin-tazobactam or ticarcillin-clavulanic acid will cover most aerobic gram-negative bacilli and *Enterococcal* spp.
- Adjust empiric therapy based on culture and sensitivity to the least toxic, cost-effective single agent.
- Start oral therapy once tolerated and after fever has resolved; continue for a total of 10–14 days.
- Cell wall synthesis inhibitors may have a higher relapse rate following completion of therapy; trimethoprim alone, trimethoprim-sulfamethoxazole, or a quinolone is preferred.
- Optimal treatment for vancomycin-resistant *Enterococcus* is not known and should be chosen in consultation with an Infectious Diseases physician.

IMAGING

- Contrast-enhanced computerized tomography (CT)
  - Initial study of choice for patients with urosepsis
  - Accurately defines renal parenchyma and surrounding anatomy
  - Improved ability to distinguish complications of upper UTI
  - Assists in placement of percutaneous drains
  - Noncontrast images help identify renal calculi
- Ultrasound (US)
  - Can be technically inadequate because of obesity, overlying bowel gas, subcutaneous emphysema, wounds, or dressings
  - Portable but results depend on the skill of the operator
  - Reliably diagnoses most causes of obstruction and perinephric collections
  - May be initial investigation in severe urosepsis when unsafe to transport patient or if at high risk for contrast-induced nephrotoxicity
- Intravenous urography (IVU)
  - Little or no role
  - Helical CT scan superior at demonstrating the collecting system, early papillary necrosis, tuberculosis, and renal scarring due to childhood reflux nephropathy
- Retrograde urography with cystoscopy
  - Can demonstrate collecting system in a nonexcreting kidney
  - Rare complications include hemorrhage, perforation, or septicemia
  - May permit relief of obstruction by passage of a stent or manipulation of a calculus

ACUTE FOCAL BACTERIAL NEPHRITIS

- Analogous to lobar pneumonia and represents infection limited to one or more lobes of the kidney.

DIAGNOSIS

- Clinical features similar to acute pyelonephritis but patients do not defervesce within 48 hours.
- *E. coli* is the most common organism isolated from patients with acute focal bacterial nephritis (AFBN).
- Differential diagnosis includes neoplasm, evolving renal infarct, and abscess.

IMAGING

- Ultrasound may be normal or may reveal a solid, hypoechoic, poorly defined mass without evidence of liquefaction.
- Noncontrast CT scanning is frequently normal.
- Contrast CT invariably reveals one or more wedge-shaped areas of decreased density: this is seen in a significant proportion of patients with acute pyelonephritis.
- Demonstration of enhancing tissue within the mass on delayed CT images excludes cancer and abscess.

TREATMENT

- Acute focal bacterial nephritis usually resolves on antimicrobial therapy.
- Increased risk of scarring and atrophy.
- Needle aspiration or percutaneous drainage not indicated.

RENAL ABSCESS

- Acute focal bacterial nephritis may progress to renal cortical abscess especially when associated with obstruction.
- Abscesses may drain spontaneously into the calyxes or rupture through the renal capsule to form a perinephric abscess.
- Usual pathogens are Enterobacteriaceae (*E. coli*, *Klebsiella pneumoniae*, and *Proteus* spp.).

PATHOGENESIS

- Organisms commonly arise via the ascending route versus hematogenous spread.

- Staphylococcal septicemia can present with renal cortical abscess with or without other features of invasive staphylococcal infection.

Diagnosis

- Clinical features can be subtle initially.
- Symptoms include chills, fever, back or abdominal pain.
- Diagnostic clues include costovertebral angle tenderness, a flank mass, or involuntary guarding of the upper lumbar and paraspinal muscles.
- Prominent abdominal features such as nausea, vomiting, and abdominal guarding may suggest another intra-abdominal cause.

Imaging

- Ultrasound usually demonstrates an ovoid mass of decreased attenuation within the parenchyma and may initially mimic AFBN, a cyst, or a tumor.
- Gas can be present within the abscess.
- Debris within a cyst or abscess strongly indicates infection.
- CT scanning shows a distinctly marginated, low-attenuation, nonenhancing mass.
- CT ring sign: surrounding rim of increased enhancement.
- CT scan has higher sensitivity for small lesions (<2 cm diameter) and gas.
- Hemorrhagic cysts and necrotic tumors can mimic an abscess. Diagnosis can be confirmed by aspiration, nuclear medicine scanning, or serial scanning that shows resolution with antimicrobial therapy.

Treatment

- Classic therapy is incision and drainage or nephrectomy for larger abscesses.
- IV antimicrobial therapy usually successful after microbial diagnosis by urine, blood, or aspirate culture.
- Closely monitor response by fever, leukocytosis, and diminution of size by US or CT.
- Larger abscesses often require guided percutaneous drainage.

EMPHYSEMATOUS PYELONEPHRITIS

- Emphysematous pyelonephritis is a fulminant disorder with a historically high mortality.
- Patients present acutely with features of pyelonephritis and severe sepsis with or without multiorgan failure.
- Gas forms in the renal parenchyma and surrounding tissues due to mixed acid fermentation of glucose by Enterobacteriaceae.
- Risk factors include uncontrolled diabetes mellitus and urinary tract obstruction.
- *E. coli* and *Klebsiella* spp. predominate.
- Pathology reveals extensive necrotizing pyelonephritis with abscess formation and papillary necrosis.
- Poor perfusion is present in most cases due to infarction, vascular thrombosis, arteriosclerosis, or glomerulosclerosis.

Imaging

- Plain radiographs
  - Early, reveals mottling of parenchyma
  - Later, one sees extensive bubbles in the parenchyma and a gas crescent surrounding the kidney within the perinephric space
- US
  - More sensitive than plain films at detecting gas
- CT
  - Identifies the gas clearly and unambiguously

Therapy

- IV antibiotics and other supportive therapies for sepsis
- ICU support including tight control of hyperglycemia
- Guided percutaneous drainage
- Nephrectomy may be required in minority of cases
- 18% mortality in one series

PERINEPHRIC ABSCESS

- Older descriptions of perinephric abscess emphasized its insidious nature, delayed diagnosis, and high mortality (50%).
- Risk factors include renal obstruction and diabetes mellitus.
- Usually confined within the renal fascia but can spread to adjacent structures and spaces.

Etiology

- Majority occur secondary to pyelonephritis caused by Enterobacteriaceae (*E. coli*, *K. pneumoniae*, *Proteus* spp.).
- Minority are bacteremic in origin due to *S. aureus* or pyogenic streptococci.
- Occasional polymicrobial infection with *Candida* and *Aspergillus* spp.

Diagnosis

- Early diagnosis commonly confirmed by US or CT.
- Most patients have fever and chills.
- Other features may include weight loss, nausea, vomiting, dysuria, flank pain, abdominal pain, pleuritic chest pain, and pain in the thigh or groin.
- Symptoms usually present for weeks to months.
- Flank mass or renal tenderness present in majority of cases.

- May present with initial diagnosis of acute pyelonephritis or as fever of unknown origin.

IMAGING
- Ultrasound demonstrates fluid that may contain debris or gas.
- CT shows loculated collections with decreased attenuation; abscess wall may enhance with IV contrast.
- May see thickened renal fascia and unilateral kidney or psoas muscle enlargement.
- Diagnosis confirmed by guided aspiration of pus.

TREATMENT
- Antimicrobial agents and percutaneous drainage.
- Multiple loculations may complicate percutaneous drainage.
- Empiric antimicrobials should cover mixed anaerobes and *S. aureus.*

PYONEPHROSIS

- Pus in collecting system with infection proximal to an obstructed hydronephrotic kidney.
- Unilateral loss of renal function is present with infection of the renal parenchyma.
- Clinical presentation similar to perinephric abscess and may be insidious.
- Initial investigations should include a plain abdominal radiograph to look for calculi.
- US will reveal a distended upper urinary tract. Sedimented echoes or dispersed internal echoes within the dilated collecting system allows distinction from simple hydronephrosis.
- Direct aspiration is indicated in septic patients with hydronephrosis.
- CT is more sensitive for detecting radiolucent calculi and will also establish perinephric infection.
- Treatment should include nephrostomy tube placement.

PYOCYSTIS

- Pus in the urinary bladder with or without gas-forming organisms.
- Can present with sepsis, lower urinary tract signs, and pneumaturia.
- Risk factors include end-stage renal disease (ESRD) and urinary diversion procedures.
- Treatment with antimicrobial therapy and bladder irrigations may be sufficient.
- Surgical resection is required in cases with bladder wall necrosis seen by CT.

INFECTED CYSTS

- Dependent debris demonstrated by CT or US suggests infection.
- Diagnosis established by aspiration of cyst fluid for Gram's stain and culture.
- Pyocysts may arise from ascending infection or by hematogenous seeding.
- Systemic responses to infection such as fever and leukocytosis are often blunted in the presence of uremia.
- May present as persistent sepsis unresponsive to IV antibiotics.
- Diagnosis complicated by polycystic renal disease:
  - US or CT frequently fails to distinguish an infected cyst from the rest of a polycystic kidney.
  - Diagnostic options include white blood cell scanning, MRI, and positron emission tomography (PET) scanning followed by percutaneous drainage of a particular cyst.

TREATMENT
- Stable patients should receive a trial of lipophilic antimicrobial therapy such as trimethoprim-sulfamethoxazole, ciprofloxacin, or ofloxacin.
- Percutaneous drainage may suffice, or unilateral nephrectomy can be done, preserving the uninfected kidney.
- Lipophobic agents such as β-lactams and aminoglycosides penetrate cysts poorly.

URINARY TRACT INFECTION DUE TO *CANDIDA*

- Diagnosis of cystitis (and possibly upper tract infection) should be suspected when $\geq 10^4$ colony-forming units/mL are present and especially when associated with pyuria.

DISSEMINATED INVASIVE CANDIDIASIS

- May originate in the urinary tract or secondarily seed it.
- Kidneys are almost universally involved.
- Renal failure may develop from bilateral renal infection.
- Risk factors include neutropenia, loss of mucous membrane integrity due to chemotherapy, burns, steroid use, diabetes mellitus, total parenteral nutrition, and upper gastrointestinal tract surgery.
- Invasion is often preceded by overgrowth on superficial tissues and often associated with prolonged broad-spectrum antibacterial therapy.
- Direct proof of deep candidal infection is frequently lacking and blood cultures are positive in only half the cases.

Primary Infection of the Kidneys

- Generally associated with indwelling urinary catheters, an obstructed urinary tract, and broad-spectrum antibacterial agents.
- Candiduria is usually present for a variable period prior to renal infection.
- Persistent candiduria can be assumed to reflect renal infection if the patient has a predisposition, is receiving broad-spectrum antibiotics, and has otherwise unexplained fever or leukocytosis.
- Search for specific features of disseminated candidiasis such as white "cotton wool" exudates in the retina and nodular skin lesions.
- Unilateral or bilateral hydronephrosis should raise suspicion of a fungus ball.
- Microscopic examination of the urinary sediment may reveal *Candida* casts.
- Careful evaluation of the clinical and laboratory data should allow selection of those patients who require early empiric antifungal therapy.

Treatment

- Renal or disseminated infection requires systemic amphotericin B therapy or fluconazole.
- Amphotericin B carries a significant risk of nephrotoxicity.
- Fluconazole is not active against many nonalbicans species but its high urinary levels may overcome such resistance.
- Outcome is superior if IV catheters are removed on or before the first day of therapy.
- To date, there are no clinical trials validating the efficacy of other agents, such as the less nephrotoxic lipid formulations of amphotericin B, 5-flucytosine, voriconazole, and caspofungin in the treatment of ascending *Candida* pyelonephritis or renal candidiasis.
- Hydronephrosis due to a fungus ball:
  - Requires percutaneous nephrostomy tube.
  - Irrigation of the ureter with an amphotericin B solution may be effective.
  - Lack of radiologic response should prompt surgical excision.

PERSISTENT CANDIDURIA IN THE STABLE INTENSIVE CARE UNIT PATIENT

- Common clinical situation that is often benign and resolves spontaneously or with withdrawal of the urinary catheter.
- Treat symptomatic candiduric patients if they have had a transplant, are neutropenic, or are preparing to undergo an invasive urologic procedure.
- Amphotericin B washouts are no longer recommended.

PROSTATIC INFECTIONS

ACUTE BACTERIAL PROSTATITIS

- Rare cause of severe sepsis or septic shock.
- Symptoms include high fever, urgency, frequency, dysuria, difficulty voiding or acute retention of urine, and suprapubic or perineal pain.
- Rectal examination reveals a tender and swollen prostate.
- Gram-negative bacilli are the most frequent pathogens.

Treatment

- Intense inflammation helps assure adequate antimicrobial levels at active site.
- Treat for a total of 6 weeks with an oral antimicrobial agent with good prostatic penetration to attempt to eradicate the organisms and prevent chronic infection.
- Choices include trimethoprim, trimethoprim-sulfamethoxazole, ciprofloxacin, and ofloxacin.

PROSTATIC ABSCESS

- Confirmed by transrectal ultrasonography or CT scan.
- Drain by transurethral resection of the prostate with unroofing, or guided perineal aspiration.

CATHETER-ASSOCIATED BACTERIURIA

GENERAL CONSIDERATIONS

- Incidence 10–20% in patients with indwelling catheters.
- One percent of patients will acquire bacteriuria from single "in-out" catheterizations.
- The per-day risk is 1–5% with higher prevalence of resistant pathogens seen in the ICU.
- Risk factors include time, age, female sex, and disconnection of the collecting tube-catheter junction.
- Systemic antimicrobials are initially protective but are associated with an increased prevalence of multidrug-resistant enterococci, coagulase-negative staphylococci, *Candida* spp., and *Pseudomonas* spp.
- Samples should always be taken by aspiration of urine through the distal catheter or collection port and after local disinfection.

PATHOPHYSIOLOGY

- Ascent of bacteria to the bladder occurs outside the lumen.
- The space between the catheter and the urethral mucous membrane is filled by a static and variable

amount of fluid, mucus, and inflammatory exudate that lacks inhibitory factors against bacterial proliferation.
- Progressive multiplication of organisms originating from the meatus accounts for the time-dependence and association with the female urethra.
- A minority of organisms originate from the collecting bag and ascend intraluminally.
- Contamination of the collecting bag can occur from one source patient to the collecting bags of others via health care personnel and is associated with most epidemics of catheter-associated bacteriuria.

PREVENTATIVE STRATEGIES

- While bladder catheterization is unavoidable in most ICU patients it should not be routinely used to avoid incontinence and contamination of the perineal skin.
- Early withdrawal of catheters in selected patients:
  - Alert, stable, and continent
  - Anuric renal failure managed with once-a-day catheterization
  - Male patients with intact voiding mechanism managed with condom drainage
- Use intermittent catheterization in stable patients with neurogenic bladders or in some patients with disturbed consciousness.
- Frequently question catheter necessity and attempt removal when feasible.
- Avoid regularly scheduled replacement.
- Studies of antimicrobial impregnated catheters have shown equivocal results.

TREATMENT

- Treat catheterized patients prior to instrumentation of the urinary tract to avoid bacteremia.
- Catheter-associated bacteriuria is generally asymptomatic but treatment can be justified to relieve symptoms of cystitis especially if the catheter removal is imminent.
- Short course treatments work well once the catheter has been removed.

BIBLIOGRAPHY

Baumgarten DA, Baumgartner BR. Imaging and radiologic management of upper urinary tract infections. *Urol Clin North Am* 1997;24:545–569.

Eggimann P, Garbino J, Pittet D. Epidemiology of Candida species infections in critically ill non-immunosuppressed patients. *Lancet Infect Dis* 2003;3:685–702.

Gordon KA, Jones RN, SENTRY Participant Groups (Europe, Latin America, North America). Susceptibility patterns of orally administered antimicrobials among urinary tract infection pathogens from hospitalized patients in North America: comparison report to Europe and Latin America. Results from the SENTRY Antimicrobial Surveillance Program (2000). *Diagn Microbiol Infect Dis* 2003;45:295–301.

Hall JB, Schmidt, GA, Wood LDH. *Principles of Critical Care*, 3rd ed. New York, NY: McGraw-Hill; 2005:1123–1136.

Huang JJ, Tseng CC. Emphysematous pyelonephritis: clinicoradiological classification, management, prognosis, and pathogenesis. *Arch Intern Med* 2000;160:797–805.

Laupland KB, Zygun DA, Davies HD, et al. Incidence and risk factors for acquiring nosocomial urinary tract infection in the critically ill. *J Crit Care* 2002;17:50–58.

Lundstrom T, Sobel J. Nosocomial candiduria: a review. *Clin Infect Dis* 2001;32:1602–1607.

Rex JH, Walsh TJ, Sobel JD, et al. Practice guidelines for the treatment of candidiasis. *Clin Infect Dis* 2000;30:662–678.

Wong AH, Wenzel RP, Edmond MB. Epidemiology of bacteriuria caused by vancomycin-resistant enterococci, a retrospective study. *Am J Infect Control* 2000;28:277–281.

60 GASTROINTESTINAL INFECTIONS

Nina M. Patel

KEY POINTS

- Gastrointestinal infections rarely proceed to a level of severity that requires ICU admission.
- More frequently, noninfectious or infectious diarrhea complicates the ICU course and leads to increased morbidity in ICU patients.
- *C. difficile*-induced infectious diarrhea remains the most common cause of infectious nosocomial diarrhea.
- A possible association between gastric stress ulceration and *H. pylori* infection is postulated.
- Immunosuppressed patients are subject to infectious esophagitis and, if myelosuppressed, typhlitis.

PATHOGENESIS

- Normal gastrointestinal (GI) host defenses are often deranged in the ICU patient.
  - Motility is often slowed by narcotics and sedatives in endotracheally intubated or postoperative patients.
  - Gastric acidity, which constitutes a barrier to the survival of pathogens, is compromised by acid suppression therapy for stress ulcer prophylaxis.

  - Antibiotics disrupt normal intestinal flora, and lead to increased susceptibility to colonization and infection by normal flora and foreign pathogens.
- Diarrhea is defined as >200 g stool output per day. Diarrhea can be classified into secretory, osmotic, and inflammatory/hemorrhagic categories, based on the pathophysiologic disturbances induced within the intestinal mucosa and intraluminally.
  - Secretory diarrheas (e.g., *Vibrio cholerae*) impair normal sodium reabsorption or promote electrolyte secretion into the lumen. Enterotoxigenic *Escherichia coli* and *V. cholerae* infections are potential causes of secretory diarrhea in the returned traveler.
  - Osmotic diarrheas result from the presence of poorly absorbed osmoles (e.g., lactate and bile) in the intestinal lumen. These osmoles introduce a gradient for movement of water into the lumen to achieve osmotic equilibrium. Osmotic diarrhea in the ICU often results from iatrogenic sources (e.g., hyperosmotic enteral feeds).
  - Inflammatory diarrheas incur significant damage within the intestinal mucosa that leads to bloody and mucus-laden stools. Hemorrhagic diarrheas manifest with frank blood in the stool and can be associated with the hemolytic-uremic syndrome (e.g., *E. coli* O157:H7).
  - Nosocomial diarrheas are frequently noninfectious (e.g., medication-induced changes in intestinal flora) or related to hospital-acquired *Clostridium difficile* colitis. *C. difficile* is a gram-positive anaerobic bacillus that has been noted to infect up to 10% of ICU patients following treatment with most antibiotics as well as some chemotherapeutic agents. Increasing use of third-generation cephalosporins in the past two decades may account for increasing rates of *C. difficile* infection. *C. difficile* infection can occur as early as 48 hours following the start of antibiotic therapy and up to months after treatment. The spectrum of *C. difficile* infection can range from asymptomatic colonization to inflammatory colitis. A most feared complication of *C. difficile* colitis is progression to toxic megacolon, which can progress to colonic perforation if not addressed early.
- Immunosuppressed patients may be afflicted by opportunistic infections of the esophagus or the intestine. Candidal species, herpes simplex virus (HSV; HSV1 > HSV2), and cytomegalovirus (CMV) are the most commonly isolated organisms in patients with esophagitis. *Cryptosporidium*, *Microsporidium*, *Cyclospora*, and *Isospora* are additional pathogens which cause diarrhea in the HIV-infected patient.
- Neutropenic patients are subject to increased risk of typhlitis (necrotizing enterocolitis). This condition is characterized by intramural infection, hemorrhage, and necrosis of the bowel wall, primarily involving the terminal ileum and cecum. A number of factors, including impaired host defenses and neutropenia, contribute to increased risk of bacterial infection within the cecal wall.

CLINICAL EVALUATION, DIAGNOSIS, AND TREATMENT

DIARRHEA

- History, when available, is an essential component in the evaluation of diarrhea. The onset, frequency, and character (bloody or nonbloody) of bowel movements as well as the presence of fever are valuable in determining the etiology and guiding the diagnostic workup. Other key features are: travel history, history of recent changes in medications or antibiotic use, food ingestion preceding illness, and illness amongst close contacts.
- Fecal leukocytes indicate the presence of an inflammatory diarrhea. In addition to history, this test is useful in guiding an initial workup. Systemic leukocytosis is also frequently seen in the setting of infectious diarrhea.
- Additional tests include the stool osmotic gap, stool culture, and *C. difficile* toxin assay. In the absence of immunosuppression or a suggestive travel history, examining stool for ova and parasites (O&P) is rarely indicated. The stool osmotic gap [2(Na + K)] facilitates differentiation between secretory and osmotic diarrheas. A gap (osmotic gap >50) will be present in patients with osmotic diarrhea (due to the presence of unmeasured osmoles) and will be absent in patients with secretory diarrhea, because their primary derangement leads to increased stool electrolyte content. Stool culture is used with variable frequency—in nontoxic patients culture results rarely change management. However, in a critically ill patient, cultures may provide valuable susceptibility data and epidemiologic data in the case of foodborne illness.
- In patients with HIV or in the returned traveler, stool should be sent for O&P to evaluate for parasitic infection, including *Cryptosporidium*, *Giardia*, and *Entamoeba histolytica*.
- Endoscopy has limited utility in the diagnosis of diarrhea, though it may help to distinguish infectious, inflammatory diarrhea from inflammatory bowel disease. If seen, pseudomembranes are confirmatory in addition to a suggestive clinical history of *C. difficile* colitis.
- Treatment of the ICU patient with diarrhea centers around supportive care with fluid and electrolyte

repletion; antibiotics as indicated; and in some situations antimotility agents or probiotics.
- In vitro fertilization (IVF) replacement can be achieved with normal saline and supplemental electrolytes or lactated Ringer solution.
- Empiric antibiotic therapy should not be instituted routinely as it infrequently improves clinical course and may lead to increased resistance or a prolonged carrier state of the intestinal pathogen. Exceptions include severely immunocompromised patients (e.g., HIV with CD4 <200) or toxic-appearing patients (prolonged fever, diarrhea, and/or significant bloody diarrhea).
- *C. difficile* colitis is treated by discontinuation of the offending agent whenever possible and metronidazole (500 mg PO q 8 h preferred or 500 mg IV q 6 h). Oral vancomycin (125–500 mg PO qid) is the first-line alternative. If the presumed responsible agent cannot be discontinued (e.g., septic patient), treatment for *C. difficile* should be added to the existing antibiotic regimen.
- High rates of recurrence (20–40%) of *C. difficile* infection have been reported. In these situations, patients should either be treated with a new agent or have a full repeat course of therapy if clinically significant diarrhea is occurring.

ESOPHAGITIS AND GASTRITIS

- The clinical evaluation for esophagitis is often limited in the ICU due to the presence of endotracheal tubes, nasogastric tubes, and sedation. If alert and able, patients may complain of dysphagia, odynophagia, or retrosternal chest burning.
- Physical examination should focus on assessment for oral thrush and oral, labial, or genital lesions consistent with HSV infection.
- Upper endoscopy with biopsy, brushing, and tissue culture facilitates achievement of a microbiologic diagnosis. Esophageal plaques or ulcers may be seen in candidal or HSV and CMV infections, respectively.
- Treatment:
  - *Candida albicans* esophagitis is treated with fluconazole (100–200 mg qd × 14–21 days). Other candidal species may be resistant to fluconazole therapy and may require the use of other antifungal agents (e.g., caspofungin or amphotericin).
  - Acyclovir (5 mg/kg IV tid × 7–14 days) is the treatment for HSV-induced esophagitis.
  - Ganciclovir (5 mg/kg IV bid) is the treatment for CMV esophagitis.
- A small, prospective evaluation of ICU patients found that *Helicobacter pylori* infection (confirmed by urea breath testing) was associated with major gastric mucosal injury on esophagogastroduodenoscopy (EGD). These findings suggest a role for *H. pylori* in the pathogenesis of stress-induced gastritis in ICU patients, but need to be confirmed in a larger population.

TYPHLITIS

- Fever and abdominal pain in the setting of neutropenia warrant attention to the possibility of typhlitis.
- Abdominal plain films often demonstrate ileus or other nonspecific findings (Fig. 60-1).
- If clinical suspicion is high, abdominal computed tomography (CT) scanning should be pursued. CT findings include cecal wall thickening; intramural air, hemorrhage, or edema; and abscess formation. CT is helpful in differentiating typhlitis from appendicitis, pseudomembranous or ischemic colitis, and colonic pseudo-obstruction.
- Medical management with bowel rest, broad-spectrum antibiotic therapy (possibly the addition of antifungal therapy), IVFs, and nasogastric decompression is the treatment of choice in nontoxic patients.
- However, in the setting of intestinal perforation, peritonitis, or severe GI bleeding, emergent surgical intervention is imperative.
- An algorithm for diagnosis and management of typhlitis is shown in Fig. 60-2.

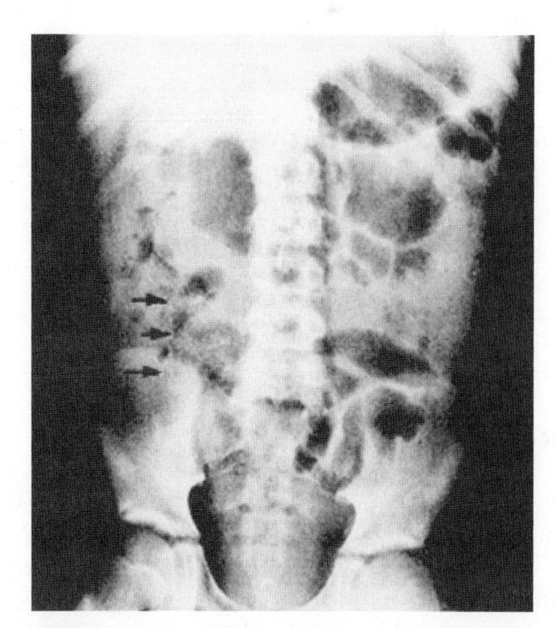

FIG. 60-1 Typhlitis. Supine film of the abdomen showing pneumatosis intestinalis of the right ascending colon (arrows) with slightly distended small bowel loops from typhlitis.
SOURCE: Reproduced with permission from Katz JA, Wagner ML, Gresik MV, et al. Typhlitis: an 18-year experience and post-mortem review. *Cancer* 1990;65:1041–1047.

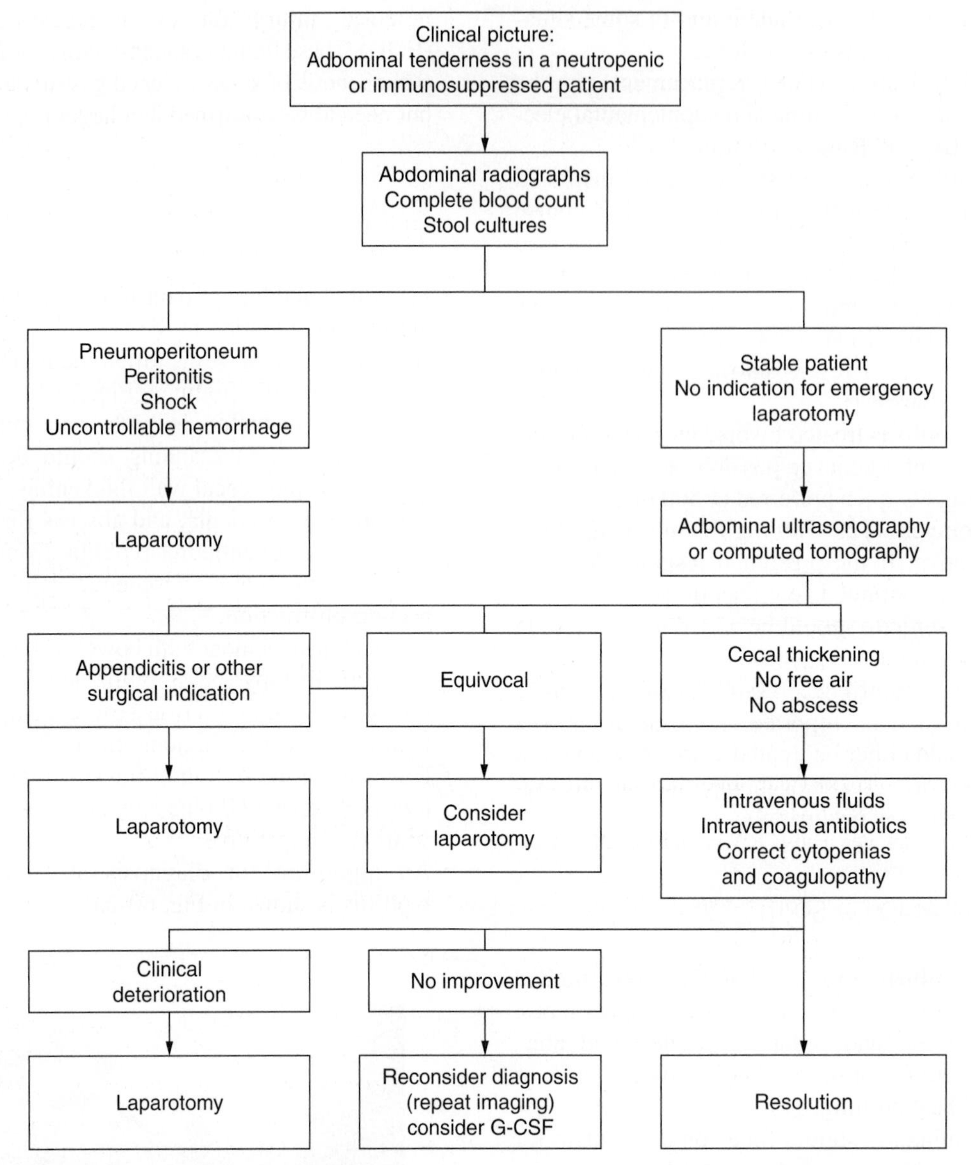

FIG. 60-2 Recommended approach to the patient with suspected typhlitis. G-CSF, granulocyte colony-stimulating factor.

SOURCE: Reproduced with permission from Canadian Medical Association. *Can J Surg* 1999;42(6):415.

PREVENTION

- Some investigators speculate that the use of probiotics may decrease rates of diarrhea and *C. difficile* infection in the ICU by reconstituting normal flora.
- Adequate hand-washing and contact precautions are essential in avoiding transmission of all infectious diarrheas. *C. difficile* spores may exist in the hospital environment for several months; therefore, aggressive infection control plays an integral role in preventing *C. difficile* transmission within the hospital.

CONCLUSIONS

- Gastrointestinal infections infrequently precipitate ICU admission but may result in significant morbidity during the ICU course.
- Since patients frequently cannot verbalize abdominal symptoms in the ICU, the intensivist must maintain a high level of vigilance to detect GI infections.
- *C. difficile* colitis is the most commonly encountered hospital-acquired infectious diarrhea.
- Electrolyte and fluid repletion is integral to the management of all infectious diarrheas. The role of antibiotic

therapy in community-acquired infectious diarrheas is variable.
- Esophagitis occurs most frequently in immunocompromised patients.
- Typhlitis is a medical emergency that will often progress through conservative therapy, requiring operative intervention.

BIBLIOGRAPHY

Baehr PH, McDonald GB. Esophageal infections: risk factors, presentation, diagnosis, and treatment. *Gastroenterology* 1994;106:509–532.

Bengmark S. Gut microbial ecology in critical illness: is there a role for prebiotics, probiotics, and synbiotics? *Curr Opin Crit Care* 2002;8:145–151.

Kyne L, Hamel MB, Polvaram R, Kelly CP: Health care costs and mortality associated with nosocomail diarrhea due to Clostridium difficule. *Clin Infect Dis* 34:346, 2002.

Quigley MM, Bethel K, Nowacki M, et al. Neutropenic enterocolitis: a rare presenting complication of acute leukemia. *Am J Hematol* 2001;66:213–219.

Riley TV. Nosocomial diarrhoea due to *Clostridium difficile*. *Curr Opin Infect Dis* 2004;17:323–327.

van der Voort PH, van der Hulst RW, Zandstra DF, et al. Prevalence of Helicobacter pylori infection in stress-induced gastric mucosal injury. *Intensive Care Med* 2001;27:68–73.

van der Voort PH, van der Hulst RW, Zandstra DF, et. al.: Suppresson of Helicobacter pylori infection during intensive care stay: Related to stress bleeding incidence? *J Crit Care* 16:182, 2001.

Wade DS, Nava HR, Douglass HO Jr. Neutropenic enterocolitis: clinical diagnosis and treatment. *Cancer*. 1992;69:17–23.

61 SEVERE MALARIA

Nathan Sandbo

KEY POINTS

- Consider malaria in any critically ill, febrile patient who has traveled recently to a malarious area.
- Begin antimalarial treatment when the diagnosis is clinically suspected or confirmed.
- Be prepared to prevent or treat complications such as hypoglycemia, seizures, pulmonary edema, renal failure, or hyperpyrexia.
- Restrict fluids when possible to reduce the risk of pulmonary edema.

EPIDEMIOLOGY

- Malaria is a leading cause of morbidity and death worldwide, with over 1 million deaths per year.
- Severe mosquito-borne protozoal infection caused by four species of Plasmodium: *P. falciparum, P. vivax, P. malariae*, or *P. ovale*. *P. falciparum* causes most life-threatening infections.
- Endemic throughout tropical countries. *P. falciparum* is the most common cause of malaria in Africa, Haiti, some parts of South America and Southeast Asia. *P. vivax* is dominant in India.
- Children from endemic areas eventually acquire immunity to severe malaria. However, immunity will lapse once recurrent exposures are discontinued.
- Malaria can be transmitted by transfusion of blood products, bone marrow, infected needles, or transplacentally.
- Eighteen human genetic polymorphisms are associated with resistance to malaria including: α and β thalassemias, hemoglobins S, E, and C, glucose-6-phosphate dehydrogenase (G6PD) deficiency, and Duffy blood group.

PATHOPHYSIOLOGY

- Sporozoites are carried in the gut of *Anopheles* mosquitoes. Transmission to humans occurs during a blood meal. After transmittal, sporozoites invade hepatocytes and mature into schizonts. After 6–16 days, merozoites are released into the bloodstream.
- In the case of *P. vivax* and *P. ovale*, sporozoites may remain dormant in the liver for months or years in the form of hypnozoites and cause relapsing infection.
- Erythrocytic cycle consists of invasion, development from rings to mature pigmented multinucleated schizonts, and rupture with the release of 4–32 merozoites, depending on species. These can reinfect erythrocytes or develop into gametocytes, which can then be taken up by a mosquito where they can complete a sexual cycle and produce more sporozoites.
- Most symptoms are related to the asexual erythrocytic cycle and the body's immune response. This response is mediated by the presence of a malarial toxin release at schizont rupture.
- Organ dysfunction is partially secondary to adherence of parasitized erythrocytes to the wall of venules, with resultant hypoxia and lactic acidosis from diminished blood flow. This most commonly occurs in brain, kidney, gut, placenta, skeletal muscle, liver, bone marrow, and retina. These effects may not become manifest until days after initiating antimicrobial therapy due to delayed increases in parasitemia.

CLINICAL FEATURES: *P. FALCIPARUM* MALARIA

- Shortest interval between mosquito bite and symptoms is 7 days, with 80% of patients developing symptoms within 1 month of leaving an endemic area.
- Presenting symptoms include headache, fever, chills, malaise, or lethargy. Myalgias, orthostasis, vomiting, and diarrhea are common.
- Signs include stigmata of anemia, jaundice, and tender hepatosplenomegaly.
- Classical tertian or subtertian fever (every 36–48 hours) is rarely seen as is the classic "paroxysm" (chill, hot phase, and diaphoresis).
- Life-threatening *falciparum* malaria is defined by the presence of any one of the following: cerebral malaria (impaired consciousness), severe normocytic anemia, renal failure, jaundice, pulmonary edema, hypoglycemia, circulatory collapse, spontaneous bleeding or disseminated intravascular coagulation (DIC), repeated generalized seizures, acidemia or acidosis, macroscopic hemoglobinuria.
- Defining characteristics of severe malaria may not be present at initial presentation. Likewise, severity of clinical syndrome at time of presentation is not a reliable indicator of development of life-threatening malaria.
- Cerebral malaria is defined as the presence of unarousable coma, *P. falciparum* parasitemia, and exclusion of other causes of coma. This syndrome should be considered in any febrile patient, possibly exposed to *P. falciparum*, with an impaired level of consciousness, coma, or seizures. Empiric antimalarial therapy should be initiated for patients with a high clinical suspicion of cerebral malaria, even if parasitemia is not present on blood smear. Other clinical features may include dysconjugate gaze, bruxism, symmetrical upper motor neuron lesion, and abnormal extensor or flexor posturing. Remarkably, survivors often are free of neurologic sequelae.
- Renal impairment occurs in one-third of patients.
- Acute pulmonary edema is common and is often fatal. Development is associated with hyperparasitemia, renal failure, lactic acidosis, excessive fluid replacement, and parturition.
- Hematologic abnormalities include anemia secondary to hemolysis of parasitized erythrocytes; thrombocytopenia from splenic sequestration or immune-mediated destruction; and DIC, which is present in about 15% of severe cases.
- Endocrine abnormalities include hypoglycemia from either quinine-induced hyperinsulinemia or inhibition of gluconeogenesis by tumor necrosis factor-alpha (TNF-α).

DIAGNOSIS

- Include malaria in the differential diagnosis of acute febrile illnesses, especially in the presence of recent travel to endemic areas, recent blood transfusion, or needlestick.
- Other travel-related febrile illnesses can present similarly, such as yellow fever, viral hemorrhagic fever, influenza, severe acute respiratory syndrome (SARS), hepatitis A and B, brucellosis, and leptospirosis.
- Diagnosis is established by microscopic examination of thin smears and thick films of patients' blood, preferably made without addition of anticoagulant, with identification and quantification of intraerythrocytic parasites. Parasitemia should be quantitated by microscopic examination, but this may not be an accurate measure of total body parasite load, due to sequestration of parasites in end organs.
- If available, antigen capture assay utilizing antibodies to *P. falciparum* PfHRP-2 antigen may be used, as it has similar sensitivity and specificity to microscopic detection.

TREATMENT

- Given complexity of clinical syndromes and propensity for multiorgan involvement, management is preferably administered in an intensive care environment.
- Maintain oxygenation, airway, and circulation.
- Initiate treatment with intravenous antimalarial agents based on weight of patient.
  - Quinine and quinidine are the first-line agents for treatment of severe malaria. In the United States, quinidine is usually used because of its widespread availability.
  - Quinidine is initiated via continuous infusion at 10 mg/kg over 1 hour followed by a continuous drip at 0.02 mg/kg/min.
  - Continuous ECG monitoring is required to assess for increased QT interval from quinine-based therapy.
  - Artemisinin derivatives (artesunate, artemether, arteether) are second-line agents useful only when quinine resistance may be a problem.
- Monitor for and aggressively treat hypoglycemia (especially after initiation of quinine-based therapy).
- Utilize antipyretics and external cooling if needed.
- Carefully administer IV fluids, and consider invasive hemodynamic monitoring to optimize therapy, as under-resuscitated patients are susceptible to circulatory collapse and shock, and over-resuscitated patients are prone to developing severe pulmonary edema.

- Perform lumbar puncture to rule out meningitis, and consider EEG to exclude subclinical seizures. Prophylactic phenobarbital may be considered, but its benefit is not fully established.
- Look for and treat concurrent bacterial infections that may complicate the clinical picture.
- Exchange transfusion should be considered in patients with substantial hyperparasitemia (>10%) or progression of disease on optimal antimicrobial therapy.
- Provide appropriate supportive care for end-organ complications such as pulmonary edema, renal failure, anemia, acidosis, and splenic rupture.
- Aggressive antimalarial and supportive therapy may reduce mortality to 10–15% in severe malaria.

BIBLIOGRAPHY

Moore DA, Jennings RM, Doherty TF, et al. Assessing the severity of malaria. *BMJ* 2003;326:808–809.

Warrell DA. Severe malaria. In: Hall JB, Schmidt GA, Wood LDH, eds., *Principles of Critical Care*, 3rd ed. New York, NY: McGraw-Hill; 2005:923–932.

White NJ. The treatment of malaria. *N Engl J Med* 1996;335:800–806.

Whitty CJ, Rowland M, Sanderson F, et al. Malaria. *BMJ* 2002;325:1221–1224.

62 TETANUS

William Schweickert

KEY POINTS

- Tetanus is a toxin-mediated disease caused by *C. tetani*, characterized by severe muscle spasm, which can progress to respiratory failure and cardiovascular instability.
- The diagnosis is made clinically.
- hTIG should be given as soon as possible.
- The site of entry should be debrided surgically and further toxin production limited by intravenous metronidazole.
- Benzodiazepines, narcotics, and intravenous magnesium may all play roles in reducing spasms and circulatory instability.
- Patients who survive should be immunized since clinical tetanus does not confer immunity.

EPIDEMIOLOGY

- Adoption of tetanus toxoid vaccination programs of children in the United States and other developed countries has resulted in dramatic decreases in the incidence of tetanus. Between 1998 and 2000, there were approximately 43 cases on average per year in the United States; similar rates have been reported in European countries.
- Although primarily a disease of the nonimmunized (underdeveloped countries) or inadequately immunized patients, tetanus can (rarely) develop in patients who had received their primary series, as well as proper "booster" doses of toxoid.
- Groups at highest risk include those aged ≥60 years, the impoverished, and intravenous drug abusers.

PATHOGENESIS

- The disease is caused by *Clostridium tetani,* an anaerobic bacterium normally present in mammalian gut and frequently isolated from soil.
- Once inoculated into injured tissue, spores transform into vegetative, pathogenic gram-negative rods which produce two toxins, tetanospasmin and tetanolysin. Tetanospasmin, a neurotoxin, is responsible for the clinical disease. Tetanolysin has hemolytic properties and is speculated to propagate local tissue damage.
- Toxin formed in a skin wound spreads to adjacent muscle, accumulates in motor fiber nerve endings, and utilizes retrograde axonal transport to track to the ventral horn of the spinal cord and brainstem.
- Tetanospasmin selectively binds inhibitory interneurons' membrane proteins, blocking neurotransmission. This irreversible blockade results in the loss of modulation of excitatory impulses from the motor cortex, translating into increased muscle tone and painful muscle spasm. Simple sensory stimuli may prompt severe spasm.
- Autonomic neurons experience disinhibition as well, and later in the course, patients may experience autonomic dysfunction.
- Tetanospasmin's irreversible binding creates effects on anterior horn cells, brainstem, and autonomic neurons that remain indefinitely. Recovery requires the growth of new axonal nerve terminals, hence the usual 4- to 6-week duration of clinical tetanus.

CLASSIFICATION

- Generalized tetanus (the most common, most severe form) is characterized by diffuse muscle rigidity.
- Localized tetanus describes rigidity of a group of muscles in close proximity to the site of injury.

- Cephalic tetanus includes trismus (lockjaw) plus paralysis of one or more cranial nerves.
- Both local and cephalic tetanus may progress to generalized tetanus, the latter occurring in approximately 65% of cases.

CLINICAL MANIFESTATIONS

- *C. tetani* most commonly enters the host through skin disruption, primarily via lacerations (especially in the setting of associated tissue necrosis or a foreign body). Other clinical settings include: neonates with an infected umbilical stump or patients with burns, animal bites, septic abortions, and rarely abdominal surgery involving necrotic infections.
- The incubation period ranges widely—days to months. The interval between injury and onset of clinical symptoms may be dictated by the proximity of the wound to the central nervous system.
- Clinical manifestations include muscular rigidity (the most prominent early symptom), specifically trismus, risus sardonicus (sardonic smile), opisthotonos, and nuchal rigidity. Rarely, cranial nerve palsy can occur (most commonly, facial nerve).
- Patients with generalized tetanus experience tonic contraction of skeletal muscles with intermittent intense muscular spasms—both are exquisitely painful. Commonly, a patient will clench fists, arch the back, and flex and abduct the arms, extend the legs, and may become apneic. Spasms may be initiated by the slightest of sensory stimuli, including touch, noise, lights, and swallowing.
- Autonomic nervous system dysfunction in severe tetanus usually occurs 1–2 weeks after the onset of the disease. Impaired sympathetic inhibition symptoms include tachycardia, labile hypertension alternating with hypotension, peripheral vasoconstriction, fever, and profuse sweating. Overactivity of the parasympathetic nervous system causes increased bronchial and salivary gland secretions, bradycardia, and sinus arrest.

LABORATORY RESULTS

- Tissue cultures are positive in fewer than 50% of patients. The organism is noninvasive, so blood cultures serve little value except in diagnosing secondary infection.
- Labs are otherwise nonspecific, including leukocytosis with lymphocyte predominance, elevated transaminases, and creatinine kinase (after the development of muscle spasm).

DIAGNOSIS

- The diagnosis of tetanus is made on clinical grounds alone, suspected when there is a history of tetanus prone injury in the setting of inadequate tetanus immunization.
- The differential diagnosis includes: neuroleptic malignant syndrome, strychnine poisoning, Stiff-man syndrome, drug-induced dystonia, meningitis, hypocalcemic tetany, or the differential of isolated trismus.

TREATMENT

- The principles of initial treatment of tetanus consist of airway management, sedation, treatment of the portal of entry, antitoxin therapy, administration of appropriate antibiotics, and general supportive measures.
- The period of onset of the disease ranges from <1 to 12 days; therefore, even patients with mild tetanus (trismus, dysphagia, and localized rigidity) should be observed in an ICU for at least 1 week.
- In severe cases, the first priority is airway management to ensure airway protection and adequate ventilation, combined with correction of hypotension related to hypovolemia or autonomic instability.
- Antibiotics are universally recommended—first-line therapy is metronidazole (15 mg/kg IVP followed by 20–30 mg/kg/day IV for 7–14 days); however, they are only effective against vegetative forms of *C. tetani.*
- The use of passive immunization to neutralize unbound toxin is associated with improved survival. Antitoxin therapy with human tetanus immune globulin (hTIG) is given intramuscularly (500 IU) as early as possible. The use of intrathecal hTIG to neutralize toxin that has entered but is not yet fixed to nervous tissue has not been fully validated (see single study outcome) and is not *routinely* recommended.[2]
- The source of toxin should be removed by wound debridement and removal of foreign bodies.
- Muscle rigidity and spasms are treated with high-dose benzodiazepines and narcotics. However, cases of refractory spasms should undergo consideration for intravenous magnesium therapy, intrathecal baclofen, or epidural blockade.

PROGNOSIS

- With modern intensive care management, mortality ranges from 10 to 15% overall. In areas without such advances, mortality rates from 25 to 50% are usual.

- Clinical tetanus does not induce immunity against further attacks of the disease and all patients should begin their primary immunization series prior to leaving the hospital. Passive immunization with hTIG does not interfere with successful active immunization.

BIBLIOGRAPHY

Pascual FB, McGinley EL, Zanardi LR, et al. Tetanus surveillance—United States, 1998–2000. *MMWR Surveill Summ* 2003;52(3):1–8.

Agarwal M, Thomas K, Peter JV, et al. A randomized double-blind sham-controlled study of intrathecal human anti-tetanus immunoglobulin in the management of tetanus. *Natl Med J India* 1998;11(5):209–212.

Gray P. Tetanus. In: Hall JB, Schmidt GA, Wood LDH, eds., *Principles of Critical Care*, 3rd ed. New York, NY: McGraw-Hill; 2005:933–937.

Hsu SS, Groleau G. Tetanus in the emergency department: a current review. *J Emerg Med* 2001;20(4):357–365.

Rhee P, Nunley MK, Demetriades D, et al. Tetanus and trauma: a review and recommendations. *J Trauma* 2005;58(5):1082–1088.

63 VIRAL HEMORRHAGIC FEVERS

D. Kyle Hogarth

KEY POINTS

- Clinical presentations may sometimes be a flu-like syndrome, but can also be abrupt: fever associated with generalized myalgias and headache is common. Severe cases progress to pulmonary edema, shock, and bleeding from mucosal surfaces.
- Clinical diagnosis is dependent on a history of potential exposure within the preceding few days up to a maximum of 4 weeks. The exposure may be to rodents, ticks, or fresh animal or human blood, or patients. Typically, the patient has been to an endemic area recently.
- Management is mainly supportive. Respiratory assistance, replacement of blood components, and support of the circulation are the mainstays of therapy. Certain infections can be treated with ribavirin.
- Prevention of transmission of infection is extremely important. Routine respiratory isolation of suspect cases in a single room, standard universal precautions for exposure to contact with blood or body fluids, and careful disinfection of exposed surfaces. With appropriate precautions the risk of nosocomial transmission is minimal.
- With prompt supportive therapy, many patients can make a rapid and complete recovery without significant long-term sequelae.

OVERVIEW OF THE VIRAL HEMORRHAGIC FEVERS

- The diseases are caused by many different enveloped RNA zoonotic viruses.
- Viral hemorrhagic fevers (VHFs) are characterized by an acute onset with high fever and the potential for high rates of mortality. These infections are endemic on every continent except Australia.
- Bleeding is a complication of severe disease, and is a manifestation of the underlying pathology of widespread capillary leak.
- Death usually results from hypovolemic shock with or without acute respiratory distress syndrome (ARDS). In survivors, recovery is rapid and usually complete.

HISTORY AND CLINICAL DIAGNOSIS

- A thorough history is essential in making the diagnosis. The zoonotic character of these infections means that they are primarily rural diseases in developing communities. An exposure and travel history must cover the maximum 4-week incubation period before the onset of fevers.
- Questions must include a thorough travel history: information on any possible contact with ticks, fresh animal blood, rodent urine or blood, wild animals, and mosquitoes and other insects, recent camping in exotic areas, possible entry into bat caves, and attendance at ceremonial funerals should be sought.
- The fever is often high and has an abrupt onset. Severe body pains and headache are prominent and may be excruciating. Other features seen can include nausea and vomiting, severe sore throat, petechiae, oozing from the gums, and bradycardia. As the disease progresses, respiratory distress secondary to pulmonary edema and hypovolemic shock from diffuse bleeding become hallmarks of the disease.

LABORATORY DIAGNOSIS

- Total peripheral white counts usually show lymphopenia and elevated neutrophil counts. Thrombocytopenia and platelet dysfunction are common. Disseminated intravascular coagulation (DIC) is not a feature of VHF except as a complication of the terminal phase.

- Serum glutamic-oxaloacetic transaminase (SGOT) is usually raised. In VHFs, the SGOT is disproportionately high compared with the serum glutamic-pyruvic transaminase (SGPT). Ratios of SGOT:SGPT may be as high as 11:1! The level of the SGOT reflects prognosis, with higher SGOT levels increasing the risk of death. The bilirubin is usually normal, the exception being yellow fever which is associated with jaundice.
- Care must be taken in collection, handling, and transport of specimens. Sera may be safely handled for immunologic tests by inactivation by heating to 60°C for 30 minutes.
- The most rapid and accurate method of diagnosis is by reverse transcriptase-polymerase chain reaction (RT-PCR).
- Virus isolation from serum requires a high level of laboratory biocontainment, and can require at least 1 week.
- Detection of high-titer IgG antibody with virus-specific IgM antibody can be diagnostic. However, the more rapid VHFs, particularly Ebola, evolve so quickly that patients may die before enough time has passed to develop antibodies.

MANAGEMENT

- Viral hemorrhagic fevers are self-limiting diseases and the majority of medical management is supportive.
- Early initiation of ribavirin therapy is useful for the following infections: Lassa, South American hemorrhagic fevers, Crimean-Congo hemorrhagic fever (CCHF), and Hantavirus pulmonary syndrome. Ribavirin does not work for Ebola, Marburg, yellow fever, Rift Valley fever, and dengue.
- Therapy with immune plasma may help in Argentine hemorrhagic fever, but has not been demonstrated to be effective in other VHFs.
- Fluid balance and volume status are the main challenges in managing patients. They will often present with a paradoxical high hematocrit due to capillary leakage aggravated by dehydration. Development of low-pressure pulmonary edema (ARDS) is common. Ventilatory support should follow low-tidal volume strategies (e.g., 6 cc/kg ideal weight).
- Pregnant patients often present with absent fetal movements. Maternal survival in Lassa fever has been shown to depend on aggressive obstetric intervention to evacuate the uterus.

PREVENTION OF SPREAD

- The key to prevention of transmission is good hospital and laboratory practice with strict isolation of febrile patients with VHF and rigorous use of gloves and disinfection. Attempts should be made to minimize the number of personnel caring for and interacting with these patients.
- Aerosol spread in hospitals has not been documented. The risk to personnel caring for a VHF patient is about equal to that of HIV transmission, if full barrier precautions are fully implemented.
- High risk of infection is associated with direct percutaneous or mucosal contact with blood or body fluids. Postexposure prophylaxis with ribavirin should be offered to contacts with high-risk exposures. People with medium- or low-risk contact histories may be safely observed for development of persistent high fever for 3 weeks from the last date of contact.

BIBLIOGRAPHY

Fisher-Hoch SP. Viral hemorrhagic fevers. In: Hall JB, Schmidt GA, Wood LDH, eds., *Principles of Critical Care*, 3rd ed. New York, NY: McGraw-Hill; 2005:939–954.

64 ANTHRAX AND SMALLPOX

Ajeet Vinayak

KEY POINTS

- The CDC classify both anthrax and smallpox among the category A agents in terms of bioterrorism potential. Category A agents include those that carry the greatest risk to public health, have the potential for widespread effect, and need extensive planning to address prevention, recognition, and treatment.
- Due to nonspecific prodromal states in these diseases, attention should be on clinical manifestations awareness, a high degree of suspicion, and preparedness (which includes resource allocation, triaging, case-reporting, and isolation/containment).
- Following a bioterrorism exposure, anthrax would probably present as an influenza-like respiratory illness, progressing to critical illness, possibly characterized by hemorrhagic mediastinitis.
- The World Health Organization (WHO) estimates mortality for 50 kg of anthrax released over a population of 5 million would approach 100,000 people.

- Smallpox is spread easily by droplets and fomites, while with anthrax human-to-human transmission probably does not occur.
- Smallpox is characterized by its rash—no effective antiviral treatment is available.

ANTHRAX

EPIDEMIOLOGY AND MICROBIOLOGY

- The causative bacteria, *Bacillus anthracis*, is a large, gram-positive, aerobic, spore-forming bacillus responsible for zoonotic infections among grazing herbivores. In nature, these animals are infected by ingestion of the hardy, resistant spores found in the soil with a minor contribution of spread due to biting insects.
- Three types of infection are possible: cutaneous, gastrointestinal, and inhalational anthrax.
- While exceedingly rare, naturally occurring human infection most commonly occurs as cutaneous anthrax resulting from contact with animal hides. Naturally occurring inhalational anthrax was reported as an occupational hazard in slaughterhouses and the textile industry (woolsorters disease).
- As a weapon, anthrax would be spread as an aerosol of spores leading to inhalational anthrax on germination in lymph nodes or cutaneous disease from direct contact.
- Two binary toxins, edema toxin and lethal toxin, along with a phagocytosis-resistant capsule are the responsible virulence factors leading to the clinical manifestations of anthrax (edema, hemorrhage, necrosis, and death).

HISTORY AND POTENTIAL

- 1876: First disease to fulfill Koch postulates (criteria used to link specific bacteria with specific disease).
- 1881: First vaccination for bacterial disease was developed for anthrax by Louis Pasteur (for sheep).
- 1940s: Only known wartime use of anthrax by the Japanese army in Manchuria.
- 1950s: Both the former Soviet Union and Iraq admit to the possession of weapon-grade anthrax.
- 1979: Release of anthrax spores in a Soviet military factory in Sverdlovsk resulted in the death of at least 66 people.
- 2001: 22 suspected bioterrorism cases (11 inhalational, 11 cutaneous) in 5 U.S. states with 5 reported deaths.

CLINICAL MANIFESTATION AND DIAGNOSIS

CUTANEOUS ANTHRAX

- This form results from direct contact of spores on an area of abraded skin. Commonly exposed areas of skin are affected.
- Disease develops usually within 2–5 days of exposure.
- The primary lesion is pruritic and maculopapular leading to a rounded ulcer, with subsequent satellite vesicles. Eventually, a large, dark eschar forms over the course of a week.
- The incidence of bacteremia and mortality are low but, without antibiotics, mortality rates can be from 5 to 15%. Cure is the usual rule with therapy.

GASTROINTESTINAL ANTHRAX

- This form occurs from ingestion of contaminated meat and is the rarest form of anthrax disease. Symptoms appear 2–5 days after ingestion.
- Germination of the spores leads to nausea, vomiting, fever, and acute abdomen. Hematemesis or hematochezia can occur.
- An oropharyngeal variant can occur if spores germinate in the upper gastrointestinal or oropharyngeal area and lead to fever, sore throat, dysphagia, and lymphadenitis.
- Mortality is very high in this form and this is likely due to late detection and frequent advancement to systemic disease with frank sepsis.

INHALATIONAL ANTHRAX

- Spores inhaled into the alveoli are ingested by macrophages and transported to mediastinal lymph nodes where germination can occur up to 60 days later. On germination in the lymph nodes, edema, hemorrhage, and necrosis can lead to hemorrhagic mediastinitis and systemic spread.
- Symptoms usually begin 1–6 days after exposure. The first phase consists of myalgia, low-grade fever, nonproductive cough, and chest pain. Rhinitis is uncommon. The chest radiograph can show a widened mediastinum.
- Usually 2–3 days following the initial phase, rapidly progressive symptoms may herald a fatal course. These symptoms include fevers, diaphoresis, dyspnea, and shock. Stridor can occur if affected lymph nodes cause tracheal obstruction. Anthrax meningitis is a rare complication after bacteremia and is characterized by hemorrhagic cerebrospinal fluid (CSF).
- Detection of bioterrorism-related inhalational anthrax will rely on recognition of clustered cases of a rapidly fulminant flu-like illness.
- Chest radiographs can show a widened mediastinum. Pneumonic processes (which were once thought to be rare) seemed to occur frequently based on the recent experience with contaminated pieces of mail in 2001.

- Presumptive diagnosis can be made on Gram's stained blood, CSF, or vesicular fluid (from a skin lesion) showing gram-positive bacilli. If anthrax is suspected, the appropriate selective media should be requested to isolate the organism. Polymerase chain reaction (PCR), enzyme-linked immunosorbent assay (ELISA), and serologic testing can be done at appropriate laboratories.

PREVENTION AND TREATMENT

- Cultures should be collected prior to initiation of antimicrobial therapy.
- Treatment for anthrax includes ciprofloxacin (400 mg IV q12) or doxycycline (100 mg IV q12). For suspected bioterrorism, the Centers for Disease Control and Prevention (CDC) has recommended adding one or two additional agents with in vitro activity against *B. anthracis*. These agents include: rifampin, vancomycin, imipenem, chloramphenicol, penicillin, ampicillin, clindamycin, and clarithromycin. The use of penicillin G or ampicillin alone is not recommended because of isolation of inducible β-lactamases in isolates recovered in 2001. (Doses of ciprofloxacin and doxycycline should be adjusted for children.)
- Routine universal precautions should be used during the care of patients with anthrax. Human-to-human transmission is not thought to occur.
- Postexposure prophylaxis with oral ciprofloxacin or doxycycline is recommended for 60 days. This duration of therapy is based on the potential of delayed germination of resistant spores based on human experience and investigation involving monkeys.
- Vaccination with a noncell vaccine is used among military personnel. The use of this vaccine in a regimen for postexposure prophylaxis is investigational only.

SMALLPOX

HISTORY AND POTENTIAL

- Spread of contaminated items to native Americans during the French and Indian Wars led to high mortality.
- A worldwide campaign that successfully eradicated smallpox by 1977 led to cessation of vaccination in 1980.
- A projection made in 1999 suggested exposure to a crowd of 1000 people in a major urban center could lead to 15,000 cases with 2000 mortalities within 2 months. Furthermore, within a year 14 countries would have re-established endemic smallpox.

EPIDEMIOLOGY AND MICROBIOLOGY

- Smallpox is an orthopoxvirus with a characteristic brick shape.
- Two clinical diseases are possible: variola major and variola minor (milder form).
- High person-to-person transmission occurs via droplet nuclei and direct contact. Spread of the disease on fomites (blankets, clothing, and so forth) can also occur.
- High infectivity occurs at the onset of the rash which predictably follows onset of constitutional symptoms by 2–3 days. The eventual scabs are considered to have a low infectious potential.

CLINIICAL MANIFESTATION AND DIAGNOSIS

- There are four types of variola major: classical (also called ordinary and accounting for 90% of cases), modified, flat (also referred to as malignant), and hemorrhagic. The characteristic manifestation of the classical type is described below.
- A 12–14 (range 7–17) day incubation period precedes the onset of constitutional symptoms which consist of malaise, high fever, nausea, abdominal pain, back ache, and headache.
- The rash follows after another 2–3 days beginning in the mouth and oropharynx then spreading to the arms, trunks, and legs.
- Initially maculopapular, the rash homogeneously becomes vesicular (with a characteristic central depression) before turning pustular. During the second week of the rash, these tense pustules become flattened and confluent.
- See Fig. 64-1 for an algorithm for evaluation by the CDC.
- Mortality of classical variola major occurs most commonly during the second week and appears to be related to the degree of confluence that develops. Overall mortality of this commonest form approaches 30%.
- Management of fluid balance, renal failure, and electrolyte abnormalities are the focus of critical care. Pulmonary edema and pulmonary hemorrhage may occur.
- Contagion risk does not stop until all scabs have fallen off.
- Modified variola major is a milder form of this disease that occurs in persons with partial protection from prior vaccination.
- The hemorrhagic variant is more severe with nearly uniform mortality. While either gender can be affected, pregnant women appear to be at higher risk. This form is characterized by a more severe, earlier prodromal phase and then skin lesions marked by petechiae and hemorrhage. Prior vaccination does not affect severity of disease.

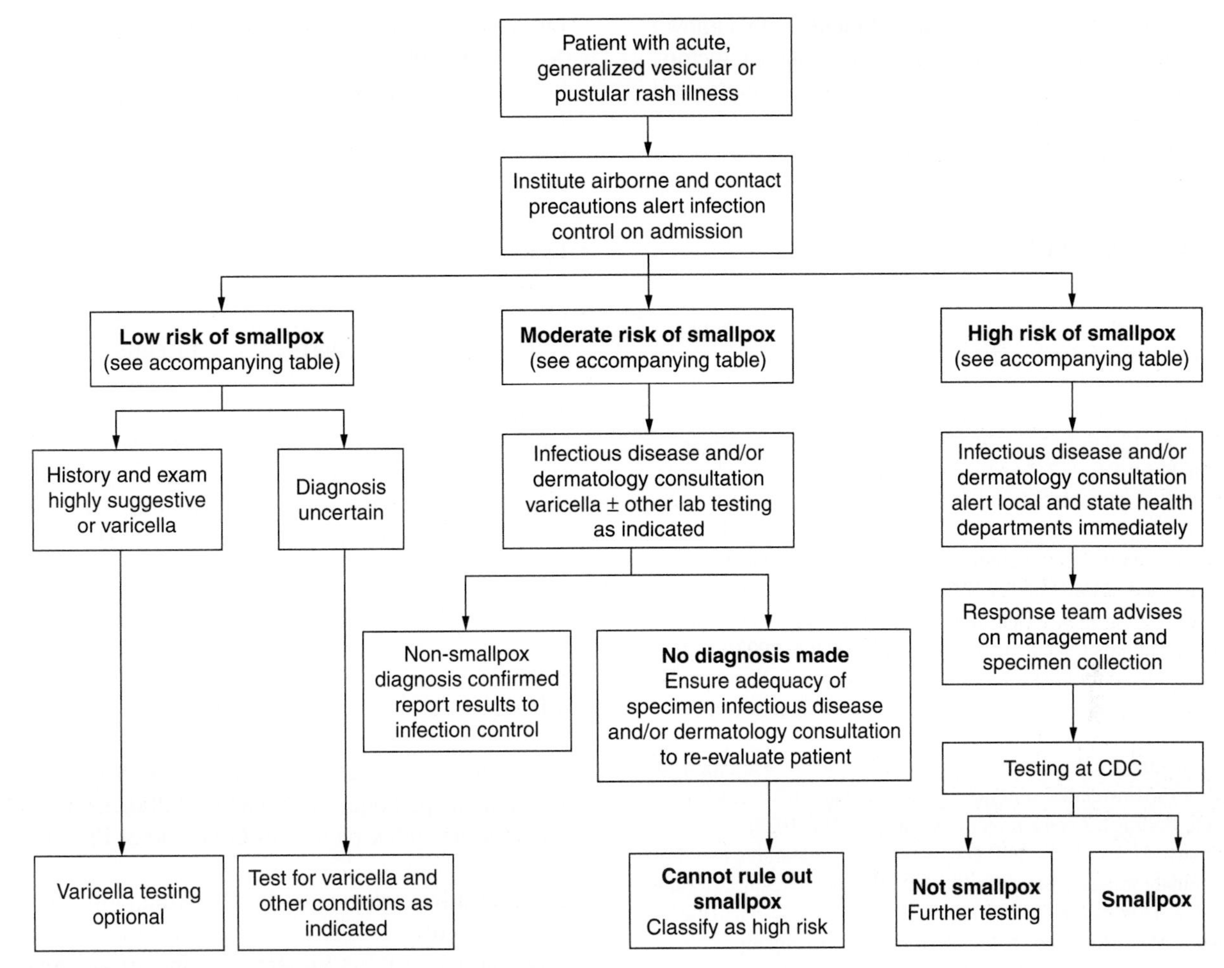

FIG. 64-1 CDC evaluation of patients for smallpox.
SOURCE: Adapted from http://www.bt.cdc.gov/agent/smallpox/diagnosis/evalposter.asp.

- Flat variola major is characterized by flat rubbery lesions rather than the tense pustules. This variant is also more severe than the ordinary disease and also seems to have a milder subtype among vaccinated individuals.
- Variola minor has fewer constitutional symptoms and a sparser rash.
- Initial cases should have laboratory confirmation. Scabs can be picked off with forceps or vesicular fluid can be sampled on cotton swabs. Samples should be appropriately packaged and sent to local or state authorities for analysis by light and electron microscopy as well as PCR methods.

PREVENTION AND TREATMENT

- Small outbreaks can be treated in isolation wards of individual hospitals. Strict airborne and contact isolation must be maintained.
- In large-scale outbreaks, entire hospitals would likely turn into treatment centers for severely ill patients with many affected people quarantined to their residences.
- No effective antiviral therapy is available.
- Antibiotic use has a role in secondary infection management.
- Postexposure vaccination within 4 days has been shown to attenuate disease course and may offer some protection.
- Groups with contraindication to vaccination include patients with HIV infection, exfoliative skin disorders, immunodeficient patients, and pregnant women.
- In these special populations vaccinia immune globulin may be used or if this is unavailable, postexposure vaccination reconsidered.
- Adverse reactions to vaccination include self-limited rashes (eczema vaccinatum and generalized vaccinia) as well as serious complications: vaccinia gangrenosa (especially in the immune compromised) and postvaccinal encephalitis (1 in 300,000).

- In addition, caution is advised in patients with a known cardiac condition or more than two cardiac risk factors.
- All cases should be reported to local, state, and national health care authorities.

BIBLIOGRAPHY

Bartlett J. Smallpox vaccination in 2003: key information for clinicians. *Clin Infect Dis* 2003;36:883–902.

CDC emergency preparedness and response site. Available at: www.bt.cdc.gov/. Accessed October 26, 2005.

Cieslak TJ, Eitzen EM Jr. Clinical and epidemiologic principles of anthrax. *Emerg Infect Dis* 1999;5:552–555.

Dixon TC. Anthrax. *N Engl J Med* 1999;341:815–826.

Henderson DA. Smallpox as a biological weapon: medical and public health management. Working Group on Civilian Biodefense. *JAMA* 1999;281:2127–2137.

Inglesby TV. Anthrax as a biological weapon, 2002: updated recommendations for management. *JAMA* 2002;287:2236–2252.

Inglesby TV. Anthrax as a biological weapon: medical and public health management. Working Group on Civilian Biodefense. *JAMA* 1999;281:1735–1745.

Jernigan DB, Raghunathan PL, Bell BP, et al. Investigation of bioterrorism-related anthrax, United States, 2001: epidemiologic findings. *Emerg Infect Dis* 2002;8:1019–1028.

Kuehnert MJ, Doyle TJ, Hill HA, et al. Clinical features that discriminate inhalational anthrax from other acute respiratory illnesses. *Clin Infect Dis* 2003;36:328–336.

Meltzer MI. Modeling potential responses to smallpox as a bioterrorist weapon. *Emerg Infect Dis* 2001;7:959–969.

O'Toole T. Smallpox: an attack scenario. *Emerg Infect Dis* 1999;5:540–546.

Pile JC. Anthrax as a potential biological warfare agent. *Arch Intern Med* 1998;158:429–434.

Swartz MN. Recognition and management of anthrax—an update. *N Engl J Med* 2001;345:1621–1626.

65 SARS

Shefali Shah

KEY POINTS

- Severe acute respiratory syndrome is caused by an infectious process and involves a febrile respiratory illness progressing, in some patients, into severe pneumonia and acute respiratory distress syndrome (ARDS).
- SARS is caused by a novel coronavirus that likely originated from an animal reservoir. The virus evolved into a human pathogen, with the first human case in November 2002, and is now capable of human-to-human transmission.
- It is responsible for the first major outbreak of the twenty-first century, and due to its rapid transmission, illustrates the need for a coordinated global effort in response to an infectious pandemic.
- Diagnosis is heavily dependent on history of exposure and clinical symptoms.
- Clinical features include high fevers, malaise, chills and rigors, cough, diarrhea and in some cases progression to ARDS and death.
- Treatment is primarily supportive. The major goals of therapy are respiratory support, circulatory support, and treatment of comorbid conditions.
- Prevention of transmission of infection is extremely important. Respiratory isolation, adherence to contact precautions, and careful disinfection of surfaces minimize the risk of transmission.

ETIOLOGY AND EPIDEMIOLOGY

- Severe acute respiratory syndrome (SARS) emerged as a human pathogen in November 2002 and can be traced to an index patient in Guangdong Province in southern China.
- The causative agent is a novel coronavirus (SARS-CoV). Coronaviruses are a family of enveloped, single-stranded RNA viruses. Coronaviruses are also the etiologic agents for the common cold.
- Precursor SARS-CoV-like viruses have been found in animals among the wild-game markets in Guangdong Province in China. The initial SARS-affected individual had contact with these animals. Human strains isolated later in the outbreak evolved from strains found early in the outbreak. This epidemiologic evidence supports the hypothesis that SARS likely originated in animals and interspecies transmission with viral evolution led to the human pathogen that caused the outbreak.
- The first major outbreak occurred in Guangzhou, China between January and March 2003, and then spread to Hong Kong, Vietnam, Singapore, Canada, and elsewhere. The subsequent outbreaks can be traced to those who had contact with the index patient.
- SARS is the first pandemic of the twenty-first century. The exceeding global economy in which we live where international air travel is commonplace combined with the highly infectious nature of the virus led to the widespread transmission of SARS. It illustrates the potential of an infectious disease to disseminate globally and cause serious health problems worldwide.

- The end of the outbreak occurred in July 2003. From December to January 2004, a small number of new cases of SARS emerged that were relatively mild and did not result in significant transmission. In these cases, the animal precursor virus was probably not adapted for efficient human-to-human transmission. However, this incident illustrates the possibility of re-emergence and a future outbreak.
- The most recent cases of SARS were found in China in April 2004 originating from a lab worker.
- To date, SARS has affected more than 8000 patients and has caused 774 deaths in 29 countries.

TABLE 65-1 Initial Clinical Symptoms in Adults with SARS*

1. Fever (99.9%)
2. Cough (65.5%)
3. Malaise (58.8%)
4. Chills/rigor (51.5%)
5. Myalgia (48.5%)
6. Shortness of breath (45.9%)
7. Headache (38.8%)
8. Dizziness (27.3%)
9. Chest pain (22.4%)
10. Diarrhea (20.1%)

*Among cases in China, Hong Kong, Canada, and Singapore, 2003.

TRANSMISSION

- The primary mode of transmission is through respiratory droplets and aerosolized infectious particles.
- The use of aerosol-generating procedures such as endotracheal intubation and bronchoscopy amplify transmission of SARS-CoV.
- SARS-CoV survives for many days when dried on surfaces and in feces. The role of fecal-oral transmission is unknown, but may be important considering the watery diarrhea that is a common clinical feature.
- Transmission is rare during the first 5 days of infection.
- Characteristic of the 2003 SARS outbreak was its "superspreading" phenomenon where a few individuals greatly augmented transmission of the virus. The reason for this phenomenon is still unclear. Researchers are currently investigating the possibility of coinfection of another entity in the role in infection and transmission of SARS-CoV.
- There have been no reports of vertical or perinatal transmission, though there is anecdotal evidence of increased pregnancy-related complications in those infected with SARS.

HISTORY AND CLINICAL CHARACTERISTICS

- A thorough travel and exposure history is essential for diagnosis.
- The incubation period lasts from 2 to 8 days and most patients develop symptoms within the first 10 days after exposure.
- The earliest symptom is high fever, usually of sudden onset. Affected individuals also initially present with myalgias, malaise, chills, and rigors. Upper respiratory complaints of rhinorrhea and sore throat are rare (Table 65-1).
- Initially, there are no obvious respiratory symptoms or chest x-ray changes.
- Within about 3–7 days, the patient usually deteriorates rapidly, with exacerbations in shortness of breath and an increase in lung infiltrates on imaging consistent with a viral pneumonitis.
- About a quarter of patients experience watery diarrhea.
- Elderly patients may be afebrile, and present with malaise, decreased appetite, or even a fall.

CLINICAL COURSE

- One-third of patients improve, with defervescence and resolution of radiographic changes.
- Two-thirds of patients have persistent fever, increasing dyspnea, tachypnea, hypoxemia, and worsening of the pulmonary physical examination. Serial chest radiographs or computed tomography (CT) scans reveal progression to unilateral or bilateral multifocal airspace consolidations in these patients.
- 20–30% require admission to an ICU, most of whom need mechanical ventilation.
- Viral load peaks at around the 10th day of illness and subsequently decreases, but some patients deteriorate during the second week of the illness despite the decreasing viral load. This observation suggests that some of the lung damage is immunopathogenic in nature.
- Diffuse alveolar damage can lead to fibrosis and formation of cysts. The rupture of these cysts can cause pneumomediastinum, an unusual complication.
- Overall mortality rate is about 15%. Terminal events include severe respiratory failure, multiple organ failure, sepsis, or intercurrent illness.
- Residual ground-glass opacifications have been noted on follow-up chest x-ray and CT scans in a majority of patients 1 month after admission.
- 6–20% of surviving patients have had some degree of residual respiratory impairment likely secondary to

pulmonary fibrosis, muscle weakness, or residual effects of the virus.

LABORATORY FINDINGS

- The most frequent initial chest radiographic finding is patchy consolidation.
- Chest radiograph and CT usually demonstrate bilateral ground-glass opacifications or consolidations. These findings can be unilateral.
- Often there is progression to bilateral bronchopneumonia over 5–10 days.
- T-cell lymphopenia and less often thrombocytopenia may be found.
- The levels of alanine aminotransferase and creatine kinase may be elevated.
- Lactate dehydrogenase is often elevated.
- Bacterial cultures of sputum yield no significant pathogens. Serum antibodies for common viruses such as adenovirus, coxsackievirus, respiratory syncytical virus (RSV), cytomegalovirus (CMV), influenza A and B are negative.
- The most rapid test for diagnosis is reverse transcriptase-polymerase chain reaction (RT-PCR) of specimens from the lower respiratory tract. In those with a productive cough, nasopharyngeal aspirates or throat swabs can be used for specimen collection. Viral RNA is also detectable in plasma, serum, leucocytes, feces, and urine.
- Identification of seroconversion remains the gold standard for diagnosis, but antibody is detectable only weeks after the illness. IgM does not aid in early diagnosis.
- Due to delayed seroconversion, the serum should be tested at least 21 days and preferably 28 days after onset of symptoms to confirm SARS.
- Mainstay of diagnosis remains history of exposure and clinical findings (Table 65-2).

TABLE 65-2 Diagnosis of SARS

1. History
   a. Recent (<20 days) close contact with an infected patient, or
   b. History of travel to an area with recent SARS within 10 days of symptom onset, or
   c. High-risk profession (e.g., laboratory worker or hospital employee during an outbreak)
2. Clinical symptoms
   a. Acute onset fever (≥38.0°C)
   b. Headache, arthralgia, myalgia, fatigue, or chest pain
   c. Cough
   d. Clinical evidence for pulmonary infection
   e. Dyspnea
   f. ARDS
3. Lymphopenia
4. Chest radiograph or CT consistent with patchy or speckled pneumonia
5. No response to antibiotic treatment for typical or atypical pneumonias

PROGNOSTIC FACTORS

- Age
  - Mortality exceeds 50% in those >65 years old.
  - Those younger than 12 years of age usually have an uneventful course and a good outcome.
- Coexisting illness, especially diabetes mellitus, chronic hepatitis B, and heart disease increase the risk of intensive care unit admission and mortality.
- High viral load in nasopharyngeal aspirates, feces, and serum during days 10–15 of the illness is predictive of poor clinical outcomes.
- Elevated lactate dehydrogenase is also correlated to a poorer outcome.

MANAGEMENT/TREATMENT

- Treatment is largely supportive.
- There is no response to antibiotics. However, early treatment with broad-spectrum antibiotics that are effective against common pathogens found in typical and atypical pneumonias can rule out the diagnosis of community-acquired pneumonia and may even serve a protective effect.
- Early nasal CPAP (continuous positive airway pressure) may be useful.
- Controversy surrounds the use of high-dose steroids, but these have been thought beneficial in some cases. Steroids should be administered with a proton pump inhibitor to prevent gastrointestinal (GI) distress and bleeding.
- At present, there is no clinical evidence for the efficacy of antiviral therapies.
- If the patient progresses to respiratory failure, then supportive care with mechanical ventilation with low tidal volume strategy is employed. Tidal volumes of 6 mL/kg of ideal body weight with target plateau pressures of <30 cm of water are generally used.
- There are a number of potential targets for antiviral drugs in the replication cycle of SARS-CoV, including fusion inhibitors and protease inhibitors. The discovery of the full genome sequence provides a basis for development of future drugs. Vaccine development and monoclonal antibodies for prophylaxis are other options that show promise for prevention and are currently under investigation.

HISTOLOGY

- Lung biopsies have shown
  - Diffuse alveolar damage
  - Inflammatory infiltration in interstitial tissue of the lung
  - Congestion with dilation, bleeding, and deformation of capillaries

- ◦ Exfoliation of the pulmonary alveolar epithelia
- ◦ Hyaline changes in some pulmonary alveoli with proliferation and fibrosis of connective tissue
- Viral RNA has also been detected at high viral loads in the lung, bowel, and lymph nodes, and also found in the spleen, liver, and kidney.

PREVENTION

- Early triage, early case detection, and isolation of affected patients are essential to prevent spread.
- Nosocomial transmission has been one of the major features of the outbreak, so rigid adherence to precautions is an essential control measure. Particularly strict adherence should be employed when an infected patient undergoes a procedure that can increase aerosol droplets in the environment, for example, endotracheal intubation or bronchoscopy.
- Protection against respiratory droplets and contact precautions can prevent the bulk of transmission. Strict hand-washing, gowning, gloving, and respiratory masks should be employed during any outbreak.
- Community containment during an outbreak is another mainstay for prevention of further transmission.

BIBLIOGRAPHY

Peiris JS, Guan Y, Yuen KY. Severe acute respiratory syndrome. *Nat Med* 2004;10:S88–S97.

Peiris JS, Yeun KY, Osterhous ADME, et al. The severe acute respiratory syndrome. *N Engl J Med* 2003;349:2431–2441.

WHO guidelines for the global surveillance of severe acute respiratory syndrome (SARS). Updated recommendations, October 2004. Available at: http://www.who.int/csr/resources/publications/WHO_CDS_CSR_ARO_2004_1/en/index.html. Accessed October 26, 2005.

Zhao Z, Zhang F, Xu M, et al. Description and clinical treatment of an early outbreak of severe acute respiratory syndrome (SARS) in Guangzhou, PR China. *J Med Microbiol* 2003;52:715–720.

66 INFLUENZA

Gordon E. Carr

KEY POINTS

- Influenza is caused by an RNA virus that displays remarkable genetic instability.
- Point mutations in the viral genome cause small antigenic changes (antigenic drift), allowing the virus to evade existing immunity in the population, producing annual epidemics which kill roughly 50,000 in the United States annually.
- Reassortment of the viral genome produces novel viral subtypes (antigenic shift), potentially changing both the ability to spread in the population and the pathogenicity, and leading sporadically to pandemics.
- Fever, cough, myalgias, and headache in the proper epidemiologic context should raise suspicion for influenza.
- Influenzal respiratory infection may be complicated by bacterial pneumonia, myocarditis, encephalitis, and rhabdomyolysis.
- Antiviral therapy is minimally effective in established infection, treatment is largely supportive.

VIROLOGY

- Two clinically important types exist: influenza A and B.
- Different nucleoprotein (NP) and matrix protein (M) antigens distinguish the viral types.
- Both types have a segmented genome consisting of single-stranded negative-sense RNA in eight fragments.
- Influenza A viruses are further characterized according to the immunologic reactivity of hemagglutinin (HA) and neuraminidase (NA) glycoproteins displayed by different subtypes, for example, H1N1, H3N2.
- 15 HA and 9 NA variants have been identified.
- Intracellular replication of the viral genome depends on a viral RNA-dependent RNA polymerase.
- Influenza A RNA polymerase is susceptible to frequent errors, with a replication error rate of $1/10^4$ bases as compared to an error rate of $1/10^9$ bases for most DNA polymerases.
- Due to its segmented genome, and the high error rate of its RNA polymerase, influenza undergoes constant genetic change.
- This constant genetic change translates into antigenic instability, contributing to a cyclical pattern of outbreaks as new viral subtypes are able to evade established immunity.
- The virus' genetic instability may also underlie changes in pathogenicity. For example, genetic mutations underlie changes in both tissue tropism and virulence in birds. However, the molecular basis of pathogenicity in human influenza infection remains to be fully elucidated.

EPIDEMIOLOGY

- Influenza persists in an animal reservoir, mainly aquatic birds, and is capable of causing infection in many species.
- In humans, two patterns of disease are described: epidemics and pandemics.

EPIDEMICS

- Both influenza A and B can cause annual epidemics, which result when the virus can evade preexisting immunity in the population.
- This ability to evade immunity results from point mutations in the viral genome (antigenic drift). Antigenic drift causes small changes to viral antigens.
- Other factors also determine the extent of viral epidemics: the virus' ability to spread among humans, the ability to replicate in the human host, and the presence or absence of immunity in the population.
- Influenza epidemics contribute to more than 200,000 hospital admissions each year in the United States, and probably contribute to more than 50,000 deaths.
- The morbidity and mortality of influenza A epidemics stem from primary viral infection as well as from the role of host factors, such as cardiovascular and respiratory disease and the patient's immune status.
- In one prospective study, epidemic or sporadic influenza A and B accounted for about 10% of cases of community-acquired pneumonia (CAP).
- However, among patients with heart disease, this study found that influenza accounted for 25% of the cases of CAP. This finding demonstrates the crucial influence of host factors in determining outcome from infection.
- The highest rates of hospitalization occur among the elderly and young children.

PANDEMICS

- Only influenza A causes pandemics.
- Pandemics can claim tens of millions of lives worldwide, and occur at unpredictable intervals.
- Pandemics may disproportionately affect younger and healthier people.
- Pandemics result from the emergence of novel viral subtypes. These novel subtypes emerge from the reassortment of genome segments (antigenic shift).
- Antigenic shift creates viral subtypes with potentially drastic immunologic novelty. Whether antigenic shift also leads to changes in viral pathogenicity requires further study.
- Currently, there is concern that the H5N1 subtype, currently circulating among birds in Asia, may lead to a pandemic. This subtype appears to be particularly novel, both in terms of pathogenicity and antigenicity.
- Furthermore, both animal-to-human and human-to-human transmission have been documented. The World Health Organization (WHO) and other agencies are actively monitoring H5N1.

PATHOPHYSIOLOGY

- Transmission occurs by three routes: inhalation of respiratory droplets, contact with fomites, and contact with infected animals such as pigs and birds.
- In humans, the viral attachment seems to be limited to the epithelial cells of the respiratory tract.
- The molecular basis of pathogenicity in humans is poorly understood, although several viral proteins have been implicated. Nonstructural protein 1, PB2, NA, and HA are important contributors.
- The virus probably does not disseminate systemically.
- Systemic illness results from the interplay between viral and host factors. The host immune response to infection and the viral ability to resist it are important determinants of the extent of disease.
- Primary infection of the respiratory tract may be catastrophic in patients with respiratory, cardiovascular, metabolic, or immunologic diseases. Likewise, the systemic consequences of infection may lead to the deterioration of other underlying comorbidities.
- Cytokines and interferons are important mediators of systemic disease. One study found a correlation between systemic cytokine levels and the extent of symptoms and viral replication.

PRESENTATION

- Signs and symptoms can be highly variable, and often include the acute onset of fever, malaise, respiratory symptoms, myalgias, and headache.
- The combination of fever and cough for <36 hours, with or without the other symptoms listed above, and in the right epidemiologic context, should prompt consideration of influenza infection.
- Infection with different subtypes can present with variable signs and symptoms. For example, in the recently reported cases of H5N1 infection in humans, there has been prominent lymphopenia and diarrhea.

DIAGNOSIS

- No symptom or set of symptoms reliably indicates influenza infection.
- The role of laboratory studies is still evolving. Physicians must rely on clinical and epidemiologic clues until well-validated and clinically practical tests for influenza are widely available.
- A two-step approach to clinical diagnosis has been proposed. First, the physician must identify an influenza-like illness (ILI): acute onset of fever and

respiratory symptoms with or without myalgias, malaise, fatigue, or other symptoms.
- Once an ILI has been identified, one should consider the epidemiologic context. During times of high prevalence and in communities with more viral presence, the likelihood of influenza infection is much more likely.
- The Centers for Disease Control and Prevention (CDC) maintains a Web site: http://www.cdc.gov/flu/weekly/fluactivity.htm. This Web site provides important information about regional and temporal patterns of influenza activity, which should assist in appropriate diagnosis of an ILI.

COMPLICATIONS

- Many complications stem from the exacerbation of chronic conditions, notably cardiovascular, pulmonary, and immunologic diseases
- Bacterial pneumonia develops in about 75% of patients with influenza who develop pneumonia
- Myocarditis, pericarditis
- Encephalitis
- Rhabdomyolysis

TREATMENT

- Two classes or drugs are available to treat influenza, but they are of limited utility: the M2 inhibitors (amantidine and rimantadine) and the NA inhibitors (oseltamivir and zanamivir). These drugs target enzymes involved in the viral life cycle.
- Anti-influenza drugs are minimally effective at treating established infection. Currently available drugs seem to shorten the length of fever or other symptoms by about a day, and may reduce the need for antibiotics if given within the first 48 hours of infection.
- There are limited settings where these drugs may be of more benefit.
  - During pandemics.
  - In the case of the high-risk patient who is not immune or has not been vaccinated, if treatment can be initiated within 48 hours of the onset of illness (zanamivir and oseltamivir).
  - In the case of infected, unvaccinated household contacts of high-risk patients.
- For the most part, care of the patient with influenza is supportive. For those progressing to acute respiratory distress syndrome (ARDS), a lung-protective ventilation strategy should be used.
- Adequate care of the patient with influenza demands close attention to the patient's cardiopulmonary and immunologic state, and the presence of other comorbidities. Patients with pneumonia should be risk-stratified based on a validated scale such as the PORT (Pneumonia Patient Outcomes Research Team) score.

PREVENTION

- Vaccines: live attenuated and inactivated vaccines are available.
  - In one meta-analysis, vaccination lead to a 50% reduction in all-cause mortality, a 47% reduction in hospital admissions for influenza and pneumonia, and 35% reduction in cases of ILI.
  - Annually revised vaccination recommendations are available on the CDC Web site: http://www.cdc.gov/flu/professionals/vaccination/#recs.
  - Some recommendations for use of inactivated vaccine (from the CDC Web site).
    - Persons aged ≥65 years
    - Residents of nursing homes and other chronic-care facilities that house persons of any age who have chronic medical conditions
    - Adults and children who have chronic disorders of the pulmonary or cardiovascular systems, including asthma (hypertension is not considered a high-risk condition)
    - Adults and children who have required regular medical follow-up or hospitalization during the preceding year because of chronic metabolic diseases (including diabetes mellitus), renal dysfunction, hemoglobinopathies, or immunosuppression (including immunosuppression caused by medications or by human immunodeficiency virus [HIV])
    - Adults and children who have any condition (e.g., cognitive dysfunction, spinal cord injuries, seizure disorders, or other neuromuscular disorders) that can compromise respiratory function or the handling of respiratory secretions or that can increase the risk for aspiration
    - Children and adolescents (aged 6 months to 18 years) who are receiving long-term aspirin therapy and, therefore, might be at risk for experiencing Reye syndrome after influenza infection
    - Women who will be pregnant during the influenza season
    - Children aged 6–23 months
  - More comprehensive and detailed recommendations are available from the CDC.
- Drugs: anti-influenza drugs may be useful for the prevention of infection in selected groups.
  - For postexposure prophylaxis of high-risk patients older than 13 years and residents of residential facilities who can begin treatment within 48 hours of exposure (oseltamivir).
  - For wider use during pandemics.

Bibliography

Bochud P, Moser F, Erard P, et al. Community acquired pneumonia: a prospective outpatient study. *Medicine* 2001;80:75–87.

Call SA, Vollenweider MA, Hornung CA. Does this patient have influenza? *JAMA* 2005;293:987–997.

Cooper NJ, Sutton AJ, Abrams KR, et al. Effectiveness of neuraminidase inhibitors in treatment and prevention of influenza A and B: systematic review and meta-analyses of randomised controlled trials. *BMJ* 2003;326:1235–1241.

Dolin R. Influenza. In: Braunwald E, Fauci AS, Kasper DL, et al., eds., *Harrison's Principles of Internal Medicine*, 15th ed. New York, NY: McGraw Hill; 2001:1125–1130.

Gerberding JL, Morgan JG, Shepard J, et al. Case 9-2004: an 18-year-old man with respiratory symptoms and shock. *N Engl J Med* 2004;350:1236–1247.

Hien TT, Liem NT, Dung NT, et al. Avian influenza A (H5N1) in 10 patients in Vietnam. *N Engl J Med* 2004;350:1179–1188.

Nicholson KG, Wood JM, Zambon M. Influenza. *Lancet* 2003;362:1733–1745.

Stiver G. The treatment of influenza with antiviral drugs. *CMAJ* 2003;168:49–57.

Thompson WW, Shay DK, Weintraub E, et al. Influenza-associated hospitalizations in the United States. *JAMA* 2004;292:1333–1339.

Ungchusak K, Auewarakul P, Dowell SF, et al. Probable person-to-person transmission of avian influenza A (H5N1). *N Engl J Med* 2005;352:333–340.

Zambon MC. The pathogenesis of influenza in humans. *Rev Med Virol* 2001;11:227–241.

67 PLAGUE: THE BLACK DEATH

Samip Vasaiwala

KEY POINTS

- Plague is caused by a gram-negative bacterium, *Y ersinia pestis*, spread by fleas from a rodent reservoir.
- The bubonic form of plague is characterized by fever, chills, and tender, erythematous lymphadenopathy (buboes).
- Septicemic plague is defined by positive blood cultures and sepsis, without lymphadenopathy.
- Pneumonic plague is acquired through droplet infection (primary pneumonic plague) or through spread to the lungs from another infected part of the body (secondary pneumonic plague) and resembles bacterial pneumonia of other causes. Strict droplet precautions are mandatory for suspected or established cases of plague.
- A high index of suspicion is required to make the diagnosis. Since antimicrobials typically used to treat severe pneumonia and sepsis do not treat plague adequately, establishing a diagnosis is especially important.
- The treatment of choice is streptomycin.

HISTORY

- The first documented mention of the plague is possibly given in the Bible in the book of *Samuel* in which an outbreak of a disease with buboes is described (I. Samuel V9-12).
- The first pandemic originated in northern Africa (Ethiopia or Egypt) around the year 532 and spread to the Mediterranean via the Nile. The pandemic started as the plague reached Constantinople (now Istanbul, Turkey) and Greece in the year 541. The most important political impact of this pandemic was the eradication of one-half of the inhabitants of the Byzantine Empire by the year 565. The prominent medical thought in this was offered by Hippocrates and Galen, who both believed in the theory of a vaporous eruption of substances into the air from swamps as the cause of these epidemics.
- The term "Black Death" was coined in England during the second pandemic because of the black spots (buboes) it produced on the skin. The devastation caused by this disease during this period is evident by a 33% drop in the population of Europe from the year 1347 to 1352. The understanding of the etiology of this disease was not more advanced than the original views of Galen and Hippocrates, with others suggesting possible unfavorable constellation of stars and comets and the wrath of God. Cities like Marseille introduced quarantine measurements to avoid these epidemics. In fact, the word "quarantine" is derived from the 40-day restriction placed on travel in Marseille in the year 1384. It was not until the year 1546 that Girolamo Fracastoro (1478–1553) and later in 1658, Athanasius Kircher implicated plague as a potential infection.
- It was not until the third pandemic that the discovery of the bacterium *Y. pestis* as the etiologic agent of the plague was made. This pandemic likely started in the Chinese province of Yunnan around 1855, spreading to Japan, Taiwan, and Mumbai, India by the year 1896 and eventually to South America, South Africa, and parts of western North America. Alexandre Yersin (1863–1943) accurately described the bacterium as a gram-negative organism in the year 1894. Based on epidemiologic data, Paul-Louis Simond (1858–1947) proposed the role of the flea in plague transmission. Ricardo Jorge was the first to implicate living rodents as a reservoir of infection as an explanation of endemic plague.

EPIDEMIOLOGY: THE LIFE CYCLE OF *YERSINIA PESTIS*

- The pathogen that causes plague belongs to the genus *Yersinia*, a member of the family Enterobacteriaceae. *Y. pestis*, a facultative anaerobe and an obligate parasite, is a gram-negative, nonmotile, nonspore-forming coccobacillus (0.5–0.8 μm in diameter and 1–3 μm long). It exhibits bipolar staining with Giemsa, Wright, or Wayson staining. The organism grows at temperatures from 4 to 40°C, with the optimum pH for growth ranges from 7.2 to 7.6.
- Plague is a zoonotic disease with no role of human infection as a part of its life cycle. Transmission between rodents happens via their associated fleas. Also, direct contact and ingestion do not play a significant role in the life cycle of *Y. pestis*, although infection is definitely possible via these routes. The main vector for transmission of the plague is the oriental rat flea (*Xenopsylla cheopis*). With each bite, this flea will ingest approximately 0.3–0.5 μL of blood from an infected rodent, with an estimated 300 *Y. pestis* organisms. The organisms multiply in the stomach of the flea and within 2–3 days they develop a dark brown mass containing bacilli, a fibrinoid material, and hemin within the flea stomach. This mass eventually obstructs the gastrointestinal tract of the flea by days 3–9. Now, as the hungry flea attempts to repeatedly feed, the blood sucked from the rodents gets mixed with the organisms and is regurgitated back into the mammalian host, with an estimated inoculation of 11,000–24,000 organisms. The infection of the mammal with subsequent bacteremia and another flea bite completes the life cycle (Fig. 67-1).

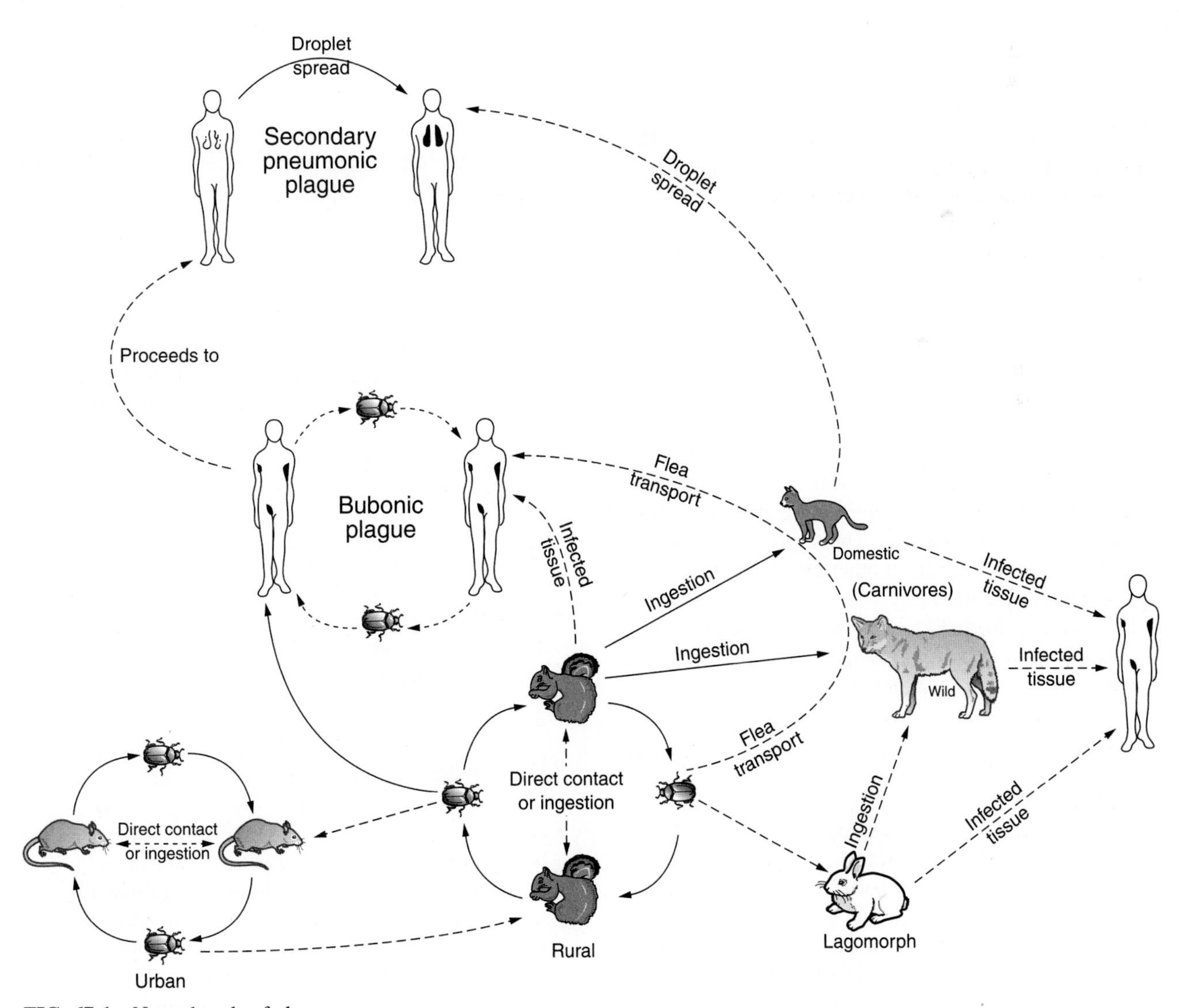

FIG. 67-1 Natural cycle of plague

- In the United States, the most common source of the human plague is through the bite of *Odontotermes montanus*, which is carried by squirrels. Cat and dog fleas (*Chlamydophila felis* and *Ctenocephalides canis*) do bite humans but are not associated with significant human disease. However, human disease associated with contact with infected cats is rising. Most of the human cases of plague in the United States are reported in the southwest and Pacific west coast.

CLINICAL MANIFESTATIONS

- Human plague usually presents in three common forms: bubonic, septicemic, and pneumonic. The less common forms of presentation like meningitis, pharyngitis, tonsillitis, and skin infections are not discussed in this chapter. The incubation period of plague is usually 2–8 days.

BUBONIC PLAGUE

- This is the most common form and presents with sudden onset of fever, chills, headache, and weakness. Also, gastrointestinal complaints such as nausea, vomiting, and diarrhea are common. The classic finding is that of a bubo, tender lymphadenopathy of usually either the inguinal or axillary lymph nodes with associated erythema and overlying skin edema but lacking fluctuance.

SEPTICEMIC PLAGUE

- This is a very difficult diagnosis to make since there may be no characteristic physical findings. The definition is positive blood cultures in a patient with no palpable lymphadenopathy. The signs and symptoms are not very different from other gram-negative sepsis syndromes. The mortality from septicemic plague is high, ranging from 30 to 50% because the antibiotics normally used to broadly cover septic patients are not very effective against *Y. pestis*.

PNEUMONIC PLAGUE

- The last case of pneumonic plague recorded in the United States that was due to a person-to-person spread was during the 1924–1925 Los Angeles plague epidemic. Primary pneumonic plague is acquired by inhalation of respiratory droplets from an infected individual, animal, or from laboratory specimens. It is more commonly seen in patients with bubonic or septicemic plague who then acquire secondary pneumonic plague. Infected cats with pneumonic plague are the most common source of primary pneumonic plague in humans. There are no obvious clinical or radiographic findings that readily differentiate plague pneumonia from other types of bacterial pneumonia. Sputum may be clear, purulent, or hemorrhagic and may contain few gram-negative rods.

DIAGNOSIS

- A high index of suspicion is needed to make a diagnosis of plague. Key questions include those that address travel to endemic areas, exposure to potential animal or rodent vectors, and classic clinical signs. Routine laboratory evaluation may reveal an elevated white blood cell count.

CULTURE

- *Y. pestis* grows well on the routine laboratory culture media and blood culture is positive in 27–96% of cases. Aspirates from buboes can also be sent for culture.

STAINING

- Gram's stain reveals small gram-negative coccobacilli. Wright-Giemsa stain of peripheral blood reveals rod-shaped organisms in 40% of cases. Wayson stain or a fluorescent antibody stain shows bipolar staining resembling a "closed safety pin."

SEROLOGY

- A fourfold rise in antibody titers to the F-1 antigen of *Y. pestis* or a single titer of >1:16 using a passive hemagglutination test is suggestive of the diagnosis.

RAPID DIAGNOSTIC TESTS

- A new test to detect the F-1 antigen of *Y. pestis* has been developed and has a sensitivity and specificity of 100% against laboratory isolates of *Y. pestis*. This test has also proved to be more sensitive than the enzyme-linked immunosorbent assay (ELISA) and culture. A polymerase chain reaction test aimed at the plasminogen activator gene of *Y. pestis* has been developed but is not yet routinely available for clinical use.

TREATMENT

- Streptomycin, which has been used against plague for the last 45 years, continues to be the treatment of choice. It is administered as an IM dose of 30 mg/kg/day (up to a total dose of 2 g/day) in two divided doses for 10 days. However, due to its toxicity, patients are usually not maintained on a full 10-day regimen and are generally switched over to tetracycline (2–4 g/day in four divided doses orally).
- Other therapies include doxycycline (100 mg bid PO or IV), chloramphenicol (25 mg/kg IV as a loading dose followed by 60 mg/kg/day in four divided doses; drug of choice for plague meningitis), and trimethoprim-sulfamethoxazole (160/800 mg bid; for bubonic plague).
- Although some outbreaks of drug-resistant plague have been reported, antibiotic-resistant strains are rare and not increasing in frequency.
- All patients diagnosed with plague are placed under strict respiratory droplet isolation until it is clear that they don't have pneumonic plague, their sputum culture is negative, and they have been treated at least for 48 hours with effective antibacterial therapy.
- Trimethoprim-sulfamethoxazole (15–30 mg/kg/day PO for 5–7 days) is also used for chemoprophylaxis for close contacts of patients suspected of having or diagnosed with pneumonic plague.

VACCINE

- Vaccination is recommended for individuals at high risk: military personnel serving in endemic areas and laboratory personnel working with fully virulent strains. A killed whole vaccine, which is no longer commercially available in the United States, is administered as a series of injections 1–3 months apart followed by a booster every 6 months until the exposure terminates.

CONCLUSION

- The recent epidemics in India remind us that plague should not be thought of as a disease of the past. Attempts have been made by the United States and the former Soviet Union at eradicating plague from certain locales; these attempts were expensive and mostly unsuccessful. Plague is here to stay.
- The diagnosis of this illness requires a very high level of suspicion.
- Recent research in the basic science and epidemiology of plague has dramatically advanced our knowledge of this infectious disease. Further arenas of research will focus on the development of a vaccine that provides long-lived immunity against plague and the modulation of virulence and drug resistance.

BIBLIOGRAPHY

Ziegler P. *The Black Death*. Wolfeboro Falls, NH: Alan Sutton Publishing, Inc.; 1991.

Campbell GL, Hughes JM. Plague in India: a new warning from an old nemesis. *Ann Intern Med* 1995;122:151–153.

Zietz B, Dunkelberg H. The history of the plague and the research on the causative agent *Yersinia pestis*. *Int J Hyg Environ Health* 2004;207:165–178.

Aberth J. *From the Brink of the Apocalypse: Confronting Famine, War, Plague, and Death in the Later Middle Ages*. New York, NY: Routledge; 2001.

Perry RD, Fetherston JD. Yersinia pestis—etiologic agent of plague. *Clin Microbiol Rev* 1997;10:35–66.

Gross L. How the plague bacillus and its transmission through fleas were discovered: reminiscences from my years at the Pasteur Institute in Paris. *Proc Natl Acad Sci U S A* 1995;92:7609–7611.

Centers for Disease Control and Prevention. Human plague—United States 1993-1994. *MMWR Morb Mortal Wkly Rep* 1994;43:242–246.

Hull HF, Montes JM, Mann JM. Septicemic plague in New Mexico. *J Infect Dis* 1987;155:113–118.

Crook LD, Tempest B. Plague: a clinical review of 27 cases. *Arch Intern Med* 1992;152:1253–1256.

Meyer KF. Pneumonic plague. *Bacteriol Rev* 1961;25: 249–261.

Craven RB, Maupin GO, Beard ML, et al. Reported cases of human plague infections in the United States, 1970–1991. *J Med Entomol* 1993;30:758–761.

Butler T. Yersinia infections: centennial of the discover of the plague bacillus. *Clin Infect Dis* 1994;19:655–663.

Chanteau S, Rahalison L, Ralafiarisoa L, et al. Development and testing of a rapid diagnostic test for bubonic and pneumonic plague. *Lancet* 2003;361:211–216.

Hinnebusch BJ, Schwan TG. New method for plague surveillance using polymerase chain reaction to detect Yersinia pestis in fleas. *J Clin Microbiol* 1993;31:1511–1514.

68 BOTULISM

David Brush

KEY POINTS

- Botulism is a clinical diagnosis that should be suspected in any adult with an acute onset of cranial nerve, gastrointestinal and autonomic dysfunction, and a history compatible with botulism exposure. Treatment should be initiated immediately, with cultures and toxin assays used to later confirm the diagnosis.
- Proper management of patients with botulism involves early diagnosis, timely antitoxin administration, careful

monitoring for respiratory compromise, and supportive care including mechanical ventilation if necessary.
- Respiratory failure is the primary cause of death in patients with botulism. Serial examination of oropharyngeal tone and frequent monitoring of spirometry can identify patients in need of mechanical ventilation before respiratory collapse is imminent.
- Patients with wound botulism need early and definitive surgical intervention.
- All suspected cases of botulism should be reported to public health authorities immediately. Prompt epidemiologic investigation helps prevent additional cases and can identify new risk factors for intoxication.

OVERVIEW

- Botulism results from intoxication with the protein neurotoxin formed by *Clostridium* bacteria, usually *Clostridium botulinum.*
- Toxins are subclassified by antigenic differences into types A through G. Types A, B, E, and F are responsible for most cases of human disease.
- Botulism neurotoxin permanently blocks alpha motor neurons from releasing acetylcholine, producing motor system paralysis and autonomic dysfunction (Fig. 68-1).

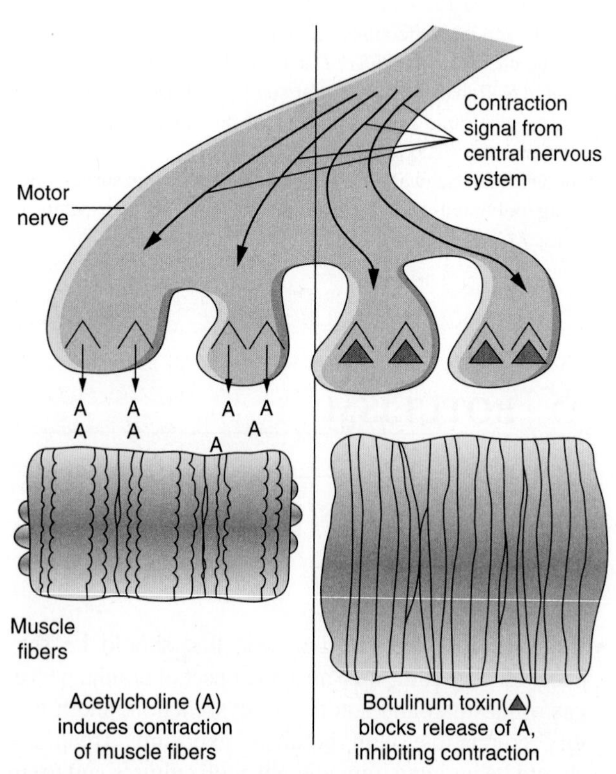

FIG. 68-1 Action of botulinum toxin.
SOURCE: Adapted from http://www.agen.ufl.edu/~chyn/age2062/lect/lect_25/FG19_011.GIF.

- Patients with the classic manifestations of botulism demonstrate acute, bilateral cranial neuropathies with symmetric descending weakness that may progress to respiratory failure.
- After treatment and toxin elimination, recovery of function occurs over the course of weeks to months as new neural synapses form.

EPIDEMIOLOGY

- Between 2001 and 2003, 425 cases of botulism were reported to the Centers for Disease Control (CDC). Of these cases, approximately 15% were foodborne botulism, 66% were infant botulism, 18% were cases of wound botulism, and 1% of cases were adult colonization botulism. Sources of botulism are listed in Table 68-1.

FOODBORNE BOTULISM

- Onset of symptoms usually occurs 12–36 hours after ingestion.
- Noncommercial food is most often implicated as the source in reported events (91%), frequently from home-canned vegetables (44%).
- In the United States, the consumption of Alaskan native foods such as fermented or smoked meats and fish are the most frequent cause of multicase outbreaks.
- Commercial food products and improper food handling at restaurants are an occasional cause of botulism, often resulting in multicase outbreaks.

WOUND BOTULISM

- Onset of symptoms varies, with reported incubations ranging from 4 to 14 days.

TABLE 68-1 Sources for Botulism

Sources
Home-canned vegetables, fruits, or fish
Noncommercial, noncanned fermented fish or meat
Home fermented beans
Commercial food improperly handled
Peyote consumption
Injection drug use
Wound infection
Sinusitis caused by cocaine inhalation
Colonization of the gastrointestinal tract with *C. botulinum*
Bioterrorism

SOURCE: Adapted from Ref. 1.

- The increased incidence of epidemics among injection drug users, especially those who use black tar heroin, has increased the occurrence of wound botulism in the United States.
- While most common among injection drug users, wound botulism can occur in any deep wound and can be a postsurgical complication.
- Sinusitis as a result of intranasal cocaine use has also been a reported cause of botulism.

ADULT COLONIZATION BOTULISM

- Rare case reports exist of adult onset "infant" botulism due to colonization of the gastrointestinal tract by *C. botulinum.*
- Factors which are thought to predispose patients to colonization include Crohns disease, achlorhydria, antimicrobial therapy, gastrectomy, intestinal surgery, and bone marrow transplantation.

BIOTERRORISM

- On at least three occasions between 1990 and 1995, botulinum toxin has been used as an aerosolized bioweapon in terrorist attacks. Other potential terrorist use of botulinum toxin includes deliberate contamination of food.

PHYSICAL SIGNS AND SYMPTOMS

- The hallmark of botulism intoxication is the acute presence of bilateral cranial neuropathies associated with symmetrical descending weakness that often progresses to involve the upper extremities and diaphragm (Table 68-2).
- Patients may experience a prodrome of gastrointestinal symptoms including nausea, vomiting, and diarrhea.
- In the absence of hypotension, the patient with botulism usually has a normal to slow heart rate. Other signs of autonomic dysfunction may include orthostasis, hypothermia, and urinary retention.
- With the exception of blurred vision, botulism does not cause sensory deficits.
- Patients with botulism remain responsive and do not usually manifest mental status changes.
- Normal pupillary function does not rule out botulism intoxication. Pupils are dilated or unresponsive in fewer than 50% of cases.
- Signs of upper airway obstruction from loss of pharyngeal tone or signs of diaphragmatic weakness require urgent intubation and mechanical ventilation.

TABLE 68-2 Signs and Symptoms in Patients with Botulism Intoxication

Common signs and symptoms (signs are usually symmetrical)
Diplopia
Blurred vision
Xerostomia
Dysphagia
Dyspnea
Dysarthria
Dizziness
Fatigue
Nausea*
Vomiting*
Diarrhea*
Sore throat
Opthalmoparesis
Pupils fixed or dilated
Facial paresis
Tongue weakness
Diminished gag reflex
Respiratory insufficiency
Upper extremity weakness
Diaphragmatic weakness
Lower extremity weakness
Uncommon signs and symptoms
Paresthesias
Ataxia
Nystagmus
Rare signs and symptoms
Lethargy or obtundation at presentation
Deep tendon hyperreflexia

*Uncommon in cases of wound botulism.

- Botulism does not cause pyrexia. A febrile patient in whom botulism is suspected should have further workup for a concomitant infectious process. Wound infections containing *C. botulinum* are often polymicrobial with other bacterial agents responsible for pyrexia.
- Wounds infected with *C. botulinum* may appear to be healing well without evidence of infection.

LABORATORY FINDINGS AND DIAGNOSTIC STUDIES

- Botulism is a clinical and epidemiologic diagnosis that can be confirmed with laboratory or electrophysiologic testing. Treatment should not be delayed pending these test results.

- Routine laboratory tests including serum electrolytes, complete blood count, liver function profiles, cerebrospinal fluid (CSF) studies, urinalysis, and electrocardiograms are normal unless secondary complications occur.
- Botulism is confirmed by the presence of botulism toxin in blood, stool, gastric contents, or wound tissue. These samples as well as implicated food items (if available) should be sent for culture and toxin identification to the appropriate state and national officials.
- Toxin typing confirming botulism is obtained in approximately 75% of cases.
- The most sensitive test for botulinum toxin is the mouse bioassay, in which serum or feces from the patient are injected into mice which are observed for signs of botulism. Toxin may also be identified through enzyme-linked immunosorbent assay (ELISA) or gel hydrolysis.
- Cultures demonstrating *C. botulinum* in serum stool or wound tissue provides good evidence for botulism infection.
- Electrophysiologic testing of clinically affected muscles shows reduced amplitude in compound muscle action potentials and a normal conduction velocity in 85% of cases.

DIFFERENTIAL DIAGNOSIS

- Classic acute inflammatory polyneuropathy (Guillain-Barré syndrome) presents with sensory deficits, rapid areflexia, and rarely begins with bulbar neuropathies. Elevated CSF protein is common.
- Miller-Fischer variant acute inflammatory polyneuropathy often produces oculomotor weakness and may involve other cranial nerves but has a characteristic ataxia lacking in patients with botulism.
- Myasthenia gravis lacks autonomic symptoms and is rarely a fulminant disease. Tensilon testing must be interpreted with caution, as some patients with botulism demonstrate increased strength after edrophonium administration.
- Eaton Lambert myasthenic syndrome can be excluded by electromyography and antibody study.
- Normal radiologic studies can help rule out stroke.
- Tick paralysis can be excluded by careful physical examination demonstrating the absence of an attached *Dermacentor* tick.
- Patients with polio are febrile and usually have asymmetric neurologic deficits.
- Magnesium intoxication can be ruled out by the absence of high serum magnesium levels.

MANAGEMENT

TOXIN NEUTRALIZATION

- Trivalent equine antitoxin (obtained from state health departments or the CDC) neutralizes only toxin molecules yet unbound to nerve endings, making early administration critical to the prevention of progression.
- Before administration of antitoxin, skin testing should be performed to test for sensitivity to serum or antitoxin.

RESPIRATORY SUPPORT

- Significant respiratory compromise can exist in the absence of symptoms. Objective measurements are needed to identify patients in need of mechanical support.
- Hypercapnia is a late finding signaling impending and rapid respiratory collapse. Most patients show signs of respiratory insufficiency requiring ventilatory support before developing hypercapnia.
- Proper assessment of oropharyngeal function for airway obstruction is critical. Loss of glossal and pharyngeal tone as well or gag impairment necessitates mechanical ventilation.
- Maximal inspiratory and maximal expiratory pressures (MEP) are the most sensitive indicators of respiratory insufficiency in neuromuscular weakness. Effective cough cannot be accomplished if the MEP is $<40\ cmH_2O$.
- Normal vital capacity (VC) in adults is usually 50 mL/kg. Patients with serial measurements demonstrating a decline in the VC by 15–20 mL/kg will need ventilatory support. Patients with a VC at or below 12 mL/kg should be immediately intubated. Noninvasive ventilation is rarely appropriate given the oropharyngeal dysfunction and expected duration of respiratory muscle weakness.
- Patients with botulism usually require extended periods of mechanical ventilation usually from 2–8 weeks. Tracheostomy should be considered early on in the patient's course to reduce the complications of long-term mechanical ventilation.

SOURCE ELIMINATION

- Unless an ileus is present, purgatives may be used in patients when there is a concern for contaminated food in the gastrointestinal tract.
- Patients with wound botulism should undergo aggressive wound debridement.

- Antibiotics against *C. botulinum* such as penicillin G (3 million units IV q4) or metronidazole (500 mg IV q8) are frequently used but are unproven in clinical trials.

BIBLIOGRAPHY

Sobel J, Tucker N, Sulka A, et al. Foodborne botulism in the United States, 1990-2000. *Emerg Infect Dis* 2004;10:1606–1611.

2001 CSTE Botulism Surveillance Summary. Centers for Disease Control and Prevention. Available at: http://www.cdc.gov/ncidod/dbmd/diseaseinfo/files/Botulism_CSTE_2001.pdf. Accessed August 28, 2005.

2002 CSTE Botulism Surveillance Summary. Centers for Disease Control and Prevention. Available at: http://www.cdc.gov/ncidod/dbmd/diseaseinfo/files/Botulism_CSTE_2002.pdf. Accessed August 28, 2005.

2003 CSTE Botulism Surveillance Summary. Centers for Disease Control and Prevention. Available at: http://www.cdc.gov/ncidod/dbmd/diseaseinfo/files/Botulism_CSTE_2003.pdf. Accessed August 28, 2005.

Bleck TP. *Clostridium botulinum* (Botulism). In: Mandell GL, Bennett JE, Dolan R, eds., *Principles and Practice of Infectious Diseases,* 5th ed. Philadelphia, PA: Churchill Livingstone; 2000:2543–2547.

Passaro DJ, Benson Werner S, McGee J. Wound botulism associated with black tar heroin among injection drug users. *JAMA* 1998;279:859–863.

Kudrow DB, Henry DA, Haake DA, et al. Botulism associated with *Clostridium botulinum* sinusitis after intranasal cocaine abuse. *Ann Intern Med* 1988;109:984–985.

Arnon SA, Schechter R, Inglesby TV. Botulinum toxin as a biological weapon: medical and public health management. *JAMA* 2001;285:1059–1070.

Hashimoto H, Clyde VJ, Parko KL. Botulism from peyote. *N Engl J Med* 1998;339:203–204.

Centers for Disease Control and Prevention: Botulism in the United States, 1899-1996. *Handbook for Epidemiologists, Clinicians, and Laboratory Workers.* Atlanta, GA: Centers for Disease Control and Prevention; 1998.

Dowell VR, McCroskey LM, Hatheway CL, et al. Coproexamination for botulinal toxin and *Clostridium botulinum.* A new procedure for laboratory diagnosis of botulism. *JAMA* 1977;238:1829–1832.

Cherington M. Electrophysiologic methods as an aid in diagnosis of botulism. A review. *Muscle Nerve* 1982;6:528–529.

Edell TA, Sullivan CP, Osborn KM, et al. Wound botulism associated with a positive Tensilon test. *West J Med* 1983;139: 218–219.

Section 5
NEUROLOGIC DISORDERS

69 CEREBROVASCULAR ACCIDENT

Nina M. Patel

KEY POINTS

- Initial history, physical examination, and noncontrast head CT are crucial elements in the diagnosis and classification of stroke.
- Diverse illnesses (e.g., hypoglycemia, intracerebral tumor, seizure, metabolic encephalopathy, and meningitis) can masquerade as stroke.
- Maintenance of adequate CPP is crucial in the management of all stroke subtypes. This often requires greater than baseline systemic blood pressure.
- t-PA should be administered to select patients who present within 3 hours of onset of ischemic CVA.
- Vigilance in providing supportive medical care to avert worsening neurologic injury and compromised cerebral perfusion is essential to management.
- Early neurosurgical consultation and evaluation is an essential component to management of SAH and ICH.

EPIDEMIOLOGY

- Cerebrovascular accident (CVA) or stroke is a leading cause of death and occurs in 200/100,000 persons/year.
- It occurs at equal rates in men and women, and the mean age of onset is 72.

PATHOPHYSIOLOGY

- Cerebrovascular accidents are caused by a decrease in cerebral perfusion and can be classified by cause into three major categories: (1) ischemia or infarction, (2) intracranial hemorrhage (ICH), and (3) subarachnoid hemorrhage (SAH). Ischemic strokes are due to atherothrombotic disease, embolic disease, or systemic hypoperfusion.
- The incidence of CVA by etiology is shown below. Ischemic etiologies account for roughly 80% of all CVAs, while hemorrhagic etiologies lead to 20%.
    - Atherothrombotic: 40–50%
    - Embolic: 30%
    - ICH: 12%
    - SAH: 8%
- Atheromatous plaques in the large vessels (e.g., ascending aorta and aortic arch) lead to 65–70% of ischemic CVAs. Embolic CVAs arise in the setting of atrial fibrillation, endocarditis (infective or noninfective), and left ventricular mural thrombus. Thrombophilic states can lead to cerebral venous thrombosis or paradoxical embolus in the setting of deep venous thrombosis with a patent foramen ovale.
- ICH occurs in patients with chronic hypertension (basal ganglia and cerebellar hemorrhage), amyloid angiopathy, coagulopathy, trauma, intracranial aneurysm, or arteriovenous malformation (AVM).
- SAH is most frequently due to the rupture of a saccular berry aneurysm or an AVM, though cocaine abuse, trauma, and pituitary apoplexy can also lead to SAH.

CLINICAL PRESENTATION

ATHEROTHROMBOTIC CEREBROVASCULAR ACCIDENT

- 10–20% of patients with atherothrombotic CVA experience a transient ischemic attack (TIA) prior to CVA.
- The majority of patients, however, do not have preceding symptoms and present with the sudden onset of a focal neurologic deficit (e.g., hemiparesis, aphasia, agnosia, and neglect). If multiple, small infarcts occur, patients may develop a global impairment, with decreased level of consciousness, as opposed to a

focal deficit. If embolic in nature, the maximal extent of neurologic deficit usually occurs at initial onset.

INTRACRANIAL HEMORRHAGE

- Intracranial hemorrhage presents as focal neurologic impairment.
- If these patients develop increased intracranial pressure (ICP), decreased mental status, vomiting, and headache may be seen.

SUBARACHNOID HEMORRHAGE

- Patients with SAH will often state that they are having "the worst headache of my life." Decreased level of consciousness and lethargy also occur frequently in the setting of severe SAH.

DIFFERENTIAL DIAGNOSIS

- Hypoglycemia, intracerebral tumor, seizures, Bell palsy, metabolic encephalopathy, meningitis, subdural hematoma, and brain abscess are other diagnostic considerations in the evaluation of a patient with focal or diffuse neurologic injury.
- History and physical examination are essential in determining the nature and distribution of the insult and time of onset.
- A complete blood count (CBC) with differential, chemistry panel, and coagulation studies are useful to evaluate for infection, metabolic encephalopathy, or coagulopathy. If the history is suggestive, urine toxicology or thrombophilia workup should also be sent.
- If ischemic CVA is a possibility, ECG should be performed to assess for atrial fibrillation, ischemia, or infarction. Echocardiography should be performed to evaluate for valvular lesions, left ventricular dysfunction, ventricular mural thrombus, atherosclerotic lesions in the aortic arch, and patent foramen ovale if the clinical history and examination are suggestive.
- Noncontrast brain computed tomography (CT) is the imaging study of choice for suspected stroke. It is a rapid and sensitive means to evaluate for ICH. If the study is negative for ICH, ischemic CVA is most likely.
- Carotid Doppler and transcranial Doppler ultrasound evaluations of extra- and intracranial vasculature are not helpful in acute management of a CVA.
- MRI is more sensitive than noncontrast CT in detecting cerebral infarction within the first 24–48 hours after onset; however, it does not improve ability to diagnose acute SAH.
- Lumbar puncture demonstrating CSF fluid with xanthochromia is highly supportive of a diagnosis of SAH. Increased ICP must be ruled out by history, examination, or CT prior to a lumbar puncture.
- Cerebral arteriography is valuable in identifying the presence and location of an aneurysm in patients with SAH.

TREATMENT AND PROGNOSIS

- Immediate goals of therapy in all patients with a CVA are to stabilize airway, breathing, and circulation. Mechanical ventilation may be necessary in patients with impaired consciousness or Glasgow Coma Scale scores <8. Supplemental oxygen should be administered if hypoxemia is present. Maintenance of an adequate mean arterial pressure (MAP) is crucial to sustaining CPP and minimizing secondary brain injury. If volume resuscitation is necessary to maintain blood pressure, normal saline or other isotonic fluid should be utilized. Hypo-osmotic fluid may exacerbate cerebral edema.
- Hyperglycemia is often observed in the setting of CVA and may contribute to neurologic injury or impaired recovery. Insulin therapy should be titrated to achieve tight glycemic control.
- Fever may exacerbate neurologic injury and should be managed aggressively.
- Thromboembolic prophylaxis with intermittent compression devices and early mobilization (as feasible) is imperative. Subcutaneous heparin may be used in patients with ischemic CVA.

ATHEROTHROMBOTIC/EMBOLIC DISEASE

- Patients with ischemic CVA often develop systemic hypertension. Lowering of systemic blood pressure in the setting of acute CVA may compromise cerebral perfusion. As such, hypertension is tolerated, unless there is evidence of resultant organ damage (e.g., congestive heart failure). In these situations, blood pressure is lowered cautiously with vigilant monitoring of neurologic status for signs of deterioration.
- The NINDS (National Institute of Neurological Disorders and Stroke) study established a role for thrombolytic therapy with alteplase (t-PA) in patients with acute ischemic CVA who present within 3 hours of onset of symptoms. CT to rule out ICH must be performed in all patients prior to administration of t-PA. t-PA was given at a dose of 0.9 mg/kg (10% in a bolus

over 1 minute, followed by a 1 hour infusion). Blood pressure was maintained at ≤185/110 and all other anticoagulant or antiplatelet therapy was held for 24 hours. t-PA improved neurologic recovery at 3 months, though it did not impact the mortality rate from ischemic CVA. t-PA increased the incidence of ICH. The inclusion and exclusion criteria for t-PA are extensive and should be reviewed closely prior to administering this therapy.

- Initiation of aspirin therapy (160–300 mg/day) within 48 hours of onset of ischemic CVA reduces the in-hospital risk of recurrent CVA and death.
- Anticoagulation with heparin in atherothrombotic CVA has not been shown to improve outcomes. Anticoagulation is indicated in the setting of acute myocardial infarction, ventricular mural thrombus, rheumatic heart disease, and cerebral venous thrombosis.
- The short-term mortality rate is 10–15% in patients with ischemic CVA due to the development of cerebral edema. Hypothermia or decompressive hemicraniectomy may be attempted to alleviate persistent cerebral edema, though neither of these techniques has proven efficacy. Twenty percent of patients require long-term care and 33–50% are left with major neurologic deficit.

INTRACEREBRAL HEMORRHAGE

- General supportive care measures as delineated above apply to patients with ICH.
- Blood pressure management in patients with ICH is a difficult issue. Up to one-third of patients will have recurrent bleeding within 24 hours. This phenomenon, however, has not been clearly associated with elevated blood pressure. As such, the goals of blood pressure management are first and foremost, to maintain adequate CPP.
- Increased ICP presents significant difficulty. This problem does not respond appreciably to corticosteroid therapy or ventriculostomy. Mannitol and hyperventilation are used acutely to lower ICP. Decompressive surgical evacuation of hematoma can be considered if conservative management fails.
- The mortality rate associated with ICH is 30–40%. Twenty percent of survivors require long-term care.

SUBARACHNOID HEMORRHAGE

- The goals of management of SAH are centered around the prevention of known life-threatening secondary complications: rebleeding, hydrocephalus, and vasospasm.
- After initial stabilization, patients are examined and graded using the Hunt-Hess scale, the Fisher grade, or other neurologic grading systems. These scales predict the risk of death and vasospasm based on the size of the lesion and the patient's neurologic status.
- Seizure and thromboembolic prophylaxis are standard therapy in the management of SAH. Corticosteroids are also used routinely, though it is unclear if they confer any benefit.
- Management of blood pressure control in SAH presents a quandary. Avoidance of significant hypertension is desired to decrease the risk of rebleeding. However, decreasing systemic pressure lowers MAP and hence, CPP. Labetalol, hydralazine, and enalapril are short-acting agents that do not increase ICP and therefore, are frequently used for blood pressure management in the setting of increased ICP. Invasive monitoring to accurately titrate therapy is recommended for the management of these patients.
- Rebleeding commonly occurs within 24 hours of initial onset. Twenty percent of patients will rebleed within 1 week. Hypertension, coughing, and Valsalva maneuvers are actively avoided to decrease the risk of increasing ICP and subsequent rebleed.
- Early surgical clipping of aneurysms is increasingly performed in patients with a Hunt-Hess score of 1–3. Timing of surgery in patients with scores of 4 and 5 is not well established.
- Ventriculostomy is performed in patients with decreased level of consciousness and evidence of acute hydrocephalus on CT scan.
- Vasospasm is a known complication of SAH that manifests as a global decline in neurologic status or a focal neurologic deficit and occurs with greatest frequency at days 5–10. Nimodipine (60 mg q 4 h × 21 days) decreases the incidence of ischemia, perhaps by affecting vasospasm. If vasospasm does occur, initial therapy consists of aggressive fluid resuscitation with a goal MAP >15–20% above the initial MAP. If there is no resolution of neurologic impairment, MAP is gradually increased with the continued use of intravenous fluids as well as vasoactive agents.
- Cardiopulmonary complications of SAH are frequent and include arrhythmias, ventricular dysfunction, neurogenic pulmonary edema, aspiration pneumonia, and pulmonary embolism.
- Cerebral salt wasting occurs in 30–50% of patients with SAH and should be treated with free water restriction.
- The prognosis for patients with SAH is grim. The mortality rate within the first 24 hours is 25% and at 1 year is 50–60%. More than one-half of survivors suffer residual neurologic deficit.

BIBLIOGRAPHY

Aiyagari V, Powers WJ, Diringer MN. Cerebrovascular Disease, In: Hall JB, Schmidt GA, Wood LDH—*Principles of Critical Care,* 3rd ed., McGraw-Hill, New York, 2005;63:985–998.

Chen SM, Sandercock P, Pan HC, et al. Indications for early aspirin use in acute ischemic stroke. *Stroke* 2000;31: 1240–1249.

de Gans K, Nieuwkamp DJ, Rinkel GJ, et al. Timing of aneurysm surgery in subarachnoid hemorrhage: a systematic review of the literature. *Neurosurgery* 2002;50:336–340.

Klijn CJM, Hankey GJ. Management of acute ischaemic stroke: new guidelines from the American Stroke Association and European Stroke Initiative. *Lancet Neurol* 2003;2:698–701.

Rinkel GJ, Feigin VL, Algra A, et al. *The Cochrane Library.* Issue 2. Oxford: Update Software; 2003.

The National Institute of Neurological Disorders and Stroke rt-PA Stroke Study Group. *N Engl J Med* 1995;333:1581–1587.

70 CNS HEMORRHAGE

Steven Q. Davis, Alex Ulitsky

KEY POINTS

- Intracranial hemorrhage is marked by high mortality and long-term neurologic morbidity.
- ICH is most often due to hypertension, but some patients have AVMs, amyloid angiopathy, or cocaine abuse.
- Supportive management includes assessment of the need for intubation; correction of hypovolemia; maintenance of modest hypertension (MAP 100–120 mmHg); reversal of coagulopathy; prevention of thromboembolism; and prompt recognition and treatment of complications.
- SAH may be complicated by rebleeding; hydrocephalus; vasospasm; or hyponatremia.
- The radiologist and neurosurgeon play key roles in diagnosis, monitoring, and management of these patients.

INTRODUCTION

- Bleeding in the central nervous system (CNS) is often a devastating neurologic event with high morbidity and mortality. Blood can extravasate anywhere within the cranial vault and spinal cord, and hemorrhages are thus classified by their location within the CNS and the vascular pathology underlying them. This chapter will focus on intracerebral (ICH) and subarachnoid (SAH) types of bleeding commonly encountered in neuro- and medical ICUs.

INTRACEREBRAL HEMORRHAGE

- Intracerebral hemorrhage is one of the most common types of CNS bleeding, accounting for 10% of all strokes and associated with a 30–40% 30-day mortality. It is defined as bleeding directly into the brain parenchyma, usually due to rupture of a penetrating vessel. This event occurs most commonly in middle aged (average age 61) people with long-standing hypertension, although other underlying processes, such as arteriovenous malformations (AVMs) and cocaine use in younger patients and amyloid angiopathy in the elderly, are often responsible. The incidence is markedly increased in African Americans, Hispanics, and Japanese, and there is a slight male predominance.
- ICH is subclassified into spontaneous, due to trauma or surgery, primary (unrelated to congenital or acquired conditions), and secondary (related to congenital or acquired conditions such as anticoagulation, neoplasia, or conversion of a thrombotic CVA; Table 70-1).

PATHOPHYSIOLOGY

- The precise mechanism of vessel rupture is unknown, but is likely related to increased vessel fragility and segmental constriction associated with long-standing hypertension. Other processes may be responsible in non-hypertension-related bleeds.

TABLE 70-1 Causes of Intracranial Hemorrhage

PRIMARY*	SECONDARY
Hypertension	Vascular malformations
Cerebral amyloid angiopathy	Arteriovenous malformations
Anticoagulant/fibrinolytic use	Dural arteriovenous fistulas
Antiplatelet use	Cavernous malformations
Drug use	Aneurysms
Amphetamines	Saccular
Cocaine	Mycotic
Phenylpropanolamine	Fusiform
Other illicit drugs	Tumors
Other bleeding diathesis	Primary brain tumors
	Secondary metastasis
	Hemorrhagic transformation of a cerebral infraction
	Venous infarction with hemorrhage secondary to cerebral venous thrombosis
	Moyamoya disease

*Primary hemorrhage unrelated to underlying congenital or acquired brain lesions or abnormalities. See text for details.

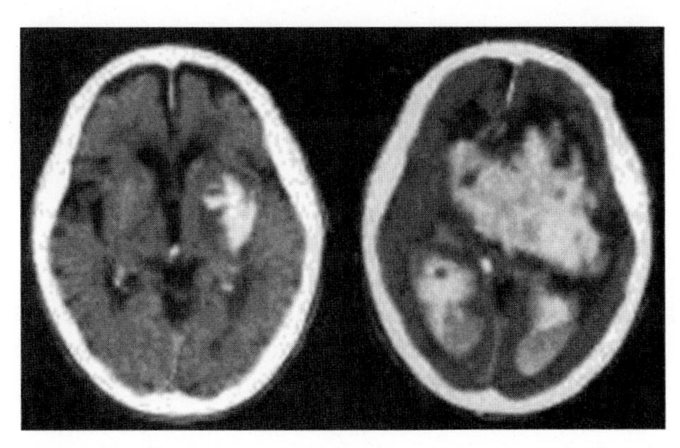

FIG. 70-1 Hematoma expansion in ICH after 3 hours.

- Most of the neurologic damage is thought to be due to edema that develops 3–7 days after the initial event, as well as hematoma expansion, which mostly occurs in the first 24 hours (Fig. 70-1).
- The size of the hematoma also appears to be the best predictor of outcome, with patients whose hematoma volume is >60 cm^3 having a 30-day mortality of over 90%.

Clinical Presentation

- Most common sites of hypertensive ICH are the basal ganglia, deep cerebellum, and pons. Since the internal capsule lies adjacent to the basal ganglia, it is invariably damaged, and thus contralateral hemiparesis is often the sentinel focal neurologic sign (Fig. 70-2).
- Numerous other possible manifestations may occur, depending on the site of damage and ranging from nausea, vomiting, and ataxia with cerebellar bleeds to deep coma and death with pontine hemorrhage.

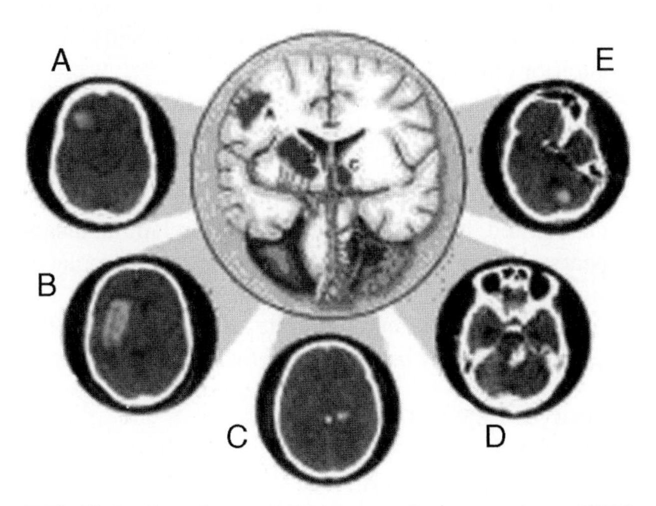

FIG. 70-2 Location and CT images of common sites of ICH with hypertension.

- Interestingly, patients are almost always awake during the event, and maybe under emotional or physical stress before the bleed happens.

Diagnosis

- After a thorough history and physical examination have been performed, noncontrast computed tomography (CT) is the study of choice in diagnosing cerebral hemorrhage. Location of the blood may also provide a clue as to the etiology. For example, bleeding into the basal ganglia, pons, or cerebellum in a patient with a history of hypertension usually results from a rupture of deep perforating arteries, whereas single or multiple hemorrhages extending to the cortical surface in an elderly person point to amyloid angiopathy as the culprit.
- MRI and angiography may be useful if the cause of hemorrhage is uncertain or a structural abnormality such as an AVM or a tumor is suspected.
- Lumbar puncture (LP) should be avoided in these patients since they often have increased intracranial pressure (ICP) and are at risk for herniation.
- A complete laboratory evaluation, particularly looking for coagulopathy, infection, and electrolyte disturbances should also be performed on every patient.

Treatment: Medical

- The initial evaluation should include global assessment of neurologic function, such as the Glasgow Coma Scale (GCS). Patients with a GCS score of <8 are at risk for airway compromise and should be electively intubated. Intubation should be performed by well-trained personnel and induction agents such as etomidate or propofol, known not to increase ICP, should be used for induction. Once mechanical ventilation is established, rate and tidal volume should be set to keep $PaCO_2$ between 30 and 35 mmHg (Table 70-2, Fig. 70-3).
- Intravenous (IV) fluids should be initiated in order to achieve euvolemia and maintain adequate intravascular volume to optimize cerebral perfusion. Hypervolemia, which can worsen cerebral edema, should be avoided.
- Any underlying coagulopathy driving the hemorrhage should be corrected as quickly as possible. This is best done with fresh frozen plasma and parenteral vitamin K (in warfarin or liver failure-associated bleeds) or protamine sulfate for heparin-induced bleeding. Activated factor VII (NovoSeven) presents an attractive alternative because of rapid onset of action and small fluid volume that needs to be delivered, but is currently limited by lack of availability and price.
- Seizure activity is frequent in intracerebral bleeding, at the time of the event or shortly after, and can increase ICP and cause further neuronal damage. Patients need to be carefully monitored for signs of seizure and

TABLE 70-2 Acute Management of ICH

TYPE	TREATMENT
Airway	Intubation and mechanical ventilation if patient has aspiration, neurogenic pulmonary edema. GCS motor score of withdrawal, or worse
Fluid	2–3 L of 0.9% NaCl per 24 h
	Fludrocortisone acetate, 0.3 mg/day if patient has hyponatremia
Blood	Accept MAP of ≤130 mmHg. If MAP is >130 mmHg, esmolol bolus, 500 μg/kg in 1 min; or labetalol, 20 mg IV in 2 min; or enalaprilat, 0.625 mg IV in 5 min
Nutrition	Enteric nutrition with continuous infusion on day 2
Additional measures	Nimodipine, 60 mg 6 times a day for 21 days
	Stool softener
	Pneumatic compression devices
	Acetaminophen with codeine or morphine, 1–2 mg, or tramadol (if no seizures), 50–100 mg, orally every 4 h for pain management
	Phenytoin, 20 mg/kg if seizures have occurred

SOURCE: Adapted from Wijdicks EF, Kallmes DF, Manno EM, et al. Subarachnoid hemorrhage: neurointensive care and aneurysm repair. *Mayo Clin Proc* 2005;80:550–559.

seizures should be controlled immediately with IV lorazepam, followed by IV phenytoin, although anticonvulsive prophylaxis is not generally recommended.
- Blood pressure management in ICH is controversial. Hypertension, sometimes severe, is common after a parenchymal bleed, but is often self-limited. The mean arterial pressure (MAP) should be kept between 100 and 120 mmHg, to maintain brain perfusion without increasing the edema surrounding the hematoma. Agents such as beta-blockers, calcium channel blockers, and angiotensin-converting enzyme (ACE) inhibitors are generally considered safe, since they do not increase ICP, while nitrates and sodium nitroprusside are generally avoided since they can suddenly increase ICP.
- ICP monitoring and management are important in taking care of ICH patients. Monitoring is accomplished by using ICP bolts or ventriculostomies. The advantage of the latter is in that they can be used to draw off cerebrospinal fluid (CSF) and decrease ICP rapidly. Several other methods for controlling ICP exist. Hyperventilation can rapidly lower ICP by inducing vasoconstriction, but its effects are short-lived, and thus it is used only to establish early and quick control of ICP. Mannitol, a hexose sugar, is commonly used to treat increased ICP. It is believed to draw interstitial fluid into the vasculature and thus decrease brain volume. It is usually administered as IV boluses whenever ICP becomes elevated—continuous infusion is generally avoided because of fear of actually increasing brain edema through leakage of mannitol into the hematoma.
- Finally, prevention and treatment of medical complications, such as gastric ulcers and infection, is essential. Fever in particular should be aggressively evaluated and treated, since hyperthermia is deleterious to neuronal function.

TREATMENT: SURGICAL

- The role of surgery in ICH is uncertain, due to lack of large randomized-controlled studies and negative results in studies that have been performed. Despite this fact, surgery is often performed, particularly in patients with large hematomas and rapid neurologic deterioration. It is generally accepted that urgent surgical removal of a hematoma is indicated for infratentorial lesions >3 cm or smaller lesions that are causing brain stem compression. However, most of the available evidence (including a recently completed STICH [Surgical Treatment of Ischemic Heart Failure] trial) tends to show that surgery is likely of little or no benefit in most ICH patients.

SUBARACHNOID HEMORRHAGE

- Spontaneous SAH is defined as bleeding into the subarachnoid space, usually due to a ruptured intracranial aneurysm, although it can also occur with a rupture of an AVM or be secondary to trauma. Its incidence is about 25,000–30,000 cases/year and the event carries a 50% 30-day mortality, with many survivors left with devastating neurologic deficits and disability.

PATHOPHYSIOLOGY

- 3–4% of the American population carries aneurysms, for a prevalence of 8–10 million people.
- Aneurysms are most commonly located at the bifurcation of arteries in the circle of Willis, usually in the anterior circulation.
- Most ruptured aneurysms are >7 mm in diameter, although it is still difficult to predict which asymptomatic aneurysms will rupture.
- As the aneurysm forms and grows, a neck and a dome are created. In the neck, internal elastic lamina disappears, media thins, and connective tissue replaces smooth muscle cells, thinning the arterial wall. The dome is the most common site of rupture, with the actual tear usually being no more than 0.5 mm in length.

CLINICAL PRESENTATION

- The classic presentation of SAH is the abrupt onset of excruciating headache, often described by patients as the worst headache of their lives. In about 50% of

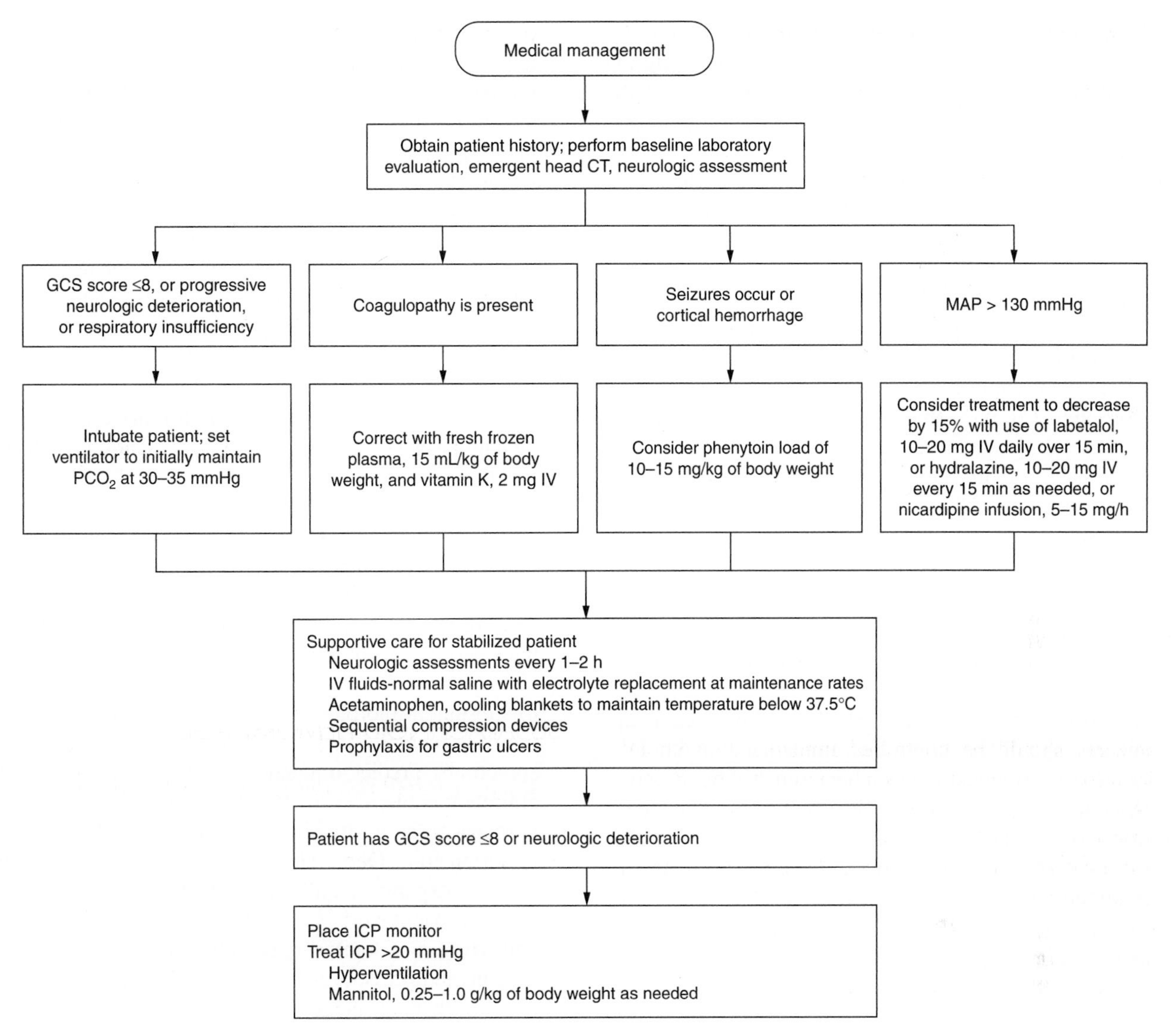

FIG. 70-3 Medical management of ICH.

patients, sudden and transient loss of consciousness follows the headache. The pain is generalized and vomiting is common.

- Although less frequent than with ICH, focal neurologic signs can occur with SAH. They range from 3rd and 6th nerve palsies (most common) to hemiparesis, nuchal rigidity, and aphasia. The cranial nerve palsies, when seen before the rupture, may cause prodromal symptoms of an enlarging aneurysm and should alert the clinician to that possibility.
- Occasionally, small leaks of blood escape from an aneurysm, causing sudden headache that is transient. These so-called sentinel bleeds often signal imminent rupture and should be immediately diagnosed and addressed.

Complications of SAH

- There are four major complications that occur in patients after SAH and which cause the majority of morbidity and mortality in those who survive the initial event. Their management will be further discussed in the Treatment section of this chapter.
  - *Rerupture*: The incidence of rerupture of an untreated aneurysm is about 30%, mostly occurring in the first 48 hours after the initial event and having a 60% mortality.
  - *Hydrocephalus*: This can occur suddenly and usually presents as stupor or coma. Alternatively, hydrocephalus can develop over several days and present as progressive drowsiness, incontinence, and slowed mentation.

- *Vasospasm*: This narrowing of the arteries at the base of the brain is a common occurrence, peaking at 7 days after initial bleed and causing infarction, with its adherent morbidity and mortality. This entity presents with sudden focal neurologic signs that vary depending on the artery involved and can usually be diagnosed with transcranial Doppler ultrasound (TCD). In general, increasing amount of blood surrounding an artery is predictive of an increasing probability of vasospasm.
- *Hyponatremia*: This can be severe and is the result of inappropriate antidiuretic hormone (ADH) secretion, developing in the first 2 weeks after the hemorrhage. The phenomenon, also known as "cerebral salt-wasting syndrome" usually clears in 1–2 weeks and occasionally requires water restriction.

DIAGNOSIS

- The hallmark of diagnosing SAH is the noncontrast CT scan, which can detect blood in CSF in 95% of cases within 72 hours of the event (Fig. 70-4).
- If CT is nondiagnostic and no mass lesions or hydrocephalus is present, an LP should be performed. The diagnostic finding in the CSF is xanthochromia, or yellow tinge of the fluid which appears within 6 hours of the hemorrhage and has a 99% sensitivity.
- Once the diagnosis of SAH is established, a conventional or CT/MR angiography is usually performed to localize the aneurysm and help in planning treatment.

TREATMENT: MEDICAL

- Medical management centers on optimizing the patient's status and minimizing neuronal damage prior to surgical intervention. In general, patients with a SAH and a GCS < 8 should be intubated for airway protection, with ventilator settings that produce mild hyperventilation ($PaCO_2$ 30–35 mmHg).
- Rebleeding is most common in the first 24 hours after the initial hemorrhage. Prevention measures include avoidance of straining, excessive stimulation, and hypertension, and thus patients should be kept in a quiet, darkened room.
- Precise blood pressure and intravascular volume control are important in maintaining brain perfusion and preventing rebleeding and vasospasm. The target MAP is between 100 and 120 mmHg, with euvolemia or slight hypervolemia preferable. Hypertension often occurs with SAH, precipitated by headache, increased ICP, and an increased catecholamine drive and must be aggressively managed with IV medications to keep MAP at goal.
- Patients must be carefully monitored for signs of hydrocephalus such as stupor or sudden change in mentation, which in the presence of enlarged ventricles on CT are an indication for urgent ventriculostomy and CSF drainage. Nonresolving hydrocephalus necessitates permanent shunting.
- Vasospasm is a major complication of SAH and leads to substantial morbidity and mortality. Daily monitoring of intracranial vessels with Doppler ultrasound can sometimes predict impending vasospasm, but is not entirely reliable. The key to prevention and treatment of vasospasm is to maintain slight hypervolemia and hypertension. Once vasospasm occurs, aggressive volume expansion and inducement of hypertension (with vasoactive drugs) should be started and invasive hemodynamic monitoring is recommended to optimize volume and pressure management. Oral nimodipine, a calcium channel antagonist, has been shown to improve neurologic outcomes after vasospasm, but can also cause hypotension. In refractory cases, balloon angioplasty of narrowed vessels may be considered, which can produce good results in experienced hands. Once begun, treatments for vasospasm should be continued for several days, and then weaned gradually while closely monitoring the patient. Vasoactive drugs should be weaned first, and then the aggressive fluid therapy may be gradually withdrawn.
- Anticonvulsants such as phenytoin decrease the frequency of seizures in the perioperative period and are often used prophylactically.
- Up to half of patients with SAH develop cerebral salt wasting, with resulting hyponatremia that can be severe. Free water should be restricted while assuring that the patient does not become hypovolemic. Occasionally, hypertonic saline is used to treat severe hyponatremia.
- Deep vein thrombosis (DVT) prophylaxis should be maintained in all patients with pneumatic compression

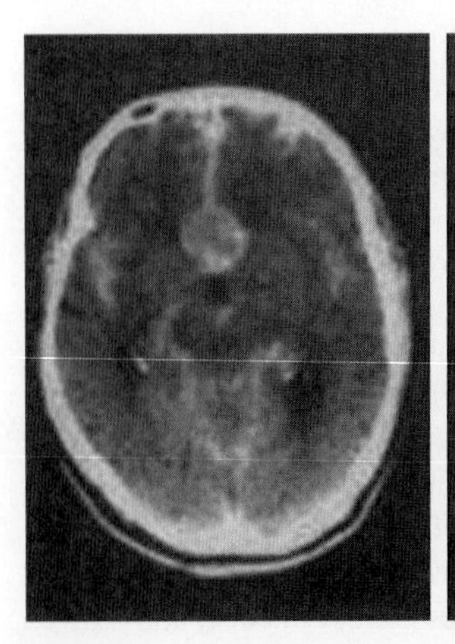
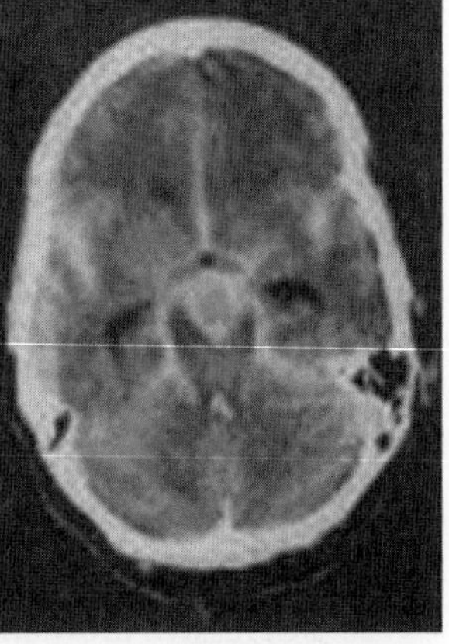

FIG. 70-4 SAH with visible giant aneurysms in anterior cerebral artery (ACA; left) and middle cerebral artery (MCA; right).

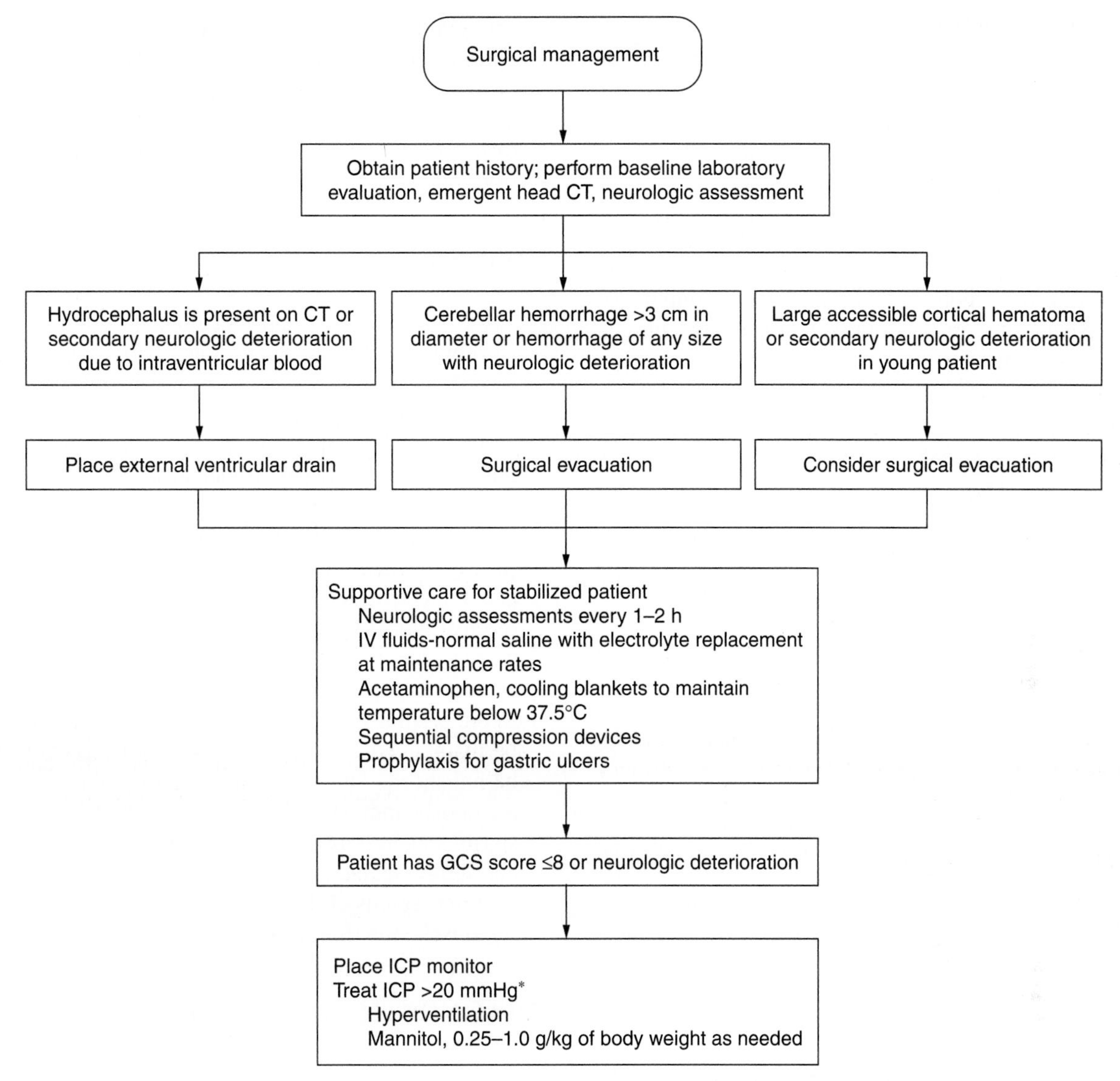

FIG. 70-5 SAH management.

devices throughout the hospitalization, and laxatives and stool softeners should be administered to prevent constipation and straining.

Treatment: Surgical

- After initial medical optimization and delineation of cerebral vascular anatomy, definitive surgical treatment of the aneurysm should be undertaken as soon as possible. Currently, two options for treatment exist—endovascular coiling or surgical clipping. The choice of technique depends on many factors, such as the location of the aneurysm, the size of the dome relative to that of the neck, clinical status of the patient, and the center's experience with the procedure. Data comparing the two approaches are scant and contradictory, therefore, necessitating patient-by-patient decision making (Fig. 70-5).

PREDICTORS OF OUTCOME

- The most important clinical factor predicting outcome is the presenting level of consciousness, graded on a World Federation of Neurosurgical Societies (WFNS) grading scale, with grades IV or V (out of five) predicting a >90% mortality, although with aggressive care up to 50% of grade IV and 20% of grade V patients can survive with favorable outcomes (Table 70-3).
- The size of the aneurysm and comorbid conditions do not seem to influence the outcomes very much,

TABLE 70-3 WFNS Grading System

WFNS GRADE	GCS SCORE	MOTOR DEFICIT
I	15	Absent
II	14–13	Absent
III	14–13	Present
IV	12–7	Present or absent
V	6–3	Present or absent

while factors such as the age, development of vasospasm, and intracerebral extension do play a significant role.

BIBLIOGRAPHY

Aiyagari V, Powers WJ, Diringer MN. Cerebrovascular disease. In: Hall JB, Schmidt GA, Wood LDH, eds., *Principles of Critical Care*, 3rd ed. New York, NY: McGraw-Hill; 2005: 985–996.

Manno EM, Atkinson JL, Fulgham JR, et al. Emerging medical and surgical management strategies in the evaluation and treatment of intracerebral hemorrhage. *Mayo Clin Proc* 2005;80:420–433.

Smith WS, Hauser SL, Easton JD. Cerebrovascular diseases. In: *Harrison's Principles of Internal Medicine*, New York, NY: McGraw-Hill, 15th ed.

Wijdicks EF, Kallmes DF, Manno EM, et al. Subarachnoid hemorrhage: neurointensive care and aneurysm repair. *Mayo Clin Proc* 2005;80:550–559.

Qureshi, Tuhrim, Broderick, et al. Medical Progress: Spontaneous intracerebral hemorrhage. *N Engl J Med* 2001;344:1450–1460.

71 ANOXIC ENCEPHALOPATHY

Maria Dowell

KEY POINTS

- Anoxic encephalopathy is the most common cause of coma in most critical care units.
- Cardiac arrest is the most common cause of global brain ischemia. Amongst early postarrest survivors, roughly 30% leave the hospital but 90% are unable to resume their former full activities due to persistent neurologic deficits.
- Other potential causes of brain ischemia or anoxia include severe hypotension, cardiac failure, strangulation, cardiopulmonary bypass, status epilepticus, diffuse cerebral atherosclerosis, increased intracranial pressure (ICP), cerebral artery spasm, closed head trauma, fat embolism, multivascular in situ clotting (disseminated intravascular coagulation [DIC]), vasculitides affecting the cerebral vessels, and hyperviscosity states.
- The degree of neuronal injury depends on the degree of mismatch between metabolic demand and delivery of oxygen and glucose to the brain.

PATHOPHYSIOLOGY

- Cerebral blood flow and metabolism during and after cardiopulmonary resuscitation (CPR) is complex. Twenty seconds after cessation of cerebral blood flow, neuronal oxygen stores are depleted and unconsciousness results. Within 5 minutes of cerebral anoxia, brain glucose and adenosine triphosphate (ATP) stores are depleted. Biochemical changes that may be involved include increased intracellular calcium, release of neurotoxic excitatory amino acids, superoxide production, and brain lactic acidosis. After cerebral anoxia, transient reactive global hyperemia resulting from vasoparalysis persists for 15–30 minutes. Thereafter, postischemic cerebral hypoperfusion is present for 2–12 hours.
- There is some evidence that if cerebral blood flow can be maintained during hyperemia, brain recovery may be enhanced. The mechanisms responsible for injury are poorly understood but may relate to diffuse arterial spasm, calcium influx, vasoconstrictor prostaglandins, and intravascular coagulation.
- Distinct regions of the brain exhibit special vulnerability to ischemia (hippocampus, neocortex, cerebellum).

DIAGNOSTIC APPROACH TO ANOXIC COMA

- *Level of consciousness*: This should initially be assessed by verbal stimulation, then if no response, a shout and gentle shake. Noxious stimuli can be applied by digital supraorbital pressure. Painful stimuli should be avoided.
- *Motor response*: The finding of flaccidity and areflexia indicate severe brainstem depression. Extensor posturing responses correlate with deep lesions of the midbrain and upper pons. Flexor posturing responses occur after damage to the hemispheres. Withdrawal and localizing responses imply voluntary behavior and obeying commands marks the return of consciousness.
- *Neurophthalmologic function*: This is assessed by pupillary size and response to light, spontaneous eye movements, oculocephalic and oculovestibular responses. Papilledema is not a reliable indicator of ICP in the post-cardiac arrest period. Absence of elicited eye movements is a grave sign. Spontaneous, roving, horizontal eye movements indicate only that midbrain and pontine

areas are intact but do not imply an intact frontal or occipital cerebral cortex.

- *Diagnostic imaging*: Imaging by computed tomography (CT) scan often fails to show abnormalities in early stages. One may see focal infarcts, edema, and atrophy days after the injury. Magnetic resonance imaging (MRI) may provide more useful detail at an earlier stage. Electroencephalogram (EEG) is a sensitive indicator in assessing the degree of cortical dysfunction and the presence of epileptic activity.

MANAGEMENT

- Clinical management involves the restoration of adequate cardiopulmonary function to prevent further cerebral injury. Neuropathologic abnormalities can continue for hours to days and no simple therapy exists that can reverse anoxic damage.
- States of reduced cerebral energy requirements such as hypothermia may prevent or reduce the extent of cerebral injury. Hyperglycemia, cerebral lactic acidosis, dysregulation of calcium homeostasis, elevated ICP, and excessive release of excitatory neurotransmitters can increase ischemic cerebral damage.
- Several clinical trials have demonstrated significant benefit in survival and neurologic outcome by the use of cooling to 32–34°C following cardiac arrest. Postarrest cooling was induced by applying cooling blankets or ice packing in a subset of patients having return of spontaneous circulation but remaining unresponsive. Cooling should be achieved as rapidly as possible and temperature should be measured every 15–30 minutes during cooling via bladder probe, pulmonary artery catheter, or tympanic probe if invasive monitoring is not available. Patients uniformly require neuromuscular blockade and sedation to minimize shivering and discomfort. Passive rewarming is then started 24 hours after the initiation of cooling. The optimal method, depth, and duration of cooling as well as the therapeutic window will likely require further investigation before this approach is widely accepted in the guidelines for resuscitation. Initiation of hypothermia induces diuresis and careful attention to intravascular volume and electrolytes during cooling and rewarming is required.
- It has been postulated that hyperglycemia contributes to cerebral damage, therefore, limiting glucose solutions in the immediate postarrest period seems prudent.
- Elevated ICP after cardiac arrest indicates a severe degree of anoxic damage and therapy to reduce ICP in this setting is controversial.
- Corticosteroids and barbiturates have no role in postarrest management.

NEUROLOGIC OUTCOMES AFTER CARDIAC ARREST

- Patients in a coma less than 12 hours after resuscitation usually make a favorable recovery. Comas lasting more than 12 hours often have neurologic deficits due to focal or multifocal infarcts of the cerebral cortex.
- Somatosensory evoked potentials (SEPs) have the highest prognostic reliability and are the most frequently applied method in clinical and experimental studies evaluating outcome after CPR. Bilateral absence of median nerve-stimulated SEPs is associated with a <1% chance of awakening from coma since it implies that widespread cortical necrosis has occurred. Importantly, the presence of cortical responses is not a guarantee for awakening from coma.
- Serum levels of molecular markers for brain injury are under study to detect the extent of cerebral damage and neurologic outcome after CPR. Increased levels of neuron-specific enolase (NSE) and the astroglial protein S100 are associated with hypoxic-ischemic brain injury and poor neurologic outcome. Interestingly, decreased levels of NSE, but not S100, was found in the majority of patients with therapeutic hypothermia and was associated with better neurologic outcome.
- Early in the course of hypoxic-ischemic encephalopathy, several neurologic signs can predict outcome with some reliability.
- Absence of pupillary responses on the first day or absence of corneal reflexes after the first day following CPR predicts poor outcome. If there are no purposeful motor responses after 3 days, there is a high risk of persistent vegetative state or severe disability.
- Verbal responses, purposeful eye movements or motor responses, normal ocular reflexes, and response to verbal commands at 1 day following CPR predict at least a 50% chance of regaining independent function. Patient age, gender, or presence of postanoxic seizure failed to correlate with outcome.

BIBLIOGRAPHY

Abella BS, Vanden Hoek TL, Becker LB. Therapeutic hypothermia. In: Hall JB, Schmidt GA, Wood LDH, eds., *Principles of Critical Care*, 3rd ed. New York, NY: McGraw-Hill; 2005: 193–200.

Bernard SA, Gray TW, Buist MD, et al. Treatment of comatose survivors of out-of-hospital cardiac arrest with induced hypothermia. *N Engl J Med* 2002;346:557–563.

Hypothermia after Cardiac Arrest Study Group. Mild therapeutic hypothermia to improve the neurological outcome after cardiac arrest. *N Engl J Med* 2002;346:549–556.

Madl C, Holzer M. Brain function after resuscitation from cardiac arrest. *Curr Opin Crit Care* 2004;10:213–217.
Meynaar IA, Straaten HM, van der Wettering J, et al. Serum neuron-specific enolase predicts outcome in post-anoxic coma: a prospective cohort study. *Intensive Care Med* 2003;29:189–195.
Robinson LR, Mickelsen PJ, Tirschwell DL, et al. Predictive value of somatosensory evoked potentials for awakening from coma. *Crit Care Med* 2003;31:960–967.
Zingler VC, Krumm B, Bertsch T, et al. Early prediction of neurologic outcome after cardiopulmonary resuscitation: a mutimodal approach combining neurobiochemical and electrophysiologic investigations may provide high prognostic certainty in patients after cardiac arrest. *Eur Neurol* 2003;49:79–84.

72 THERAPEUTIC HYPOTHERMIA

John E.A. Blair, Raina M. Merchant

KEY POINTS

- Hypothermia is thought to blunt the effects of neurologic damage from ischemia-reperfusion injury.
- Several methods of cooling exist, with external cooling being inexpensive but slow, cumbersome, and difficult to control. Several invasive methods exist such as extracorporeal cooling and cold intravenous fluids, each with their characteristic features.
- Hypothermia places patients at increased risk for arrhythmias, coagulopathies, infection, and metabolic derangements. The incidence and severity of these complications increases when core temperature is <30°C, but careful monitoring is necessary for any degree of hypothermia.
- Hypothermia may improve mortality and neurologic outcomes after cardiac arrest. Clinical trials are conflicting regarding its use in traumatic brain injury, with some suggestion that benefits may derive from maintaining the hypothermic state for longer than 48 hours. Its use in stroke and neurologic fever still requires further investigation.
- There are other clinical situations where therapeutic hypothermia may prove beneficial such as subarachnoid hemorrhage, neuroprotection during invasive surgeries, myocardial infarction, and acute liver failure. It is important for staff in intensive care units to be aware of the complications of this potentially useful intervention.

HISTORY

- The use of hypothermia for clinical purposes originates in ancient times, with use by Egyptians, Greeks, and Romans. Hippocrates advocated packing wounded patients in snow to reduce hemorrhage. In the nineteenth century, Napoleon's Surgeon General Baron Larrey found that injured soldiers who became hypothermic were more likely to die if they were placed close to the fire than those with more gradual rewarming.
- Case reports of successful resuscitation of hypothermic drowning victims despite long periods of asphyxia in the 1930s and 1940s led to animal experiments in the 1950s demonstrating benefit from hypothermia during or after focal brain ischemia and traumatic brain injury.
- Several small trials were conducted in the 1960s using hypothermia for various brain injuries, but were discontinued due to side effects, uncertain benefit, and management problems.
- Research in therapeutic hypothermia was rekindled in the 1980s when animal studies showed benefits from mild (defined as core body temperature of 32–35°C in most studies) hypothermia with fewer side effects than deeper hypothermia used earlier. In addition, larger clinical trials became more feasible as the capabilities of intensive care units grew.

RATIONALE

- Therapeutic hypothermia is thought to preserve neuronal function in several types of brain injury. Much of what is known about the neuroprotective mechanisms is based on animal models.
- Hypothermia has been clearly shown to be neuroprotective if applied early enough in many animal experiments involving both global ischemia (simulating the clinical circumstance of cardiac arrest or near drowning), and focal ischemia models (simulating the clinical circumstance of stroke).
- Favorable neurologic outcome after brain injury depends on rapid restoration of circulation followed by blunting or prevention of the reperfusion response.
- Hypothermia is thought to suppress the reperfusion response by suppressing many of the chemical reactions associated with reperfusion injury, including destructive enzymatic reactions, free radical production, inflammatory cell invasion, excitatory amino acid release, and mitochondrial damage that may subsequently cause primary necrosis and/or trigger apoptosis (programmed cell death). Hypothermia may also reduce cerebral edema and enhance cellular membrane integrity.

COOLING METHODS

- Two general methods of cooling are available: external surface cooling and invasive cooling. The optimal method has yet to be determined, as neither method combines ease of use with efficacy.
- External cooling methods include cooling blankets, cooling helmets, specially designed cooling beds, wet towels, sprays, ice packs, fans, and immersion. These methods are easily applied, but slow in reducing core temperature.
- Invasive cooling methods range from the very complex and expensive extracorporeal cooling to the simple large-volume cold intravenous fluid infusions. These methods are not as well studied as the external cooling methods (Table 72-1).

SIDE EFFECTS

- There are several potential side effects of therapeutic hypothermia that if encountered may counteract any benefit from the intervention itself. Awareness of potential complications is essential. Generally, hypothermia has effects in almost every organ system, but special attention must be paid to the cardiovascular, hematologic, immunologic, and metabolic systems.
- *Cardiovascular*: Initially, hypothermic patients develop sinus tachycardia followed by bradycardia. Most malignant arrhythmias develop after the temperature drops below 30°C, when atrial fibrillation may soon lead to ventricular arrhythmias. To complicate matters, arrhythmias become more difficult to treat at lower temperatures. In addition to arrhythmias, hypothermia reduces cardiac output by approximately 25%. Below 30°C, contractility decreases, causing both systolic and diastolic dysfunction.
- *Hematologic*: Hypothermia increases bleeding time due to a reduction in platelet count and function and alteration of coagulation enzyme kinetics. Coagulation tests such as prothrombin time and partial thromboplastin time will remain normal unless performed at the patient's actual core temperature. Despite these abnormalities, none of the clinical trials studying patients with traumatic brain injury (TBI), subarachnoid hemorrhage, or cardiac arrest experienced intracranial bleeding with cooling.
- *Immunologic*: Hypothermia inhibits release of several inflammatory cytokines and suppresses leukocyte migration and phagocytosis. Clinically, this may present as delayed wound healing and respiratory tract infections.
- *Other effects*: Hypothermia seems to cause a reduction in circulating volume through diuresis, which is often profound. Low levels of the electrolytes magnesium, potassium, inorganic phosphate, and calcium have also been observed. Hypothermia can also impair insulin sensitivity and secretion, often inducing hyperglycemia.

MONITORING

- Younger patients have a higher capacity to counteract changes in temperature and are therefore more difficult to cool and require higher doses of sedatives than older patients, who have a lower basal metabolic rate, lower body mass index, and less effective vasoconstriction. Obese patients are more difficult to cool through external cooling methods due to the insulating properties of fat.

TABLE 72-1 Cooling Methods

	ADVANTAGE	DISADVANTAGE
External cooling		
Cooling blanket		Special equipment needed, cumbersome
Cooling helmet	Fast cooling times	Special equipment needed
Specially designed cooling beds		Special equipment needed
Wet towels, ice packs, alcohol or water sprays	Simple, no special equipment needed	Slow, difficult to titrate, cumbersome
Fans		Associated with increased infection rates
Immersion		Cumbersome
Invasive cooling		
Extracorporeal venovenous cooling, peritoneal lavage		Very invasive, cumbersome, requires specialist to initiate and administer
Cooling catheter	Temperature easily titrated and maintained	Special equipment needed
Ice water nasal lavage		Difficult to titrate
Large-volume ice-cold IV fluids	Simple	Short duration of effect
Antipyretic drugs		May not induce hypothermia

- All patients receiving therapeutic hypothermia should be comatose, intubated, and sedated, as these patients are most likely to benefit from a therapy that improves neurologic outcome.
- Shivering during cooling can generate heat and lead to increases in oxygen consumption by 40–100%, both of which are prevented by administration of neuromuscular blocking agents, sedatives, anesthetics, and opiates.
- Paralysis and sedation may make it difficult to assess neurologic status and presence of seizures, so careful monitoring for any new neurologic signs is warranted.
- Diligent monitoring for complications of hypothermia along with early aggressive therapy against these complications is necessary. For example, early electrolyte supplementation and intensive insulin administration may prevent arrhythmias and infections, respectively.
- Hospitals should develop specific protocols and strict guidelines for the initiation and monitoring of therapeutic hypothermia, with extensive education for all members of the medical staff involved.

CLINICAL APPLICATIONS OF HYPOTHERMIA

CARDIAC ARREST

- Two recent randomized, controlled trials have demonstrated favorable neurologic outcomes after induction of mild hypothermia in comatose patients surviving out-of-hospital ventricular fibrillation (VF) arrest.
- The hypothermia after cardiac arrest (HACA) group randomly assigned the use of a cooling blanket to cool 137 of 235 comatose survivors in out-of-hospital VF in 9 European centers to a target temperature of 32–34°C for 24 hours. Primary and secondary outcomes were favorable 6-month neurologic function and mortality, respectively, which were significantly improved in the hypothermia group.
- An Australian group randomly cooled 43 of 77 cardiac arrest victims in 4 centers to a goal temperature of 33°C for 12 hours by applying cold packs to the head, neck, torso, and limbs. The primary outcome of favorable neurologic function at discharge was significantly improved in the patient undergoing therapeutic hypothermia.
- A recent meta-analysis of these studies found that patients in the hypothermia group were more likely to have no or minimal neurologic damage at discharge (relative risk [RR] 1.68, 95% confidence interval [CI] 1.29–2.07, number needed to treat [NNT] 6). There was a trend toward improved survival at discharge in the hypothermia group.
- The HACA trial reported 6-month outcomes. Being alive at 6 months with favorable functional neurologic recovery was more likely in the hypothermia group (RR 1.40, 95% CI 1.08–1.81, NNT 6). There was also improved survival at 6 months in the hypothermia group (RR 0.74, 95% CI 0.58–0.95, NNT 7).
- Current recommendations from the International Liaison Committee on Resuscitation (ILCOR) and American Heart Association (AHA) state that unconscious adult patients with spontaneous circulation after out-of-hospital cardiac arrest should be cooled to 32–34°C for 12–24 hours when the initial rhythm was VF.
- Such cooling may also be beneficial for other rhythms or for in-hospital cardiac arrest. Studies regarding these types of arrests are ongoing.

TRAUMATIC BRAIN INJURY

- Traumatic brain injury (TBI) is any brain injury sustained from externally inflicted trauma. Common causes include motor vehicle crashes, falls, acts of violence, and sports injuries. In the United States, TBI accounts for approximately 270,000 hospitalizations, 52,000 deaths, and 80,000 patients with permanent neurologic deficits.
- In treating TBI, the majority of neurologic damage occurs not at the initial impact, but at later stages during the hospitalization. Most interventions for TBIs are focused on prevention of this secondary neurologic injury.
- The secondary injury from TBI often stems from cerebral edema and increased intracranial pressures (ICP) which damage injured areas of the brain, as well as the release of substances such as glutamate, nitric oxide, and free radicals, both thought to be mitigated by hypothermia.
- There have been several clinical studies using hypothermia for TBI reliably demonstrating a reduction in ICP. However, the studies were conflicting as to whether this reduction translates to improvement in mortality and neurologic outcome.
- A thorough meta-analysis of the literature demonstrated a small but statistically significant mortality (RR for death 0.81; 95% CI 0.69–0.96) and neurologic (RR for a poor neurologic outcome 0.81; 95% CI 0.69–0.96) benefit in TBI survivors who were cooled to a target temperature of 32–35°C. These benefits seemed to be even greater in patients cooled for >48 hours.
- Since the meta-analysis, two large single-center trials reported favorable mortality and neurologic outcomes when mild hypothermia was applied for >48 hours,

and the rate of rewarming was slower compared to previous studies. In contrast, the only multicenter trial studying hypothermia for TBI patients showed no mortality or neurologic benefits.
- The differences in outcomes between studies seem to be multifactorial, related to the length of time spent cooled, rate of rewarming, expertise in specific centers, and procedural variations between studies.
- Therapeutic hypothermia for TBI is a complex undertaking and should be performed with caution in tertiary care centers with expertise in the area. Since mortality and survival benefit seem to appear after cooling for 48 hours, careful monitoring and management of complications from hypothermia should be performed.

STROKE

- There is strong evidence in animal models that therapeutic hypothermia is an effective strategy in controlling stroke. Despite these data, very few clinical trials have been conducted using hypothermia for human stroke patients.
- A focal ischemic event causes necrosis in a central core region nearest the occluded vessel. Surrounding that core is an area of hypoperfused but functional neurons at risk of necrosis called the penumbra. The penumbra will become necrotic unless perfusion is restored or other interventions initiated.
- Hypothermia is thought to reduce the damage caused by hypoperfusion and therefore the size of the ischemic penumbra through mechanisms previously described. It also may reduce resultant cerebral edema caused by the stroke.
- To date, there are no published randomized, controlled trials using hypothermia as part of therapy for stroke. There have been several uncontrolled feasibility trials with varying protocols for patients with middle cerebral artery (MCA) infarction, confirming the safety of hypothermia in this setting. Outcomes after cooling are yet to be determined.
- Although a promising strategy for neuroprotection, hypothermia for stroke remains experimental. Randomized, controlled trials need to be performed in order to define the role of hypothermia for stroke in the future.

NEUROLOGIC FEVER

- Fever is a very common phenomenon among neurologic patients in the intensive care unit, affecting many patients with ischemic stroke, head injury, intracranial hemorrhage, and subarachnoid hemorrhage.
- Several studies have found a significant association between fever and outcomes after TBI, intracerebral hemorrhage, subarachnoid hemorrhage, and stroke independent of other factors such as extent of neurologic injury and comorbidities.
- Animal studies have demonstrated that elevated brain temperatures may lead to greater release of excitatory amino acids and free radicals, breakdown of the blood-brain barrier, inhibition of protein kinases, and cytoskeletal proteolysis leading to more profound neuronal death in global and focal brain ischemia models.
- Theoretically, keeping core body temperature and therefore brain temperature normothermic in patients with neurologic injury slows the destructive processes associated with brain hyperthermia.
- Administration of antipyretics such as acetaminophen or cooling blankets for fever in neurologic patients has not proven efficacious in lowering temperature, indicating a role for more intense forms of cooling in these settings.
- Randomized, controlled trials have not been conducted to assess outcomes after cooling for fever in neurologic patients, but a trial is underway by the Copenhagen Stroke Study.
- Cooling neurologic patients with fever remains of theoretical benefit. In managing these patients, it is important to rigorously search for foci of infection.

OTHER POTENTIAL USES OF HYPOTHERMIA

- *Subarachnoid hemorrhage*: Data are limited to animal studies which show a reduction of cerebral vasospasm and decrease in ICP.
- *Intraoperative hypothermia*: Small clinical studies have shown neurologic protection using hypothermia in patients undergoing cerebral aneurysm clipping, cardiac surgery, and spinal cord protection in thoracoabdominal aortic aneurysm repair.
- *Myocardial infarction*: A pilot study demonstrated that hypothermia is feasible in the setting of percutaneous coronary intervention after myocardial infarction.
- *Acute liver failure*: Animal models demonstrate that hypothermia may be beneficial in lowering ICP in hepatic encephalopathy.

CONCLUSIONS

- Therapeutic hypothermia is a promising strategy for controlling the neurologic damage that follows many injuries to the brain.

- Intensivists should be aware of the side effects of hypothermia and take great care to prevent and treat them.
- Future research will help determine the clinical scenarios in which therapeutic hypothermia should be used, as well as the specifics of effective cooling protocols.

BIBLIOGRAPHY

Holzer M, Bernard SA, Hachimi-Idrissi S, et al. Hypothermia for neuroprotection after cardiac arrest: systematic review and individual patient data meta-analysis. *Crit Care Med* 2005;33:414–418.

McIntyre LA, Fergusson DA, Hebert PC, et al. Prolonged therapeutic hypothermia after traumatic brain injury in adults: a systematic review. *JAMA* 2003;289:2992–2999.

Nolan JP, Morley PT, Vanden Hoek TL, et al. Therapeutic hypothermia after cardiac arrest: an advisory statement by the advanced life support task force of the International Liaison Committee on Resuscitation. *Circulation* 2003;108: 118–121.

Polderman KH. Application of therapeutic hypothermia in the ICU: opportunities and pitfalls of a promising treatment modality. Part 1: Indications and evidence. *Intensive Care Med* 2004;30:556–575.

Polderman KH. Application of therapeutic hypothermia in the intensive care unit. Opportunities and pitfalls of a promising treatment modality. Part 2: Practical aspects and side effects. *Intensive Care Med* 2004;30:757–769.

73 STATUS EPILEPTICUS

D. Kyle Hogarth

KEY POINTS

- Status epilepticus (SE) is defined as a protracted seizure episode or multiple frequent seizures lasting 30 minutes or longer. There is no interictal return to baseline mental status.
- Single seizures that persist longer than 5–7 minutes should be treated to prevent progression to SE.
- Recommended treatment is lorazepam 0.1 mg/kg intravenously.
- Delay in recognition and treatment of seizures is associated with increased mortality, and prolonged seizure duration is a negative prognostic factor.

EPIDEMIOLOGY

- The incidence of generalized convulsive status epilepticus (GCSE) in the United States is estimated to be up to 195,000 episodes per year.
- In adults, cerebrovascular disease and noncompliance of anticonvulsive medications are the most common causes of SE. Central nervous system (CNS) infection, neoplasm, and metabolic disturbances can also cause SE.
- Three major factors determine the outcome of patients with SE: the type of SE, the etiology, and the duration of seizure.
- Causes associated with increased mortality included anoxia, intracranial hemorrhage, tumor, infection, and trauma.
- SE in the setting of acute ischemic stroke has a very high mortality, approaching 35%.

CLASSIFICATION

- The simplest classification scheme divides SE into GCSE and nonconvulsive SE (NCSE), depending on whether convulsive movements are present.
- Inadequately treated GCSE can become NCSE. After prolonged generalized convulsions, visible motor activity may stop, but the electrochemical seizure continues. The patient is still seizing!
- Patients who do not start to awaken after 20 minutes of GCSE should be assumed to have entered NCSE.
- Management of NCSE should be guided by the electroencephalogram (EEG).
- A high suspicion for NCSE should be maintained in patients with unexplained alteration in level of consciousness.

PATHOPHYSIOLOGY

- The systemic manifestations of early phase GCSE result from an adrenergic surge and excessive muscle activity. The adrenergic surge causes tachycardia, hypertension, and hyperglycemia.
- The systemic manifestations of late phase GCSE relates to complications of extreme muscle activity; hyperthermia, acidosis, rhabdomyolysis, and secondary acute renal failure.

CLINICAL MANIFESTATIONS

- Seizure recognition in the ICU can be difficult to diagnose for the following reasons:
  - Nonconvulsive seizures in the setting of depressed consciousness

- Masking of seizures by pharmacologically induced paralysis or sedation
- Misinterpretation of other abnormal patient movements as seizures

- Tachycardia, tachypnea, and hypertension are often signs of seizure that can be misinterpreted as evidence of inadequate sedation.
- Patients with metabolic disturbances, anoxia, and other types of nervous system injury may demonstrate abnormal movements that can be confused with seizure. Myoclonus in postanoxic coma can occur in the presence and absence of epileptiform discharges.

INITIAL MANAGEMENT

- The initial approach to seizure management involves the ABCs: airway, breathing, and circulation. Medication to treat tachycardia and hypertension before the seizure activity stops is not warranted.
- The conventional agents used for first-line treatment of SE are the benzodiazepines, phenytoin, and phenobarbital. Lorazepam is more efficacious than phenytoin, and easier to use than phenobarbital for GCSE.
- A single intravenous dose of 0.1 mg/kg of lorazepam is recommended therapy.
- If lorazepam is not available, a single intravenous dose of 0.15 mg/kg diazepam can be given, but phenytoin or phenobarbital should also be started as the duration of action of diazepam against SE is only about 20 minutes.
- If there is no intravenous access, 0.2 mg/kg of midazolam administered intramuscular will be rapidly and reliably absorbed.
- Phenytoin is useful in SE, but the prolonged loading time limits its usefulness acutely. However, a 20 mg/kg dose of phenytoin produces an adequate serum level for the next 24 hours and should be begun for the patient in SE.
- Phenobarbital in the management of acute SE is not routinely recommended.

OTHER MANAGEMENT ISSUES

- Seizures in ICU patients have many potential causes that must be investigated. Medications are a major cause of seizures in critically ill patients, especially in the setting of renal or hepatic dysfunction.
- Recreational drugs are frequently overlooked but can cause seizures. Acute cocaine or methamphetamine intoxication is characterized by a state of hypersympathetic activity followed by seizures. Ethanol withdrawal can obviously cause seizures and narcotic withdrawal may produce seizures in the critically ill.
- Serum glucose, electrolyte concentrations, and serum osmolality should be measured. Dextrose and thiamine should be administered if hypoglycemia is present.
- New-onset seizures warrant brain imaging. Computed tomography (CT) scanning is rapid and can detect acute blood, swelling, large tumors or abscesses, and subacute or remote ischemic strokes.
- When CNS infection is suspected, empiric antibiotic treatment should be started while imaging studies are being obtained.

REFRACTORY STATUS EPILEPTICUS

- In refractory SE (RSE), cessation of EEG seizure activity is the goal.
- High-dose barbiturates, most commonly pentobarbital, are extremely useful in RSE, but side effects of hypotension can be severe and may limit use.
- If successful in stopping RSE, barbiturate anesthesia should not be rapidly discontinued. Therapy should be continued for at least 48 hours after cessation of EEG seizure activity. Then, a gradual taper of the dose should occur with the administration of phenobarbital during the drug taper.
- Pentobarbital is loaded at 5–12 mg/kg followed by an infusion of 1–10 mg/kg/h. Thiopental sodium may be given in 75–125 mg IV boluses followed by infusion rates of 1–5 mg/kg/h as an alternative agent.
- Midazolam can be loaded at 0.2 mg/kg followed by continuous infusion of 0.05–2.0 mg/kg/h for RSE.
- There are only case report data supporting propofol use in SE.

BIBLIOGRAPHY

Bassin SL, Fountain NB, Bleck TP. Seizures in the intensive care unit. In: Hall JB, Schmidt GA, Wood LDH, eds., *Principles of Critical Care*, 3rd ed. New York, NY: McGraw-Hill; 2005: 997–1006.

Lowenstein DH, Alldredge BK. Status epilepticus. *N Engl J Med* 1998;338:970–976.

74 ACUTE SPINAL CORD COMPRESSION

Nuala J. Meyer

KEY POINTS

- Acute and subacute spinal disorders are frequently the result of extramedullary compression of the spinal cord.

- Compression may result from trauma, tumor, infection, or spondylosis.
- In the multiple injured trauma patient, a spinal injury should be assumed present and unstable until adequately assessed. A stable injury is one in which only one of the columns (anterior, middle, or posterior) is involved, and no further neural structures are in danger.
- The hallmark of spinal cord disease is the presence of a *level* below which sensory, motor, or autonomic nervous function is impaired, and the determination of this level may be invaluable in localizing the site of injury.
- Outcome of spinal injury is extremely dependent on the extent of injury at the time of diagnosis; complete cord injuries have no potential for functional recovery, whereas incomplete injuries have recovery potential. Evolving spinal injuries must be recognized early in order to maximize the potential for recovery. After 48 hours, fixed paralysis is unlikely to be reversed.

PATHOPHYSIOLOGY

- Anatomically, the spinal column is surrounded by a ring of bones made up of vertebral bodies anteriorly and spinous processes and pedicles posteriorly. Within the ring lies the epidural space, the dura, and the thecal sac. Compression of the thecal sac may be asymptomatic, or may progress to complete paraplegia, strangulating the spinal cord.
- The pattern of cord compression determines the pattern of injury.
  - Anterior cord syndrome results in loss of all spinal cord function—motor, sensory, and autonomic—below the level of the lesion, with only positional and vibratory sense preserved. This occurs most frequently from clot, compression, or ischemia of the anterior spinal artery or from anterior compression of the cord.
  - Central cord syndrome, caused by hemorrhage within the cord, classically incites arm weakness worse than leg weakness, with variable sensory deficits.
  - Brown-Séquard syndrome is the result of complete or partial transaction of the cord, typically from blunt trauma or penetrating injury. It involves the loss of motor function below the level on the ipsilateral side, with loss of contralateral pain and temperature function.

LOCALIZING SIGNS

- High cervical cord injuries are frequently life threatening due to weakness of respiratory muscles and diaphragm (C3-C5).
  - When injury is extensive and involves the junction of the cervical cord with the medulla, the outcome is usually fatal from medullary cardiopulmonary collapse.
  - C4-C5 lesions lead to quadriplegia, but usually with preserved breathing function due to a functional C3 lesion.
  - Midcervical (C5-C6) lesions will cause loss of biceps and brachioradialis reflexes.
  - C7 injuries spare the biceps but weaken the hand and wrist, whereas C8 lesions cause loss of wrist and digit flexion.
- Thoracic cord lesions are mapped by their sensory dermatomes. Landmarks include the nipple (T4) and umbilicus (T10).
  - Thoracic injuries may causes weakness of the lower extremities, along with bowel, bladder, and sexual dysfunction. Midline back pain is common.
  - Upper and lower abdominal wall musculature is paralyzed by lesions above T9, whereas below this level only the lower muscles are affected.
- Lumbar cord injuries paralyze thigh flexion and adduction at L2-L4, and cause loss of foot and ankle motor function at L5-S1. The cremasteric reflex reflects intact function at L1-L2.
- Sacral cord injuries or conus syndrome tend to spare lower extremity motor function but cause saddle anesthesia with bowel, bladder, and sexual dysfunction.

NEOPLASTIC CORD COMPRESSION

- Most neoplasms affecting the spinal column in adults are extramedullary, arising from metastases to the vertebrae with epidural compression, as opposed to neoplasms of neural origin.
- Almost any malignancy has the potential to metastasize to vertebrae, but the most common to do so include breast, lung, prostate, and renal cell cancer, along with lymphoma and myeloma.
- Approximately 20% of patients with malignant spinal cord compression are presenting with their initial manifestation of cancer.
- Metastatic cord compression is most common in the thoracic spine, followed by lumbosacral vertebrae.
- Bone destruction by tumor may cause vertebral collapse, which in turn may compress the cord, cauda equine, or individual nerve roots.
- Intradural tumors—mainly meningiomas and neurofibromas—tend to be slow growing and benign.
- Primary tumors of the spinal cord are uncommon and typically present as hemicord or central cord symptoms.

CLINICAL PRESENTATION

- Pain is the common initial symptom in the vast majority of patients.
  - It may be nerve root pain or localized back pain.
  - Most patients rate their pain as severe and progressive, and worse with movement.
  - In one study, patients had pain on average 3 months prior to being diagnosed with cord compression.
- Motor weakness is present in more than 60% of patients at diagnosis, and is classically symmetric lower extremity weakness.
- Sensory complaints are common and often begin 1–2 weeks before the diagnosis of cord compression.
- Bowel and bladder dysfunction are late findings in cord compression, and while common at the time of diagnosis, point to advanced compression.
- Ataxia or inability to walk is frequently present at diagnosis, either due to weakness or spinocerebellar dysfunction. One study found that only 18% of patients were able to walk at the time of diagnosis.

DIAGNOSIS

- Plain radiographs or bone scan are inadequate studies to diagnose compression of the thecal sac, as they are insensitive—missing approximately 20% of cases—and delay the definitive diagnostic study, the MRI or myelogram.
- While MRI is less invasive and spares the patient a lumbar puncture, myelogram may be especially helpful for a patient with intractable pain who is unable to lie still. The two tests performed equivalently well in studies of sensitivity and specificity.

TREATMENT

- Corticosteroids improved the percentage of patients ambulatory at 3 and 6 months in one trial, and are generally used in high doses (Decadron 30 mg daily in divided doses). Slightly lower doses may be used for less severe symptoms, for example, when no weakness is present.
- Radiation therapy is the definitive therapy for most patients with malignant cord compression.
- Surgery—decompression or vertebral resection—should be considered if compressive symptoms are worsening despite radiotherapy, if the patient has received his or her maximal allowable dose of radiation already, or if a vertebral compression contributes to the cord compression.
- Pain control with both opioids and nonopioid analgesics is a mainstay of therapy.

EPIDURAL ABSCESS

- The classic triad for an infected fluid collection in the epidural space is fever, back pain, and progressive weakness.
  - Back pain is almost invariably present, and may be subacute or chronic.
  - As the abscess expands, it induces edema and thrombosis, compressing the spinal cord and potentially leading to irreversible spinal injury.
- Risk factors for epidural abscess are immunocompromised states, IV drug abuse, or skin infections. Infection may arise from hematogenous spread (approximately two-thirds of cases) or by direct extension from vertebral osteomyelitis or decubitus ulcers (one-third).
- *Staphylococcus aureus* and other gram-positive organisms are the most common to cause epidural abscess, but tuberculosis remains an important cause in the developing world.
- MRI is the diagnostic study of choice.
- Treatment is emergency decompressive laminectomy and long-term antibiotic therapy.

BIBLIOGRAPHY

Abrahm JL. Management of pain and spinal cord compression in patients with advanced cancer. *Ann Intern Med* 1999;313:37–46.

Johnson GE. Spine injuries. In: Hall JB, Schmidt GA, Wood LDH, eds., *Principles of Critical Care*, 3rd ed. New York, NY: McGraw-Hill; 2005:1409–1420.

Levack P, Graham J, Collie D, et al. Don't wait for a sensory level—listen to the symptoms: a prospective audit of the delays in diagnosis of malignant cord compression. *Clin Oncol* 2002; 14:472–480.

75 DELIRIUM IN THE INTENSIVE CARE UNIT

Joseph Levitt

KEY POINTS

- Delirium is present when there is an acute change or fluctuation in mental status, inattention, and either disorganized thinking or altered level of consciousness.
- Delirium is extremely common in the ICU but often goes unrecognized.

- Development of delirium is associated with increased mortality, prolonged hospital stay, and discharge to long-term care facilities.
- Screening for delirium is simple and reliable and should be a routine part of daily patient care.
- Many known risk factors exist but it is unclear if altering these factors can prevent delirium or its long-term sequelae.
- Psychoactive drugs are major risk factors for developing delirium in the ICU. However, clinical data are lacking to support detailed recommendations, other than close monitoring for adverse effects and avoiding oversedation.

PATHOPHYSIOLOGY

- Delirium should be considered a form of unrecognized organ dysfunction.
- Delirium results from an imbalance of neurotransmitters controlling cognitive function. Dopamine increases excitability of neurons while gamma aminobutyric acid (GABA) and acetylcholine suppress neuronal activity. Excesses in dopamine and depletion of acetylcholine are felt to be important in the development of delirium. Other neurotransmitters, such as serotonin, endorphins, and noradrenalin, also play a role.
- Factors leading to neurotransmitter imbalance include reduction in cerebral metabolism, primary intracranial disease, systemic illness, secondary infection of the brain, exogenous toxic agents, withdrawal from substances of abuse such as alcohol or sedative-hypnotics, hypoxemia, metabolic disturbances, and the administration of psychoactive medications such as benzodiazepines and narcotics.
- Hyperactive delirium is more frequently recognized by care providers but is much less common than hypoactive or mixed forms.
- Delirium encompasses and should replace other terms describing recognized entities such as "ICU psychosis" and "toxic confusional state."

PREVALENCE AND IMPACT

- Delirium is exceedingly common, occurring in from 20 to 80% of ICU patients depending on risk factors and screening modality; however, it may go unrecognized by clinicians in up to 66–84% of cases.
- Delirium is not a normal "transitional state" between coma and normal consciousness and has been found to occur as often in patients without prior coma and frequently persists beyond hospital discharge.
- The occurrence of delirium has been found to be an independent risk factor for increased mortality, prolonged hospitalization, and discharge to skilled nursing facility in both ICU and non-ICU hospitalized patients. In mechanically ventilated patients, it is associated with increased aspiration, nosocomial pneumonia, self-extubation, and reintubation.
- Overall, a three times greater mortality has been found in ICU patients who develop delirium compared with those who don't, even when controlling for other independent risk factors.
- Health care costs directly attributable to delirium have been estimated in the billions of dollars.

MONITORING AND RISK FACTORS

- Delirium may be the presenting sign of a serious underlying disorder including evolving sepsis, impending respiratory failure, alcohol withdrawal, or hypoglycemia; recognition of delirium necessitates an evaluation for underlying etiology.
- Recently, the Society of Critical Care Medicine's guidelines recommended routine daily monitoring for delirium, as well as sedation levels in all critically ill patients.
- Many validated sedation scales exist in clinical practice, but less attention has been paid to monitoring for delirium. The Confusion Assessment for the ICU (CAM-ICU) can be performed at the bedside in about a minute, has good interoperator reliability, is designed to include mechanically ventilated patients, and has a sensitivity and specificity of 95% of detecting delirium.
- Risk factors for developing delirium can be divided into host (older age, prior mild cognitive impairment, smoking, hypertension), underlying illness (sepsis, organ dysfunction, metabolic derangements, mechanical ventilation), and iatrogenic (psychoactive medications, notably benzodiazepines and opiates) categories.

MANAGEMENT

- Initial management should focus on correcting reversible organic etiologies and risk factor modification.
- While many risk factors have been identified, it is unclear whether altering these risk factors can prevent occurrence of delirium in the ICU.
- A study of general medicine patients showed a 40% reduction (15–9.9%) in incidence of delirium through a protocol of
  - Repeated reorientation
  - Cognitively stimulating activity three times daily

  - Imposing a sleep protocol preserving day and night rituals
  - Early mobilization exercises
  - Early removal of catheters
  - Avoiding restraints
  - Use of regular eyewear and hearing aides
- While some risk factors are unavoidable and clinical data are lacking for detailed guidelines in the ICU, attention should be paid to minimizing iatrogenic causes.
- Psychoactive medications are exceedingly common and to some degree necessary in the ICU. However, frequent monitoring of sedation levels is critical in avoiding excessive use and oversedation.
- Benzodiazepines and their metabolites are particularly implicated in provoking delirium. Substituting haloperidol for benzodiazepines in the treatment of agitation, particularly in nonmechanically ventilated patients, may decrease rates of delirium.
  - A study of postcardiac surgery patients showed that dexmedetomidine for agitation led to better outcomes compared to benzodiazepines or propofol, but more experience is needed before it can be recommended.
- While no drugs have Food and Drug Administration (FDA) approval for the treatment of delirium, haloperidol has the most clinical experience in the ICU.
  - Haloperidol is a dopamine (D_2) antagonist and should be particularly effective in hyperactive delirium.
  - While non-ICU doses start at 0.5–1 mg, ICU doses should start at 5 mg (IV or PO) every 12 hours with maximal effective dose usually 20 mg/day.
  - Potential adverse effects are rare but significant and include torsades de pointes (should be avoided in patients with long QT intervals on ECG), dystonia, and extrapyramidal side effects, hyperthermia (associated with malignant hyperthermia), laryngeal spasm, and anticholinergic effects.
  - Newer atypical neuroleptics (e.g., risperidone and olanzapine) may be effective and have fewer adverse effects, but more experience is needed.

BIBLIOGRAPHY

Ely WE. Delirium in the intensive care unit. In: Hall JB, Schmidt GA, Wood LDH, eds., *Principles of Critical Care.* New York, NY: McGraw-Hill, 2005.

Jacobi J, Fraser GL, Coursin DB, et al. Clinical practice guidelines for the sustained use of sedatives and analgesics in the critically ill adult. *Crit Care Med* 2002;30(1):119–141.

Truman B, Ely EW. Monitoring delirium in critically ill patients. Using the confusion assessment method for the intensive care unit. *Crit Care Nurse* 2003;23(2):25–36; quiz 37-28.

76 NEUROMUSCULAR WEAKNESS IN THE ICU

Michael Moore

KEY POINTS

- Neuromuscular disorders (NMDs) both precipitate and complicate critical illness.
- Maximal inspiratory and expiratory pressures and the VC are readily available measures assisting the clinician in assessing the impact of NMDs on the adequacy of ventilation.
- Critical illness myopathy and neuromyopathy complicates many patients with protracted critical illness, regardless of cause.

NEUROMUSCULAR DISORDERS IN CRITICAL CARE

- Neuromuscular weakness can be attributed to disorders involving the peripheral nerves, neuromuscular transmission, or skeletal muscles.
- Weakness can be divided into disorders that result in ICU admission and disorders acquired during treatment of critical illness.
- Common disorders that lead to ICU admission include Guillain-Barré syndrome (GBS), myasthenia gravis (MG), dermatomyositis/polymyositis (DM/PM), and metabolic myopathies related to mitochondrial disease.
- Common clinical scenarios that result in weakness after admission to the ICU include persistent blockade of the neuromuscular junction from neuromuscular blocking agents (NMBA), sensorimotor axonal polyneuropathy, and acute myopathies.

REVIEW OF RESPIRATORY MUSCLE IMPAIRMENT

- Requires objective testing as symptoms can be subtle.

SYMPTOMS

- Orthopnea
- Sleep disturbance
- Tachypnea
- Exercise intolerance

OBJECTIVE TESTING

- Most important respiratory muscle parameters:
  - Maximal inspiratory pressure (MIP)
  - Maximum expiratory pressure (MEP)
  - Vital capacity (VC)
  - Assessment of oropharyngeal function
- Frequent assessment and attention to serial changes is required in patients with an evolving neuromuscular disorder (NMD).
- MIP and MEP:
  - Most sensitive measure of respiratory muscle strength
  - Measurement requires a bedside manometer fitted with a mouthpiece
  - MIP
    - Maximal inspiratory effort at residual volume
    - Normal values
      - −70 cmH_2O in women
      - −100 cmH_2O in men
    - Hypercapnia more likely when MIP less negative than −20 cmH_2O
  - MEP
    - Maximal expiratory effort at total lung capacity
    - Normal values
      - 100 cmH_2O in women
      - 150 cmH_2O in men
    - Effective cough unlikely when MEP <40 cmH_2O
- VC:
  - Normal VC is approximately 50 mL/kg
  - Clearance of secretions with coughing is impaired when VC <30 mL/kg
  - Risk of respiratory failure increased with serial decline in VC <15–20 mL/kg
- Arterial blood gases and VC are commonly normal in the early stages of respiratory muscle weakness.
- Sleep-related deterioration in ventilation and oxygenation is common.

BULBAR MUSCLE IMPAIRMENT

- Increased risk of aspiration-related respiratory failure.
- Symptoms:
  - Nasal speech
  - Protruding tongue
  - Difficulty swallowing
- Intact musculature involving the mouth, pharynx, palate, tongue, and larynx are necessary for effective oropharyngeal function.
- Assessment is primarily based on clinical observation (i.e., swallow study).
- Early consultation with an experienced speech pathologist is recommended.

NEUROMUSCULAR DISORDERS LEADING TO INTENSIVE CARE UNIT ADMISSION

- Respiratory failure is the most common reason patients with a primary NMD are admitted to the ICU.
- Most will have a previously defined NMD but the recent onset of acute or subacute bilateral muscle weakness should elicit a broad differential diagnosis (Table 76-1).
- The differential diagnosis is initially based on the patient's history and a careful neurologic examination (Table 76-2).
- Additional diagnostic tests such as nerve conduction studies and electromyogram (EMG) are often required (Table 76-2).
- Upper and lower motor neuron disease may occasionally be responsible for new-onset weakness that necessitates ICU admission.

TABLE 76-1 Causes of Acute and Subacute Bilateral Weakness

SYNDROME/LEVEL OF ABNORMALITY	REPRESENTATIVE DISORDER
Basilar artery occlusion	Embolic
	Thrombotic
	Vasculitic
Myelopathy	Cord compression (e.g., abscess, neoplasm, disc herniation, and trauma)
	Transverse myelitis
Central nervous system infections	Poliomyelitis
	West Nile virus
Central nervous system toxins	Neurotoxic fish poisoning
Peripheral nerve disorders	GBS
	Diphtheria
	Heavy metal toxicity
	Vasculitic neuropathy
Disorders of neuromuscular transmission	MG
	Eaton-Lambert syndrome
	Botulism
	Tick paralysis
	Organophosphate poisoning
	Penicillamine toxicity
Myopathic disorders	DM/PM
	Metabolic myopathy (e.g., mitochondrial disease)
	Toxic myopathy (e.g., corticosteroid injury and rhabdomyolysis)
Electrolyte disorders	Periodic paralysis
	Hypophosphatemia
	Hypokalemia

TABLE 76-2 Differential Diagnosis of NMDs Leading of ICU Admission

LEVEL OF ABNORMALITY	PRESENTATION	REPRESENTATIVE DISORDER	NERVE CONDUCTION	EMG
Upper motor neuron	Weakness	Cortical	Normal	Normal
	Spasticity	Subcortical		
	Hyporeflexia	Brainstem		
	Sensory/autonomic changes	Spinal cord lesions		
Lower motor neuron	Weakness	Poliomyelitis	Normal	Denervation
	Flaccidity	Postpolio syndrome		
	Hyporeflexia	Amyotrophic lateral sclerosis		
	Fasciculations			
	Bulbar changes			
	No sensor changes			
Peripheral nerve	Weakness	GBS	Reduced	Denervation
	Flaccidity	Diphtheria		
	Hyporeflexia	Heavy metal toxicity		
	Bulbar changes	Vasculitic neuropathy		
	Sensory/autonomic changes			
Neuromuscular junction	Fluctuating weakness	MG	Normal	Abnormal repetitive stimulation
	Fatigability	Eaton-Lambert botulism		
	Normal reflexes	Tick paralysis		
	No sensor changes	Organophosphate		
	+/- Autonomic changes	Penicillamine		
Muscle	Weakness	DM/PM	Normal	Small motor units
	Normal reflexes	Metabolic myopathies		
	No sensory/autonomic changes	Muscular dystrophy		
	+/- Pain			

SOURCE: Modified from Luce J. Neuromuscular diseases care. In: Hall JB, Schmidt GA, Wood LDH, eds. Principles of Critical Care 2nd ed. New York, NY: McGraw-Hill; 1998: 995–1004.

GUILLAIN-BARRÉ SYNDROME

- Acute inflammatory demyelinating polyneuropathy that most often presents with ascending symmetrical weakness and depressed or absent reflexes.
- Typically evolves over days to weeks but a subset of patients have a rapid decline in function over hours.
- Sensory involvement is common and paresthesias may be the initial complaint.
- Other early symptoms include an aching discomfort in the lower back and legs.
- Autonomic dysfunction is common and results in brady- or tachyarrhythmias, orthostatic hypotension, hypertension, or abnormal sweating.
- Bowel and bladder function are usually preserved.
- The Miller-Fischer variant presents with ataxia, ophthalmoparesis, and areflexia.

EPIDEMIOLOGY

- More common in young adults and elderly patients.
- Approximately two-thirds of patients have a preceding gastrointestinal (GI) or respiratory infectious syndrome.
- Most common triggers are infections with *Campylobacter jejuni* and cytomegalovirus.

DIAGNOSIS

- Based on clinical presentation and electrodiagnostic studies compatible with a demyelinating polyneuropathy
- Cerebrospinal fluid
  - Elevated protein levels after the first week of symptoms
  - Limited mononuclear pleocytosis (<10 cells/cm^3)
- Signs or symptoms that suggest alternative diagnoses
  - Intact reflexes despite generalized weakness
  - Asymmetric weakness
  - Fever during the initial presentation
  - Electrodiagnostic features inconsistent with an acquired demyelinating polyneuropathy
- Important to rule out a rapidly progressive spinal lesion

CLINICAL COURSE

- Monophasic illness with a fairly predictable natural history
- 90% reach nadir of neuromuscular impairment by 4 weeks

- Respiratory failure
  - 10% of patients present with and up to 43% will eventually develop respiratory failure
  - Predictors of respiratory failure
    - "20/30/40 rule"
      - VC <20 mL/kg
      - MIP less negative than −30 cmH_2O
      - MEP <40 cmH_2O
    - Inability to cough
    - Time from onset to admission <7 days
    - Inability to stand or lift head or elbows
    - Autonomic dysfunction
- Morbidity and mortality
  - Strongly associated with the need for and duration of mechanical ventilation
  - Two-thirds experience mild residual deficits
  - 10–20% have complete recovery
  - Mortality reported to be between 3 and 8%
    - Causes of mortality
      - Pneumonia
      - Acute respiratory distress syndrome (ARDS)
      - Sepsis
      - Pulmonary emboli
      - Cardiac arrest

TREATMENT

- Plasma exchange:
  - Improved strength and reduced the incidence of respiratory failure in three multicenter trials conducted in the 1980s.
  - Two to four exchanges may be needed depending on severity.
- Intravenous immune globulin:
  - Also effective.
  - Mechanism is unclear but may be related to neutralizing neuromuscular blocking antibodies.
  - May be superior to plasmapheresis in patients with *C. jejuni* infections and antibodies to peripheral nerve gangliosides.
- A randomized, multicenter, international trial that compared plasma exchange, IVIg, and plasma exchange followed by IVIg concluded that IVIg and plasmapheresis are equally effective without additional benefit with combined therapy.
- IVIg may be preferred because of ease of administration and acceptable side effect profile.
- Corticosteroids have not been shown to be beneficial.

MYASTHENIA GRAVIS

- Acquired autoimmune disorder of neuromuscular junction transmission characterized by muscle weakness, progressive muscle fatigue with repetitive use, and improvement in strength after rest.
- Clinical presentation:
  - 85% have generalized weakness with fatigability involving the trunk and extremities.
  - Ocular muscle involvement including ptosis and diplopia are common.
  - Bulbar muscle impairment results in dysphonia and dysphagia.
- Incidence highest in younger women and older men.
- Neuromuscular weakness results from autoantibodies to acetylcholine receptors that impair neuromuscular transmission.
- Respiratory muscle function:
  - Isolated respiratory muscle impairment can occur but typically presents along with generalized muscle weakness.
  - VC, MIP, and MEP are significantly reduced.
- Upper airway obstruction with abnormal vocal cord adduction during inspiration has been described.

DIAGNOSIS

- Relies on a compatible clinical presentation and three principal studies:
  - Positive anticholinesterase test
  - Presence of serum acetylcholine receptor antibodies
  - Electrophysiologic (EP) studies indicative of a neuromuscular junction disorder that show decrement in response to repetitive nerve stimulation
- Acetylcholine receptor-binding antibodies are identified in approximately 71–93% of patients.
- Single fiber EMG may be useful if the diagnosis remains undefined.

ASSOCIATED CONDITIONS

- Thymic hyperplasia or thymoma.
- Autoimmune conditions including rheumatoid arthritis, lupus, thyroiditis, and Graves' disease.
- Thyroid function testing should be obtained in all patients with MG.
- Thymic abnormalities are common and chest computed tomographic (CT) or magnetic resonance imaging (MRI) has been used as a screening tool in MG.

MYASTHENIC CRISIS

- 15–27% of patients experience myasthenic crisis.
- Defined as a rapid and severe decline in respiratory muscle function.
- Associated with a mortality of 4–13%.
- Cardiac dysrhythmias are a common cause of death.
- 73 episodes of myasthenic crises and respiratory failure were described in a retrospective study.
  - 50% of patients were extubated within 2 weeks.
  - Median ICU and hospital stays were 14 and 35 days, respectively.

- Independent predictors of prolonged intubation:
  - Preintubation serum bicarbonate >30 mg/dL
  - Peak VC <25 mL/kg on day 1–6 postintubation
  - Age >50 years

Treatment

- First line of therapy
  - Anticholinesterase agents, most commonly pyridostigmine
  - Respiratory muscle function improves in approximately 50% of patients
  - Side effects of therapy
    - Muscarinic effects include abdominal cramping with frequent defecation, increased urinary frequency, bronchospasm, bradycardia, fasciculations, and increased oral secretions
    - Cholinergic crisis
      - Usually occurs during initiation of therapy
      - Can be difficult to differentiate from myasthenic crisis
      - Treatment for both usually requires withholding anticholinesterase medications for 4–10 days
- Second line of therapy
  - Majority of patients require additional immunosuppressive therapy
    - Response to anticholinesterase therapy is usually incomplete and relapse is common
    - Dose escalation often leads to significant side effects
  - Corticosteroids
    - Most commonly used agents
    - Result in remission or marked improvement in approximately 75% of patients
  - Azathioprine
    - Delayed onset of action
    - Usually requires at least 3 months of therapy
  - Cyclosporine
    - Reduces acetylcholine receptor antibody production
    - Toxicity limits use
  - Cyclophosphamide
    - Beneficial in refractory patients
    - Also limited by toxicity
- Third line of therapy
  - Plasma exchange and IVIg commonly used for intensive short-term therapy
  - Plasma exchange
    - Rapidly removes acetylcholine receptor antibodies
    - Usually improves strength within several days
    - Typical treatment is with 2- to 4-L exchanges two to three times per week over a 10- to 14-day period
    - First-line therapy for myasthenic crisis
  - Intravenous immune globulin
    - Results in a rapid improvement in most patients
    - Usually reserved for use after a course of plasma exchange
- Thymectomy
  - Has been associated with clinical improvement and remission
  - Generally recommended for patients <60 years
  - Preoperative plasma exchange is recommended in patients with significant ventilatory impairment

Differential Diagnosis

- Disorders of neuromuscular transmission that mimic MG
  - Eaton-Lambert syndrome
  - Botulism
  - Tick paralysis
  - Organophosphate toxicity
  - Myasthenic-like syndrome induced by penicillamine
- Botulism
  - Toxin-mediated irreversible inhibition of neuromuscular transmission
  - Causes an acute symmetric descending paralysis that begins with bulbar impairment
  - Early bulbar involvement of botulism may initially be confused with the Miller-Fischer variant of GBS which predominantly involves the bulbar musculature
  - Most commonly associated with food-borne and intestinal sources
- Tick paralysis
  - Tick-borne neurotoxin that causes an ascending paresis or paralysis
  - Typically affects children
  - Diagnosis requires a high index of clinical suspicion
  - Treatment
    - Careful physical examination to identify and remove all ticks and their body parts
    - Close observation and supportive care
  - Significant improvement in neuromuscular strength usually occurs within several hours of tick identification and removal

DERMATOMYOSITIS AND POLYMYOSITIS

- Idiopathic inflammatory disorders which usually present with progressive symmetrical muscle weakness over several months.
- An acute presentation with rapidly evolving muscle weakness is less common.
- Shoulder and pelvic girdle muscles are most often affected.
- Neck flexion muscles are weakened in up to 50% of patients with sparing of facial muscles.
- Pharyngeal muscle involvement may present with dysphonia or dysphagia.

- Myalgias and muscle tenderness occur in up to 50% of patients.
- Etiology is likely related to an immune-mediated mechanism.
- Clinical predictors of poor outcome:
  - Symptom duration >6 months before diagnosis
  - Severe symptoms
  - Presence of dysphagia

DIAGNOSIS

- Diagnostic criteria include
  - Presence of symmetrical proximal muscle weakness
  - Elevated skeletal muscle enzymes
  - Compatible findings on electromyography and skeletal muscle biopsy
  - Characteristic dermatologic findings in DM
  - Heliotropic changes of the eyelids
  - Gottron sign
- Muscle enzymes
  - Creatine phosphokinase is most consistent indicator of muscle inflammation
  - Others include aldolase, aspartate aminotransferase, alanine aminotransferase, and lactate dehydrogenase
- Electromyography
  - Typically reveals features of a generalized myopathic disorder
  - May be normal in 10–15% of patients
- Muscle biopsy is most definitive and demonstrates variable degrees of type I and II fiber necrosis and inflammation

IMPORTANT COMPLICATIONS

- Respiratory and cardiovascular complications are main concern in the ICU
- Respiratory complications
  - Infectious pneumonia from immunosuppression
  - Aspiration pneumonia
    - Dysphagia suggests pharyngeal muscle dysfunction and increased risk of aspiration
    - Most common pulmonary complication
  - Respiratory muscle weakness
    - Both inspiratory and expiratory muscles are involved
    - Reported in up to one-third of patients
  - Interstitial lung disease
    - Identified in nearly one-third of patients
    - Nonspecific interstitial pneumonitis is most common underlying histopathologic lesion
- Cardiac complications
  - Tachyarrhythmias and other conduction abnormalities
  - Myocarditis
  - Dilated cardiomyopathy
  - Chronic pulmonary hypertension

TREATMENT

- Corticosteroids
  - Most patients respond over weeks to months
  - Requires high-dose therapy (0.5–1.5 mg/kg prednisone) that can be gradually tapered after patient response
- Alternative immunosuppressive agents
  - Considered in patients with poor prognostic markers or limited response to corticosteroids
  - Options include methotrexate, azathioprine, and cyclophosphamide
  - Methotrexate or azathioprine may be particularly useful for corticosteroid intolerance and long-term maintenance therapy
- Alternative therapies
  - Refractory patients have been treated with IVIg, cyclosporine, tacrolimus, alkylating agents, and tumor necrosis factor inhibitors
  - IVIg
    - 71% of patients refractory to combination immunosuppressive therapy showed significant improvement in strength after treatment with IVIg
    - IVIg also reported to be beneficial for life-threatening esophageal involvement
  - Surgical division of the cricopharyngeal muscle has been used for severe refractory cricopharyngeal achalasia
  - A pacemaker-defibrillator should be considered for serious conduction abnormalities or ventricular dysrhythmias

MITOCHONDRIAL DISEASE

- Metabolic myopathies result from acquired mutations in genes coding for critical proteins in glycolysis, fatty acid oxidation, or oxidative phosphorylation.
- Increasingly recognized disorders that may present with diverse manifestations in the critical care setting including respiratory muscle dysfunction.
- Possible indicators of an underlying mitochondrial disorder:
  - Unexplained dyspnea progressing to respiratory failure
  - Sedative-related respiratory failure out of proportion to sedative dose
  - Respiratory failure with persistent unexplained lactic acidosis
  - Prolonged paralysis following neuromuscular blockade
  - Unexplained difficulty weaning from mechanical ventilation

DIAGNOSIS

- Glycolytic disorders suggested by lactate-to-pyruvate ratio >20.

- Disorders of fatty acid oxidation suggested by low carnitine levels.
- Muscle biopsies are usually diagnostic and have characteristic findings on light and electron microscopy.

TREATMENT
- Primarily supportive.
- Includes treatment of precipitating infections and withholding sedatives and neuromuscular blockers.
- High carbohydrate diet may be beneficial in fatty acid oxidation disorders.

NEUROMUSCULAR DISORDERS ACQUIRED IN THE INTENSIVE CARE UNIT

- Acquired NMDs are the most common cause of severe generalized weakness in the ICU.
- While the neuromuscular dysfunction is generally reversible, respiratory muscle involvement can lead to prolonged mechanical ventilation and delayed weaning.
- After successful extubation patients often require prolonged physical rehabilitation and may be unable to perform basic activities of daily living for weeks to months.
- Recent studies have documented significant weakness up to several years after hospital discharge suggesting the possibility of permanent disability.
- Increased awareness over the past two decades has brought into focus the major medical, economic, and psychosocial costs of ICU-acquired neuromuscular dysfunction.

CAUSES OF INTENSIVE CARE UNIT-ACQUIRED WEAKNESS

- Three basic causes of ICU-acquired neuromuscular weakness:
  - Persistent blockade of the neuromuscular junction after NMBA
  - Sensorimotor axonal polyneuropathy
  - Acute myopathy
- Diagnosis is usually made by EP studies and muscle and nerve biopsy.
- Elucidation of the underlying cause of weakness can be difficult and combined disorders of muscle and nerve may occur.

PERSISTENT NEUROMUSCULAR JUNCTION BLOCKADE

- Paralysis with NMBAs can result in residual blockade of the neuromuscular junction after discontinuation.
- Rare cause of persistent neuromuscular weakness.
- The use of vecuronium in patients with renal failure may result in accumulation of the active metabolite 3-desacetylvecuronium and prolonged paralysis.
- Diagnosis can be made by EP studies with repetitive nerve stimulation protocol.

CRITICAL ILLNESS POLYNEUROPATHY

- First described in the 1980s by Bolton and colleagues who reported a group of critically ill patients who developed generalized weakness after several weeks in the ICU.
- Most patients had underlying sepsis and underwent neurologic evaluation for diffuse limb weakness or because of difficulty weaning from mechanical ventilation.
- Neurologic examination findings:
  - Distal muscles affected most prominently
  - Sparing of the cranial nerves
  - Reduced or absent deep tendon reflexes
- Electroneurography (ENG) and EMG suggested an axonal sensorimotor polyneuropathy.
- Survivors had parallel improvement in EP studies and clinical examination over several months.
- Pathogenesis:
  - Mechanism is not understood.
  - The peripheral nervous system may be a target for tissue damage in the setting of sepsis.
  - Sepsis-induced loss of effective vascular autoregulation, increased microvascular permeability, and cytokine-mediated neuronal injury may be involved.

INTENSIVE CARE UNIT-ACQUIRED MYOPATHY (CRITICAL ILLNESS MYOPATHY)

- A severe ICU-acquired myopathy was first reported 25 years ago, with numerous individual case reports and case series having been published subsequently.
- Myopathy was most often described in the setting of ventilated status asthmaticus patients who were treated with corticosteroids and NMBAs.
- However, myopathy has also been documented in patients treated with corticosteroids without paralysis and in critically ill septic patients who received neither corticosteroids nor NMBAs.
- Some authors have attempted to subdivide ICU-acquired myopathies but it is not clear that distinct subtypes exist.
- A recent editorial suggested the term critical illness myopathy be used as the sole descriptor for all instances of ICU-acquired myopathy.

SYMPTOMS

- Typically not recognized until withdrawal of sedation allows neuromuscular assessment.
- Generalized muscle weakness with variable manifestations based on severity:
  - Less severe—predominantly distal weakness with foot and wrist drop.
  - More severe—quadriplegic paresis that may resemble a "locked in" state or even coma.
  - Reflexes may be depressed or absent.
- Sensation is intact.
- Respiratory muscle function is relatively preserved even in setting of near-quadriplegic limb weakness.

DIAGNOSIS

- Serum creatine kinase (CK) levels
  - Elevated or normal
  - Neither establish nor exclude an underlying myopathy
- EMG
  - Normal or decreased compound muscle action potential (CMAP) amplitudes depending on severity
  - Spontaneous fibrillations and positive sharp waves in resting muscle similar to critical illness polyneuropathy
  - Voluntary contractions elicit a characteristic myopathic pattern of abundant low amplitude, short duration polyphasic units with early recruitment
- Muscle biopsy
  - Pathologic findings are variable
  - Most common finding is fiber atrophy and vacuolization without inflammation
  - Electron microscopy
    - Selective loss of myosin with relative sparing of actin and Z bands
    - Highly characteristic of ICU-acquired myopathy

PATHOGENESIS

- Pathophysiology is uncertain.
- Myosin loss may interfere with normal contractility.
- May also be related to temporary muscle inexcitability detected by direct muscle stimulation.
  - Documented in patients with severe ICU-acquired myopathy related to corticosteroids and NMBAs.
  - Also found in a heterogenous group of patients with ICU weakness who had not received either corticosteroids or NMBAs.

POLYNEUROPATHY, MYOPATHY, OR "POLYNEUROMYOPATHY"

DIAGNOSTIC DILEMMA

- ICU-acquired neuromuscular weakness often presents a diagnostic dilemma: polyneuropathy, myopathy, or both.
- Studies using standard ENG/EMG and muscle histopathology have failed to differentiate a primary neuropathy from a myopathy.
- EMG differentiation between an axonal motor polyneuropathy and severe myopathy requires patient cooperation and the inability to cooperate may preclude reliable diagnosis.
- Sensory ENG studies might be limited by tissue edema.
- Routine histopathologic findings in muscle biopsy specimens may be similar.
- Recent evidence suggests that both polyneuropathy and myopathy may coexist.

CLINICAL IMPLICATIONS

- A purely clinical approach that defines the presence of a "critical illness weakness syndrome" may be adequate.
- Since there is no specific therapy, clarification of the underlying mechanisms of ICU-acquired weakness may only be important from a research perspective.
- However, EP studies may detect rare cases of GBS triggered by acute nonneurologic critical illness.
- In addition, the prognosis for recovery may be different with a pure myopathy and severe axonal polyneuropathy (see below).

INTENSIVE CARE UNIT-ACQUIRED WEAKNESS: INCIDENCE AND RISK FACTORS

- Studies have generally focused on two types of patient cohorts:
  - Status asthmaticus
  - Heterogeneous ICU population in which sepsis, systemic inflammatory response syndrome (SIRS), and multiorgan failure were dominant

STATUS ASTHMATICUS

- In studies of asthma patients who acquire a myopathy in the ICU systemic corticosteroid use has been universal and most received NMBAs.
- Ventilated and paralyzed asthmatic patients have a 30% incidence of myopathy.
- The risk increases with duration of paralysis and the incidence is similar with steroidal and nonsteroidal NMBAs.
- Myopathy has also been reported in mechanically ventilated patients with airflow obstruction who received corticosteroids and deep sedation without paralysis.
- This suggests that prolonged paralysis increases the risk of myopathy in status asthmaticus but avoidance of NMBAs does not eliminate the risk of neuromuscular weakness.

SEPSIS, SIRS, AND OTHER CAUSES OF CRITICAL ILLNESS

Incidence of Intensive Care Unit-Acquired Paresis

- The reported incidence has varied widely due to differences in diagnostic criteria and case mix.
- In studies of patients with sepsis and multiorgan failure, the reported incidence has been 70–82%.

Risk Factors for Intensive Care Unit-Acquired Paresis

- Most studies involving mixed ICU populations (primarily sepsis, SIRS, and multiorgan dysfunction) have not found a relationship between corticosteroid and/or NMBA use and persistent muscle weakness.
- Multiple risk factors have been identified in this population:
  - Sepsis
  - Higher APACHE (Acute Physiology, Age, Chronic Health Evaluation) III score and presence of SIRS
  - Duration of mechanical ventilation
  - Presence of multiorgan dysfunction
- One multicenter prospective study, however, found corticosteroid therapy to be a significant risk factor for ICU-acquired paresis.

Outcomes

- Recovery rates from ICU-acquired weakness have varied greatly.
- Resolution of severe quadriparesis in the setting of severe asthma treated with corticosteroids and NMBAs has occurred within 10–14 days but may require several weeks.
- In studies in mixed ICU populations significantly longer recovery times have been reported.
- Two prospective studies found that all survivors recovered by 2–3 months with a median recovery time of 21 days.
- Recent evidence suggests that ICU-acquired weakness may be prolonged and potentially permanent.
  - A study in 109 ARDS survivors found significant functional limitation at 1 year largely attributed to muscle wasting and weakness.
  - Another study found that one-third of patients with ICU stays >1 month had persistent weakness 1–5 years after discharge.
  - An evaluation of 19 rehabilitation patients with severe ICU-acquired weakness found that 33% had persistent quadriparesis 2 years after discharge.
  - Finally, 85% patients in one study had incomplete recovery 1–2 years after ICU discharge.
- The data combined suggest that patients with ICU-acquired weakness may never fully recover with potentially profound effects on functional capacity and quality of life.

Treatment and Prevention

- There is no specific treatment other than physical rehabilitation.
- The risk of neuromuscular weakness may be largely determined by the severity and duration of the underlying illness and may not be easily preventable.
- Unproved but potentially beneficial preventative strategies:
  - Maintaining as much muscle activity as is safely possible during critical illness
  - Avoidance of oversedation and decreased duration of ventilatory support by daily period of sedation withdrawal
  - Tight glycemic control in ICU

BIBLIOGRAPHY

Bednarik J, Lukas Z, Vondracek P. Critical illness polyneuromyopathy: the electrophysiological components of a complex entity. *Intensive Care Med* 2003;29:1505–1514.

De Jonghe B, Sharshar T, Lefaucheur JP, et al. Paresis acquired in the intensive care unit: a prospective multicenter study. *JAMA* 2002;288:2859–2867.

DiMauro S, Schon EA. Mitochondrial respiratory-chain diseases. *N Engl J Med* 2003;348:2656–2668.

Fletcher SN, Kennedy DD, Ghosh IR, et al. Persistent neuromuscular and neurophysiologic abnormalities in long-term survivors of prolonged critical illness. *Crit Care Med* 2003;31:1012–1016.

Hall JB, Schmidt, GA, Wood LDH. *Principles of Critical Care*, 3rd ed. New York, NY: McGraw-Hill; 2005:1123–1136.

Henderson RD, Lawn ND, Fletcher DD, et al. The morbidity of Guillain-Barre syndrome admitted to the intensive care unit. *Neurology* 2003;60:17–21.

Herridge MS, Cheung AM, Tansey CM, et al. One-year outcomes in survivors of the acute respiratory distress syndrome. *N Engl J Med* 2003;348:683–693.

Laghi F, Tobin MJ. Disorders of the respiratory muscles. *Am J Respir Crit Care Med* 2003;168:10–48.

Ragette R, Mellies U, Schwake C, et al. Patterns and predictors of sleep disordered breathing in primary myopathies. *Thorax* 2002;57:724–728.

Schnabel A, Reuter M, Biederer J, et al. Interstitial lung disease in polymyositis and dermatomyositis: clinical course and response to treatment. *Semin Arthritis Rheum* 2003;32:273–284.

Sharshar T, Chevret S, Bourdain F, et al. Early predictors of mechanical ventilation in Guillain-Barre syndrome. *Crit Care Med* 2003;31:278–283.

Tobin MJ, Brochard L, Rossi A. ATS/ERS statement on respiratory muscle testing. Assessment of respiratory muscle function in the intensive care unit. *Am J Respir Crit Care Med* 2002;166:610–623.

van den Berghe G, Wouters P, Weekers F, et al. Intensive insulin therapy in the critically ill patients. *N Engl J Med* 2001;345: 1359–1367.

Ward NS, Hill NS. Pulmonary function testing in neuromuscular disease. *Clin Chest Med* 2001;22:769–781.

77 HEAD TRAUMA

Nina M. Patel

KEY POINTS

- Injury from head trauma can be potentiated by subsequent hypoxia and ischemia, which should be avoided if at all possible.
- Invasive monitoring of ICP should be considered in carefully selected patients with head trauma.
- Prophylaxis of and further aggressive treatment of seizures after head trauma should be instituted.
- Systemic sepsis is often a late complication of head trauma and early empiric antibiotics coupled to source control should be pursued.

INTRODUCTION

- Traumatic brain injury (TBI) occurs in 3/1000 people per year in the United States.
- Motor vehicle accidents (MVA) are the most common cause of TBI, followed by falls, assault, and penetrating trauma.
- Alcohol intoxication is a causal or contributory factor in 10–50% of head trauma occurrences.

NORMAL CEREBRAL PHYSIOLOGY

- Cerebral blood flow (CBF) is determined by the equation:

$$\text{CBF} = \frac{\text{Cerebral perfusion pressure (CPP)}}{\text{Cerebral vascular resistance}}$$

(normal = 50 mL/100 g brain tissue/min)

- CPP is determined by the equation:
    - CPP = mean arterial pressure (MAP) − intracranial pressure (ICP) (normal CPP = 70–100 mmHg, ICP = 0–10 mmHg)
    - In a range of CPP of 50–150 mmHg, autoregulation of cerebrovascular resistance occurs to maintain CBF.
    - Significant decreases in MAP or increases in ICP can lead to a CPP that is too low to be corrected by autoregulation.

PATHOPHYSIOLOGY

- Primary brain injury results from direct mechanical injury to the brain parenchyma. Injury may be focal or diffuse. Leading etiologies of primary brain injury include:
    - *Skull fracture*—depressed or nondepressed, linear or stellate
    - *Epidural hematoma*—between skull and dura mater, often temporal or temporoparietal, results from middle meningeal artery tear, often lenticular in shape
    - *Subdural hematoma*—between dura mater and brain, results from tear of bridging vein, often crescent-shaped, occurs in up to 30% of severe head injuries
    - *Intracranial hemorrhage*—intraparenchymal hematoma, frontal or temporal lobes, may not appear until >24 hours following injury
    - *Diffuse axonal injury*—acceleration-deceleration (most often with a MVA) leads to shearing forces with resultant axonal injury
- Secondary brain injury is the consequence of altered physiologic responses in reaction to primary brain injury.
    - Two major contributing factors to secondary brain injury are hypotension and hypoxia.
    - Intracranial hypertension (ICH), dysregulation of total body sodium and water content, infection and coagulopathy are potential manifestations of secondary brain injury.
    - Many aspects in the management of primary brain injury are directed toward preventing or controlling secondary brain injury.

DIAGNOSIS

- Evaluation of the patient with head trauma begins with a thorough history (when available), physical examination assessing sites of injury, and a neurologic examination (including appraisal of brainstem reflexes).
- The gross neurologic examination focuses on identifying the presence or absence of a focal deficit and the level of consciousness.
- Level of consciousness is assessed with the Glasgow Coma Scale (GCS; see Table 77-1):
    - 13–15 = mild head injury
    - 9–12 = moderate head injury
    - ≤8 = severe head injury

TABLE 77-1 The GCS Score

FINDING	SCORE
Eye opening	
Spontaneous	4
To voice	3
To pain	2
None	1
Verbal response	
Oriented	5
Confused speech	4
Inappropriate words	3
None	2
Inappropriate words	1
Motor response	
Obeys commands	6
Localizes pain	5
Withdraws	4
Abnormal flexion	3
Extension	2
None	1

- If there is concern for cervical spine injury, cervical spine films should be performed prior to manipulating the cervical spine.
- Head computed tomography (CT) should be performed in all patients with a depressed GCS score to evaluate for intracranial hematoma, cerebral edema, intracerebral hemorrhage, or cerebral infarction.

MANAGEMENT

- The goals of acute and continued management of TBI center upon: (a) preservation of cerebral oxygenation, (b) maintenance of cerebral perfusion, (c) avoidance of secondary brain injury, and (d) prompt neurosurgical evaluation.

INITIAL

- Airway stabilization with either orotracheal or nasotracheal intubation is essential in all patients with GCS ≤8 (coma).
- Short-term modest hyperventilation (PCO_2 to 30–35 mmHg) to acutely decrease ICP is indicated, though continuous and aggressive hyperventilation (PCO_2 <25 mmHg) may increase risk of cerebral vasoconstriction and decrease CBF.
- Volume resuscitation with normal saline should be instituted to achieve a stable circulation with a target CPP >70 mmHg. Hypotonic solutions should be avoided. Hypertonic saline may effectively increase intravascular volume while decreasing cerebral edema.
- Timely neurosurgical consultation to determine if lesion is amenable to surgical therapy.

MEDICAL MANAGEMENT IN INTENSIVE CARE UNIT

- Intracranial hypertension is defined as an ICP >20 mmHg for >5–10 minutes. The presence of elevated ICP implies decreased CBF and is associated with poorer outcomes in patients with TBI. ICP monitoring is often used to indirectly measure CBF, as there is no direct means to measure CBF.
  - Aggressive monitoring of ICP with an intraventricular or subdural pressure monitor is recommended in patients with GCS scores of <10. Alternative methods of monitoring CBF include evoked potentials, electroencephalography, and jugular venous oximetry.
  - Aggressive control of fever, titrated mechanical ventilation with goals of PO_2 >70 mmHg and mild hypocapnia (PCO_2 30–35 mmHg) at minimal levels of positive end-expiratory pressure, elevation of the head of the bed to 30° to maximize jugular venous drainage, and sedation to minimize acute increases in ICP are all integral components in the medical management of ICH.
  - Mild hypothermia (32–34°C) has not been consistently shown to confer significant neuroprotective benefit in randomized, controlled trials.
  - Paralysis, osmotic diuresis with mannitol (0.5–1.0 g/kg of 20% solution q 2-6 h, m goal serum osmolality 310–320 mOsm/kg H_2O), and/or drainage of CSF with an intraventricular catheter is pursued if elevated ICP persists despite conservative measures. Overdiuresis without volume repletion in patients receiving mannitol will lead to hypovolemia and may compromise CPP.
  - If all of the above measures fail to control ICP, a pentobarbital (10 mg/kg bolus over 10 minutes, 1–3 mg/kg/h with invasive blood pressure monitoring) coma may be utilized as a last resort.
- Adjunctive aspects of management of patients with TBI include: seizure prophylaxis (phenytoin), nutritional support (enteral feeding), stress ulcer prophylaxis, deep vein thrombosis (DVT) prophylaxis, and rehabilitation.
- Abnormal free water regulation in TBI may give rise to syndrome of inappropriate antidiuretic hormone (SIADH) or diabetes insipidus, thus complicating management of fluid and electrolyte status. Serum and urine osmolarity and sodium measurements are useful

in determining which disorder is present. If SIADH is present, free water restriction should be implemented. Diabetes insipidus is treated with desmopressin.

PROGNOSIS AND CONCLUSIONS

- There is a 30–50% mortality rate associated with TBI.
- Factors associated with a poor outcome include: older age, initial low GCS, significant intracranial bleed, hypotension, hypoxia, elevated ICP, and/or significant associated systemic injury.
- Meticulous initial evaluation, early neurosurgical consultation, aggressive vigilance in managing secondary brain injury, and maintaining adequate CBF are essential to improve outcomes in TBI.

BIBLIOGRAPHY

Mouton RJ, Pitts LW. Head injury and intracranial hypertension. In: Hall JB, Schmidt GA, Wood LDH, eds., *Principles of Critical Care*, 3rd ed. New York, NY: McGraw-Hill; 2005:1395–1408.

Narayan RK, Michel ME, Ansell Bet, et al. Clinical trials in head injury. *J Neurotrauma* 2002;19:503–507.

Polderman KH, Tjong Tjin Joe R, Peerdeman SM, et al. Effects of therapeutic hypothermia on intracranial pressure and outcome in patients with severe head injury. *Intensive Care Med* 2002;28:1563–1566.

78 COMA AND PERSISTENT VEGETATIVE STATE

Nathan Sandbo

KEY POINTS

- An essential aspect of management of the comatose patient is to assure a stable circulation and oxygenation while evaluation is conducted to avoid secondary damage to the central nervous system.
- Therapeutic hypothermia should be considered in carefully selected patients following anoxic or other brain injuries.
- A focused history, neurologic examination, and brain imaging coupled to laboratory examinations create the essential database for diagnosis of causes of coma.
- The vegetative state is a chronic condition of preserved sleep-wake cycles but with an absence of cognitive function and no awareness of self or environment.
- The longer a vegetative state persists, the less likely significant recovery of brain function becomes.

COMA

EPIDEMIOLOGY

- In the intensive care unit, the presence of coma is associated with poor outcome. Up to 61% of patients are dead within 2 weeks.
- The ability to successfully resuscitate cardiac arrest patients has increased the prevalence of nontraumatic coma in the intensive care unit.

DEFINITION AND PHYSIOLOGY

- Defined as a state of unarousable, psychological unresponsiveness, implicating a disorder in the two primary components of consciousness, arousal, and awareness.
- Coma should be distinguished from other similar disorders:
  - Hypersomnia—characterized by excess drowsiness
  - Akinetic mutism—defined by a silent, alert, and awake appearance, with no response to environmental stimuli
  - Locked-in syndrome—a state of paralysis of all somatic musculature, but with preserved consciousness. Occurs mainly with pontine infarction or may be mimicked by neuromuscular paralysis from pharmacologic agents
- Most sensory stimuli pass through the ascending reticular activating system (ARAS), which lies in the center of the brain stem. Damage to this system from ischemia, infection, or compression can result in coma.

EVALUATION

- Coma of both traumatic and nontraumatic etiologies can be graded using the Glasgow Coma Scale (GCS). A patient's score can be from 3 to 15, and is determined by the sum of three components: motor response, verbal response, and eye opening. Although this scoring system provides prognostic information, it is not as reliable as a thorough assessment of individual components of brain stem reflexes.
- Neurologic examination should focus on:
  - Assessment of response to different degrees of external stimuli: verbal command, touch (such as light shaking), and finally noxious stimulation such as nail bed pressure or supraorbital pressure.

- All responses should be recorded:
  - Purposeful attempts to remove the stimuli implies preservation of brain stem function and connection to the cerebral hemisphere.
  - Decorticate (flexor) posturing indicates cerebral damage or toxic depression.
  - Decerebrate (extensor) posturing indicates destructive lesion of the midbrain and upper pons or severe metabolic insults.
  - Absence of motor function as shown by flaccid paralysis indicates severe brain stem damage.
- Eye opening to varying degrees of stimuli (spontaneous, speech, pain, or none):
  - Any eye opening indicates preserved function of the ARAS.
- Size and reactivity of pupils:
  - Small reactive pupils may indicate metabolic brain disease. Pinpoint pupils suggest narcotic overdose.
  - Bilateral fixed and dilated pupils are due to sympathetic overactivity from endogenous catecholamines (seizure, anoxic ischemia), exogenous catechols (norepinephrine, dopamine), or atropine like drugs.
  - Midposition and fixed pupils imply both sympathetic and parasympathetic failure at the level of the midbrain and is found in brain death.
  - Unilateral dilated pupil suggests third nerve compression due to a space-filling defect (mass, herniation).
- Assessment of eye movements:
  - Deep coma usually has no spontaneous eye movement.
  - Roving pupils suggest brain stem function without cortical input.
  - When cortical input is depressed, but brain stem function remains, passive head motion will result in conjugate deviation to the side opposite the direction of motion (doll's eye reflex). Absence of this reflex is suggestive of brain stem injury.
  - Confirmation can be made by the cold coloric test, in which ice-cold water is infused into the external auditory canal. Comatose patients have tonic deviation toward the side of infusion, normal patients have deviation toward the side of infusion and additionally have nystagmus away from that side. Brain death results in the absence of any response.
- Pattern of breathing:
  - Cheyne-Stokes breathing: a crescendo-decrescendo pattern of rate and depth of respiration.
  - Central neurogenic hyperventilation is sustained hyperpnea found in patients with upper brain stem damage.
- Assess for presence of focal neurologic deficits, such as unilateral muscle weakness. Note presence of myoclonus, or evidence of seizure activity.

- As well as assessing for focal neurologic syndromes, a thorough assessment of systemic disorders which can cause coma is warranted. Common syndromes that cause coma should be sought such as hypothermia, drug ingestion, metabolic derangements present on the laboratory panel, evidence of sepsis syndrome in the circulatory examination.
- Laboratory assays of serum looking for infection, electrolyte abnormalities, and toxic ingestion should be sent.
- Imaging of the brain is most quickly and reliably achieved by computed tomography (CT) looking for structural lesions or hemorrhage.
- Acquisition of cerebrospinal fluid (CSF) for cell count and electroencephalogram (EEG) looking for subclinical seizures or diffuse slowing suggestive of a metabolic encephalopathy are also indicated in almost all cases, although exclusion of a mass lesion or other cause of intracranial hypertension must precede lumbar puncture.

DIFFERENTIAL DIAGNOSIS

- Metabolic and toxic etiologies are the most common causes of depressed consciousness. Metabolic coma usually results in preservation of the pupillary response, as opposed to structural etiologies. Metabolic coma may be accompanied by asterixis, myoclonus, tremor, or seizures.
- Head trauma and cerebrovascular disease are also common causes of coma.
- Hypoxic-ischemic encephalopathy is a devastating cause of coma in the intensive care unit. Cardiac arrest is the most common cause. Other causes include severe hypotension, status epilepticus, increased intracranial pressure, head trauma, and hyperviscosity syndromes.
- Supratentorial mass lesions usually are accompanied by focal neurologic signs.

TREATMENT

- Maintenance of adequate cerebral perfusion and oxygenation is the mainstay of therapy in coma.
- Identification and, if possible, correction of the underlying etiology, such as metabolic derangements.
- Airway protection is paramount as coma patients lack protective reflexes.
- Empiric initial treatment with intravenous glucose, usually accompanied by thiamine.
- Identification and treatment of seizures.
- Identification and treatment of intracranial hypertension, especially in traumatic head injury and hemorrhagic or ischemic cerebrovascular accident (CVA).

- Identification and prompt treatment of systemic infections.
- Treatment of hyperthermia with antipyretics.
- Consideration for therapeutic hypothermia in selected patients (closed head trauma, anoxic-ischemic injury secondary to cardiac arrest).

PERSISTENT VEGETATIVE STATE

- Chronic condition characterized by preserved sleep wake cycles, with an absence of evidence of cognitive function, and lack of awareness of self and environment. Usually results from severe, diffuse brain injury secondary to anoxic damage. Brain stem functions remain intact.
- The presence of this state for more than a few weeks is termed a "persistent" vegetative state; whereas the term "permanent" vegetative state is a clinical diagnosis made when the likelihood of recovery is exceedingly small.
- May develop in 1–14% of patients with coma.
- Most pathologic patterns consist of either diffuse laminar cortical necrosis or diffuse axonal injury.
- Prognosis depends on cause:
    - In acute traumatic and nontraumatic brain injuries up to 33% of patients in persistent vegetative state (PVS) at 1 month regained some level of consciousness by 3 months, and 52% at 12 months. Lack of recovery at 12 months portended a bleak prognosis, with <5% regaining consciousness.
    - Nontraumatic causes of coma have a significantly worse prognosis, with <15% of patients regaining consciousness at 1 year.
    - In degenerative and metabolic brain disorders recovery after several months is unlikely.

BIBLIOGRAPHY

Booth CM, Boone RH, Tomlinson G, et al. Is this patient dead, vegetative, or severely neurologically impaired? Assessing outcome for comatose survivors of cardiac arrest. *JAMA* 2004;291:870–879.

Laureys S, Owen AM, Schiff ND. Brain function in coma, vegetative state, and related disorders. *Lancet Neurol* 2004;3:537–546.

Rosengart AJ, Frank JI. Coma, persistent vegetative state, and brain death. In: Hall JB, Schmidt GA, Wood LDH, eds., *Principles of Critical Care*, 3rd ed. New York, NY: McGraw-Hill; 2005: 1037–1053.

Wijdicks EF, Cranford RE. Clinical diagnosis of prolonged states of impaired consciousness in adults. *Mayo Clin Proc* 2005;80:1037–1046.

79 BRAIN DEATH

Nathan Sandbo

KEY POINTS

- The Uniform Determination of Death Act states that an individual who has sustained either irreversible cessation of circulatory and respiratory functions, or irreversible cessation of all function of the entire brain, including the brain stem is dead.
- The determination of death by brain criteria is based on clinical examination; importantly, the cause of coma must be known, and the cause must be sufficient to explain irreversible cessation of whole brain function.

INTRODUCTION

- The advent of mechanical ventilation and improved ability to support the circulation has led to patients with complete cessation of all brain function and cerebral blood flow, but with preserved cardiopulmonary function.
- Importantly, observational series from the 1950s detailed the eventual circulatory deterioration of these patients.
- Making the diagnosis of brain death is important not only for the patient and his/her family, but now entails the opportunity for organ donation for transplantation.
- As a result, it is of critical importance to distinguish between the severely brain injured patient and brain death.
- Currently, the primary etiologies leading to brain death in adults are traumatic head injury and subarachnoid hemorrhage.

DECLARATION OF DEATH USING NEUROLOGIC CRITERIA

- Guidelines have been established by the President's Commission in 1981 and are accepted by the American Medical Association, American Academy of Neurology, and the American Bar Association.
- The Uniform Determination of Death Act states that an individual who has sustained either irreversible cessation of circulatory and respiratory functions, or irreversible cessation of all function of the entire brain, including the brain stem is dead.
- The determination of brain death is a clinical diagnosis, and the clinical examination is the primary tool to gather the relevant data. The practitioner performing

the examination must be competent to perform the requisite tests to exacting standards. He/she must also be free of any conflict of interest.

- The core feature in establishing the diagnosis is demonstrating unresponsiveness, brain stem areflexia, and apnea.
- Prior to making the diagnosis, two preconditions must be met: (1) the etiology of the coma must be known and (2) the etiology must be adequate to explain the coma. Conversely, reversible metabolic, toxic, endocrine, or pharmacologic derangements must not be present at the time of evaluation.
- Imaging of the brain by either computed tomography (CT), magnetic resonance imaging (MRI), or both is required in the vast majority of patients as part of the workup to determine the etiology of coma.
- Confirmatory tests include electroencephalogram (EEG) and cerebral perfusion studies; however, these should be used only when the underlying etiology or the reversibility of coma is uncertain.

CRITERIA FOR BRAIN DEATH

- An individual with irreversible cessation of all function of the entire brain, including the brain stem, is dead.
- The patient must be in deep coma and unresponsive to all external stimuli, including pain, bright light, or loud noises.
- Brain stem reflexes must be absent:
    - Pupils must be unreactive to light. The size of the pupils is most often midposition (4–6 mm) although this is not required.
    - Ocular movement must be absent to passive head turning (i.e., absent oculocephalic reflex) and to irrigation of ear canals with 30 mL of iced water at head elevation of 30°.
    - Corneal reflexes must be absent.
    - Oropharyngeal reflexes (gag, cough) must be absent (if testable).
    - Apnea testing is a critical part of brain stem assessment. Patient must have a normal blood pressure and be ventilated with 100% oxygen prior to testing. A maximum stimulus for breathing is attained when PCO_2 is >60 mmHg. This usually occurs by 10–15 minutes of apnea. Arterial blood gas (ABG) should be sent to confirm the appropriate level of PCO_2 stimulus.
    - Decerebrate or decorticate posturing require intact brain stem structures at and below the level of the vestibular nuclei, and are inconsistent with brain death.
    - Spontaneous reflex movements have been well described in patients and can confuse the diagnosis of brain death. The Lazarus sign, gooseflesh followed by upper extremity extensor movements and flexion of arms and hands to the sternum; undulating toe flexion, and hip flexion have all been described. If present, a careful reassessment of the neurologic examination and confirmatory tests may be used to reassure caregivers and family of the certainty of the diagnosis.
- The cause of coma must be known and irreversible.
    - If not immediately ascertainable by clinical data and neuroimaging, confirmatory studies, such as EEG, and cerebral perfusion studies (Doppler ultrasound, cerebral angiography, or technetium scintigraphy) should be performed.
    - If present, hypothermia, hypotension, and metabolic derangements should be corrected. If a toxic ingestion is suspected, identification of the agent should be made, if possible. An observation period of four times the elimination half-life should be used prior to making the diagnosis of brain death. If an unknown agent is suspected, an observation period of 48 hours may be used.
    - After determination of brain death, family and/or legal surrogate decision-maker should be notified. Appropriate organ-procurement agencies should be contacted to facilitate approaching the legal surrogate for organ donation (Table 79-1).

TABLE 79-1 Criteria for Determination of Brain Death

1. Coma, unresponsive to stimuli above the foramen magnum.
2. Apnea off ventilator (with oxygenation) for a duration sufficient to produce hypercarbic respiratory drive (usually 10–20 min to achieve PCO_2 50–60 mmHg).
3. Absence of cephalic reflexes, including papillary, oculocephalic, oculovestibular (caloric), corneal, gag, sucking, swallowing, and extensor posturing. Purely spinal reflexes may be present, including tendon reflexes, plantar reflexes, and limb flexion to noxious stimuli.
4. Body temperature above 34°C.
5. Systemic circulation may be intact.
6. Diagnosis known to be structural cause or irreversible metabolic disturbance; absence of drug intoxication, including ethanol, sedatives, potentially anesthetizing agents, or paralyzing drugs.
7. In adults with known structural cause and without involvement of drugs or ethanol, at least 6 h of absent brain stem function; for others, including those with anoxic-ischemic brain damage, at least 24 h observation plus negative drug screen.
8. Diagnosis of brain death inappropriate in infants younger than 7 days of age. Observation of at least 48 h for infants aged 7 days to 2 months, at least 24 h of observation for those aged 2 months to 1 year, and at least 12 h for those aged 1–5 years (24 h if anoxic-ischemic brain damage). For other children, adult criteria apply.
9. Optional confirmatory studies include:
    a. EEG isoelectric for 30 min at maximal gain
    b. Absent brain stem evoked responses
    c. Absent cerebral circulation demonstrated by radiographic, radioisotope, or magnetic resonance angiography

BIBLIOGRAPHY

Guidelines for the determination of death. Report of the medical consultants on the diagnosis of death to the President's Commission for the Study of Ethical Problems in Medicine and Biomedical and Behavioral Research. *JAMA* 1981;246: 2184–2186.

Morenski JD, Oro JJ, Tobias JD, et al. Determination of death by neurological criteria. *J Intensive Care Med* 2003;18:211–221.

Rosengart AJ, Frank JI. Coma, persistent vegetative state, and brain death. In: Hall JB, Schmidt GA, Wood LDH, eds., *Principles of Critical Care*, 3rd ed. New York, NY: McGraw-Hill; 2005: 1037–1053.

Wijdicks EF. The diagnosis of brain death. *N Engl J Med* 2001;344:1215–1221.

Section 6
HEMATOLOGY AND ONCOLOGY

80 ANEMIA, TRANFUSION, MASSIVE TRANFUSION

Maria Dowell

KEY POINTS

- Anemia developing in the ICU often has a contribution from phlebotomy, but other causes of red cell loss, as well as red cell destruction or underproduction should be explored.
- For patients without active blood loss or cardiac disease, a transfusion target of 7–9 g/dL of hemoglobin appears safe.
- Massively transfused patients may develop hypothermia or coagulopathy, each of which may accelerate their further blood loss.

ANEMIA

- Common in critically ill patients and often multifactorial.
- Oxygen delivery to tissues depends on hemoglobin concentration, hemoglobin saturation, and cardiac output. Compensatory mechanisms for anemia include increasing cardiac output (overall blood flow), peripheral vascular changes (individual organ perfusion), and increased oxygen extraction.
- Evaluation of the anemic patient should determine whether or not there is active bleeding and any need for urgent transfusion. Consideration should then be given to the pathophysiologic process responsible for the anemia. Besides a careful history and examination, examination of the blood smear and evaluation of the red cell indices and reticulocyte count may provide clues to the possible pathophysiology involved.
- The differential diagnosis includes blood loss, hemolysis, sequestration, and underproduction.
  - *Blood loss*: Generally through hemorrhage or phlebotomy. Gastrointestinal bleeding is the most common site of blood loss, but retroperitoneal, intrapleural, intramuscular, or mediastinal hemorrhage may result from invasive procedures. Compensation for the daily phlebotomy that tends to occur in the ICU roughly requires a twofold increase in erythropoiesis.
  - *Hemolysis*: May be diagnosed by anemia, increased erythroid production (reticulocytosis, polychromasia, basophilic stippling, nucleated red blood cells [RBCs]), and increased RBC turnover (hemoglobinemia/uria, hyperbilirubinemia, increased lactate dehydrogenase [LDH], decreased haptoglobin). Intravascular destruction causes hemoglobinemia and may be due to glucose-6-phosphate dehydrogenase (G6PD) deficiency (Heinz bodies), microangiopathic hemolytic anemia, transfusion reaction, or erythrocytic infection. Extravascular destruction may arise from sickle cell disease and immunohemolytic anemia. Patients in the ICU may also experience microangiopathic hemolytic anemia with schistocytes (disseminated intravascular coagulation [DIC], thrombotic thrombocytopenic purpura [TTP], hemolytic uremic syndrome [HUS], valve prosthesis) or iatrogenic hemolysis from intra-aortic balloon pumps, left ventricular assist devices, and extracorporeal membrane oxygenation.
  - *Sequestration*: Splenic sequestration may arise from any causes of spleen enlargement. Anemia and mild thrombocytopenia are common and blood smears may reveal spherocytes, giant platelets, and reticulocytosis. Splenectomy may be performed if underlying disorder cannot be completely corrected.
  - *Underproduction*: An absolute reticulocyte count is a simple way to evaluate bone marrow function and an anemic patient with a low or normal reticulocyte count has at least some degree of underproduction.

Underproduction may manifest as megaloblastic anemia (folate or B_{12} deficiency), hypochromic anemia (iron deficiency), marrow infiltration (tumor, fibrosis, granulomata, miliary tuberculosis), or primary reduction in erythroid activity (chronic renal failure).

- Critically ill patients may be at increased risk for the immunosuppressive and microcirculatory complications of RBC transfusion; therefore, erythropoietin was evaluated in several studies and has been shown to reduce the number of RBC transfusions during hospitalization. As the dosing regimens varied considerably among these studies, defining the optimal dosing regimen and route of administration remains the subject of ongoing investigation. There is general agreement, however, that iron should be administered concurrently.

TRANSFUSION

- *Indications/contraindications*: In the face of increased awareness of infectious diseases transmitted by blood transfusion, in general there is no justification for transfusing anemic patients with adequate cardiovascular compensation and whose anemia will respond to medical therapy. Many critically ill patients, however, have severely limited oxygen delivery in the face of increased oxygen demand and transfusion may improve oxygenation to critical organs. Other indications include major trauma with bleeding, shock due to blood loss, intraoperative blood loss, and anemia. The Transfusion Requirements in Critical Care trial determined that a restrictive strategy of RBC transfusion (hemoglobin <7 g/dL to preserve a level of 7–9 g/dL) was at least as effective and likely superior to liberal transfusion (hemoglobin <10 g/dL to preserve level of 10–12 g/dL). The possible exception to this was the setting of acute myocardial infarction (MI) and unstable angina.
- *Blood components*: One unit (approximately 200–250 mL) of packed RBCs will increase the hemoglobin by 1 g/dL and hematocrit by 3% in an average-sized adult.
- *Adverse effects/immunologic considerations*: The most common adverse effect, but associated with few clinical consequences, is allergic, nonhemolytic, febrile transfusion reaction. Also commonly seen are RBC alloimmunization and leukocyte/thrombocyte alloimmunization. RBC transfusions are associated with higher rates of infectious complications probably related to exogenous iron availability to the bacteria and immunosuppressive effects related to leukocyte exposure and sensitization. Hepatitis A/B/C, human immunodeficiency virus (HIV), human T-cell lymphotropic viruses (HTLV), and parvovirus B19 infections occur rarely. In several hematologic conditions (aplastic anemia, acute leukemia, myelodysplasia), transfusion should be avoided if possible to reduce the risk of alloimmunization in bone marrow transplant candidates or those requiring long-term blood product support.
- *Iron overload*: It is generally advisable to avoid transfusions in stable patients with chronic anemia to avoid the complications of iron overload (cardiac failure, arrhythmias, cirrhosis). Diagnosis of iron overload requires elevated serum iron content, transferrin saturation, ferritin, and evidence for increased hepatic iron stores.
- *Transfusion therapy*: Workup for transfusion requires RBC typing and an antibody screen and crossmatch (30–45 minutes). If the situation requires extremely urgent transfusion, a blood sample must be delivered to the blood bank before blood is administered after which group O, Rh-negative packed RBC may be given. If time permits in emergent situations or massive transfusions, an abbreviated immediate spin crossmatch (5 minutes) can be done and involves reaction of the recipient's serum with donor red cells to look for IgM to ABO blood groups.

MASSIVE TRANSFUSION

- Generally refers to volume transfused within a 24-hour period that approximates the patient's normal blood volume.
- Clinical results depend on the effects of shelf storage and the dilutional effects on platelet number and coagulation factors. Theoretically, aged RBC packs experience seepage of K^+ into the plasma, reduced plasma bicarbonate levels, rise in lactate concentration, and deterioration of some of the coagulation factors. With the rise in serum K^+ during storage, massive transfusion could lead to hyperkalemia, however, this rarely occurs except in patients with shock, acidosis, and reduced renal perfusion. Hypokalemia may actually be more common as a result of the hypokalemic RBCs uptake of K^+ after transfusion.
- Due to the rise in lactic acid content of stored RBCs, massive transfusion may result in a temporary shift of the oxygen dissociation curve of hemoglobin with tighter binding of O_2 to hemoglobin and impaired tissue oxygenation. The temporary increase in O_2 affinity can be compensated for by increases in cardiac output and regeneration of 2,3-bisphosphoglycerate (2,3-DPG) by RBCs.

- Normal functioning platelets are virtually absent in stored blood. Useful tests in guiding management of coagulopathy during massive transfusion are platelet count, fibrinogen level. Prothrombin time (PT), partial thromboplastin time (PTT), and bleeding time may also be useful.
- Hypocalcemia may result from the binding of calcium by the citrate anticoagulant in stored blood. However, citrate is rapidly metabolized by the liver and clinically significant hypocalcemia does not usually develop. Nevertheless, the serum ionized calcium level and an ECG to assess QT interval should be monitored during massive transfusion.
- Massive transfusions may result in lowering of the patients' core body temperature as the rapidly administered products may not have been fully warmed to body temperature. Hypothermia can cause a coagulopathy (see Chap. 72).

BIBLIOGRAPHY

Givens M, Lapointe M. Is there a place for epoetin alpha in managing anemia during critical illness? *Clin Ther* 2004;26: 819–829.

Hebert PC, Wells G, Blajchman A, et al. A multicenter, randomized, controlled clinical trial of transfusion requirements in critical care. *N Engl J Med* 1999;340:409–417.

Luce J. Anemia and blood transfusion. In: Hall JB, Schmidt GA, Wood LDH, eds., *Principles of Critical Care*, 3rd ed. New York, NY: McGraw-Hill; 2005: 1055–1064.

MacLaren R, Gasper J, Jung R, et al. Use of exogenous erythropoietin in critically ill patients. *J Clin Pharm Ther* 2004;29:195–208.

81 SICKLE CELL DISEASE

D. Kyle Hogarth

KEY POINTS

- Sickle cell disease is a disease of chronic hemolytic anemia.
- The acute manifestation of the disease is the VOC.
- Sickle cell patients will require ICU management for the ACS, very severe anemia, sepsis, stroke, priapism, and splenic sequestration.
- Red cell transfusion is an important treatment for most sickle cell patients requiring ICU management. Aggressive initiation of rapid exchange transfusion is indicated for CNS events, serious respiratory disease, or multiorgan failure in sickle cell patients.
- Patients requiring surgery should undergo preoperative red cell transfusion and attentive supportive care postoperatively.
- Secondary pulmonary hypertension is an underrecognized complication of the disease and occurs in 30% of patients.

INTRODUCTION

- Sickle cell anemia affects 1 in 500 African American births in the United States. It is an autosomal recessive disease.
- Sickle hemoglobin will form rod-like polymers in deoxygenated red cells. This occurs in areas with low oxygen tension, acidosis, or hyperosmolarity (see Fig. 81-1).
- The consequence of the polymerization of the hemoglobin is impaired blood flow and tissue damage. The subsequent ischemia and reperfusion of the tissue leads to generalized inflammation, organ dysfunction, and the potential for organ infarction.
- Fever and leukocytosis are common consequences of the tissue ischemia.
- The tissue ischemia and infarction produce severe pain. These episodes are referred to as "acute pain crisis" but are better referred to as vaso-occlusive crisis (VOC). Depending on the organ location and syndrome, the vaso-occlusive crisis sometimes has other names, for example, acute chest syndrome (ACS).

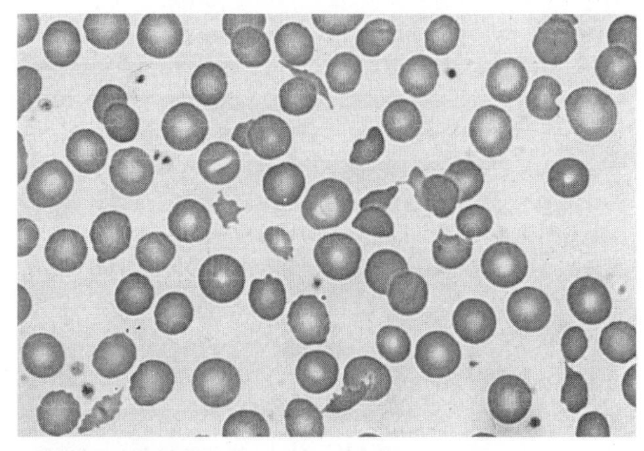

FIG. 81-1 Sickle cells. Homozygous sickle cell disease. SOURCE: Lichtman MA, Beutler E, Kipps TJ, eds., *Williams Hematology*, 7th ed. New York, NY: McGraw Hill.

- The microcirculation can be acutely or chronically impaired in virtually any organ in the body. Typically, chronic dysfunction of organs follows after damage done from a lifetime of acute attacks.
- Sickle cell disease is essentially a severe hemolytic anemia. The hemolysis is mostly extravascular and is due to mechanical injury and destruction of erythrocytes that are no longer pliable or flexible due to intracellular hemoglobin S polymerization.
- Labs at baseline typically demonstrate a normocytic, normochromic anemia with reticulocytosis.
- Hydroxyurea reduces disease severity and mortality rate.

PHYSIOLOGY

- As a consequence of the chronic anemia and diminished oxygen-carrying capacity, the cardiac output is increased.
- Most adult patients are functionally asplenic due to subclinical infarctions of the spleen.
- The baseline glomerular filtration rate is elevated, leading to hyperfiltration. Thus, a low baseline serum creatinine range is normal and typically ranges from 0.5 to 0.6 mg/dL. This is due to the increased cardiac output and higher plasma content. Therefore, a serum creatinine level >0.6 mg/dL raises the concern about renal insufficiency.
- Sickle cell patients have a baseline hyperdynamic cardiovascular examination. They have relatively low blood pressure, low systemic and pulmonary vascular resistance, and high cardiac output. Baseline sickle cell patient examinations are very similar to septic patients.
- Leukocytosis is commonly present, but reticulocytes are often miscounted as white blood cells (WBCs) in the complete blood count and may give an artificially elevated WBC count.

VASO-OCCLUSIVE PAIN CRISIS

- The VOC is the most common manifestation of sickle cell anemia.
- The attacks are severely painful and result from impaired microvascular flow, and affect the bones most commonly (Fig. 81-2).

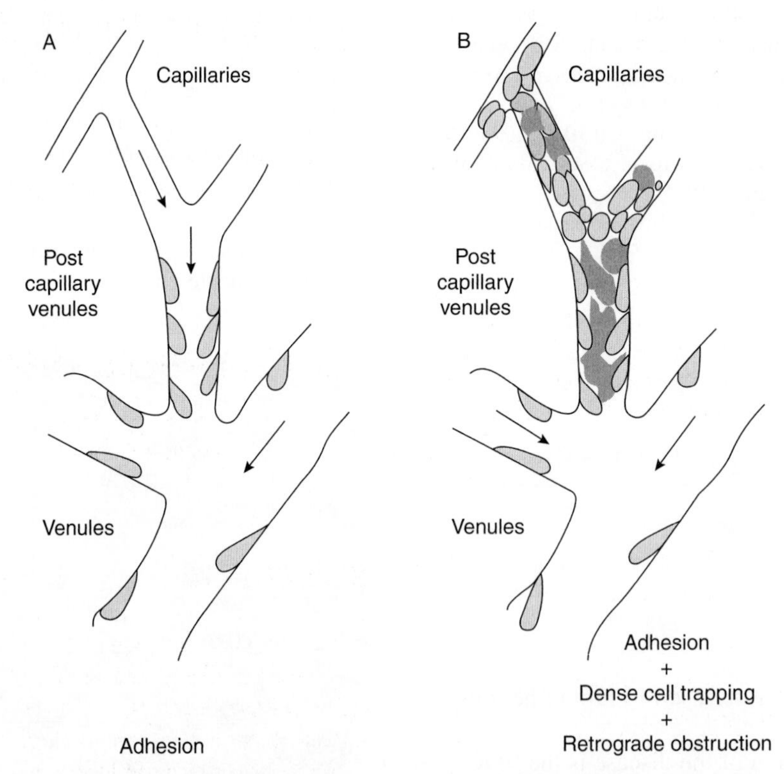

FIG. 81-2 Proposed mechanisms of vascular occlusion in sickle cell disease. Panel A (on left) illustrates adhesion of sickle cells to the vascular endothelium in postcapillary venules and venules. Panel B (on right) illustrates the subsequent trapping of dense red cells in the partially obstructed postcapillary venules, followed by retrograde obstruction.

- Management involves analgesics, including nonsteroidal anti-inflammatory medications and/or opioids. Hydration should be maintained with isotonic saline.
- Hypoxemia should be corrected immediately.
- All patients should be evaluated for and monitored for development of the ACS.

ACUTE CHEST SYNDROME

- A dreaded complication of sickle cell disease is the ACS. This VOC of the lung leads to an acute lung injury syndrome, and in extreme states is similar to the acute respiratory distress syndrome.
- ACS should be considered present in patients with a new pulmonary infiltrate, fever, and chest pain.
- Laboratory findings often include an acute drop in the hemoglobin level and elevated WBC count.
- 25% of patients with ACS will require mechanical ventilation.
- Mortality for adults with this syndrome is 9%.
- Management is pain control, IV hydration, mechanical ventilation if necessary, and antibiotics covering for both typical and atypical community-acquired organisms.
- Simple transfusion of 2–4 units of packed red blood cells (RBCs) should be initiated once ACS is diagnosed. Simple transfusion is as effective as a complete RBC exchange. However, during ACS the hemoglobin should be kept below 10 g/dL during the transfusion. As the hemoglobin tends to decline during ACS, this is usually easy to do.

SEPSIS

- Sickle cell patients are at increased risk of sepsis and meningitis from encapsulated organisms, such as *Haemophilus influenzae* and *Streptococcus pneumoniae*.
- This increased risk is due to the progressive loss of the spleen due to microinfarctions in the splenic circulation.

STROKE

- Stoke will occur in about 7% of sickle cell patients over a lifetime, with a peak incidence in adults over 50 years old.
- The strokes commonly affect large vessels.
- Management of stroke in sickle cell patients is emergency exchange transfusion.

PRIAPISM

- Prolonged erection of the penis is extremely painful and is a potential complication of sickle cell disease.
- Therapy has only been evaluated in case reports and case controls. Exchange transfusion is considered the accepted management, though it has not been rigorously tested.
- Others have tried adrenergic agonists, nitrates, percutaneous drainage and irrigation of the corpus cavernosum, and a urologic procedure called a Winter shunt.

BIBLIOGRAPHY

Charache S, Terrin ML, Moore RD, et al. Effect of hydroxyurea on the frequency of painful crises in sickle cell anemia. Investigators of the Multicenter Study of Hydroxyurea in Sickle Cell Anemia. *N Engl J Med* 1995;332:1317–1322.

Frenette PS. Sickle cell vaso-occlusion: multistep and multicellular paradigm. *Curr Opin Hematol* 2002;9:101–106.

Kato GJ and Gladwin MT, Sickle cell disease in Hall JB, Schmidt GA, Wood LDH, eds., *Principles of Critical Care*, 3rd ed. New York, NY: McGraw-Hill; 2005:1655–1670.

Ohene-Frempong K, Weiner SJ, Sleeper LA, et al. Cerebrovascular accidents in sickle cell disease: rates and risk factors. *Blood* 1998;91:288–294.

Steinberg MH, Barton F, Castro O, et al. Effect of hydroxyurea on mortality and morbidity in adult sickle cell anemia: risks and benefits up to 9 years of treatment. *JAMA* 2003;289:1645–1651.

Vichinsky EP, Neumayr LD, Earles AN, et al. Causes and outcomes of the acute chest syndrome in sickle cell disease. National Acute Chest Syndrome Study Group. *N Engl J Med* 2000;342:1855–1865.

Vichinsky EP. Current issues with blood transfusions in sickle cell disease. *Semin Hematol* 2001;38:14–22.

82 BLEEDING DISORDERS IN THE ICU

Michael Moore

KEY POINTS

- Bleeding disorders can be subdivided into vascular disorders, platelet disorders, fibrin generation disorders, fibrinolytic disorders, and complex coagulopathies.
- Brisk bleeding is rarely from spontaneous bleeding due to coagulopathy: look for another cause.
- Vascular and platelet disorders usually lead to immediate bleeding that is prolonged.
- Fibrin generation disorders usually lead to delayed bleeding after initial hemostasis.

- TTP is a serious disorder suggested by the classic pentad of fever, mental status changes, microangiopathic hemolytic anemia, low platelets, and renal dysfunction.
- Consultation with hematology is suggested for complex bleeding issues in the critically ill patient.
- General guidelines for invasive procedures in coagulopathic patients include: perform invasive procedures only when necessary, limit planned intervention as much as possible, perform under direct vision by most experienced operator available, coordinate the procedure with appropriate support staff (i.e., blood bank and pharmacy), and carefully monitor for immediate and delayed bleeding complications.

INTRODUCTION

- Generalizations to help direct workup and treatment:
  - Exclude uncomplicated vascular injury amenable to surgical hemostasis.
  - Brisk bleeding is almost never secondary to spontaneous bleeding from a coagulopathy alone.
  - Clinically significant bleeding is most often seen in the setting of a potential or known bleeding site.
  - Use initial and follow-up laboratory screening to predict and prevent bleeding complications in critically ill patients prior to procedures.
- Diagnosis of bleeding disorders in the ICU:
  - Determine history of congenital and acquired bleeding diathesis, recent surgery, pregnancy/abortion, transfusion, medications, and/or current organ dysfunction.
  - Determine by physical examination if bleeding is consistent with a known vascular injury or trauma or suggestive of a systemic disorder.
  - Mechanism of bleeding disorder and clinical presentation:
    - Vascular and platelet disorders are characterized by immediate bleeding that is prolonged after onset with petechial and mucosal abnormalities.
    - Fibrin generation disorders (coagulation cascade defects) and fibrinolysis are characterized by delayed bleeding after initial hemostasis with prominent ecchymoses or deep muscle and joint hemorrhage.
    - Complex coagulopathies may have features of both vascular/platelet disorders and coagulation cascade defects.
- Screening labs:
  - Complete blood count (CBC)
  - Peripheral smear
  - Platelet function screen and bleeding time
  - Prothrombin time (PT)/partial thromboplastin time (PTT)
  - Thrombin time
  - Functional fibrinogen level
  - Fibrin-degradation products (FDP)/D-dimer assay

VASCULAR DISORDERS

- Vascular disorders consist of vasculitides, vascular malformations, and microcirculatory obstructions.
  - Vasculitis of any cause results in increased bleeding risk secondary to vascular fragility.
  - Vascular malformations may bleed when traumatized or unintentionally biopsied.
  - Diagnosis of vasculitides is suspected by palpable purpura and absence of systemic coagulopathies.

PLATELET DISORDERS

- Platelet disorders are divided into thrombocytopenias, thrombocytosis/thrombocythemias, and thrombocytopathies.

THROMBOCYTOPENIA

- The platelet count reflects the balance between platelet production and the rate of platelet removal from the circulation and thrombocytopenia can be secondary to underproduction states, shortened platelet survival, or sequestration.

UNDERPRODUCTION THROMBOCYTOPENIAS

- Etiology—generalized decrease in marrow mass or a selective decrease in megakaryocyte number secondary to infectious states, drugs/toxins, immune mechanisms, prior radiation injury, and occasionally idiopathic hypoplastic or aplastic marrow.
- Diagnosis—history and bone marrow biopsy.
- Ineffective marrow states as a subgroup of underproduction are characterized by normal or increased blood cellularity with abnormal release of precursors into the circulation. These states are found in megaloblastic anemia with thrombocytopenia, marrow replacement by tumor or granulomas, and in metabolic states such as hypothyroidism and azotemia.

SHORTENED PLATELET SURVIVAL

- Common in critically ill patients.
- Etiology—fever, consumption of platelets secondary to bleeding, sepsis, and specific disease states.
- Specific disease states leading to shortened platelet survival include immune thrombocytopenic purpura (ITP), posttransfusion purpura (PTP), thrombotic thrombocytopenic purpura (TTP), disseminated

intravascular coagulation (DIC), and heparin-induced thrombocytopenia (HIT).

SEQUESTRATION

- Hypersplenism may result in thrombocytopenia alone or in thrombocytopenia with anemia and neutropenia.
- Can be acute or chronic; secondary to chronic liver disease, splenic venous occlusion, or leukemia/lymphoma involving the spleen.
- Diagnose an enlarged spleen by physical examination or ultrasonography.
- Treatment is splenectomy in some cases.

SPECIFIC DISEASES

Immune thrombocytopenic purpura

- Associated with exposure to specific drugs, connective tissue diseases, lymphomas, and viral infections.
- Diagnosis confirmed by finding antiplatelet antibodies in serum or on platelets.
- Therapy consists of general measures such as discontinuing offending agents and avoidance of drugs that interfere with platelet function.
- Directed therapy may involve corticosteroids, IVIG, splenectomy, or IV human anti-Rh_o (D) IgG.
- Platelet transfusion is often limited by the short survival of transfused platelets.

Posttransfusion purpura

- Diagnosis suggested by an otherwise unexplained, abrupt onset of severe thrombocytopenia following transfusion.
- Treatment—IVIG.

Thrombotic thrombocytopenic purpura

- Typical triggers—infections, drugs (especially ticlopidine and clopidogrel), chemotherapy, and malignancies.
- Intravascular clumping of platelets results in thrombocytopenia and vascular occlusion of arterial beds.
- Diagnosis—suggested by classic pentad of fever, mental status changes, microangiopathic hemolytic anemia, low platelets, and renal dysfunction.
- Important diagnostic considerations—schistocytes on a peripheral smear, negative direct Coombs' test in the setting of hemolysis.
- Standard therapy—corticosteroids and plasma exchange.
- Platelet transfusion has been shown to worsen the vaso-occlusive state.

Heparin-induced thrombocytopenia

- Heparin-induced thrombocytopenia can occur with any heparin product including low molecular weight heparin (LMWH) given or exposed by any route including heparin-coated catheters.
- Small, reversible decrease in platelet number 1–2 days after initiation of unfractionated heparin is common.
- Immune-mediated HIT is uncommon (<1% of patients) but a potentially serious complication of heparin exposure.
- After initial exposure, platelet numbers usually drop 5–7 days later with a more rapid drop over 1–2 days on re-exposure.
- Clinical consequences range from asymptomatic to life-threatening venous or arterial thrombosis.
- Clinical diagnostic criteria include otherwise unexplained thrombocytopenia <150,000/μL or a 50% decrease 2–7 days after heparin exposure.
- Treatment—discontinue all heparin products.
- Normalization of platelet count after stopping heparin confirms the presence of HIT.
- All patients with HIT are hypercoagulable and require immediate alternative anticoagulation.

Mechanical surface-related thrombocytopenia

- Platelets passing over or through mechanical surfaces can result in a decrease in platelet number.
- Common examples include cardiopulmonary bypass (CPB) and intra-aortic balloon pumps.

THROMBOCYTOSIS

- An elevated platelet count >350,000/μL is common is the ICU.
- Can be complicated by thrombosis or bleeding.
- Can be reactive or secondary to myeloproliferative states.
- Reactive thrombocytosis:
  - Most common in ICU.
  - Associated with common clinical states including inflammation, bleeding, surgery, hemolysis, severe injury, and cancer.
  - Usually uncomplicated and does not require treatment.
- Myeloproliferative states:
  - Thrombocytosis secondary to myeloproliferative states can be associated with either bleeding or thrombosis especially when the platelet count is $>1 \times 10^6$/μL.
  - Diagnosis is usually known prior to presentation.
  - Suspected by an abnormal peripheral smear or after bone marrow biopsy.
  - No definitive test is available to predict complications but a prolonged bleeding time may indicate risk. Risk is greatest in older patients with fixed vascular disease.

- Treatment for symptomatic patients:
  - Plateletpheresis
  - Avoid splenectomy
  - Anagrelide or hydroxyurea

THROMBOCYTOPATHY

- Qualitative platelet abnormalities are common in the ICU.
- Frequent contributor to other bleeding abnormalities and can be independently associated with increased bleeding risk.
- Thrombocytopathy can result from a number of clinical states including uremia, drugs, myeloproliferative disorders, dysproteinemias, cardiopulmonary disorders, and active DIC.

Uremia

- Common in ICU patients.
- Interferes with platelet function and prolongs the bleeding time.
- Hemodialysis is the most effective treatment.
- Other therapies include corticosteroids, cryoprecipitate, platelet transfusions, and intravenous estrogens.
- DDAVP will correct bleeding time but its usefulness decreases over 1–2 days.

Drugs

- Aspirin (ASA), nonsteroidal anti-inflammatory drugs (NSAIDs), ethanol, and glycoprotein (GP) IIb/IIIa platelet inhibitors are common offenders.
- ASA is a classic platelet inhibitor and irreversibly inhibits cyclooxygenase resulting in net decrease in thromboxane A_2 and prolongation of the bleeding time. After discontinuation of ASA therapy, newly formed platelets function normally and the significant effects on bleeding time usually resolve after 3 days. DDAVP or platelet transfusion will rapidly reverse significant platelet abnormalities in cases of acute bleeding.
- NSAIDs reversibly inhibit cyclooxygenase and result in shorter periods of platelet dysfunction after discontinuation.
- GP IIb/IIIa platelet inhibitors affect the bleeding time in a less predictable fashion.
- Treatment:
  - Discontinue offending agent.
  - Avoid surgery or invasive procedures for several days after the offending agent has been discontinued and new unaffected platelets are released into the circulation.
  - Platelet transfusion or DDAVP for acute bleeding or emergent procedures.

Dysproteinemias

- Abnormally increased immunoglobulins can interfere with platelet function and prolong bleeding time.

Cardiopulmonary Bypass

- Platelet contact with membranes used in CPB causes an acquired thrombocytopathy.
- Can contribute to significant bleeding in post bypass.
- Rule out hypofibrinogenemia and inadequate heparin neutralization.

FIBRIN GENERATION DISORDERS

- The coagulation cascade involves a series of events that ultimately lead to the generation of a stable fibrin clot.
- Assess the coagulation cascade by PT and activated partial thromboplastin time (aPTT).
- Bleeding can result from specific factor deficiencies, inhibitors to factors, and combined deficiency states.

FACTOR DEFICIENCIES

Hypofibrinogenemia

- Low functional fibrinogen levels are most commonly from decreased hepatic synthesis or increased consumption during DIC in ICU patients.
- Risk of spontaneous bleeding:
  - Increases when levels fall below 100 mg/dL.
  - Significantly increases when levels fall below 50 mg/dL.
  - Bleeding risk is increased by high titers of fibrin split products.
- Treatment:
  - Fresh frozen plasma (FFP) or cryoprecipitate (less volume).
  - One cryopack will increase fibrinogen level 4–10 mg/dL.
  - Measuring serial fibrinogen levels every 6–12 hours.

Hemophilia A

- Sex-linked recessive deficiency of factor VIII.
- Most common hereditary disorder of coagulation occurring in 1:10,000 live births.
- Laboratory features:
  - Elevated aPTT
  - Normal PT
  - Normal von Willebrand factor (VWF)

- Critically ill patients with hemophilia A require careful correction of factor VIII levels.
- Treatment:
  - Concentrated factor VIII.
  - Dose and frequency is dependent on degree of bleeding or need for invasive procedures.
  - Rule out a factor VIII inhibitor prior to major surgery.
- Monitor levels before invasive procedures or surgery and after replacement.

HEMOPHILIA B

- Sex-linked recessive deficiency of factor IX.
- Clinical and laboratory features are similar to hemophilia A.
- Treatment considerations are the same except replace factor IX with FFP, factor IX concentrates, prothrombin complex, or recombinant factor IX.

FACTOR VII DEFICIENCY

- Non-X-linked disorder of variable severity.
- Can present with a severe hemophilia-like condition.
- Laboratory feature—prolonged PT.
- The half-life of factor VII is short and replacement therapy may require frequent dosing.

VON WILLEBRAND FACTOR

- Inherited abnormality of factor VIII-related antigen that results in abnormal platelet function.
- Clinical features—bleeding disorder similar to other quantitative or qualitative platelet disorders.
- Classification:
  - Type I—most common; characterized by abnormal secretion of normal VWF from vascular endothelial cells.
  - Type II—abnormal structure and function of VWF.
  - Type III—severely decreased synthesis of normal VWF.
- Diagnosis:
  - Prolonged bleeding time, moderately prolonged PTT, and depression of factor VIII coagulant (VIII:C) level.
  - Low ristocetin cofactor and von Willebrand antigen.
  - In vitro platelet function analyzer allows rapid diagnosis.
- Treatment:
  - Normalize VWF levels during active bleeding and prior to surgery or invasive procedures.
  - Type I patients may respond to DDAVP infusion.
  - Tachyphylaxis develops after 1–2 days and is not indicated for long-term use or as monotherapy for major surgical procedures.
  - Factor VIII concentrate can be used for tachyphylaxis because of its high VWF content.
  - Factor VIII-related antigen level (VIII:C) can be used to assess bleeding tendency and effect of treatment.

INHIBITORS

- Factor inhibitors can result in a life-threatening bleeding diathesis during critical illness.
- Diagnosis is made when normal plasma mixed with patient's plasma fails to correct the PT or PTT.
- Inhibitor potency can be determined by titration studies.

FACTOR VIII INHIBITORS

- Most common inhibitor.
- Patient groups at risk: hemophilia, advanced age, postpartum, lymphoma, or autoimmune disease.
- Treatment:
  - Potency of inhibitors is measured in Bethesda units
  - Potent inhibitors (>10 Bethesda units):
    - Prothrombin complex concentrate (PCC)
    - Combination immunosuppressive regimes including steroids, cytotoxic agents, IVIG, and plasmapheresis
  - Nonhemophiliacs:
    - Require less intense immunosuppressive therapy
    - Treat underlying malignancy or autoimmune disease
  - Treat for 10 days after major invasive procedures

LUPUS ANTICOAGULANTS

- Phospholipid inhibitor associated with prolonged aPTT but indicates an underlying thrombophilia in about 25% of patients.
- First described in systemic lupus erythematosus (SLE) patients who clinically present with a thrombophilia in the setting of a prolonged aPTT.
- Also seen in drug-induced lupus, other autoimmune diseases, and de novo in otherwise normal patients.
- Diagnosis:
  - Prolonged PTT
  - Prolonged Russell viper venom time with evidence of an inhibitor
  - Tissue thromboplastin inhibition (TTI) test with steep rise in PT
- Treatment:
  - Long-term anticoagulation in patients with deep vein thrombosis (DVT) or pulmonary embolism (PE)
  - Inhibitor potency may decrease with immunosuppressive therapy or after discontinuation of offending drug

COMBINED FACTOR DEFICIENCY STATES

VITAMIN K DEFICIENCY

- Common in ICU patients.
- Risk factors include poor nutritional status, antibiotics, and biliary obstruction.

- Diagnosis:
  - Suggested by clinical setting
  - Prolonged PT with low factor VII level
  - Absence of liver disease or warfarin effects
- Treatment:
  - Vitamin K supplementation
  - Oral or SQ route preferred
- Complications:
  - Hematoma (IM)
  - Anaphylaxis (IM, IV)

FIBRINOLYTIC DISORDERS

PRIMARY FIBRINOLYSIS

- Abnormal breakdown of fibrinogen induced from a circulating activator of plasminogen in plasma.
- This is pathologic when secondary to states of tissue injury or therapeutic when induced by exogenous activators of plasminogen (e.g., urokinase or streptokinase).
- Euglobulin lysis time:
  - Measures plasmin generated by circulating activators
  - Abnormal in primary fibrinolysis

SECONDARY FIBRINOLYSIS

- Normal mechanism of clot degradation.
- Plasminogen activators present in formed clots generate plasmin.
- Euglobulin lysis time is normal.
- D-dimer levels:
  - Unique to the breakdown of cross-linked fibrin
  - Elevated in states of increased clot formation
  - Helps differentiate fibrinogenolysis (primary fibrinogenolysis) from fibrinolysis (secondary fibrinogenolysis)

COMPLEX COAGULOPATHIES

ACUTE DISSEMINATED INTRAVASCULAR COAGULATION

- Most important complex coagulopathy in the ICU.
- Clinical features/pathophysiology:
  - Generally a state of increased propensity for clot formation.
  - May present with clinical and laboratory evidence of hypercoagulability.
  - Acutely can present with a consumptive coagulopathy and bleeding.
  - Laboratory findings include thrombocytopenia, prolonged clotting times, low levels of cascade factors (especially factor VIII), and increased fibrinolysis (high FDP, D-dimer. and hypofibrinogenemia).
  - Microangiopathic hemolysis is common.
  - Hemorrhagic or vaso-occlusive complications can cause multiple organ dysfunction.
- Triggers include sepsis, tissue injury, neoplasm, burns, giant hemangioma, retained products of conception.
- Diagnosis is made by presence of a complex coagulopathy in the appropriate clinical setting.
- Treatment:
  - Correct the underlying cause.
  - Supportive care with transfusion of RBCs, platelets, and FFP.
  - Cryoprecipitate to correct hypofibrinogenemia.
  - Monitor therapy by following clotting times, platelet count, fibrinogen level, and FDPs.
- Heparin therapy:
  - May be beneficial in severe purpura fulminans, massive thromboembolism, and acute promyelocytic leukemias.
  - Gage success of therapy based on evidence of less bleeding with rising platelet counts and increased fibrinogen levels.
  - Contraindicated if evidence of bleeding in critical sites (e.g., intracranial hemorrhage).

MASSIVE TRANSFUSION

- Transfusion of 1–2 blood volumes of stored RBCs in a 24-hour period increases risk of a complex coagulopathy.
- Pathophysiology:
  - Dilutional and consumptive thrombocytopenia
  - Thrombocytopathy
  - Low factor V and VIII levels
  - Cold-induced coagulopathy
  - Citrate-induced hypocalcemia
- Diagnose secondary or recurrent bleeding in appropriate clinical setting.
- Treatment:
  - Transfuse adequate amounts of platelets and FFP
  - Blood warmers may be useful
  - Replete calcium

ANTIBIOTIC THERAPY

- Multiple or broad-spectrum antibiotics may predispose to a complex coagulopathy.
- Mechanisms:
  - Vitamin K deficiency
  - Penicillin-induced platelet dysfunction

LIVER DISEASE

- Hepatic function is vital for most clotting factor and thrombopoietin synthesis and predisposes to a complex coagulopathy.
- Pathophysiology:
  - Multifactorial thrombocytopenia ± thrombocytopathy.
  - Hepatocyte injury can trigger primary fibrinolysis (mimics DIC).
  - DIC superimposed on liver failure results in a severe complex coagulopathy.
- Treatment:
  - Replete clotting factors, platelets, and correct vitamin K deficiency.
  - FFP is first-line therapy.
  - Other options include prothrombin complex (vitamin-K-dependent factors), fibrinolysis inhibitors, and rVIIa.

RENAL DISEASE

- Prolongs bleeding time from uremia-induced thrombocytopathy.
- Nephrotic syndrome increases risk of acquired factor deficiencies.
- Treatment:
  - Hemodialysis
  - Platelet transfusion
  - FFP

DYSPROTEINEMIAS

- Multiple myeloma and Waldenström macroglobulinemia can result in significant coagulopathies.
- Pathophysiology:
  - Thrombocytopenia (disease or therapy related)
  - Thrombocytopathy
  - Impaired conversion of fibrinogen to fibrin
- Laboratory manifestations:
  - Low platelet count
  - Increased bleeding time
  - Prolonged thrombin time
- Treatment—decease paraprotein levels via chemotherapy or plasmapheresis.

INVASIVE PROCEDURE GUIDELINES FOR COAGULOPATHIC PATIENTS

GENERAL GUIDELINES

- Perform invasive procedures only when necessary.
- Limit planned intervention as much as possible and perform under direct vision by most experienced operator available.
- Carefully define the coagulopathy to gauge risk and plan therapy.
- Evaluate success of preprocedure therapy prior to procedure.
- Coordinate procedure with appropriate support staff, that is, blood bank and pharmacy.
- Carefully monitor for immediate and delayed bleeding complications.

SPECIFIC COAGULOPATHIES

VASCULITIS

- Avoid skin incisions over sites of vasculitic rashes.
- Platelet transfusion is not indicated without concomitant thrombocytopenia or thrombocytopathy.

THROMBOCYTOPENIA

- Platelet counts of 50,000–80,000/μL are generally adequate for procedures performed under direct vision.
- Platelet counts of 80,000–100,000/μL are preferred for major surgical procedures, insertion of central lines, or closed-space needle biopsies.
- Lumbar punctures generally safe with platelet count of 50,000/μL.

THROMBOCYTOPATHY

- An attempt to normalize the bleeding time is generally warranted despite the poor predictive value of an elevated bleeding time.
- Discontinue thrombocytopathy-inducing drugs and wait.
  - Acutely transfused normal platelets will correct a prolonged bleeding time in this setting.
  - DDAVP infusions may temporarily override the thrombocytopathic effects of aspirin and ticlopidine in urgent situations.

THROMBOCYTHEMIA

- Platelet counts in excess of 1×10^6/μL in myeloproliferative disorders predispose to excessive bleeding.
- Avoid or minimize invasive procedures.
- Normalize platelet count.

FIBRIN GENERATION DEFECTS

- A normal PT and PTT is mandatory, when achievable, for procedures in critical sites (e.g., neurosurgery).
- Correct known factor deficiency states.

- Clotting times should not exceed 1.2–1.3 times the baseline for procedures done under direct vision or line placements.
- Evaluate for delayed onset bleeding.

Fibrinolytic States

- Avoid any invasive procedures.
- Hyperfibrinolytic states with short clot survival, hypofibrinogenemia, and elevated levels of FDPs may result in serious bleeding during and after procedures.
- Intracranial bleeding, thrombotic events, and recent major surgical procedures are contraindications to the initiation of fibrinolytic therapy.
- If bleeding occurs during therapeutic fibrinolysis, discontinue and provide blood product support including cryoprecipitate as source of fibrinogen.

ANTICOAGULANT DRUG EFFECTS

Unfractionated Heparin

- Discontinue heparin approximately 6 hours before invasive procedures.
- Protamine sulfate is antidote for emergencies.

Low Molecular Weight Heparin

- Relatively long half-life.
- No predictably effective antagonist.
- Can measure LMWH levels prior to procedure.

Warfarin

- Prothrombin time normalizes in 2 or more days after discontinuation.
- FFP or prothrombin complex (less volume) will immediately correct the PT for emergent situations.
- Oral or intravenous vitamin K (1–5 mg):
  - Onset of effect approximately 8–12 hours after administration.
  - High-dose vitamin K may lead to warfarin resistance.
- Temporary heparinization for flexible planning of interventions after stopping warfarin therapy.

Direct Thrombin Inhibitors

- Discontinue
- Follow PTT until normal prior to invasive procedures
- No effective antagonist

Drotrecogin Alfa (Xigris)

- Recombinant activated protein C product with antithrombotic and profibrinolytic properties used in the management of patients with severe sepsis.
- Major side effect is bleeding.
- Most serious bleeding events are seen in patients with coexisting thrombocytopenia ≤30,000/μL.
- Discontinue 2 hours prior to procedure and maintain platelet count above 30,000/μL.
- Wait 12 hours after major invasive procedures before cautiously restarting the infusion.

Bibliography

Bernard GR, Vincent J-L, Laterre RF, et al. The recombinant human activated protein C world-wide evaluation in severe sepsis (PROWESS) study group, efficacy and safety of recombinant human activated protein C for severe sepsis. *N Engl J Med* 2001;344:699–709.

Bussel JB, Kimberly RP, Inman RD, et al. Intravenous gammaglobulin treatment of chronic idiopathic thrombocytopenic purpura. *Blood* 1983;62:480–486.

Furie B. Acquired coagulation disorders and dysproteinemias. In: Colman RW, Hirsh J, Marder VJ, et al., eds., *Hemostasis and Thrombosis*, 2nd ed. Philadelphia, PA: Lippincott; 1987:841.

Hall JB, Schmidt, GA, Wood LDH. *Principles of Critical Care*, 3rd ed. New York, NY: McGraw-Hill; 2005:1123–1136.

Harrigan C, Lucas CE, Ledgerwood AM, et al. Primary hemostasis after massive transfusion for injury. *Am Surg* 1982;48:393–396.

Hewson JR, Neame PB, Kumar N, et al. Coagulopathy related to dilution and hypotension during massive transfusion. *Crit Care Med* 1985;13:387–391.

Hirsh J, Warkentin TE, Shaughnessy SG, et al. Heparin and low-molecular weight heparin: mechanisms of action, pharmacokinetics, dosing, monitoring, efficacy, and safety. *Chest* 2001;119(Suppl 1):64S–94S.

Joist JH, George JN. Hemostatic abnormalities in liver and renal disease. In: Colman RW, Hirsh J, Marder VJ, et al., eds., *Hemostasis and Thrombosis*, 4th ed. Philadelphia, PA: Lippincott Williams & Wilkins; 2001:995.

Mannucci PM, Remuzzi G, Pusineri F, et al. Deamino-8-D arginine vasopressin shortens the bleeding time in uremia. *N Engl J Med* 1983;308:8–12.

Marder VJ, Feinstein DI, Colman RW. Consumptive thrombohemorrhagic disorders. In: Colman RW, Hirsh J, Marder VJ, et al., eds., *Hemostasis and Thrombosis*, 4th ed. Philadelphia, PA: Lippincott Williams & Wilkins; 2001:1197.

Roberts HR, Stinchcombe TE, Gabriel DA. The dysfibrinogenaemias. *Br J Haematol* 2001;114:249–257.

Sadler JE, Blinder M. von Willebrand's disease: diagnosis, classification, and treatment. In: Colman RW, Hirsh J, Marder VJ, et al., eds., *Hemostasis and Thrombosis*, 4th ed. Philadelphia, PA: Lippincott Williams & Wilkins; 2005:905–921.

Shapiro SS, Thiagarajan P. Lupus anticoagulants. *Prog Hemost Thromb* 1982;6:263–285.

Shapiro SS. Acquired inhibitors to the blood coagulation factors. *Semin Thromb Hemost* 1975;1:336–385.

Thompson AR, Harker LA. *Manual of Hemostasis and Thrombosis*, 3rd ed. Philadelphia, PA: Davis; 1983:175–185.

83 THROMBOLYTIC THERAPY

Amit Pursnani

KEY POINTS

- Thrombolytic therapies may be employed in the management of selected patients with pulmonary embolus, acute stroke, and MI.
- Stringent inclusion and exclusion criteria must be applied to properly select patients who may benefit.
- Early treatment is important and for each clinical entity the window of opportunity for benefit may close, leaving the patient with only risk of treatment.

THROMBOLYTIC AGENTS

- Thrombolytic agents are proteins or other substances that activate a blood proenzyme, plasminogen, to its active enzyme form plasmin. Plasmin then solubilizes fibrin and degrades a number of other plasma proteins, including fibrinogen.
- Applications for thrombolytic therapy include acute myocardial infarction (AMI), acute pulmonary embolism (PE), and acute ischemic stroke.
- A number of thrombolytic agents are available and described below.

STREPTOKINASE

- Streptokinase (SK) is derived from group C, β-hemolytic streptococci. This agent activates adjacent plasminogen by forming a noncovalent SK-plasminogen activator complex. Its half-life in plasma is 30 minutes.

UROKINASE

- Urokinase (UK) is derived from cultured human cells. It activates plasminogen directly by enzymatic action. Its half-life in plasma is 20 minutes.

TISSUE PLASMINOGEN ACTIVATOR

- Tissue plasminogen activator (t-PA) is derived by recombinant genetic technology from human DNA. It is fibrin-specific unlike the agents above. It works by activating plasminogen associated with fibrin directly by enzymatic action. It has a very short half-life. The following are preparations of tPA that are available:
  - *Alteplase (t-PA)* is the glycosylated protein of 527 amino acids produced by recombinant DNA technology. There are two derivatives of tPA:
    - *Reteplase* (sometimes called rPA) is a 39,571 molecular weight deletion mutant of tPA. It contains 355 of the 527 amino acids of native tPA.
    - *Tenecteplase* is a 527 amino acid protein produced by recombinant technology. It differs from alteplase (tPA) by only 6 amino acids.

PRECAUTIONS WITH USE OF THROMBOLYTICS

- *Bleeding* is the major complication of thrombolytic therapy. Consequently, *absolute* contraindications include dissecting aortic aneurysm, pericarditis, hemorrhagic stroke, or neurosurgical procedures within 6 months or known intracranial neoplasm. *Relative* contraindications include major surgery or bleeding within 6 weeks, known bleeding diathesis, and severe uncontrolled hypertension.
- *Allergic reactions*: SK and the related agent anistreplase are potentially allergenic. Patients are usually pretreated with intravenous hydrocortisone 100 mg and antihistamines.
- *Antibody production*: SK and anistreplase induce antibody production, which makes re-treatment with either of these agents less effective.

THERAPY FOR PULMONARY EMBOLISM

BACKGROUND AND INDICATIONS

- Traditionally, thrombolysis has been reserved for massive PE resulting in cardiogenic shock. However, recent evidence suggests a role for thrombolysis in stable patients (normal systemic arterial pressure) with *submassive PE* and subsequent right ventricular dysfunction.
- One study has shown that the combination of heparin and t-PA decreased the need for escalation of treatment due to clinical deterioration of patients with submassive PE more often than patients on heparin and placebo. Escalation of treatment included the use of pressors, mechanical ventilation, or use of open-label t-PA. Results of this study are summarized in Table 83-1.
- The goal of thrombolytic therapy is rapid clot lysis, which hastens reperfusion of lung tissue and prevents

TABLE 83-1 Comparison of t-PA to Placebo in the Treatment of Pulmonary Embolus with Right Heart Strain

THERAPY	MORTALITY*	ESCALATION OF TREATMENT*
Placebo and heparin	3.4%	24.6%
t-PA and heparin	2.2%	10.2%

*The *P*-value for mortality difference was .71 and *P*-value for escalation of treatment difference was significant at .006.

SOURCE: Adapted from Goldhaber SZ. Perspective: thrombolysis for pulmonary embolism. *N Engl J Med* 2002;347:1131–1132.

chronic complications of PE such as pulmonary hypertension and the more acute complication of right ventricular infarction. A secondary goal is decreasing the risk of subsequent pulmonary emboli by diminishing the source of embolization.
- Prior to thrombolytic administration, objective evidence of pulmonary embolization must be obtained by some imaging modality—most typically computed tomography (CT) angiography or ventilation-perfusion scanning, and on rare occasion pulmonary angiography. For unstable patients, a bedside echocardiogram may give inferential information in the form of right heart strain and pressure overload, but it must be considered as less compelling diagnostic information than visualization of the pulmonary circulation by some modality.

EXCLUSION CRITERIA

- Cerebrovascular accident, intracranial trauma, or surgery within past 2 months
- Active intracranial disease (neoplasm, aneurysm, vascular malformations)
- Major internal bleeding within past 6 months
- Uncontrolled hypertension (systolic blood pressure [SBP] >200 mmHg, diastolic blood pressure [DBP] >110 mmHg)
- Bleeding diathesis/coagulopathies
- Recent major surgery, organ biopsy, or obstetric delivery (within 10 days)
- Recent trauma
- Infective endocarditis/pericarditis
- Pregnancy
- Aortic aneurysm
- Hemorrhagic retinopathy

DOSING AND USE OF THROMBOLYTICS

- Agents that have been used include SK, UK, and alteplase (t-PA). t-PA is infused at 100 mg over 2 hours. Postinfusion partial thromboplastin time (PTT) monitoring is necessary to ensure value 2.5 times control. If <2.5, heparin infusion should be adjusted to maintain goal PTT. Patients should preferably be in a closely monitored setting (i.e., intensive care unit). Patients should be anticoagulated with heparin (and eventually warfarin) immediately after thrombolytic agent is completely infused. One should not administer heparin concomitantly; check PTT every 6 hours until therapeutic (1.5–2 times value of upper limit of normal). Blood for laboratory tests should not be drawn during thrombolytic infusion. If bleeding occurs, thrombolytic infusion should be immediately stopped and blood products should be given as needed.
- There is a larger time window of opportunity for thrombolysis for PE compared to stroke or MI. That is, there is a persistent but attenuated benefit from using thrombolytics up to 14 days after the diagnosis of PE is made. But clearly, most benefit is derived if these agents are used early.

THROMBOLYTIC THERAPY FOR ACUTE ISCHEMIC STROKE

BACKGROUND AND INDICATIONS

- Acute ischemic stroke is the result of a sudden interruption of cerebral blood flow. The goal of reperfusion therapy is to reperfuse potentially salvageable tissue around the core of infarcted brain tissue. Thrombolytic therapy is typically used after imaging (usually CT) to rule out hemorrhagic infarct.
- Indications and exclusions for thrombolytic therapy for stroke:
  - Age ≥18 years
  - Diagnosis of ischemic stroke causing clinical neurologic deficits
  - Symptom onset <3 hours prior to treatment initiation
  - No history of stroke in last 14 days
  - No history of intracerebral hemorrhage (ICH)
  - SBP <185 mmHg
  - DBP <110 mmHg
  - No rapidly resolving symptoms
  - No subarachnoid hemorrhage or suggestive symptoms thereof
  - No gastrointestinal (GI) or urinary tract hemorrhage in last 14 days
  - No arterial puncture at noncompressible site within last 7 days
  - No seizure at onset of stroke
  - Prothrombin time (PT) <15 or international normalized ratio (INR) <1.7 without use of anticoagulation
  - PTT in normal range (if previous use of heparin)

- Platelet count >100,000/mm^3
- Blood glucose >50 mg/dL
- No aggressive measure to decrease blood pressure in limits above

INTRAVENOUS THROMBOLYTIC THERAPY

- tPA is given at a dose of 0.9 mg/kg (max 90 mg) over 60-minute period with the first 10% of dose given over 1 minute as bolus.
- Neurologic examinations should be performed every 15 minutes during infusion of t-PA, followed by assessments q 30 min for next 6 hours, and q 60 min for next 16 hours.
- Blood pressure checks should be performed q 15 min for 2 hours, then q 30 min for 6 hours, then q 60 min for 16 hours. If SBP >180 or DBP >105, antihypertensive drugs should be administered to maintain blood pressure below those levels.
- In the NINDS (National Institute of Neurological Disorders and Stroke) t-PA study, 31–50 % of patients receiving t-PA had complete or near-complete recovery at 3 months versus 20–38% of patients receiving placebo. The incidence of symptomatic brain hemorrhage was 6.4% of t-PA group and 0.6% of placebo group. Mortality rates similar in both groups at 3 months and 1 year.

INTRA-ARTERIAL THROMBOLYTIC THERAPY

- Local arterial thrombolysis can be performed with a catheter placed at the site of arterial occlusion.
- It has not yet been compared head-to-head with intravenous thrombolytic therapy. There is a high rate of arterial canalization—approximately 40% with full arterial canalization and 35% with partial canalization.
- The PROACT (Prourokinase for Acute Ischemic Stroke) trial showed benefit of intra-arterial thrombolysis in stroke caused by occlusion of middle cerebral artery (MCA)—identified either on brain CT or CT angiography.

THERAPY FOR ACUTE MYOCARDIAL INFARCTION

- Thrombolytics prevent recurrent thrombus formation and rapidly restore hemodynamic stability in selected patients with MI. These agents can dissolve pathologic intraluminal thrombus or embolus not yet dissolved by the endogenous fibrinolytic system. When given within 12 hours of symptom onset, they restore patency of occluded arteries, salvage myocardium, and reduce morbidity and mortality of AMI.
- Thrombolytic agents studied for MI include *SK* and *alteplase* (recombinant tPA). Alteplase is more expensive but has shown a greater benefit in the GUSTO-1 (Global Utilization of Streptokinase and Tissue Plasminogen Activator for Occluded Coronary Arteries) trial with a 15% relative risk reduction (1% absolute risk reduction) compared to SK. Newer agents like tenecteplase and reteplase are as effective as alteplase.
- Benefit from thrombolytic therapy is largely correlated with time to therapy. Early therapy has the greatest impact on infarct size and left ventricular ejection fraction. Thrombolytic treatment should be started within 30 minutes of arrival (door-drug time). Maximum benefit occurs when administered within 1–3 hours of symptom onset.
- American College of Cardiology/American Heart Association (ACC/AHA, 2004) guidelines recommend thrombolytic therapy for patients without contraindications within 12 hours of symptom onset. It is reasonable to give thrombolytic therapy within 12–24 hours after symptom onset if persistent ST elevations or continuing symptoms are present.
- Achievement of TIMI-3 (Thrombosis in Myocardial Infarction Trial 3) flow (normal flow which fills distal coronary bed completely) after thrombolytic therapy occurs in only 50–60% of patients—much less than that achieved with percutaneous coronary intervention (PCI) which is almost 90%. TIMI-3 flow postintervention is highly correlated with long-term survival.
- Risks of thrombolytic therapy for MI include bleeding—with the most worrisome complication being hemorrhagic stroke. In this light, the absolute and relative contraindications for thrombolytic therapy in MI are summarized below:
  - Absolute contraindications include prior ICH, cerebral vascular lesion, malignant intracranial neoplasms, ischemic stroke in last 3 months, significant head or facial trauma in last 3 months, suspected aortic dissection, and active bleeding.
  - Relative contraindications are hypertension (SBP >180), ischemic stroke more than 3 months old, dementia, major surgery in last 3 weeks, prolonged cardiopulmonary resuscitation (CPR, >10 minutes), internal bleeding in last 2–4 weeks, noncompressible vascular puncture, pregnancy, active peptic ulcer, current anticoagulant use, and prior exposure or allergic reaction to SK/alteplase (if these are the drugs being considered).

TABLE 83-2 Thrombolytic Therapy Vs. PCI

ENDPOINT (AT 30 DAYS)	ANGIOPLASTY	FIBRINOLYSIS
Mortality	8.5%	14.2%
Nonfatal reinfarction	1.6%	6.3%

SOURCE: Adapted from Andersen HR, Nielsen TT, Rasmussen K, et al., for the DANAMI-2 Investigators. A comparison of coronary angioplasty with fibrinolytic therapy in acute myocardial infarction. *N Engl J Med* 2003;349:733–742.

PERCUTANEOUS CORONARY INTERVENTION VERSUS THROMBOLYTICS FOR MYOCARDIAL INFARCTION

- Trials that have compared thrombolytic therapy to angioplasty suggest an advantage of PCI or angioplasty in terms of mortality, especially if performed early—within 90 minutes of symptom onset. Primary PCI is also preferable if transfering to neighboring institution with cardiac catheterization lab within 30–60 minutes.
- PCI does not have the risk of ICH that is inherent to thrombolytic therapy.
- Table 83-2 summarizes the results of thrombolytic therapy versus PCI for mortality and nonfatal reinfarction rate. There is both a clear mortality benefit and a benefit with respect to nonfatal reinfarction when comparing PCI to thrombolytic therapy.

BIBLIOGRAPHY

Adams HP, Adams RJ, Brott TG, et al. Guidelines for the early management of patients with ischemic stroke: a scientific statement from the Stroke Council of the American Heart Association. *Stroke* 2003;34:1056–1064.

Andersen HR, Nielsen TT, Rasmussen K, et al., for the DANAMI-2 Investigators. A comparison of coronary angioplasty with fibrinolytic therapy in acute myocardial infarction. *N Engl J Med* 2003;349:733–742.

Brott T, Bogousslavsky J. Treatment of acute ischemic stroke. *N Engl J Med* 2000;343:710–722.

Goldhaber SZ. Perspective: thrombolysis for pulmonary embolism. *N Engl J Med* 2002;347:1131–1132.

Konstantinides S, Geibel A, Heusel G, et al., for the Management Strategies and Prognosis of Pulmonary Embolism-3 Trial Investigators. Heparin plus alteplase compared with heparin alone in patients with submassive pulmonary embolism. *N Engl J Med* 2002;347:1143–1150.

Thrombolytic therapy with streptokinase in acute ischemic stroke. The Multicenter Acute Stroke Trial—Europe Study Group. *N Engl J Med* 1996;335:145–150.

84 THROMBOTIC THROMBOCYTOPENIC PURPURA-HEMOLYTIC UREMIC SYNDROME

Shashi Kiran Bellam, Joyce Tang

KEY POINTS

- Demographically, peak incidence of TTP-HUS is in the third decade. Certain stereotyped populations that develop TTP-HUS include HIV-infected individuals, postchemotherapy patients, and patients receiving cyclosporine postorgan transplantation.
- TTP is characterized by the following classic pentad: fever, microangiopathic hemolytic anemia, thrombocytopenia, neurologic symptoms, and renal impairment.
- Diagnosis of TTP, however, requires only two of these five findings: microangiopathic hemolytic anemia and thrombocytopenia that are both otherwise unexplained.
- To diagnose TTP, it is essential to rule out other conditions that may result in hemolytic anemia and thrombocytopenia, including DIC and malignant hypertension.
- Treatment should include early plasmapheresis.

CLARIFICATION OF TERMINOLOGY

- Thrombotic thrombocytopenic purpura (TTP) and hemolytic uremic syndrome (HUS) share a common pathologic basis, overlap in terms of the organ systems they affect, and are treated in a similar fashion. Classically, the term TTP is used in states where neurologic symptoms predominate the clinical picture, whereas HUS refers to conditions in which renal dysfunction predominates. The term TTP-HUS, however, can be used more generally to encompass the full spectrum of conditions.

PATHOPHYSIOLOGY

- Etiologies of TTP-HUS include the following:
  - Drugs (platelet inhibitors, quinine, bleomycin, mitomycin, gemcitabine, cisplatin, cyclosporine, valacyclovir, others reported)
  - Autoimmune diseases (antiphospholipid antibody syndrome, systemic lupus erythematosus [SLE], scleroderma)
  - Pregnancy and postpartum state
  - HIV/AIDS

    ◦ Enterohemorrhagic *Escherichia coli* with bloody diarrhea
    ◦ Idiopathic
- TTP-HUS has numerous etiologies, but a single common pathologic endpoint:

Inciting event → platelet aggregation → thrombi formation

- Vessels in the kidneys and brain are disproportionately affected.

CLINICAL PRESENTATION

- Thrombotic thrombocytopenic purpura is characterized by pentad of fever, microangiopathic hemolytic anemia, thrombocytopenia, neurologic symptoms, and renal impairment.
- Symptoms of TTP vary with the extent and severity of the thrombotic lesions. Neurologic findings can be nonspecific and mild (such as a headache) or severe (such as seizures or coma). Renal dysfunction may range from mild insufficiency to acute renal failure.
- Even in the absence of characteristic physical findings, however, the existence of characteristic laboratory findings of hemolytic anemia and thrombocytopenia should be sufficient to arouse suspicion and workup for TTP.

DIAGNOSIS

- Differential diagnosis includes disseminated intravascular coagulation (DIC), malignant hypertension, preeclampsia, and vasculitis.
- Key lab findings for diagnosis of TTP include the following:
    ◦ Evidence for a hemolytic anemia
        ▪ Schistocytes on smear (usually >1%)
        ▪ Elevated indirect bilirubin, lactate dehydrogenase (LDH), severely reduced haptoglobin
    ◦ Thrombocytopenia (often <50,000/μL, but the range is wide)
    ◦ Absence of coagulation abnormalities
        ▪ Normal prothrombin time (PT)/partial thromboplastin time (PTT)
        ▪ Normal fibrinogen level
        ▪ Normal level of fibrin-degradation products
    ◦ Negative direct Coombs' test
- DIC may be distinguished from TTP-HUS by the following:
    ◦ Different precipitating factors: DIC is more common in the setting of sepsis or peripartum situations, while TTP-HUS will evolve without evidence of infection and often earlier in pregnancy when it is pregnancy related
- Patients with malignant hypertension and preeclampsia may have supporting pertinent histories and physical findings suggesting these as diagnoses. TTP is rare in pregnant patients.
- Patients with vasculitis may have other signs/symptoms of systemic involvement including rash and arthralgias.

TREATMENT AND OUTCOMES

- Therapy for TTP should be approached as a hematologic emergency.
- Plasma exchange (plasmapheresis) is the therapy of choice for TTP.
- Plasma exchange should occur daily until evidence that disease is in remission (platelet count >150,000/μL, afebrile, normal mental status, normal renal function, and normal urinary sediment).
- The usual length of plasma exchange treatment is 5–10 days.
- In patients not improving with plasma exchange, splenectomy should be considered.
- Steroids and vincristine are used but there is no proven role for them.
- The mortality rate is 20–30%.

BIBLIOGRAPHY

Goodnough LT. Thrombotic thrombocytopenic purpura, hemolytic syndromes, and the approach to thrombotic microangiopathies. In: Hall JB, Schmidt GA, Wood LDH, eds., *Principles of Critical Care*, 3rd ed. New York, NY: McGraw-Hill;2005.

Moake JL. Mechanisms of disease: thrombotic microangiopathies. *N Engl J Med* 2002;347:589–600.

85 DISSEMINATED INTRAVASCULAR COAGULATION

Steven Q. Davis, Sandy Nasrallah

KEY POINTS

- Disseminated intravascular coagulation is a syndrome resulting in both thrombosis and hemorrhage.
- DIC is the most important coagulopathy in critical illness, as it complicates several disease states commonly seen in the intensive care unit setting.

- It is an acquired disorder, resulting from an underlying condition.
- Multisystem organ failure can occur.
- Diagnosis is based on clinical presentation in conjunction with a panel of blood tests.
- The complete picture of DIC is characterized by thrombocytopenia, prolonged clotting times, low levels of clotting factors and fibrinogen, and increased fibrin degradation products and D-dimer.
- Treatment of DIC is aimed at treating the primary disorder.
- Transfusion of blood products may be required to counteract the hemorrhagic complications while the primary disorder is being treated.

PATHOPHYSIOLOGY

- Widespread activation of the clotting cascade is initiated by the increased presence of tissue factor, which can result from (Fig. 85-1):
  - Enhanced expression by inflammatory cells
  - Vascular epithelial injury
  - Release of thromboplastins into the systemic circulation
- Inflammatory cytokines can initiate clotting, which, in turn, can stimulate inflammation, resulting in a self-perpetuating cycle.
- Counteracting, homeostatic systems are disrupted in disseminated intravascular coagulation (DIC), leading to an imbalance favoring clot formation:
  - Dysregulation and excessive production of thrombin and subsequent fibrin deposition causes widespread activation of the clotting cascade.
  - The normal anticoagulant mechanisms are perturbed, resulting from decreased concentrations and activation of antithrombin III and protein C, as well as insufficient levels of tissue factor pathway inhibitor to prevent coagulation.
  - Impaired fibrinolysis occurs via enhanced production of plasminogen-activator inhibitor (PAI) type 1.

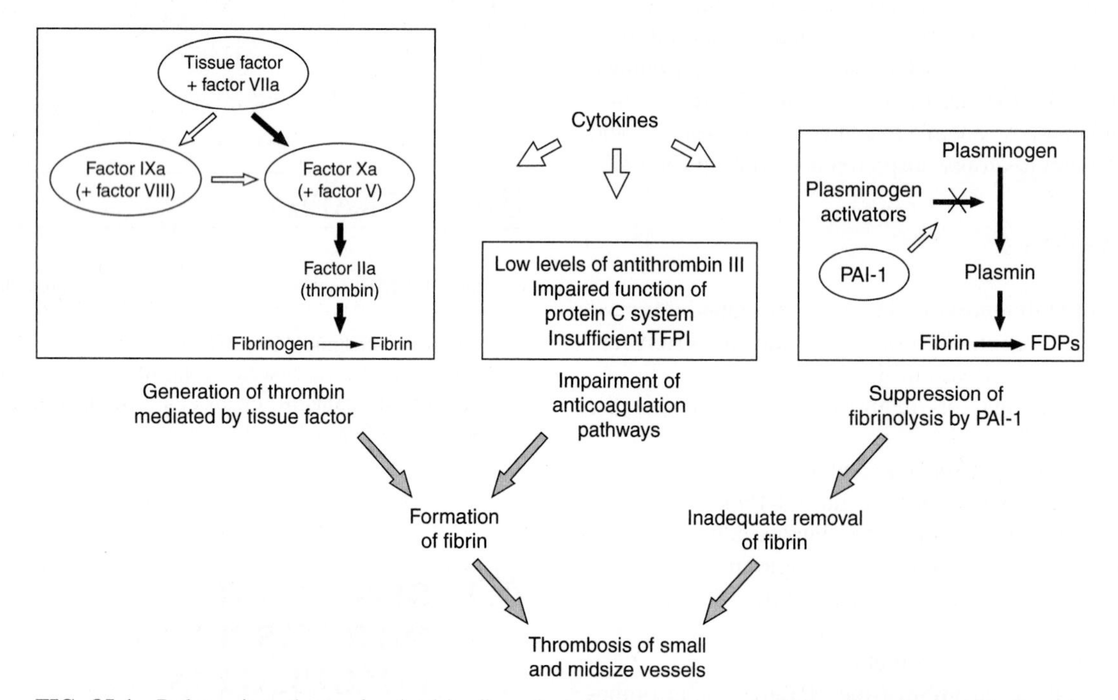

FIG. 85-1 Pathogenic pathways involved in disseminated intravascular coagulation. In patients with disseminated intravascular coagulation, fibrin is formed as a result of the generation of thrombin mediated by tissue factor. Tissue factor, expressed on the surface of activated mononuclear cells and endothelial cells, binds and activates factor VII. The complex of tissue factor and factor VIIa can activate factor X directly (black arrows) or indirectly (white arrows) by means of activated factor IX and factor VII. Activated factor X, in combination with factor V, can convert prothrombin (factor II) to thrombin (factor IIa). Simultaneously, all three physiologic means of anticoagulation—antithrombin III, protein C, and tissue factor pathway inhibitor (TFPI)—are impaired. The resulting intravascular formation of fibrin is not balanced by adequate removal of fibrin because endogenous fibrinolysis is suppressed by high plasma levels of PAI-1. The high levels of PAI-1inhibit plasminogen-activator activity and consequently reduce the rate of formation of plasmin. The combination of increased formation of fibrin and inadequate removal of fibrin results in disseminated intravascular thrombosis. FDPs denote fibrin-degradation products. SOURCE: Adapted from Levi M, ten Cate H. Current concepts: disseminated intravascular coagulation. *N Engl J Med* 1999;341:586–592.

- Systemic clotting occurs within the microvasculature, which can then lead to multisystem organ failure.
- Overconsumption of clotting factors and platelets exhausts the coagulation system, therefore, leading to widespread bleeding.

COMMON UNDERLYING CONDITIONS

- *Sepsis*-induced DIC can occur with any type of microorganism infection. The pathogen promotes a generalized inflammatory response by the host immune system, resulting in a widespread release of cytokines. These cytokines may then stimulate circulating granulocytes and macrophages to produce and release more tissue factor.
- *Trauma* can lead to DIC by hemolysis, endothelial damage, and the release of fats and phospholipids from damaged tissues.
- The mechanism by which *malignancy* causes DIC is unclear, but is possibly related to expression of tissue factor on tumor cell surfaces.
- During *obstetrical emergencies*, thromboplastin-like products can seep into the maternal circulation, activating widespread clot formation. This can occur with several obstetrical conditions, including amniotic fluid embolism and abruptio placentae.
- *Vascular disorders*, including giant hemangiomas and large aortic aneurysms, may mediate DIC by the local activation of coagulation with systemic depletion of clotting factors.

CLINICAL PRESENTATION

- DIC can be acute or chronic.
  - Acute DIC develops when a large amount of tissue factor is released within the circulation in a short amount of time, overcoming the natural anticoagulant and fibrinolytic mechanisms.
  - Chronic DIC occurs when there is a continuous, slow release of tissue factor within the circulation. When this process is gradual enough, the body is able to compensate by adequately repleting clotting factors and platelets, which results in more thrombosis than bleeding.
- Bleeding is the most common clinical manifestation of acute DIC, occurring in about 60% of patients.
  - Ecchymoses, petechiae, and diffuse oozing of blood from line sites, surgical wounds, and mucosal surfaces may occur. If widespread, this bleeding can be life-threatening.
  - Bleeding within the central nervous system (CNS) can present with mental status changes, coma, or focal neurologic deficits.
  - Pulmonary hemorrhage occurs in approximately 15% of patients with DIC, resulting from pulmonary vascular endothelial damage. This can lead to tachypnea and dyspnea and, if severe enough, may cause the acute respiratory distress syndrome (ARDS).
  - Gastrointestinal (GI) bleeding may lead to significant blood loss secondary to the large amount of GI mucosal endothelium subject to injury.
- Acute renal failure (ARF) is also commonly seen with DIC.
  - ARF is likely directly caused by DIC via clotting of the renal microvasculature, leading to ischemia of the renal parenchyma.
  - Indirectly, severe hypotension, as may occur with sepsis or trauma, can also lead to acute tubular necrosis concomitant with DIC.
- Jaundice is frequently present in patients with DIC.
  - This is caused by an unconjugated hyperbilirubinemia, resulting from hemolysis. Deposits of intravascular fibrin cause lysis of red blood cells by shear stress forces.
  - Hepatic dysfunction from an underlying disorder, such as sepsis, may also contribute to this presentation.

DIAGNOSIS

- There is no single test that can diagnose DIC.
- One of the clinical conditions known to trigger DIC *must* be present to make this diagnosis.
- There are several blood tests that can be used in conjunction with the clinical presentation to identify the presence of DIC:
  - Low platelets, defined as <100,000, or an abrupt drop in the platelet count
  - Prolongation of prothrombin time (PT) and activated partial thromboplastin time (aPTT), representing the overconsumption of coagulation factors
  - Elevated concentration of fibrin degradation products, indicative of increased fibrinolysis
  - Elevated D-dimer, resulting from cross-linked fibrin degradation
  - Decreased circulating fibrinogen concentration, reflecting its massive deposition within the blood vessels
  - Decreased levels of specific coagulation factors, including factors V, VII, and VIII
  - Decreased levels of anticoagulant factors, such as antithrombin, protein C, and protein S
  - Schistocytes seen on peripheral blood smear, signifying the presence of hemolysis

TREATMENT

- The paramount therapy for DIC is treatment of the underlying, driving condition.
- Supportive (replacement) therapy may positively impact morbidity and mortality when the patient is significantly bleeding or at risk for bleeding.
    - *When active bleeding occurs*, platelets, fresh frozen plasma (FFP), and cryoprecipitate can be given to replace the exhausted platelets and coagulation factors.
    - These blood products should also be given in situations where an invasive procedure must be performed.
- In theory, the use of anticoagulants could disrupt the massive clotting that occurs during DIC, but there has been little clinical evidence to support this presumption. In specific clinical situations, however, the use of anticoagulants, such as heparin, may be appropriate.
    - For catastrophic thromboembolism or purpura fulminans, heparin therapy is appropriate together with the aforementioned blood product support.
    - In chronic, low-grade DIC, subcutaneous heparin may help to prevent thrombotic complications.
    - Heparin dosing is variable, depending on the clot burden generated by the coagulopathy. In general, the dose is lower than that given for anticoagulation for more routine purposes (i.e., venous thromboembolism).
- Replacement of anticoagulant factors, such as antithrombin and protein C, has been used with variable success and is not routinely recommended.
- Clotting times, platelet count, and fibrinogen level are all used to follow the progress of therapy. Fibrinogen-degradation product (FDP) levels lag behind clinical improvement.

BIBLIOGRAPHY

Baron JM, Baron BW. Bleeding disorders. In: Hall JB, Schmidt GA, Wood LDH, eds., *Principles of Critical Care*, 3rd ed. New York, NY: McGraw-Hill; 2005:1065–1080.

Franchini M, Manzato F. Update on the treatment of disseminated intravascular coagulation. *Hematology* 2004; 9:81–85.

Levi M, ten Cate H. Current concepts: disseminated intravascular coagulation. *N Engl J Med* 1999;341:586–592.

Levi M. Current understanding of disseminated intravascular coagulation. *Br J Haematol* 2004;124:567–576.

Toh CH, Dennis M. Disseminated intravascular coagulation: old disease, new hope. *BMJ* 2003;327:974–977.

86 THROMBOCYTOPENIA IN CRITICALLY ILL PATIENTS

Daniel A. Pollyea

KEY POINTS

- Thrombocytopenia is a common occurrence in the ICU and increases risk for bleeding complications.
- Common skin findings from low platelets include petechiae, purpura, or ecchymosis, particularly in dependent areas.
- Causes of thrombocytopenia can be classified into one of four broad categories, including: pseudothrombocytopenia, dilution, increased platelet destruction, and decreased platelet production.
- Sepsis is the most common cause of thrombocytopenia in ICU patients.
- Drug-induced thrombocytopenia is not uncommon in the ICU. Heparin is the most common ICU medication responsible for thrombocytopenia, but others include thiazide diuretics, valproic acid, and trimethoprim/sulfamethoxazole.

DEFINITION

- Thrombocytopenia is defined as a platelet count <150,000/mm^3.
- The risk of bleeding complications increases as platelet counts decrease (Table 86-1).

INCIDENCE AND PROGNOSIS

- Thrombocytopenia is common in intensive care unit (ICU) patients.
- Twenty-three percent reach a nadir platelet count <100,000/mm^3.

TABLE 86-1 Bleeding Risk Stratification According to Platelet Count*

PLATELET COUNT (CELLS/MM^3)	BLEEDING RISK
>100,000	No increase in risk
50,000–100,000	Increased risk with major trauma
10,000–50,000	Increased risk with minor trauma
<10,000	Risk of spontaneous bleeding

*As platelet counts decrease the risk of bleeding increases.
SOURCE: Adapted from Reed ed, Steven EW. Thrombocytopenic disorders in critically ill patients. *Am J Respir Crit Care Med* 2000; 162:347–351.

- Ten percent have a nadir platelet count <50,000/mm^3.
- Patients with thrombocytopenia were found to have increased length of ICU stays and increased mortality.
- Mortality increases as platelet counts decrease.

PATHOPHYSIOLOGY

- Platelets are small, anucleated blood elements that are derived from megakaryocytes in the bone marrow.
- The average adult has 250 billion platelets per liter of blood, for a total body platelet count of over 1 trillion.
- Platelets survive in the circulation for 8 days, requiring the production of roughly 250 billion platelets each day.
- Injury results in a disruption of the vascular endothelium. Platelets that are subsequently exposed to the subendothelium release the contents of their cytoplasmic granules, which cause platelet aggregation and activation of the coagulation cascade, allowing a thrombus to form.
- For these reasons, low platelet counts can result in uncontrolled bleeding.

CLINICAL PRESENTATION AND EVALUATION

- A thorough history and physical, in concert with a measured low platelet count, is essential for the diagnosis of thrombocytopenia.
- Patients with symptomatic thrombocytopenia most commonly present with bleeding, typically from cutaneous and mucosal sources.
- Skin findings can include petechiae, purpura, or ecchymoses, particularly in dependent areas.
- An ocular fundoscopic examination should be employed if a central nervous system bleed is suspected.
- Stool samples should be tested for evidence of occult gastrointestinal bleeding.
- Metrorrhagia or menorrhagia are occasionally presenting complaints.
- Splenomegaly may be present (see "Dilutional Causes of Thrombocytopenia," below).

DIFFERENTIAL DIAGNOSIS AND MANAGEMENT

- It is often difficult to identify one discrete etiology for thrombocytopenia in ICU patients, as multiple causes often exist.

TABLE 86-2 Differential Diagnosis of Thrombocytopenia

Pseudothrombocytopenia	Laboratory error
Dilutional causes	Aggressive transfusion of blood products
Increased destruction	Sepsis/DIC
	Drug-induced
	Thrombotic microangiopathies (TTP/HUS)
	HELLP
	ITP
Decreased production	• Bone marrow failure
	◦ Bone marrow replacement
	◦ Leukemia
	◦ Lymphoma
	◦ Chemotherapy
	◦ Radiation
	• Bone marrow infection

- However, thrombocytopenia can be classified into one of four broad categories.
- These include pseudothrombocytopenia, dilutional causes, increased platelet destruction, and decreased platelet production (Table 86-2).

PSEUDOTHROMBOCYTOPENIA

- If the blood sample has been inadequately anticoagulated, clumps of platelets can be improperly counted by automated cell counters.
- If thrombocytopenia seems inappropriate given the clinical context, a repeat sample should always be evaluated.

DILUTIONAL CAUSES

TRANSFUSION RELATED

- Often ICU patients require massive donor blood transfusions.
- Platelets are only viable in donor blood for 24 hours.
- Therefore, the transfusion of large amounts of platelet-free blood can result in a dilutional thrombocytopenia.

SPLENOMEGALY

- Up to one-third of all circulating platelets can be found in the spleen.
- Patients with splenomegaly can sequester up to 90% of the total platelet volume in the spleen, resulting in peripheral platelet counts that appear low.
- No intervention is necessary for splenomegaly-associated thrombocytopenia.

PLATELET DESTRUCTION

DISSEMINATED INTRAVASCULAR COAGULATION-RELATED SEPSIS

- Sepsis is the most common cause of thrombocytopenia in ICU patients.
- It is estimated that 50% of septic patients experience thrombocytopenia.
- The mechanism by which this occurs is not entirely known, but it often involves disseminated intravascular coagulation (DIC).
- DIC results from an activation of the coagulation pathways, leading to excessive thrombin formation. This is thought to be partially due to endothelial damage associated with widespread infection.
- The resultant consumption of coagulation factors can cause a combination of bleeding and clotting complications, as well as thrombocytopenia from the platelet consumption involved in thrombosis.
- Prolonged prothrombin time (PT) and activated partial thromboplastin time (aPTT), as well as decreased fibrinogen and coagulation factors are also seen.
- Management requires identification and treatment of the underlying disorder, which in ICU patients is often gram-negative sepsis, meningococcemia, or viremia.

DRUG-INDUCED

- Common culprits include quinine, thiazide diuretics, valproic acid, trimethoprim/sulfamethoxazole, and heparin.
- Heparin is by far the most common ICU medication responsible for thrombocytopenia.
- An antibody against platelet factor 4 in 1–3% of the population leads to a consumptive thrombocytopenia in the presence of heparin.
- Patients can experience venous as well as arterial thromboses as a result of the platelet aggregation.
- Thrombocytopenia is usually apparent within 14 days of administration of heparin, but it can occur more quickly.
- Even minimal exposure to heparin, such as from line flushes or placement of heparin-coated catheters, can cause thrombocytopenia in susceptible patients.
- Diagnosis of heparin-associated thrombocytopenia is possible with an assay for heparin-induced IgG antibodies.
- Management includes immediate discontinuation of heparin and heparin products.
- If anticoagulation remains necessary, substitution with lepirudin, argatroban, or Coumadin is possible.

THROMBOTIC MICROANGIOPATHIES (THROMBOTIC THROMBOCYTOPENIC PURPURA/HEMOLYTIC UREMIC SYNDROME)

- These are multisystem diseases characterized by thrombocytopenia, fevers, and microangiopathic hemolytic anemia.
- Those who have predominant neurologic symptoms are classified as having thrombotic thrombocytopenic purpura (TTP), while those with predominant symptoms of renal failure are considered to have hemolytic uremic syndrome (HUS). These microangiopathies are characterized by fevers, acute renal failure, thrombocytopenia, anemia, and neurologic symptoms.
- TTP and HUS often overlap.
- A prognosis for these conditions can be made based on the extent of symptoms and the severity of laboratory values (Table 86-3).
- The pathophysiology involved is still largely unclear, but platelet activation from endothelial injury, *Escherichia coli* Shiga toxins, and autoimmunity have all been suggested.
- In TTP, deficiency of a protease that cleaves von Willebrand factor (VWF) results in deposition of VWF in the vessels, causing platelet aggregation and shearing of red blood cells.
- Schistocytes should be visualized on the peripheral blood smear.
- Without treatment, mortality approaches 90%.
- Plasma exchange with fresh frozen plasma until the platelet counts recover is required for management of TTP/HUS.
- Platelet transfusion has been considered contraindicated due to concerns that it could worsen the consumptive process. However, in practice, if platelet

TABLE 86-3 Severity Score for HUS/TTP*

SCORE	NEUROLOGIC SYMPTOM	RENAL INVOLVEMENT	PLATELET COUNT (mm^3)	HEMOGLOBIN (g/dL)
0	None	None	>100,000	>12
1	Confusion	Creatinine 120–150 mmol/L Proteinuria Hematuria	20,000–100,000	9–12
2	Seizures Coma Focal deficits	Creatinine >250 mmol/L Requires dialysis	<20,000	<9

*Poor outcome if score >6 at presentation.

SOURCE: Adapted from Michal R, Amiram E. High incidence of relapses in thrombotic thrombocytopenic purpura. *Am J Med* 1987;83:437–444.

transfusions are necessary for management of an acute bleed or in preparation for an invasive procedure, they may be administered with caution.

HELLP Syndrome

- HELLP is an uncommon obstetric complication characterized by **h**emolysis, **e**levated **l**iver enzymes and **l**ow **p**latelets.
- It ordinarily presents in the third trimester, but can also be seen within a week after delivery.
- HELLP is often associated with severe preeclampsia or eclampsia.
- Besides the noted laboratory abnormalities, patients also have schistocytes on peripheral blood smears.
- Management requires immediate delivery of the fetus and platelet transfusions as needed.

Idiopathic Thrombocytopenic Purpura

- Patients with idiopathic thrombocytopenic purpura (ITP) have isolated thrombocytopenia with normal red blood and white blood cell counts, and an unremarkable peripheral blood smear.
- ITP is a diagnosis of exclusion, thought to be the result of an autoantibody-mediated platelet destruction.
- Prednisone, intravenous immunoglobulins (IVIG), immunosuppressive agents, splenectomy, and platelet transfusions can be used to manage ITP.

DECREASED PLATELET PRODUCTION

Bone Marrow Failure

- This condition results from decreased or absent hematopoietic precursors in the bone marrow.
- In addition to thrombocytopenia, these patients can have anemia or neutropenia, depending on the cell lines affected.
- A variety of etiologies can account for bone marrow failure (Table 86-4).
- Relevant causes in ICU patients include:

TABLE 86-4 Causes of Bone Marrow Failure in the ICU

Bone marrow replacement
Leukemia
Lymphoma
Myelodysplastic syndrome
Chemotherapy
Radiation
Bone marrow infection
Varicella
Parvovirus
Hepatitis C
Epstein-Barr virus
HIV

  - Leukemia and lymphoma, which can invade the bone marrow and reduce or extinguish megakary- ocytes.
  - Some forms of chemotherapy or radiation which can poison the bone marrow and prevent platelet production.
  - Viral infections, including varicella, parvovirus, hepatitis C, Epstein-Barr, and HIV, which can infect and damage the bone marrow.

BIBLIOGRAPHY

Drews R, Weinberger S. Thrombocytopenic disorders in critically ill patients. *Am J Respir Crit Care Med* 2000;162:347–51.

Marino PL. Platelet disorders and replacement. *The ICU Book*, 2nd ed. Philadelphia, PA: Lippincott Williams & Wilkins; 1998:710–717.

Pene F, Vigneau C, Auburtin M, et al. Outcome of severe adult thrombotic microangiopathies in the intensive care unit. *Intensive Care Med* 2005;31:71–78.

Rose M, Eldor A. High incidence of relpases in thrombotic thrombocytopenic purpura. *Am J Med* 1987;83:437–44.

Vanderschueren S, De Weerdt A, Malbrain M, et al. Thrombocytopenia and prognosis in intensive care. *Crit Care Med* 2000;28:1871–1876.

Vincent J, Yagushi A, Pradier O. Platelet function in sepsis. *Crit Care Med* 2002;30:S313–S317.

87 PLASMAPHERESIS IN THE ICU

Nuala J. Meyer

KEY POINTS

- "Therapeutic apheresis" refers to a blood processing technique designed to remove large molecular weight substances from the circulation.
- Apheresis techniques employed in the ICU include therapeutic plasma exchange and therapeutic cytoreduction. Both techniques require high-flow venous access, typically a central catheter with two lumens for blood removal and return. Cytapheresis is the selective removal of a specific cell type—such as defective red cells or excess platelets or leukocytes. Plasmapheresis employs a highly permeable filter and dialysis equipment to remove a specific protein or to exchange the plasma volume.
- Apheresis is most helpful when the substance to be removed has a relatively large molecular weight, a

long half-life, and is toxic yet resistant to conventional therapy.

- The most common disorders for which apheresis is performed are hematopoietic, immunologic, or neurologic disorders.
- The American Society for Apheresis (ASFA) and American Association of Blood Banks (AABB) have issued guidelines for therapeutic apheresis which classify the use of apheresis as category I—first-line therapy with efficacy based on published trials or extensive clinical experience or category II—therapeutic apheresis is generally accepted in a supportive role. We will not discuss the many disorders for which apheresis has been attempted but without good supporting evidence for its role (categories III and IV). The more commonly encountered ICU situations are discussed below.

HEMATOLOGIC DISORDERS EMPLOYING PLASMA EXCHANGE

THROMBOTIC THROMBOCYTOPENIC PURPURA

- Thrombotic thrombocytopenic purpura (TTP) is a syndrome characterized by the pentad of microangiopathic hemolytic anemia, thrombocytopenia, renal failure, neurologic changes, and fever. All five features are rarely present, but the diagnosis relies on the presence of an intravascular hemolytic anemia.
- Once considered universally fatal, more than 90% of patients now survive when plasmapheresis is instituted early.
- Plasmapheresis has a category I indication for TTP.
- Hemolytic uremic syndrome (HUS) shares many pathologic similarities with TTP, but is considered a category II indication for plasmapheresis, as data for it have been less conclusive.

HYPERVISCOSITY SYNDROME

- Hyperviscosity syndrome results from circulating paraproteins in high titers which are capable of raising the serum viscosity, and typically stems from multiple myeloma (IgG, IgA, or light chain disease) or Waldenström macroglobulinemia (IgM).
- Clinical findings include headache, visual impairment, mental status changes, and epistaxis, thought to represent compromised cerebral microcirculation as well as platelet dysfunction.
- The diagnosis is made by measuring serum viscosity. Normal values are between 1.4 and 1.8; symptoms are rarely present until viscosity is measured above 5.
- Plasma exchange has a category II indication for neurologic impairment due to paraprotein-driven hyperviscosity, and a category II indication for acute myeloma renal failure.

COAGULATION FACTOR INHIBITORS

- Circulating anticoagulants, or inhibitors, are antibodies which interfere with and inactivate coagulation factors, and can often cause severe, life-threatening hemorrhage.
- Patients with a circulating inhibitor will fail to correct their coagulopathy in a mixing study.
- Acquired factor VIII inhibitor is the most frequent abnormality described, although any factor can be a target of antibody production.
- Plasma exchange is given a category II indication for the treatment of severe coagulation inhibitors.

CATASTROPHIC ANTIPHOSPHOLIPID SYNDROME

- "Catastrophic" antiphospholipid syndrome (APS) is the term used to describe an accelerated form of APS resulting in multiorgan failure from occlusion of multiple small vessels in the presence of antiphospholipid antibodies.
- Catastrophic APS is rare but life threatening, with a mortality rate approaching 50%.
- Optimal treatment remains empiric in the absence of large clinical trials, but a recent international consensus statement recommends plasma exchange along with anticoagulation and high-dose steroids for catastrophic APS whenever the patient's condition is deemed life threatening.

NEUROLOGIC DISORDERS EMPLOYING PLASMA EXCHANGE

- Neurologic conditions are among the most common indications for plasma exchange in the United States.
- *Guillain-Barré syndrome* and *chronic inflammatory demyelinating polyradiculoneuropathy (CIDP)*—the acquired demyelinating neuropathies—are thought to be immune-mediated although their precise immunopathogenesis is not known. Both are considered category I indications for plasmapheresis.
- *Myasthenia gravis (MG)* is a neuromuscular disorder of skeletal muscle weakness, caused by autoantibodies to the acetylcholine receptor (AChR). In an acute myasthenic crisis, when the patient may have ventilatory failure due to profound muscle weakness,

plasmapheresis may induce dramatic reductions in anti-AChR antibodies and in symptomatology. MG is a category I indication for plasma exchange.

- *Lambert-Eaton myasthenic syndrome*, a presynaptic disorder of the neuromuscular junction which presents with symptoms similar to MG, is also believed to be immune-mediated and can respond to plasmapheresis. It is given a category II status.

RENAL DISORDERS EMPLOYING PLASMA EXCHANGE

- As mentioned above, multiple myeloma with acute renal failure is a category II indication for plasmapheresis.
- *Goodpasture disease*, or antiglomerular basement membrane (anti-GBM) antibody disease, is a category I indication for plasmapheresis, whereby anti-GBM antibody is removed from the circulation.

HEMATOLOGIC DISEASES EMPLOYING CYTAPHERESIS

LEUKOSTASIS

- Leukostasis arises when excess white blood cells aggregate and cause microvascular infarcts, resulting in end-organ ischemia, hemorrhage, or infarction.
- Patients may present with acute dyspnea, mental status changes, or visual changes, and on examination may demonstrate pulmonary infiltrates, renal or hepatic insufficiency, priapism, or even cerebral infarct.
- Patients at highest risk for leukostasis are those with acute leukemia, especially acute myelogenous leukemia, or the blast phase of chronic myelogenous leukemia (CML) with blast counts >50,000. Despite blast counts of >500,000, patients with chronic lymphocytic leukemias have a much lower risk for leukostasis.
- Acute leukemia is considered a medical emergency, and if a patient is exhibiting symptoms consistent with leukostasis, primary consideration should be given to emergent reduction in the white cell count by leukapheresis, chemotherapy, or a combination of the two.
- Leukapheresis has a category I indication for acute leukemia in blast crisis.

THROMBOCYTOSIS

- In myeloproliferative disorders such as essential thrombocytosis, the platelet count can occasionally exceed 1 million. These abnormal platelets contribute to a bleeding diathesis characterized by both hemorrhage and thrombosis.
- Symptoms of excess platelets mimic those of hyperviscosity, with headache, visual changes, and epistaxis.
- Cytapheresis to selectively decrease the platelet count to below 1 million has a category I indication in myeloproliferative syndromes.
- In contrast, cytapheresis is not indicated for reactive thrombocytosis, such as may accompany an infectious or rheumatologic process.

RED BLOOD CELL EXCHANGE

- In severe sickle cell crises, the abnormal red cells can aggregate and contribute to microvascular or macrovascular thrombosis, ischemia, or infarct.
- Clinically, vaso-occlusive crises can present as severe pain crises, acute chest syndrome, cerebrovascular accident or transient ischemic attack (TIA), or sequestration crisis.
- Exchanging the patient's sickled red blood cells (RBCs) for normal morphology cells can greatly reduce morbidity, and should be undertaken emergently in these circumstances. It may be helpful to follow the patient's fraction of sickled cells as a marker for improvement.
- RBC exchange has a category I indication in severe sickle cell crisis.

COMPLICATIONS OF APHERESIS

- Therapeutic apheresis procedures are generally safe and well tolerated, with approximately a 5% incidence of adverse events. The majority of adverse events are reversible.
- Possible reactions include transfusion reaction, nausea, pallor, rigors, fever, and rarely seizure.
- Complications may also arise from the placement of central venous catheters.

BIBLIOGRAPHY

Asherson RA, Cervera R, de Groot PG, et al. Catastrophic antiphospholipid syndrome: international consensus statement on classification criteria and treatment guidelines. *Lupus* 2003;12:530–534.

Lamont EB, Hoffman PC. Oncologic emergencies. In: Hall JB, Schmidt GA, Wood LDH, eds., *Principles of Critical Care*, 3rd ed. New York, NY: McGraw-Hill; 2005:1099–1110.

Larson RA, Hall MJ. Acute leukemia. In: Hall JB, Schmidt GA, Wood LDH, eds., *Principles of Critical Care*, 3rd ed. New York, NY: McGraw-Hill;2005:1089–1098.
McLeod BC, Sniecinski I, Ciavarella D, et al. Frequency of immediate adverse effects associated with therapeutic apheresis. *Transfusion* 1999;39:282–288.
Smith JW, Weinstein R, Hillyer KL. Therapeutic apheresis: a summary of current indication categories endorsed by the AABB and the American Society for Apheresis. *Transfusion* 2003;43:820–822.

88 ACUTE LEUKEMIA

Shashi Kiran Bellam

KEY POINTS

- Acute leukemia is uniformly fatal if untreated, but many patients can be cured with the combination of chemotherapy and aggressive supportive care.
- Critical care is often required for either the complications of the disease or of the treatment.
- Blood transfusions should be used to maintain a hemoglobin of 10 g/dL and a platelet count >10,000/μL.
- Extreme leukocytosis may lead to leukostasis, which is a medical emergency and requires immediate leukopheresis and chemotherapy.
- Many complications occur from the infiltration of leukemic cells into various organs.
- Infection and bleeding are predisposed by the severe pancytopenia and resolve with supportive care and restoration of normal bone marrow production.
- Rapid cellular turnover, often precipitated by chemotherapy, can lead to hyperuricemia and renal failure.

GENERAL CLINICAL FEATURES

- *Etiology*: Leukemia occurs when a genetic alteration occurs in a hematopoietic stem cell leading to the proliferation of a clone of cells in the bone marrow; ultimately, the normal bone marrow elements are replaced by neoplastic cells.
- *Diagnosis*: White blood cell (WBC) counts are frequently elevated with abnormal cell types (especially blasts), but some patients have normal or low WBC counts. Anemia and thrombocytopenia are common. More precise diagnosis and classification depends on bone marrow aspirate and biopsy, with subsequent cytochemical tests (e.g., presence of myeloperoxidase), immunochemical tests (e.g., flow cytometry), and cytogenetic analyses allowing for a more precise classification. Arterial blood gases may reveal low oxygen content due to consumption of oxygen by blast cells after sampling. This "pseudohypoxemia" may be minimized by transport on ice and prompt laboratory measurements.

THERAPY

- Primarily chemotherapy; the successfulness of chemotherapy depends on the individual response to therapy and the ability of the patient to survive the complications that occur with treatment. Chemotherapy can be split into several stages (remission, consolidation, and maintenance).
- The goal of remission therapy is to induce a complete remission (defined as absence of leukemic cells in the bone marrow and blood, return of normal bone marrow cells, and return of normal peripheral blood counts).
- For induction chemotherapy, anything less than complete remission does not improve survival. After induction chemotherapy and complete remission, most patients would relapse within 2–4 months without further therapy.
- Consolidation chemotherapy aims to destroy any residual leukemic cells (undetected) after induction chemotherapy, and usually consists of 1–4 monthly cycles. Patients who relapse after acute leukemia can undergo a repeat of the induction chemotherapy regimen to attempt to achieve a second remission, though the likelihood of a second remission is lower than a first remission, and patients who relapse usually do not have a long survival. Bone marrow or peripheral stem cell transplantation can be an option for some patients who suffer a relapse of their leukemia.
- Patients with evidence of peripheral organ hypoperfusion may benefit from red blood cell (RBC) transfusions to maintain a hemoglobin concentration >10 g/dL. The significance of potential additional immunosuppression due to RBC transfusion on patients who have leukemia and/or are neutropenic is unknown.
- All transfusions should be leukocyte depleted to decrease the rate of alloimmunization.
- Platelets should be transfused to maintain a platelet count of >10,000/μL. All transfusions should be single-donor platelets collected by apheresis to decrease the rate of alloimmunization.
- Severely neutropenic patients who remain bacteremic despite antibiotics may benefit from granulocyte transfusions, though complications such as rapid alloimmunization, worsening respiratory status due to granulocyte agglutination or infiltration into the lung, and transmission of cytomegalovirus (CMV) infection are potential complications.

COMMON COMPLICATIONS OF LEUKEMIA

HYPERVISCOSITY SYNDROME

- *Etiology*: Hyperviscosity syndrome is a condition of decreased blood movement through small capillaries leading to physical occlusion and hypoxemia (leukostasis). RBC transfusions can precipitate leukostasis by increasing blood viscosity.
- *Clinical features*: Include respiratory distress, cardiac arrhythmias, and altered mental status, including coma.
- *Diagnosis*: Hyperviscosity occurs in the setting of hyperleukocytosis, is defined as >100,000 blast cells/μL. However, risks of hyperviscosity can occur at levels between 50,000 and 100,000 blast cells/μL. Immature myelocytes are much larger than immature lymphocytes; thus, the incidence of leukostasis is more common in chronic myeloid leukemia (CML) in blast phase or acute myeloid leukemia (AML) than acute lymphocytic leukemia (ALL). Chronic lymphocytic leukemia (CLL) rarely leads to leukostasis.
- *Treatment*: Hydration, leukopheresis to directly remove blast cells from the circulating blood volume, and prompt use of chemotherapeutic agents such as hydroxyurea to decrease the blast count. Central nervous system (CNS) abnormalities can be treated with cranial irradiation (200–400 cGy). Pulmonary abnormalities may respond to thoracic radiation.

MYELOID SARCOMA

- *Etiology*: Myeloid blast cells may form a solid tumor, most commonly in CML with blast phase. These solid tumors (aka myeloid sarcoma) may occur in the bone, lymph nodes, skin, soft tissues, and gastrointestinal (GI) tract.
- *Clinical features*: Common symptoms include pain, neuropathy, and intestinal obstruction.
- *Treatment*: Local radiation (1000–2000 cGy) in addition to chemotherapy (which often treats these masses quickly).

CENTRAL NERVOUS SYSTEM LEUKEMIA

- *Definition*: Penetration of leukemic cells into the CNS, more commonly in children, in ALL, and with elevated circulating blast counts.
- *Clinical features*: Presentations include cranial or spinal nerve defects (neuropathy or radiculopathy). The most common symptoms occur due to increased intracranial pressure and include headache, nausea, papilledema, and lethargy. Facial nerve palsies, diplopia, spinal radiculopathy, and the cauda equina syndrome can also occur. Mass lesions, seizures, and meningismus are uncommon.
- *Diagnosis*: Finding of leukemia cells in the cerebrospinal fluid (CSF). In that setting, usually the opening pressure is elevated, the glucose concentration is low, and the protein level is elevated. Thrombocytopenia should be treated with platelet transfusion prior to attempting lumbar puncture.
- *Treatment*: Radiation (2400 cGy to the whole brain in 12 fractions) and intrathecal chemotherapy (methotrexate 12 mg/m^2 to a maximum dose of 15 mg every 3 days intrathecal for at least 6 doses along with hydrocortisone 50 mg to prevent an inflammatory arachnoiditis). Spinal column radiation is appropriate for patients with symptomatic radiculopathy, but risks damage to underlying bone marrow. Dexamethasone (4 mg qid) can be an adjunctive treatment to lower intracranial pressure. Chronic chemotherapy once the CSF is clear of malignant cells should occur monthly. An Ommaya reservoir is often used to allow for repetitive intraventricular administration of chemotherapy.

HEPATOSPLENOMEGALY

- *Etiology/clinical features*: Leukemic infiltration with blast cells (usually in ALL or CLL) into the liver and spleen can cause symptoms of acute hepatitis (jaundice, hepatomegaly, transaminitis). Splenic infiltration may lead to vascular infarction, clinically presenting as a painful subcapsular hematoma; rarely, spleen rupture may occur leading to shock with intraperitoneal hemorrhage.
- *Diagnosis*: Biliary ultrasound to rule out bile duct obstruction should be performed, auscultation of the left upper quadrant (LUQ) demonstrating a rub with respiratory variation can be seen in splenic subcapsular hematoma, and diagnostic peritoneal lavage may reveal intraperitoneal hemorrhage.
- *Therapy*: Liver infiltration usually responds to chemotherapy; however, initial drug options may be limited as many chemotherapeutics are metabolized in the liver. Spleen rupture may require surgical repair.

KIDNEY INFILTRATION AND URETERAL OBSTRUCTION

- *Etiology/clinical features*: Leukemic infiltration into the kidney is more common in ALL and presents as oliguric acute renal failure; enlarged retroperitoneal lymph nodes may cause ureteral obstruction.
- *Diagnosis*: Renal ultrasound reveals kidney enlargement but no ureteral obstruction.

- *Therapy*: Kidney infiltration resolves with chemotherapy, but decreased urinary function may not allow adequate excretion of products of tumor lysis. Radiation (200–400 cGy) to the kidneys or ureters can reestablish renal excretory function prior to chemotherapy in the case of obstructing lymphadenopathy.

TYPHLITIS (NECROTIZING ENTEROCOLITIS)

- *Etiology*: Typhlitis usually affects the terminal ileum, appendix, cecum, and right colon in granulocytopenic patients.
- *Clinical features*: Mimics inflammatory bowel disease, with nausea, vomiting, abdominal pain, and tenderness, watery or bloody diarrhea, and fever. Intestinal mucosal ulceration allows for the loss of proteins and electrolytes as well as the translocation of enteric organisms into and through the bowel wall, potentially leading to ileus, bowel perforation, and peritonitis. Bacterial seeding of the portal vein can lead to jaundice and hepatitis.
- *Therapy*: Includes antibiotics, transfusion of blood products as needed, repletion of serum electrolytes, and bowel rest. Agents that decrease bowel peristalsis (e.g., narcotics) should be avoided. Granulocyte transfusions can be lifesaving. Bowel perforation requires surgical evaluation.

LYSOZYMURIA AND RENAL TUBULAR DYSFUNCTION

- Lysozyme is a protein in granulocytes that is capable of lysis of bacterial cells walls. It is excreted in the urine, but is toxic to renal tubule cells and can lead to marked hypokalemia. Treatment of the underlying leukemia is usually adequate.

DISSEMINATED INTRAVASCULAR COAGULATION

- *Etiology/clinical features*: Disseminated intravascular coagulation (DIC) universally occurs in acute promyelocytic leukemia and can occur with any type of leukemia. Clinical presentations include diffuse bleeding or oozing from venipuncture sites, thrombosis within the renal vasculature leading to mild renal insufficiency (potentially exacerbated by aminoglycoside antibiotics, leading to acute renal failure at normal antibiotic serum concentrations).
- *Therapy*: Chemotherapy to reduce the tumor burden leads to improvement in the DIC. Blood product or factor repletion and/or heparin administration is not well validated and usage is institution and/or physician dependent.
- All-trans retinoic acid (ATRA) is an effective agent for acute promyelocytic leukemia, but can lead to hyperleukocytosis and the retinoic acid syndrome. ATRA induces differentiation of leukemic blasts in the bone marrow leading to leukocytosis in the peripheral blood. Concomitant chemotherapy and/or leukopheresis may be useful in reducing the WBC count. The retinoic acid syndrome occurs in 25% of patients receiving ATRA and presents as fever, progressive respiratory distress with diffuse infiltrates on chest x-ray (CXR), pleural effusions, and weight gain anytime from 2 days to 4 weeks after ATRA treatment. Untreated, retinoic acid syndrome can lead to death. Prompt treatment with steroids (dexamethasone 10 mg bid for 3 days) is effective in most patients.

LACTIC ACIDOSIS

- Elevated blood lactate or pyruvate concentrations are common in patients with leukemia due to a variety of causes. Occasionally, hemodialysis or peritoneal dialysis to remove lactic acid may be useful.

COMMON COMPLICATIONS OF THERAPY

INFECTION AND SEPSIS

- *Etiology/clinical features*: Severe immunosuppression may occur due to both the effect of leukemia and the effect of therapy. Chemotherapy leads to cellular death of mucosal barriers, leading to invasion of endogenous organisms, such as gram-negative enteric bacteria, gram-positive cocci, and fungi (such as *Candida* and *Aspergillus*). Patients with ALL also have specific susceptibility to Pneumocystis pneumonia, mycobacterial, and viral infections due to lymphocyte dysfunction. Clinical features include fever (temperature >101.5°F) and neutropenia.
- *Therapy*: Cultures of blood, urine, and sputum, and empiric therapy with either ceftazidime or imipenem (either as a single agent therapy) or a combination of antipseudomonal penicillin with an aminoglycoside. Antibiotic regimen depends on renal function, allergy history, and individual physician preference. Empiric vancomycin can be indicated depending on prevalence of methicillin-resistant gram-positive bacteria. Transfusions of blood products as described above should be used. Granulocyte-stimulating factors (granulocyte colony-stimulating factor [G-CSF] or granulocyte-macrophage colony-stimulating factor

[GM-CSF]) can reduce the risk of febrile neutropenia when used prophylactically.

TUMOR LYSIS SYNDROME

- *Etiology/clinical features*: Uric acid, a product of cell turnover, is excreted by the kidneys and elevated levels may cause nephropathy, either due to the high cell turnover of the underlying leukemia, or as a response to therapy. Urate crystals precipitate in the collecting system due to dehydration and aciduria. Phosphate levels may be elevated due to cellular death leading to calcium phosphate precipitation in the calyces and tubes.
- *Therapy*: Hydration to maintain urine flow, correction of acidosis, including usage of sodium bicarbonate and acetazolamide to alkalinize the urine to a pH of 7.0–7.5. Allopurinol (300 mg/day) will inhibit the conversion of cellular byproducts to uric acid. The combination of allopurinol, hydration, and alkalinization of the urine is usually adequate to prevent uric acid nephropathy. Rasburicase (0.20 mg/kg) rapidly metabolizes serum uric acid and can be given intravenously for 1–5 days. Allopurinol should be held during that time and can be restarted after the hyperuricemia resolves.

BIBLIOGRAPHY

Larson RA, Hall MJ. Acute leukemia. In: Hall JB, Schmidt GA, Wood LDH, eds., *Principles of Critical Care*, 3rd ed. New York, NY: McGraw-Hill; 2005:1089–1098.

Lowenberg B, Downing JR, Burnett A. Acute myeloid leukemia. *N Engl J Med* 1999;341:1051–1062.

Pui CH, Relling MV, Downing JR. Acute lymphoblastic leukemia. *N Engl J Med* 2004;350(15):1535–1548.

89 SUPERIOR VENA CAVA SYNDROME

Nuala J. Meyer

KEY POINTS

- Superior vena cava syndrome occurs when blood flow through the SVC is obstructed by direct compression or thrombus.
- SVC obstruction is most frequently caused by malignancy or thrombosis. Infections are an infrequent cause.
- Patients typically present with edema of the face, neck, and upper extremities, but may demonstrate airway obstruction, esophageal obstruction, dyspnea, dysphonia, or even cardiovascular compromise.
- Treatment of SVCS depends on the severity of the patient's symptoms as well as the underlying cause.

DEFINITION

- Superior vena cava syndrome (SVCS) is the name given to the symptoms and signs of obstruction to blood flow through the SVC.
- SVC obstruction occurs as a consequence of external compression or invasion of the vessel—most commonly by tumors of the lung or mediastinum—or of thrombosis within the SVC.

ETIOLOGY

- Malignancy is the most common cause of SVC obstruction, accounting for approximately 85% of cases.
  - Lung cancer is the most common malignant cause of SVCS, and among primary lung neoplasms, small cell carcinoma is an especially frequent cause.
  - Lymphoma is the second leading malignant cause of SVCS, and may occur in 2–4% of cases of non-Hodgkin lymphoma (Figs. 89-1, 89-2, and 89-3).
  - Other malignancies rarely implicated in SVC obstruction include the tumors of anterior mediastinum (teratoma or germ cell tumors and thymoma) or metastatic disease to the mediastinal lymph nodes.
  - SVCS may be the presenting symptom of cancer.

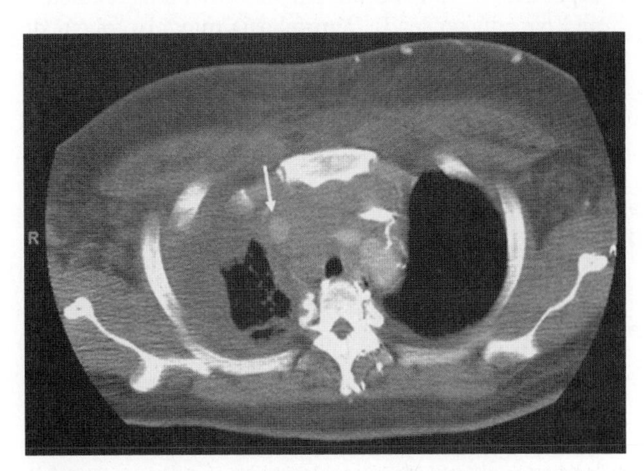

FIG. 89-1 Demonstrate SVCS on the CT scan of a patient with an anterior mediastinal mass. The arrow points to the SVC, which is moderately narrowed from Fig. 89-1.

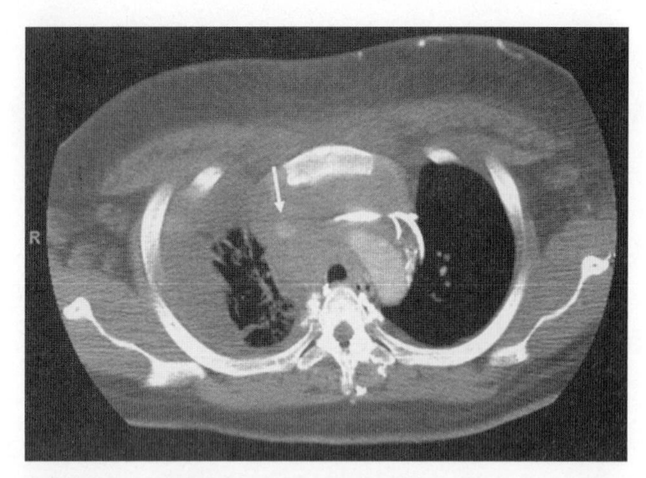

FIG. 89-2 The SVC is further narrowed.

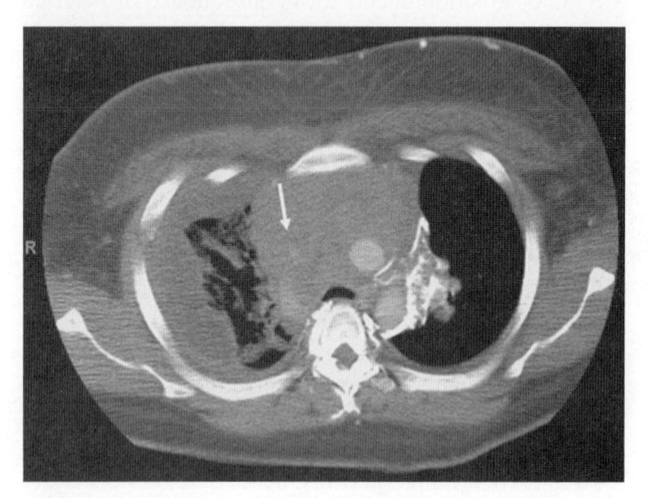

FIG. 89-3 Here the SCV, surrounded and compressed is barely recognized.

- Thrombosis is a rapidly expanding cause of SVCS, especially given the advent of indwelling catheters and pacemaker leads. Thrombosis may also occur de novo in patients with hypercoagulable states.
- Infectious complications—especially syphilitic aortitis or fibrosing mediastinitis associated with histoplasmosis—were historically important causes of SVCS. These complications are relatively rare in the industrialized world.

PATHOPHYSIOLOGY

- Tumors tend to involve the SVC by extrinsic compression or by direct invasion. Enlarged mediastinal lymph nodes or tumors arising from the central airways are classically at fault.
- Rare intravascular lymphomas may arise within the SVC itself.
- Thrombosis results from the typical risk factors of stasis, vascular injury, or hypercoagulability, but most often forms around a nidus for clot such as indwelling lines.
- The more rapid the SVC obstruction, the more acute the symptoms due to the lack of time to form collateral venous channels.

CLINICAL FEATURES

- Obstruction of the SVC raises the central venous pressure and impedes venous outflow from the head and neck, reducing venous return to the right atrium.
- Depending on the extent of mediastinal compression, airway or esophageal obstruction may also be present, causing dyspnea or dysphagia.
- Laryngeal edema, airway obstruction, and stridor are the most ominous complications of SVCS and represent true medical emergencies requiring rapid treatment.
- In patients with chronic or indolent obstruction of the SVC, venous collaterals form and may cause impressive distention of the azygos, internal mammary, intercostal, and long thoracic veins.
- Patients report dyspnea as the most frequent symptom; facial swelling and fullness, arm edema, and cough are also common. Symptoms may worsen with lying supine or bending forward.
- On examination, one typically finds facial plethora with obvious venous distention of the neck and chest.
- Especially when the cause is thrombotic, SVCS may coexist with pulmonary embolism.

DIAGNOSTIC EVALUATION

- Early recognition and diagnosis is critical to appropriately manage patients with obstruction of the SVC. Malignant compression must be distinguished from thrombotic occlusion, as these represent distinct therapeutic categories.
- As malignancy is the leading cause of SVCS, the most helpful initial test is typically a chest radiograph. Abnormalities may include mediastinal mass or widening, pleural effusion, or lung mass.
- Infused chest computed tomography (CT) is helpful to confirm the diagnosis of SVCS, to define the extent of venous blockage, and to evaluate collateral drainage. CT is also helpful in elucidating the ultimate cause of SVC obstruction.
- Venography or ultrasonography of upper extremity veins may also permit diagnosis of SVCS, but frequently do not reveal the etiology of obstruction.
- When malignancy is suspected without a known primary cancer, tissue biopsy should be obtained.

- Depending on the clinical presentation, minimally invasive procedures such as sputum cytology, pleural fluid analysis, or excisional lymph node biopsy may yield a diagnosis in a majority of cases.
- If lymphoma is suspected, bone marrow biopsy may prove diagnostic.
- Bronchoscopy with transbronchial needle aspiration from paratracheal lymph nodes may prove diagnostic.
- When less invasive measures fail to make a histologic diagnosis, consideration should be given to mediastinoscopy, thoracoscopy, or thoracotomy.
- Symptomatic obstruction occurs over weeks, and the delay of therapy until a diagnosis has been obtained is both safe and appropriate for most patients with malignant SVCS. Radiation therapy without first obtaining a diagnosis is NOT recommended as it may preclude definitive diagnosis.

INTENSIVE CARE UNIT MANAGEMENT

- Treatment of an occluded SVC is directed at the underlying pathologic process.
- In the case of iatrogenic or thrombotic SVCS resulting from indwelling vascular hardware, treatment is generally a combination of anticoagulation, percutaneous transluminal angioplasty, and/or metallic wall stents.
  - Some authors advocate the use of thrombolytic therapy with or without angioplasty if the clot has been symptomatic for fewer than 5 days.
  - Subsequent oral anticoagulant therapy is generally indicated for at least the short term.
- Malignant SVCS is treated based on the severity of symptoms and the knowledge of the underlying histology.
  - In emergent cases, such as stridor, hypotension, or cardiopulmonary collapse, the patient should receive either emergent endovascular wall stenting or emergent radiotherapy. Wall stenting may be superior in this instance, both for its faster resolution (72 hours vs. 1–3 weeks for radiotherapy) and for its preservation of diagnostic ability.
  - For less emergent symptoms, treatment is based on the knowledge of the specific tumors response to treatment.
  - Treatment-responsive tumors with relatively good prognoses, such as non-Hodgkin lymphoma, germ cell tumors, or early small cell lung cancer, respond well to chemotherapy with or without the addition of radiotherapy.
  - Less responsive tumors—nonsmall cell lung cancer or primary mediastinal B-cell lymphoma—may respond as well to endovascular stents or radiotherapy/chemotherapy at presentation.
- Benign SVCS, as may occur following fibrosing mediastinitis related to prior infection with histoplasmosis, tuberculosis, or other indolent infections, often occurs over many years with ample time for the formation of extensive collateral venous drainage. Such patients rarely require any intervention. If the syndrome develops rapidly, consideration should be given to endovascular stenting or even SVC bypass surgery.
- No trial has demonstrated a benefit of corticosteroids in SVCS.

BIBLIOGRAPHY

Kvale PA, Simoff M, Prakash UB. Palliative care. *Chest* 2003;123:284S–311S.

Parish JM, Marschke RE, Dines DE, et al. Etiologic considerations in superior vena cava syndrome. *Mayo Clin Proc* 1981;56:407–413.

Rowell NP, Gleeson FV. Steroids, radiotherapy, chemotherapy and stents for superior vena cava obstruction in carcinoma of the bronchus: a systematic review. *Clin Oncol* 2002;14:338–351.

Selcuk ZT, Firat P. The diagnostic yield of transbronchial needle aspiration in superior vena cava syndrome. *Lung Cancer* 2004;42:183–188.

Urruticoechea A, Mesia R, Dominguez J, et al. Treatment of malignant superior vena cava syndrome by endovascular stent insertion: experience of 52 patients with lung cancer. *Lung Cancer* 2004;43:209–214.

90 BONE MARROW TRANSPLANTATION

Joseph Levitt

KEY POINTS

- Stem cell transplantation is the reconstitution of a patient's hematopoietic stem cells after myeloablative chemotherapy with previously harvested stem cells.
- During the period prior to engraftment of the stem cells, the patient is functionally without an immune system.
- Reintroduction of the patient's native stem cells is an autologous bone marrow transplant (BMT). Introduction of another person's stem cells is an allogeneic BMT.
- Allogeneic BMT carries the risk of GVHD.

- The various disease syndromes associated with BMT will be discussed below, and include GVHD, HVOD, infections, and bronchiolitis.
- Allogeneic BMT requires immune suppression of the patient, predisposing them to serious infectious complications even after successful transplant.

BACKGROUND

- Hematopoietic stem cell transplantation (SCT) consists of infusing previously harvested patient bone marrow or peripheral stem cells (autologous or auto-SCT) or a donor's cells (allogeneic or allo-SCT) following myeloablative chemoradiation therapy.
- Donors are matched by their human leukocyte antigen (HLA) pattern. Identically matched siblings (25% chance per sibling) have the best results. When no matched sibling exists, donors can be selected from a registry. Many antigen interactions other than HLA exist but are not screened for. Unrelated donors are likely to have more mismatches in unmeasured antigens and thus more graft-versus-host disease (GVHD).
- Auto-SCT patients suffer many of the same complications as allo-SCT but do not develop GVHD. However, they also don't benefit from the beneficial graft-versus-malignancy effect and show higher relapse rates.
- Understanding the time course of recovery of immune function is essential in diagnosing various clinical syndromes following SCT.
  - Engraftment of stem cells and return of granulocytes usually occurs 3 weeks following chemoradiation therapy.
  - Lymphocyte numbers may normalize at 1 month but antibody levels are reduced for >3 months and secretory IgA may be permanently suppressed.
  - Abnormal T-cell antigen production (important for vaccine-mediated immunity) may persist for a year.
- The incidence of many opportunistic infections has been dramatically altered by effective prophylactic regimens.
- Morbidity and mortality following SCT result from rejection, relapse of underlying condition, infection, toxicity (hepatic, gastrointestinal [GI], cardiac, lung, and central nervous system [CNS]) of chemotherapeutic conditioning regimens, and GVHD.

RELAPSE AND REJECTION

- Rejection is rare (<1%) in HLA identical recipients conditioned with total body irradiation (TBI), but risks rise with increasing HLA mismatching and prior history of receiving multiple transfusions.
- Relapse of hematologic malignancies occurs in about 20% of cases transplanted after first relapse or in chronic phases but increases to 50–70% of transplants after relapse or in blast crisis.
- Less experience exists for relapse rates in solid tumor malignancy.

INFECTIONS

- Serious bacterial infections occur in up to 50% of patients; most during the 30 days of neutropenia following transplant. Most common sources are indwelling central catheters, lung, and translocation from the GI tract.
- Sepsis syndromes in the posttransplant period may have many etiologies but treatment should include efforts to identify a source (careful examination including skin and catheter sites, blood and urine cultures, chest x-ray, and computed tomography [CT] scan) and early empiric broad-spectrum antibiotics (including *Pseudomonas* and methicillin-resistant *Staph aureus* coverage).
- Invasive hemodynamic monitoring and vasoactive drugs, including inotropes are often necessary for management due to the tendency for transplant patients to become whole body volume overloaded and many have occult cardiac dysfunction secondary to cardiotoxic therapies.
- Fungal infections are also common during neutropenia. *Aspergillus* is the most common in lung and sinuses with *Candida* frequently invading the GI tract and blood stream via indwelling catheters. The development of new antifungal therapies with improved side effect profiles (voriconazole and caspofungin) has increased the prevalence of empiric treatment in unexplained fever.
- Viral infections are most common between 30 and 100 days posttransplant. Cytomegalovirus (CMV) is the most common, particularly in seropositive patients or seronegative recipients with a seropositive donor. Routine ganciclovir prophylaxis is practiced by many centers for these high-risk patients. Use of seronegative or leukocyte-filtered blood products in seronegative patients reduces rates of CMV transmission. Routine screening for CMV viremia and treatment with ganciclovir at first sign of positivity is also recommended even in absence of symptoms.
- Incidence of herpes simplex virus (HSV) and varicella (VZV) infections are markedly reduced with the routine use of acyclovir prophylaxis.
- Respiratory syncytial virus (RSV) and parainfluenza virus are common causes of diffuse pulmonary infiltrates and may occur in the early posttransplant phase, especially during endemic months.

- Pneumocystis (PCP) infections are rare when trimethoprim-sulfamethoxazole prophylaxis is complied with.

GRAFT-VERSUS-HOST DISEASE

ACUTE

- Acute GVHD occurs in the first 3 months following allo-SCT and consists of lymphatic infiltration of skin, liver, and GI tract.
- Incidence of at least mild GVHD is 20–50% in HLA identical patients and 80% with nonidentical or unrelated donors despite the routine use of prophylactic immunosuppressive regimens of methotrexate and cyclosporine. T-cell depleted donor stem cells are also used to reduce GVHD rates in some protocols.
- Presentation may include fever, macular dermatitis, cramping abdominal pain, watery or bloody diarrhea, jaundice, cholestasis, and hepatocellular necrosis.
- Associated mortality depends on severity and site of organ involvement. Hepatitis is the most serious complication but desquamative dermatitis and severe mucositis predisposing to GI bleeding (in setting of low platelets and liver dysfunction) and malnutrition can cause significant morbidity.
- Clinical diagnosis can be difficult because of the many other conditions (veno-occlusive disease, viral- and drug-induced hepatitis) that may mimic the presentation in this population. Biopsy, particularly of skin, is recommended when it can be performed safely. Endoscopic biopsy of the GI tract and even transjugular liver biopsy (percutaneous procedures are too high risk) may be necessary, even with positive skin biopsy, to rule out other etiologies.
- Hepatitis due to GVHD is characterized by extremely high alkaline phosphatase levels.
- Acute GVHD has variable response to increased immunosuppression. Treatment consists of corticosteroids (methylprednisolone 2 mg/kg/day) and antithymocyte globulins. Steroid refractory disease is often fatal.

CHRONIC

- Chronic GVHD may involve the lung as well as skin, liver, and GI tract.
- It usually occurs following a history of acute GVHD but 20–30% of cases can develop de novo.
- It usually follows an indolent course but adversely affects long-term survival.
- Chronic GVHD suppresses host immunity independent of the immunosuppressive therapy used to treat it and infection is the most common cause of death.

HEPATIC VENO-OCCLUSIVE DISEASE

- Hepatic veno-occlusive disease (HVOD) results from occlusion of hepatic venules by thrombosis and cellular debris that is likely due to endothelial injury related to the chemoradiation-conditioning regimen.
- Incidence is as high as 20–60% in transplantation following TBI.
- Onset occurs 14 days posttransplant and is characterized by the triad of weight gain, painful hepatomegaly, and jaundice. Ascites, elevated transaminases, and progression to hepatorenal syndrome may occur.
- Diagnosis is clinical and criteria are based on degree of hyperbilirubinemia and weight gain plus or minus the presence of ascites.
- No definitive diagnostic test exists but CT and ultrasound can confirm the hepatomegaly and ascites and may help rule out other diagnoses (i.e., Budd-Chiari). Doppler ultrasound criteria for pulsatile hepatic vein flow and reversal of portal flow exist but are not specific for HVOD. Wedge hepatic venous pressure gradient during transvenous liver biopsy may be diagnostic but is not generally indicated.
- Overall mortality is 30% but is >90% in severe (graded by degree of hyperbilirubinemia and weight gain) cases.
- No effective treatment exists, although experimental therapies with anticoagulants and thrombolytics are being tried.

PULMONARY COMPLICATIONS

- Pneumonia syndromes develop in 40–60% of patients with the etiology heavily dependent on the time course posttransplant.

INFECTIOUS ETIOLOGIES

- Bacterial or fungal infections are the most common etiologies of focal opacities particularly during neutropenia. Typical appearing nodules with cavitation or enhancing rings (halo sign) on CT scan are highly suggestive of fungal infection, (although septic emboli from indwelling catheters may also appear nodular and cavitate).
- *Aspergillus* is the most common fungal infection of the lung, although mucormycosis, *Fusarium*, histoplasmosis, and other endemic fungi are seen.
- *Candida* is often found on airway sampling (sputum or lavage) but is thought to only cause invasive infection in the lung through hematogenous spread. Isolating *Candida* from other sites (blood, urine, GI tract) is recommended before initiating therapy.

- As previously mentioned, CMV, HSV, and VZV are more common between 30 and 100 days posttransplant and usually cause a diffuse infiltrate.
- RSV and parainfluenza virus are the most common infectious causes of diffuse infiltrates in the first 30 days.

NONINFECTIOUS ETIOLOGIES

- Pulmonary hemorrhage, high-pressure pulmonary edema, acute respiratory distress syndrome (ARDS), and drug toxicity are all frequent causes of diffuse infiltrates in first 30 days.
- The idiopathic pneumonia syndrome (IPS) is a common clinical entity of nonspecific lung injury likely related to drug toxicity but may be multifactorial.
  - Diagnostic criteria are (1) signs and symptoms of pneumonia, (2) hypoxemia or restrictive defect of pulmonary function testing, (3) bilateral infiltrates, and (4) a nondiagnostic bronchoscopy with bronchoalveolar lavage (BAL).
  - Onset is a mean of 45 days posttransplant.
  - Overall mortality is 60% but when it progresses to respiratory failure, mortality approaches 100%.
- Pulmonary GVHD presents >100 days posttransplant and is highly associated with CMV infection and bronchiolitis obliterans.
- Bronchiolitis obliterans occurs in 10% of patients but, depending on diagnostic criteria, incidence may be >30% in chronic GVHD. Onset is >100 days posttransplant and is characterized by breathlessness due to progressive airflow obstruction.
  - Definitive diagnosis is made by surgical biopsy which shows cellular infiltration compressing small airways. However, diagnosis can be made on clinical grounds and spirometry showing airflow obstruction that doesn't respond to bronchodilators.
  - Chest x-ray may show hyperinflation or be normal. High-resolution CT scans show mosaic attenuation on expiratory views highlighting air-trapping in terminal airways.
- Airflow obstruction may be progressive and rapidly fatal or may stabilize but rarely resolves. Treatment consists of increasing immunosuppression but is of unclear benefit.

DIAGNOSIS AND MANAGEMENT

- Bronchoscopy with BAL is the diagnostic procedure of choice and can be performed safely even with profound thrombocytopenia.
- Diagnostic yield is high for bacterial, PCP, and viral infections and pulmonary hemorrhage but less so for fungal infections and other noninfectious etiologies. BAL fluid should be processed for:
  - Bacterial, viral, and fungal cultures and stain
  - Rapid detection for viral pathogens including polymerase chain reaction (PCR), direct fluorescent antibodies, or shell viral culture for CMV
  - Cell count and cytologic review
- Transbronchial biopsy adds little to diagnostic yield and can often not be performed due to thrombocytopenia. CT-guided percutaneous biopsy of peripheral nodules may be possible.
- Surgical lung biopsy is necessary for diagnosis of most noninfectious etiologies including IPS. However, experience shows that even this can be nonspecific and often does not alter therapy or outcomes and should only be performed in highly selected patients who can safely tolerate the procedure and have a high probability of clinical benefit.
- Treatment is often empiric with broad-spectrum antibiotics, antifungal and antiviral therapies, and immunosuppression.
- Early use of noninvasive positive pressure ventilation may improve mortality in neutropenic patients with respiratory failure.
- Transplant patients who progress to respiratory failure often do so despite maximal therapy to prevent it. Mechanical ventilation in the setting of multisystem organ failure is universally fatal. Standard of care is to restrict protracted intensive care in such cases.

BIBLIOGRAPHY

Crawford SW, Folz RJ, Sullivan KM. Hematopoietic stem cell transplantation and graft-versus-host disease. In: Hall JB, Schmidt GA, Wood LDH, eds., *Principles of Critical Care*, 3rd ed. New York, NY: McGraw-Hill; 2005:1111–1122.

Wadleigh M, Ho V, Momtaz P, et al. Hepatic veno-occlusive disease: pathogenesis, diagnosis and treatment. *Curr Opin Hematol* 2003;10:451–462.

Yen KT, Lee AS, Krowka MJ, et al. Pulmonary complications in bone marrow transplantation: a practical approach to diagnosis and treatment. *Clin Chest Med* 2004;25:189–201.

91 TOXICITIES OF CHEMOTHERAPY

Michael Moore

KEY POINTS

- Complications of chemotherapy should be in the differential diagnosis of all cancer patients admitted to the ICU.

- Fever, hypersensitivity reactions, mucositis, gastritis, and myelosuppression are the most common toxicities.
- Not all toxicities of chemotherapy agents are known, especially with newer agents.
- Certain agents have known toxicity syndromes (e.g., bleomycin pulmonary toxicity).

INTRODUCTION

- As more intensive anticancer regimens are being used to achieve cure, an increasing number of oncology patients are admitted to intensive care units (ICUs) for complications of treatment.
- A thorough oncologic and chemotherapy history is an integral component of managing the cancer patient admitted to the ICU.

PRINCIPLES OF DRUG-INDUCED TOXICITY

- Drug toxicity is often a diagnosis of exclusion:
  - Antineoplastic drug toxicity is frequently clinically and pathologically nonspecific.
  - Always consider other causes like infection, tumor effects, and other drug toxicities.
- Dose, schedule, and combination make a difference:
  - Antineoplastic drugs are often given in combination and combined with radiation.
  - Toxicities of combination therapy may be more severe than individual drugs.
  - Different drug schedules may have a different spectrum of side effects for the same agent.
  - Very high-dose chemotherapy with colony-stimulating factor or stem cell support has exposed new toxicities.
- Not all toxicities are known:
  - New drugs and drug combinations are often tried before all toxicities are known.
  - Diagnosis of sporadic versus dose-related drug toxicity is often difficult.
- Treatment is supportive:
  - Treatment-related toxicity is important to diagnose to avoid additional exposure.
  - Specific therapy is rarely indicated or available.

COMMON REACTIONS: FEVER AND HYPERSENSITIVITY REACTIONS

- Acute hypersensitivity reactions:
  - Most common with L-asparaginase, taxanes (paclitaxel and docetaxel), and platinum agents.
  - Antianaphylaxis medications should be readily available.
  - Paclitaxel is routinely administered with corticosteroids and antihistamines.
- Hypersensitivity from platinum agents often occurs during second or third exposure.
- Hypersensitivity reactions associated with rituximab and trastuzumab can be managed with a slower infusion rate and premedication.
- Febrile reactions are common with bleomycin and cytarabine.

COMMON REACTIONS: MYELOSUPPRESSION

- Complications of myelosuppression account for most therapy-related ICU admissions.
- Cell lines are variably suppressed:
  - Granulocytes (half-life 6 hours) affected early and most severely.
  - Platelets (half-life 5–7 days) affected next.
  - RBCs (half-life 120 days) relatively spared.
- Nitrosoureas and mitomycin C typically produce a late, severe thrombocytopenia.
- Rule out bleeding and other causes of anemia before very low hemoglobin levels are attributed to chemotherapy alone.
- For most agents, granulocyte counts nadir at 7–14 days and recover by 21–28 days after administration of a single dose.
- Pelvic or spinal irradiation and multicourse chemotherapy may be associated with severe and prolonged myelosuppression.
- Bone marrow biopsy helps characterize cytopenias in critically ill patients.
- Hematopoietic growth factors (i.e., granulocyte colony-stimulating factor) may be useful to ameliorate bone marrow suppression.
- Empiric institution of broad-spectrum antibiotic therapy has been shown to improve mortality in febrile neutropenic patients in some clinical situations.

COMMON REACTIONS: MUCOSITIS AND DIARRHEA

GENERAL CONSIDERATIONS

- Gastrointestinal tract epithelial cells proliferate rapidly and are particularly susceptible.
- Toxicity ranges from mild mouth sores to ulcerative stomatitis and severe bloody diarrhea.
- Loss of the protective mucosal barrier contributes to patient morbidity and mortality especially in neutropenic hosts.

TABLE 91-1 Antineoplastic Drugs That Cause Stomatitis or Diarrhea

DRUG	EFFECT
Anthracyclines	Stomatitis
Bleomycin	Stomatitis
5-FU	Stomatitis, anal sores, diarrhea
Capecitabine	Stomatitis, diarrhea
Cytarabine	Stomatitis, diarrhea
Cyclophosphamide	Stomatitis
Dactinomycin	Stomatitis, diarrhea
Taxanes	Stomatitis
Vinca alkaloids	Stomatitis
Methotrexate	Stomatitis
Irinotecan (CPT-11)	Diarrhea
Gefitinib	Diarrhea

- Table 91-1 lists agents that commonly cause stomatitis or diarrhea at standard doses.
- High-dose chemotherapy regimens prior to bone marrow transplantation frequently cause severe mucositis.

TREATMENT

- *Candida* and herpes viruses commonly cause or worsen stomatitis and esophagitis.
- Always consider *Clostridium difficile* infections in hospitalized patients with diarrhea.
- Aggressive mouth care with soft swabs and saline or peroxide rinses is imperative.
- Stomatitis pain can be severe and should be treated with topical anesthetics and/or systemic narcotics.
- Consider early use of intravenous alimentation when enteral feeding is compromised.

SPECIFIC AGENT: IRINOTECAN (CPT-11)

- Causes severe diarrhea in the absence of mucositis.
- Two distinct types of diarrhea have been described:
  - Early-onset:
    - Occurs during or within 30 minutes of infusion
    - Acute cholinergic response
    - Controlled with IV atropine, 0.5–1.0 mg
  - Late-onset:
    - Appears 6–10 days after administration
    - May be linked to a secretory process in the small intestine
    - Can be massive (10 L/day)
  - Treatment:
    - Early recognition
    - Aggressive treatment with loperamide and octreotide

COMMON REACTIONS: PULMONARY TOXICITY

OVERVIEW

- A large number of antineoplastic drugs can cause pulmonary toxicity (Table 91-2).
- Pulmonary toxicity syndromes include:
  - Acute pleuritic chest pain
  - Hypersensitivity lung disease
  - Noncardiogenic pulmonary edema
  - Pneumonitis/fibrosis: This is classically associated with the "three B's": busulfan, bleomycin, and carmustine (BCNU)

CLINICAL PRESENTATIONS

- Onset of pneumonitis/fibrosis:
  - Usually subacute over several weeks but acute presentations occur.
  - Busulfan: after prolonged, continuous treatment.
  - Bleomycin: after a few cycles of therapy.
  - BCNU: can occur many years after therapy.
- Signs and symptoms:
  - Frequently nonspecific but dyspnea is invariably present.
  - Dry cough, fatigue, fever, and end-expiratory crackles are common.
  - Hemoptysis is atypical and suggests an alternative diagnosis.
- Differential diagnosis includes infection, irradiation, cardiogenic edema, pulmonary embolus, hemorrhage, leukoagglutinin reaction, and progressive tumor.
- May be reversible or can progress in the absence of additional exposures.

DIAGNOSTIC TESTING

- Chest x-ray can be normal or reveal a basilar or diffuse reticulonodular pattern:
  - Bleomycin occasionally produces a nodular appearance that can mimic recurrent tumor.
  - Methotrexate can be associated with a pleural effusion or hilar adenopathy.
- Pulmonary function tests reveal restriction and reduced DLCO (diffusing capacity of the lung for carbon monoxide).
- Lung biopsy:
  - Histologic findings are not specific.
  - May not definitively establish the diagnosis.
  - Patient selection and timing of biopsy is controversial.

TABLE 91-2 Antineoplastic Drugs That Have Pulmonary Toxicity

AGENT	TYPE OF TOXICITY	INCIDENCE (%)	COMMENT
Bleomycin	Pneumonitis/fibrosis	2–40	Chest x-ray may be atypical
	Hypersensitivity pneumonitis	Rare	Eosinophilia may be seen on lung biopsy; steroids felt to be useful
	Acute chest pain	Rare	Substernal pressure or pleuritic pain; self-limited over 4–72 h
Busulfan	Pneumonitis/fibrosis	4	Insidious onset after prolonged therapy; poor prognosis
Carmustine (BCNU)	Pneumonitis/fibrosis	20–30	Toxicity is dose related; common in pretransplantation regimens; effects may appear years after therapy has ended
Cyclophosphamide	Pneumonitis/fibrosis	<1	May potentiate toxicity of bleomycin, BCNU
High-dose cytarabine	Noncardiogenic pulmonary edema	4–20	Care is supportive, but corticosteroids are occasionally helpful; prognosis is variable
Gemcitabine	Noncardiogenic pulmonary edema	1–5	Care is supportive, but corticosteroids are occasionally helpful: prognosis is variable
Methotrexate	Hypersensitivity pneumonitis	8	Prognosis is good; dramatic response to corticosteroids reported
	Acute pleuritic pain	Rare	May be associated with pleural effusion or friction rub; subsides over 3–5 days
	Noncardiogenic Pulmonary edema	Rare	Few reports, most with intrathecal injection
Mitomycin C	Pneumonitis/fibrosis	3–12	High mortality reported
Procarbazine	Acute hypersensitivity		Onset within hours after drug dose; recovery rapid
Tretinoin (ATRA)	Retinoic acid syndrome	10–20	Corticosteroids suggested
Vinorelbine	Acute dyspnea	5	Readily reversible chest pain
Gefitinib	Interstitial lung disease	1–3	One-third of the cases can be fatal
Trastuzumab	Organizing pneumonia	Rare	Case reports only

TREATMENT

- Generally supportive
- Discontinue precipitating agent
- Empiric trial of corticosteroid therapy is supported by anecdotal reports

SPECIFIC AGENTS

BLEOMYCIN

- Believed to directly injure the pulmonary capillary endothelium and type I pneumocytes stimulating an inflammatory cascade.
- Sporadic rather than dose related below a threshold cumulative total dose of 450–500 mg.
- Incidence dramatically increases above threshold dose.

MONITORING THERAPY

- Serial DLCO measurements have been used to predict and prevent pulmonary toxicity.
- Stopping therapy when a significant decrease in DLCO is shown is recommended but has not been shown to alter the incidence of fatal toxicity.
- Patients may present with an acute decline in pulmonary function weeks to months after a normal DLCO.

RISK FACTORS

- Age over 70
- Prior or concurrent pulmonary radiation therapy
- Concurrent treatment with cyclophosphamide or methotrexate
- Oxygen therapy:
  - Small studies have reported a high incidence of severe postoperative respiratory distress in bleomycin-treated patients attributed to a high intraoperative concentration of inspired oxygen.
  - Limiting intra- and perioperative FiO_2 to the lowest safe concentrations is recommended.

TRETINOIN (ALL-TRANS-RETINOIC ACID, ATRA)

- Derivative of vitamin A used for acute promyelocytic leukemia (APL).
- Retinoic acid syndrome:
  - Unique pulmonary toxicity
  - Symptoms include high fever, fluid retention, pulmonary infiltrates, and respiratory distress.

- Incidence as high as 25%.
- Occurs as soon as 2 days after therapy.
- Treatment with dexamethasone may be helpful.

GAITANIS

- Oral inhibitor of epidermal growth factor receptor (EGFR) tyrosine kinase approved for treatment of refractory lung cancer.
- Results in interstitial lung disease in about 1% of the patients worldwide.
- Approximately one-third of reported cases have been fatal.
- Patients present with acute dyspnea, with or without cough, and low-grade fevers.
- Prompt discontinuation of the agent with adequate supportive care is recommended.

CARDIOVASCULAR TOXICITY

OVERVIEW

- The majority of cardiac events in cancer patients are related to preexisting heart disease or secondary to tumor effects as opposed to anticancer drugs (Table 91-3).
- Anthracyclines are an exception to this rule:
  - Doxorubicin and daunorubicin have very similar effects on the heart.
  - Doxorubicin is more commonly used and its cardiac effects better studied.
  - Trastuzumab also reported to cause a cardiomyopathy similar to the effects anthracycline therapy.
- Immunomodulatory agents such as interferon and interleukin (IL)-2 also have cardiotoxic effects.

ECG CHANGES AND ARRHYTHMIA

- Cisplatin and others may produce secondary effects through alterations in plasma potassium, calcium, and magnesium levels.
- Direct effects appear limited to the anthracyclines and paclitaxel and can occur up to 40% during infusions.
- Acute anthracycline-induced fatal arrhythmia has been reported and is very rare:
  - Cardiac monitoring during drug infusion not warranted.
  - ECG changes usually transient and do not necessitate stopping therapy.
  - No association with cardiomyopathy.
- Doxorubicin:
  - Incidence up to 40% during infusion.
  - Most common effects are nonspecific ST-T-wave changes.
  - Premature atrial and ventricular contractions, sinus tachycardia, and decreased QRS voltage are also common.
- Paclitaxel:
  - Causes asymptomatic, reversible sinus bradycardia:
    - Heart rates ranging from 30–50 beats per minute (BPM)
    - Incidence 29% during a 24-hour infusion
  - Third-degree heart block is rare.
  - Myocardial infarction and tachyarrhythmias have been reported.

MYOCARDIAL ISCHEMIA AND INFARCTION

- Rarely caused by antineoplastic agents.
- Radiation therapy to the heart may result in accelerated atherogenesis.

TABLE 91-3 Antineoplastic Drugs That Have Cardiac Toxicity

DRUG	EFFECT	INCIDENCE (%)	COMMENT
Anthracyclines	Acute ECG changes	Common	Almost always benign and reversible
	Acute myocarditis/pericarditis syndrome	Rare	
	Chronic cardiomyopathy	1–2	May appear years after treatment
Cyclophosphamide	Acute hemorrhagic cardiac necrosis	Unusual	Only in very high doses
5-FU (Capecitabine—oral prodrug of 5-FU)	Angina/myocardial infarction	Rare	Usually within hours of drug dose; asymptomatic ECG changes more common
Mitoxantrone	Cardiomyopathy	1–2	Drug is structurally related to anthracyclines, but incidence of cardiomyopathy is probably somewhat less; risk is <1% if cumulative dose <120 mg/m^2
Paclitaxel	Arrhythmias	10–20	Most common is asymptomatic bradycardia
Vinca alkaloids	Angina/myocardial infarction	Rare	Scattered case reports
Trastuzumab	Cardiomyopathy	More common when combined with chemotherapy	Often managed medically

- Vinca alkaloids:
  - Reported to precipitate myocardial infarction in a few instances.
  - Concomitant use of bleomycin may be a risk factor.
- 5-Fluorouracil (5-FU):
  - Up to 4% of patients have reported anginal symptoms.
  - Transient asymptomatic ECG changes suggestive of ischemia are more common.
  - Nitrates and calcium channel blockers may reverse vasospasm.
- Capecitabine:
  - Orally administered prodrug of 5-FU
  - Similar toxicities associated with prolonged infusion of 5-FU

CARDIOMYOPATHY AND PERICARDITIS

ANTHRACYCLINES

- Can cause a myocarditis-pericarditis syndrome:
  - An acute drop in ejection fraction seen in the hours to weeks after drug administration
  - Associated with pericardial effusion
  - May result in sudden death
  - Exceedingly rare
- Cardiomyopathy:
  - Classically, the presentation is subacute (doxorubicin)
  - Develops in 1–10% of patients receiving 550 mg/m^2
  - Increased incidence with cumulative doses >600 mg/m^2
  - Total dose most important risk factor
  - No cutoff dose below which treatment is conventional heart failure therapy
- Late presentation of cardiomyopathy:
  - Clinical course:
    - Symptoms appear around 30–60 days after administration.
    - Symptoms include tachycardia, dyspnea, cardiomegaly, peripheral and pulmonary edema.
  - Treatment is conventional congestive heart failure (CHF) therapy.
- Late presentation:
  - 57% of anthracycline-treated survivors of childhood cancers have abnormalities of left ventricular afterload or contractility:
    - Trastuzumab is associated with moderate cardiomyopathy
    - No specific therapy after onset
    - Care is supportive
    - Seems to be worse with the coadministration of anthracyclines

TRASTUZUMAB

- Cardiotoxicity greatest with combination chemotherapy (especially anthracyclines).
- Clinical symptoms are well controlled with CHF therapy.

CYCLOPHOSPHAMIDE

- Minimal cardiac toxicity at standard doses.
- Higher doses can cause severe myopericarditis and arrhythmias:
  - Hemorrhagic myopericarditis is the major nonhematologic dose-limiting toxicity.
  - Usually seen at doses higher than 1.5 g/m^2.
  - Virulent form:
    - Symptoms appear within 48 hours after last dose.
    - Cardiogenic shock usually results in rapid death.
  - Typical presentation:
    - Toxicity develops 7–10 days after therapy.
    - Usually preceded by a decrease in QRS amplitude.
    - Symptoms include edema, tachycardia, and tachypnea.
  - Hemorrhagic or serosanguineous pericardial effusion is common:
    - Tamponade may be present.
    - Pericardiocentesis usually does not result in clinical improvement.
- Treatment is supportive.
- Prognosis is good if patients survive the acute phase.
- Ifosfamide at higher doses can cause severe myopericarditis and arrhythmias:
  - Toxicity associated with total doses in excess of 1000 mg/m^2.
  - Symptoms generally develop within 2 weeks of receiving the drug.

NEUROTOXICITY

GENERAL CONSIDERATIONS

- Rare primary reason for ICU admission.
- Neurologic problems are common and most are produced by local tumor effects.
- Rule out neurologic changes from commonly used medications including high-dose corticosteroids, narcotics, and benzodiazepines (Table 91-4).

PERIPHERAL NEUROPATHY

- Common side effect of some widely used anticancer drugs
- Paclitaxel and docetaxel:
  - Glove-stocking paresthesias
  - Rarely, motor

CISPLATIN

- Primarily sensory but may progress to disabling ataxia.
- Symptoms may worsen after treatment is completed and persist for years.

TABLE 91-4 Antineoplastic Drugs That Have Neurologic Toxicity

DRUG	INCIDENCE (%)	COMMENT
Encephalopathy		
L-Asparaginase	25–50	Ranges from drowsiness to stupor; onset usually on the day after start of therapy; generally resolves rapidly when therapy is over
High-dose busulfan	15	Acute obtundation, seizures; prophylactic anticonvulsants often used
High-dose carmustine (BCNU)	10	Severe acute or chronic encephalomyelopathy; time of onset variable; usually not reversible
High-dose cytarabine	10–20	Ranges from disorientation to coma; onset usually 5–7 days after start of therapy; prognosis variable
Fludarabine	Rare at conventional doses	Optic neuritis, altered mental status, paralysis. May appear weeks after treatment
Hexamethylmelamine	Variable	Toxicity ranges from depression to hallucinations; usually reversible when drug is withdrawn
Ifosfamide	5–30	Frequency greater with higher doses; ranges from mild somnolence to coma; onset hours after infusion, recovery usually within days; use of methylene blue might reverse or shorten the duration of toxicity
High-dose methotrexate	2–15	Onset usually 1 week after administration; most common presentation is a stroke-like syndrome; usually reversible
Mitotane	40	Lethargy, somnolence, dizziness, vertigo
Pentostatin	Rare at conventional doses	Lethargy, seizures, coma
Procarbazine	10	Usually mild drowsiness or depression, rarely stupor or manic psychosis
High-dose thio-TEPA	Dose-dependent	Somnolence, seizures, coma; dose-limiting extramedullary toxicity
Vincristine/vinblastine	Rare	SIADH
Acute cerebellar syndrome		
High-dose cytarabine	10–20	Ranges from mild dysarthria to disabling ataxia; onset is 5–7 days after start of therapy; prognosis is variable
5-FU	<1	Usually seen with large bolus doses; reversible in 1–6 weeks
Acute paraplegia		
Intrathecal administration of cytarabine, methotrexate, thio-TEPA	Rare	These are the only drugs normally given intrathecally; all cause acute reversible arachnoiditis fairly often, paralysis exceedingly rarely; paralysis may or may not be reversible
Peripheral neuropathies		
Cisplatin	Dose-dependent	Ototoxicity; distal sensory neuropathy
Oxiliplatin	Common	Acute and chronic sensory neuropathy; reversible pharyngolaryngeal dysesthesias; cold exposure may exacerbate symptoms
Hexamethylmelamine	Variable	Peripheral paresthesias and weakness
Procarbazine	10–20	Decreased tendon reflexes, mild distal paresthesias
Paclitaxel, docetaxel	Common	Distal sensory neuropathy
Vinca alkaloids	See text	Symmetrical areflexia and distal paresthesias; symmetrical motor weakness starting with dorsiflexors; jaw pain; cranial nerve palsies; paralytic ileus
Thalidomide		Peripheral neuropathy

ABBREVIATIONS: thio-TEPA, *N,N′N′*-triethylenethiophosphoramide; SIADH, syndrome of inappropriate antidiuretic hormone.

- Other toxicities include tinnitus, deafness, Lhermitte sign, autonomic neuropathy, seizures, transient cortical blindness, and retinal injury.

OXALIPLATIN

- New platinum agent.
- Can cause dose-limiting acute and chronic neuropathy.
- Acute and reversible sensory neuropathy in up to 95% of patients.
- Chronic neuropathy:
    - Develops in 15–20% of patients treated with cumulative doses >780 mg/m^2.
    - Doses >1000 mg/m^2 may cause Lhermitte sign and urinary retention.
    - Usually reversible.
- Pharyngolaryngeal dysesthesias:
    - Acute and reversible syndrome.
    - Reported in 1–2% of patients.
    - Causes a distressing and overwhelming sensation of difficulty with breathing and swallowing.
    - Symptoms frequently triggered or exaggerated by cold exposure.

- Education is required to avoid panic and unnecessary medical interventions.

VINCA ALKALOIDS

- Tubulin poisons that disrupt microtubule function in neuronal axons.
- Vincristine most neurotoxic.
- Symmetric mixed sensorimotor neuropathy:
  - Most common toxicity.
  - Can progress to quadriparesis in severe cases.
  - Symptoms are dose related and gradual in onset.
  - Deep tendon reflexes are lost.
  - Peripheral nerve conduction velocities are characteristically normal despite severe clinical deficits.
  - Paresthesias and motor weakness may or may not gradually improve.
- No known treatment for vinca-related neuropathies.
- Vincristine has accidentally been administered intrathecally and is invariably fatal.

THALIDOMIDE

- Causes reversible and irreversible sensory neuropathies with chronic use in 60% of patients.
- Symptoms range from mild reversible paresthesias to severe irreversible sensory neuropathies.
- Central nervous system (CNS) manifestations are common and include sedation, dizziness, muscle incoordination, fatigue, unsteady gait, tremulousness, mood changes, confusion, and weakness.

CRANIAL NERVE PALSIES

- Cranial nerve palsies include vocal cord paralysis, dysphagia, optic atrophy (rare), ptosis, ophthalmoplegias, and facial nerve paralysis.
- Occur in up to 10% of vincristine-treated patients.
- Cranial neuropathies may be abrupt in onset and mimic a brain stem stroke.
- Symptoms are usually bilateral and reversible with discontinuation of the drug.

AUTONOMIC NEUROPATHY

- Symptoms include ileus, bladder atony, impotence, and orthostatic hypotension.
- May occur in patients without signs of peripheral nerve toxicity.
- Severe paralytic ileus:
  - Can presents as an acute abdomen.
  - Occurs acutely or following long-term administration of vincristine, vinblastine, or vinorelbine.
  - Usually reversible over the course of several days.
  - Treatment:
    - Nasogastric tube drainage is standard therapy.
    - Metoclopramide in patients without suspicion of mechanical obstruction.

SPECIFIC AGENTS

L-ASPARAGINASE

- Twenty-five to 50% incidence of cerebral dysfunction.
- Toxicity ranges from mild depression and drowsiness to confusion, stupor, and coma.
- Encephalopathy:
  - Often occurs on the first day after administration and usually clears rapidly after the end of therapy.
  - Resembles hepatic encephalopathy and may be associated with high ammonia levels.
  - Electroencephalogram (EEG) shows diffuse slowing with resolution after drug therapy.
- Clotting abnormalities:
  - Thrombotic and hemorrhagic cerebrovascular accidents
  - Severe decrease in fibrinogen levels associated with elevated prothrombin time

CYTARABINE (ARA-C)

- Neurotoxic at high doses (2–3 g/m^2 twice daily).
- 10–20% incidence of cerebellar and cerebral toxicity.
- Risk factors:
  - Large cumulative doses
  - Age over 55
- Cerebellar toxicity:
  - Most common and severe.
  - Onset usually 5–7 days after the start of therapy.
  - Symptoms include intention tremor, dysarthria, horizontal nystagmus, limb and truncal ataxia.
- Cerebral toxicity:
  - Symptoms range from mild somnolence to disorientation, memory loss, seizure, and coma.
  - EEGs show diffuse slowing.
  - Lumbar puncture and computed tomography (CT) are normal.
  - Symptoms last days to weeks and may be irreversible.
  - Rarely fatal.
  - Treatment is supportive care.

METHOTREXATE

- Systemic administration:
  - Neurotoxic at high doses (1–7 g/m^2).
  - 2–15% incidence of various transient CNS syndromes.
  - Onset is abrupt after several hours to several weeks of treatment.

- Clinical syndromes:
  - Stroke-like syndrome with hemiplegia and speech disorder.
  - Findings may fluctuate.
  - Focal or generalized seizures are common.
  - Recovery occurs completely over several days.
  - May or may not recur with subsequent courses.
- Diagnostic studies:
  - Electrolyte levels and radiologic studies are normal.
  - EEG shows a variety of abnormalities.
  - CSF may reveal elevated protein levels.
  - Treatment is generally supportive.
- Intrathecal methotrexate:
  - Clinical syndromes:
    - Acute arachnoiditis:
      - Most common.
      - Resolves over 12–72 hours without sequelae.
      - May mimic bacterial meningitis if severe.
    - Acute reactions:
      - Rare.
      - Symptoms include paralysis, cranial nerve palsies, and seizure.
    - Necrotizing leukoencephalopathy:
      - Occasionally seen with concomitant cranial irradiation.
      - Delayed effect with insidious onset months after treatment.
  - Cerebrospinal fluid (CSF) may show increased pressure, high protein concentrations, and a reactive pleocytosis.
  - Recovery is often complete.

IFOSFAMIDE

- Can cause an encephalopathy.
- Associated with high-dose therapy.
- Symptoms range from subtle sensorimotor deficits to severe mental status changes and death.
- Treatment:
  - Early recognition with discontinuation
  - Intravenous methylene blue
  - Symptoms usually resolve over 24–48 hours

RENAL AND URINARY TOXICITY

- Common renal abnormalities are listed in Table 91-5.

CISPLATIN

- Renal injury is a dose-limiting toxicity
- Renal dysfunction:
  - Mild to acute renal failure
  - Creatinine levels rise over days, peak at 3–14 days; then decline toward pretreatment levels
- Risk factors
  - Coexisting aminoglycoside therapy
  - Preexisting renal dysfunction
  - Dehydration
- Vigorous pretreatment hydration minimizes renal dysfunction:
- Electrolyte disorders are a common consequence of toxicity, including magnesium, calcium, potassium, and sodium:
  - May be refractory to treatment if serum magnesium levels are not first corrected
  - Use aminoglycosides with extreme caution
  - Replete magnesium via IV or IM route
- Sodium:
  - Hyponatremia from renal salt wasting
  - Symptomatic orthostatic hypotension

METHOTREXATE

- Associated with high-dose methotrexate (>50 mg/kg).
- Renal failure usually reversible over 2–3 weeks following drug withdrawal.
- Preventions/treatment:
  - Careful hydration.
  - Urinary alkalinization promotes drug excretion.
  - Follow levels and give leucovorin rescue:
    - Leucovorin is continued until the drug concentration has fallen to a safe level.

TABLE 91-5 Antineoplastic Drugs Producing Renal and Electrolyte Abnormalities

AGENT	TOXICITY	COMMENT
Cisplatin	Magnesium, calcium, potassium, sodium wasting; renal insufficiency	
Cyclophosphamide	Impaired free water excretion	Transient; seen with doses >50 mg/kg
Ifosfamide	Proximal tubular defect	—
High-dose methotrexate	Acute renal failure	Usually reversible
Mitomycin C	Renal failure with microangiopathic hemolytic anemia (HUS/TTP)	Common with cumulative dose >60 mg
Nitrosoureas (BCNU, CCNU, methyl-CCNU)	Progressive renal failure appearing After large cumulative doses	Decrease in renal size may be noted; effect may occur years after therapy
Streptozotocin	Renal failure, proximal renal tubular acidosis, nephrotic syndrome	Transient proteinuria is earliest manifestation

- Goal methotrexate level is $<5 \times 10^{-8}$ M.
- Will not completely prevent toxicity.
  - Hemodialysis with high-flux membranes.
  - Carboxypeptidase-G2 on compassionate emergent use basis.
- Toxic levels persist in the setting of acute renal failure.
- Renal dysfunction contributes to other morbidities including cytopenias and mucositis.
- Toxic methotrexate may also persist in patients with large third-space fluid reservoirs (e.g., pleural effusions or ascites).

CYCLOPHOSPHAMIDE AND IFOSFAMIDE

- Urologic complications include bladder fibrosis, bladder cancer, and hemorrhagic cystitis.
- Can be difficult to manage.
- See "Hemorrhagic Cystitis," below.

THROMBOTIC AND HEMORRHAGIC TOXICITY

GENERAL CONSIDERATIONS

- All myelosuppressive agents potentially cause thrombocytopenia and bleeding.
- Thrombotic microangiopathies occur with various chemotherapeutic agents.

HEMORRHAGIC CYSTITIS

- Well-described complication of cyclophosphamide and ifosfamide.
- Can be idiosyncratic but increased incidence with prolonged or high-dose therapy.
- Acrolein, a metabolite of cyclophosphamide, is believed to cause local bladder irritation.
- Clinical presentation:
  - Acute form appears within days after treatment.
  - Symptoms range from minimal hematuria with mild dysuria, urgency, and frequency to massive hemorrhage requiring transfusion.
  - Thrombocytopenia with high-dose cyclophosphamide increases morbidity.
  - Bleeding usually self-limited with a median duration of 1 month.
- Prevention:
  - Sodium 2-mercaptoethane sulfonate (mesna):
    - Provides free sulfhydryl groups to neutralize acrolein in urine.
    - Required with ifosfamide therapy.
    - Not useful in treating established cystitis.
  - Adequate prehydration with frequent voiding:
    - Decreases contact time of acrolein in bladder.
    - Avoid hypotonic solutions for hydration.
- Treatment:
  - Stop therapy. No other treatment for mild episodes.
  - Severe cases:
    - Vigorous hydration to promote urine flow and maintenance of adequate platelet counts (50,000/mL).
    - Continuous bladder irrigation:
      - Use large-bore catheter.
      - Avoid obstructing clots.
    - Other therapies:
      - Intravesical instillation of formalin
      - Urinary diversion
      - Hypogastric artery embolization and cystectomy with urinary diversion

MICROANGIOPATHIC HEMOLYTIC ANEMIA

- Can be effect of cancer or cancer therapy.
- Most closely associated with mitomycin C.
- Other agents include bleomycin, cisplatin, interferon, and gemcitabine.
- Thrombotic thrombocytopenic purpura/hemolytic-uremic syndrome (TTP/HUS) is a late complication of allogeneic and autologous bone marrow transplantation.
- The severity of the presentation and the prognosis in transplant patients is variable.
- The prognosis in mitomycin C-associated HUS may be poor.
- Treatment:
  - Staphylococcal protein A immunoadsorption may be useful for mitomycin C-associated HUS.
  - Other therapies including plasma exchange with cryosupernatant, IVIg, and glucocorticoids are of uncertain benefit.

THROMBOEMBOLISM

- Thalidomide is associated with significant risk of thromboembolic complications.
- Increased risk when administered with other chemotherapeutic agents.

HEPATOTOXICITY

- Many cytotoxic agents can result in hepatotoxicity but few do so regularly or severely (see Tables 91-6 and 91-7).
- Veno-occlusive disease (VOD) of the liver is a major toxicity of high-dose regimens given before transplantation.

TABLE 91-6 Cytotoxic Agents That Have Hepatic Toxicity

DRUG	FREQUENCY OF TOXICITY	COMMENT
L-Asparaginase	Common	Fatty metamorphosis; decreased synthetic function; reversible
Azathioprine	Uncommon	Cholestasis/necrosis; hyperbilirubinemia; variable prognosis
High-dose cytarabine	Common	Elevated bilirubin and transaminases; reversible
Floxuridine (FUDR)	Common	Biliary sclerosis with hepatic intra-arterial infusion; chemical hepatitis
Methotrexate	Common	Cirrhosis, fibrosis, fatty metamorphosis; laboratory data may be normal; seen with prolonged daily therapy; variable prognosis
High-dose methotrexate	Common	Elevated transaminase levels, usually reversible in weeks
6-Mercaptopurine	Common	Cholestasis or necrosis; usually reversible
Mithramycin	Common	Necrosis; rarely seen with lower doses used for hypercalcemia
Nitrosoureas (BCNU, CCNU)	Occasional	Generally mild and reversible
Vincristine	Rare	May produce severe damage when combined with radiation to the liver

VENO-OCCLUSIVE DISEASE OF THE LIVER

- Rare and sporadic with cytotoxic drugs at conventional doses.
- High-dose chemotherapy or chemoradiotherapy for bone marrow transplant:
  - Most common cause
  - Incidence up to 20%
  - Common cause of death
- Clinical picture:
  - Resembles Budd-Chiari syndrome
  - Symptoms begin at mean of 10 days after marrow reinfusion
  - Death or recovery occurs by day 35 after transplantation
  - Late-onset VOD occurs with some regimens
- Diagnosis:
  - Largely clinical
  - Presence of at least two of the triad of jaundice, hepatomegaly, or right upper quadrant pain, and ascites or unexplained weight gain
  - Hyperbilirubinemia is usually out of proportion to transaminase concentrations
  - Major differential diagnosis:
    - Graph-versus-host disease
    - Abdominal catastrophe:
      - Suggested by acute, severe abdominal pain
      - Includes pancreatitis, bowel infarction, biliary obstruction, peritonitis, and pyogenic liver abscess
    - Cyclosporine-induced hepatotoxicity
    - Sepsis
  - Liver biopsy:
    - Percutaneous approach usually contraindicated
    - Transvenous can still result in fatal hemorrhage
    - Histopathology:
      - Early disease characterized by subintimal edema, hemorrhage within small central venules, and centrilobular congestion
      - Late disease characterized by fibrous obliteration of central venule lumina and centrilobular sinusoidal fibrosis
  - Ultrasound studies may show increased mean hepatic artery resistive index or reversal of portal venous flow.

TABLE 91-7 Toxicities of IL-2

TOXICITY	COMMENT
Febrile reaction complex	Dose-dependent fever and chills are ameliorated with antipyretics and meperidine
Cardiovascular toxicity	Capillary leak syndrome; see text. Rare cases of eosinophilic myocarditis
Toxicity CNS	Dose-dependent reversible somnolence Disorientation, cognitive deterioration Appears several days after beginning of a treatment course
Hematopoietic toxicity	Frequent anemia, occasional thrombocytopenia, rare neutropenia; lymphopenia with rebound lymphocytosis, dramatic eosinophilia
Gastrointestinal toxicity	Mild nausea, vomiting, diarrhea. Mucositis is unusual, but may be severe. Profound, reversible cholestasis with hyperbilirubinemia and elevated alkaline phosphatase but normal transaminases
Infectious complications	Increase in staphylococcal bacteremia, often catheter related
Renal toxicity	Oliguria and prerenal azotemia reversible when infusion discontinued
Cutaneous toxicity	Rash ranging from discrete nonpruritic maculopapular lesions to diffuse erythroderma with flaky exfoliation after resolution of redness
Other	Hypo- and hyperthyroidism, decrease in vitamin-K-dependent coagulation factors, severe myalgias

- Treatment is supportive:
  - No prospective randomized studies
  - Supportive

BIOLOGIC AGENTS

- A variety of cytokines are available for widespread use.
- Each has a unique toxicity profile dependent on dose, schedule, and combination therapy.
- "Cytokine cascade" is a shared feature:
  - Typical features include fever and myalgia.
  - Capillary leak syndrome:
    - Can lead to hypotension and cardiovascular collapse.
    - Fluid resuscitation may lead to pulmonary edema.
    - Vasopressors often required.
    - Resolves rapidly after discontinuation of therapy.
- Arrhythmias and myocardial infarction have been reported.
- CNS toxicity is frequent:
  - Usually reversible
  - May persist for days after cessation of treatment
- Side effects of IL-2 treatment seen at recommended dose for renal cancer (600,000 U/kg every 8 hours for 14 doses) listed in Table 91-7 as an example.

TOXICITIES OF "TARGETED" AGENTS

- "Targeted therapies" include agents that inhibit specific targets such as surface receptors or intra- and extracellular proteins that play role in tumor progression.
- Many are monoclonal antibodies and small molecule kinase inhibitors.
- Increasing use has resulted in new clinical toxicities being recognized and reported.
- Clinical experience with the newer targeted agents is still limited.

MONOCLONAL ANTIBODIES

- Toxicities such as acute infusion reactions are common to the drug class.
- Specific toxicities likely related to the modulation of the targeted pathway by each specific antibody.
- Rituximab (Rituxan):
  - Chimeric anti-CD20 antibody routinely used in various lymphoid malignancies.
  - Case reports support role in various dermatologic and systemic toxicities.
  - Toxicity ranges from mild cutaneous reactions to Stevens-Johnson syndrome and serum sickness.
  - Generally resolve with discontinuation of therapy, corticosteroids, and supportive care.
- Radioisotope-labeled antibodies are frequently associated with prolonged myelosuppression.

ANTIANGIOGENIC AGENTS

- Thalidomide and bevacizumab (Avastin) are the only agents currently approved for cancer therapy.
- Toxicities include bleeding, thromboses, hypertension, and proteinuria.
- Treatment:
  - Discontinue treatment
  - Appropriate medical therapy
- Thalidomide is associated with high rates of thromboembolic complications in several trials:
  - Combination with other chemotherapeutic agents appears to be greatest risk factor.
  - Management approaches are evolving.

SMALL MOLECULE TYROSINE KINASE INHIBITORS

- Predominant toxicities dictated by the pathways inhibited by each agent.
- Imatinib mesylate:
  - Inhibits the Bcr-Abl protein-tyrosine kinase.
  - Approved for chronic myeloid leukemia (CML) and active against gastrointestinal stromal tumors.
  - Common toxicities include mild nausea, emesis, edema, and rash.
  - 2–4% of patients develop pleural and pericardial effusions and severe cutaneous reactions.
  - Severe events more common with high-dose therapy (>600 mg/day).
- Gefitinib:
  - EGFR tyrosine-kinase inhibitor approved for the treatment of lung cancer.
  - Mild to moderately severe skin rash and diarrhea in most patients
  - Mild toxicity managed with dose reduction or supportive care.
  - Severe symptoms (5–10% of patients) require discontinuation of therapy and aggressive supportive care.

BIBLIOGRAPHY

Hall JB, Schmidt, GA, Wood LDH. *Principles of Critical Care*, 3rd ed. New York, NY: McGraw-Hill; 2005:1123–1136.

Patterson WP, Reams GP. Renal toxicities of chemotherapy. *Semin Oncol* 1992;19:521–528.

Perry MC. Chemotherapy agents and hepatotoxicity. *Semin Oncol* 1992;19:551–565.

Weiss RB. Miscellaneous toxicities in cancer. In: DeVita VT, Hellman S, Rosenberg SA, eds., *Principles and Practice of Oncology*, 6th ed. Philadelphia, PA: Lippincott-Raven; 2001: 2964–2976.

92 RADIATION PNEUMONITIS

Peter H. O'Donnell

KEY POINTS

- Radiation pneumonitis can occur in any patient receiving radiation to the thorax, though certain factors predispose patients to develop this syndrome.
- The clinical syndrome is varied, but usually includes symptoms of dyspnea and cough.
- Radiographic changes can include opacification or fibrotic changes. Often these changes will not follow anatomic lines but instead the radiation field.
- The diagnosis is usually made clinically.
- Steroids are typically used to manage the disease, but there are no prospective trials demonstrating their effectiveness.

OVERVIEW OF RADIATION PNEUMONITIS

- Radiation pneumonitis is an acute, inflammatory, injury-response of the lung, occurring usually 1–3 months following thoracic irradiation, which may produce a clinical syndrome of pulmonary symptoms primarily characterized by dyspnea and cough (Table 92-1).
- The clinical symptoms are often accompanied by chest radiographic changes, most often manifested as a hazy opacification of areas of lung which have been irradiated. Virtually pathognomonic for radiation pneumonitis on chest x-ray is the appearance of sharp boundary lines for the haziness, which do not correspond to anatomic lung lobes but rather to the prior radiation field.

TABLE 92-1 Overview of Radiation Pneumonitis

History	Thoracic radiation 1–3 months prior
Clinical symptoms	Dyspnea, cough
Confirmatory studies	Chest radiograph with haziness having sharp boundary lines, which do not correspond to anatomic lung lobes
Differential diagnosis	Tumor recurrence or progression, lymphangitic spread of cancer, infection, aspiration
Predisposing factors	Large total or fraction radiation doses; large volume of lung irradiated; concurrent chemotherapy; recent withdrawal of steroids
Severity	Can range from mild symptoms to fatal syndrome; may progress to pulmonary fibrosis
Treatment	Supportive, oxygen, bronchodilators, prednisone

- Diagnosis can often be made by history plus chest radiography. Historical cues which suggest the diagnosis—besides (1) a recent history of thoracic irradiation—include: (2) lack of symptoms of infection; (3) recent withdrawal of steroids; (4) multiple courses of lung or thoracic irradiation; (5) recent concomitant chemotherapy; and (5) a history of previous radiation pneumonitis.
- The incidence of symptomatic radiation pneumonitis among patients receiving thoracic irradiation is approximately 7–8%, whereas the total number with radiation-induced chest radiograph changes, whether symptomatic or not, is much higher at about 40%.
- Factors associated with increased incidence of radiation pneumonitis include: (1) larger volumes of irradiated lung; (2) higher total dose of radiation; (3) higher daily fraction doses; (4) concomitant chemotherapy; and (5) recent withdrawal of steroids.
- The clinical severity of radiation pneumonitis can be scored according to several proposed scales, where, in general, 0 = no radiation pneumonitis; 1 = mild; 2 = steroid therapy may be indicated; 3 = patient requires supplemental oxygen; 4 = life threatening; and 5 = death from radiation pneumonitis.
- Radiation pneumonitis, therefore, can present a variable clinical spectrum. In addition, it should be realized that radiation pneumonitis represents an acute manifestation of pulmonary radiation injury; the related chronic form, radiation fibrosis, also exists as an important but distinct clinical syndrome.

CLINICAL PRESENTATION

- The primary symptoms are dyspnea (frequency ~ 90%) and cough (~60%), the latter more commonly nonproductive.
- Some patients demonstrate low-grade fever, but most will be without fever.
- Patients sometimes also describe a feeling of chest fullness.
- Physical examination is often without specific abnormality. Radiation changes of the skin, in the area of the thorax, might be a helpful clue in patients who are unable to provide a verbal history.
- Laboratory tests, such as the complete blood count and arterial blood gas, usually add little toward making the diagnosis, since abnormalities, if present, are usually nonspecific.
- The chest radiograph remains as one of the cornerstones, along with the history, in making the diagnosis. Radiation pneumonitis on chest x-ray is most often manifested as a hazy opacification of areas of lung which have been irradiated. The appearance of

sharp boundary lines for the haziness, which do not correspond to anatomic lung lobes but rather to the prior radiation field, is virtually pathognomonic. Less common findings also include fuzziness of the pulmonary vasculature in affected areas, and sometimes, the presence of air bronchograms. However, symptoms can precede radiographic changes. While usually not necessary for diagnosis, chest computed tomography (CT) will also demonstrate radiation-induced lung changes.
- In considering the differential diagnosis, possibly the most important distinction is to determine whether the symptoms and radiographic changes could represent tumor recurrence or progression, rather than radiation-induced injury. Specifically, lymphangitic spread of tumor may present similarly.
- The differential diagnosis of these patients also includes infection, especially given the particular susceptibility of cancer patients—and even more specifically those with thoracic disease—for pulmonary infectious diseases. In addition to the usual bacterial, viral, and fungal pathogens, *Pneumocystis carinii* (PCP) should be considered.
- An aspiration event, with either chemical pneumonitis or aspiration pneumonia, is possible.
- Finally, the differential diagnosis should also contain the possibility of chemotherapy-induced pneumonitis.

MECHANISMS OF RADIATION-INDUCED LUNG INJURY

- Radiation can cause both direct cellular injury and DNA damage to dividing cells.
- Direct cellular damage by ionizing radiation involves initiation of apoptotic signal transduction pathways, including breakdown of cellular membrane sphingomyelin with resultant generation of the apoptotic second-messenger ceramide.
- Additionally, irradiated cells cause cellular activation of "stress response" cytokines, including transforming growth factor-beta (TGF-beta) and basic fibroblast growth factor.
- These inflammatory cellular activations, whether apoptotic or directed at tissue repair, explain how such pneumonitis at the alveolar-capillary interface could cause clinical manifestations.
- Similarly, from the standpoint of radiation-induced DNA damage, type II pneumocytes and capillary endothelial cells—which share comparatively high mitotic indices compared to other cells in the lung—are thus particularly subject to radiation-induced injury and are the fundamental cellular locations of DNA damage in radiation pneumonitis. Radiation-induced DNA injury likely involves generation of DNA-damaging reactive oxygen species.
- The turnover rate of these mitotic cells (e.g., 20–35 days for type II pneumocytes based on studies in mice) might partially explain the delay between the administration of radiation and the occurrence of clinical symptoms in radiation pneumonitis.

FACTORS WHICH INCREASE THE RISK OF RADIATION PNEUMONITIS

- Several well-studied factors have been shown to be associated with a higher incidence of developing radiation pneumonitis. Chiefly, the development of radiation pneumonitis seems to obey a "threshold phenomenon," where both the percentage of irradiated lung and the total radiation dose can determine a threshold at which radiation pneumonitis is more likely to occur.
- Though very high doses in small lung fields can cause symptoms, larger irradiated lung volumes (especially at or above 50%), especially when both lungs are irradiated, correlate with a higher incidence of symptomatic radiation pneumonitis.
- Similarly, larger total radiation doses correlate with a higher incidence, but the relationship does not appear to be linear. Risk increases at partial-lung total doses above 25–30 Gy. For comparison, 64–70 Gy are typically used to treat stage III nonsmall cell lung cancer (NSCLC).
- While total radiation dose matters, evidence suggests that fraction dose is equally important in conferring risk. Daily fraction doses above 2.67 Gy have been associated with increased incidence of pneumonitis, and some suggest the daily fraction threshold is at or below 2 Gy.
- Chemotherapy alone can cause clinical pneumonitis, but concurrent chemoradiation has been shown to be associated with an even greater incidence of pneumonitis, particularly with certain drugs. While many chemotherapeutic agents have been implicated, the best known include dactinomycin, doxorubicin, cyclophosphamide, and bleomycin, the latter most commonly associated with pulmonary fibrosis.
- One study in breast cancer patients receiving radiation demonstrated the synergistic effect of concomitant chemoradiation on the incidence of pneumonitis as opposed to sequential treatment. In that study, the incidence of radiation pneumonitis was 8.8% when chemoradiation was concurrent, compared to 1.3% when sequential.
- Of note, some chemotherapeutic agents have been associated with radiation "recall" pneumonitis. In these situations, patients who have had prior thoracic

irradiation will develop pneumonitis on administration of the chemotherapeutic agent. This phenomenon has been best characterized with doxorubicin and dactinomycin.

- Even more well-described is the phenomenon of radiation recall pneumonitis on withdrawal of steroids, a clinical scenario which can arise in patients who receive corticosteroids as part of chemotherapeutic regimens, or who receive steroid treatment for other clinical indications. In these patients, symptomatic radiation pneumonitis can develop shortly after withdrawal of the steroid. Given the inflammatory underlying mechanism of radiation pneumonitis (see above), it follows that steroid withdrawal could unmask and precipitate an acute pneumonitis initiated by prior radiation damage.

TREATMENT

- Given the inflammatory nature postulated for radiation-induced lung injury, it is not surprising that corticosteroids comprise the mainstay of therapy for radiation pneumonitis.
- Interestingly, no prospective clinical trials have demonstrated the utility of steroids in humans, but a wealth of clinical experience has shown their effectiveness.
- Prednisone, given at 1 mg/kg daily, is the standard therapy for symptomatic radiation pneumonitis if the clinical scenario warrants treatment. This dose is continued, usually for weeks, and then gradually reduced in a protracted taper, with clinical alertness for rebound of symptoms.
- Prophylactic steroids have not been shown to decrease the incidence of radiation pneumonitis.
- Of note, many cases of radiation pneumonitis will be clinically mild, and can be managed supportively (oxygen, bed rest) and with bronchodilators.

FUTURE DIRECTIONS

- Several novel prophylactic and therapeutic strategies have been proposed which attempt to target the reactive oxygen and cytokine cascades which underlie the mechanisms of radiation lung injury.
- One promising intravenous agent, amifostine, a reactive oxygen species scavenger, has been shown in two phase III trials to decrease the incidence of radiation pneumonitis in patients undergoing radiation for NSCLC.
- In the first study, 146 patients with advanced stage NSCLC were randomized to receive either radiation alone or radiation plus amifostine (given just prior to each radiation treatment). At 2 months follow-up, the group receiving amifostine had an incidence of pneumonitis of 9% compared to 43% in those receiving radiation alone ($P < .001$). There was no difference between the groups in the number of patients showing complete or partial response to the radiation treatment.
- In the second study, 60 patients with NSCLC were randomized to receive a regimen of etoposide plus cisplatin plus radiation with or without concurrent amifostine. Again, the incidence of pneumonitis was lower in the amifostine group (3.7%) compared to the standard-treatment group (23%) ($P = .037$), and median survival was not significantly changed for the two groups, though the amifostine group did experience a significantly higher incidence of hypotension.
- Other novel strategies under preclinical investigation include whether inhibitors of tumor necrosis factor-alpha (TNF-alpha) or TGF-beta, molecules implicated in the lung injury cytokine pathway, could be clinically useful.
- Finally, continued improvements in the ability to preferentially deliver radiation energy to tumor with sparing of normal surrounding tissue, via advances in radiation physics and radiation-delivery techniques, should only decrease the incidence of radiation lung injury while preserving or increasing the therapeutic effect of ionizing radiation.

BIBLIOGRAPHY

Abid SH, Malhotra V, Perry MC. Radiation-induced and chemotherapy-induced pulmonary injury. *Curr Opin Oncol* 2001;13:242–248.

Choi NC. Radioprotective effect of amifostine in radiation pneumonitis. *Semin Oncol* 2003;30(Suppl 18):10–17.

Movsas B, Raffin TA, Epstein AH, et al. Pulmonary radiation injury. *Chest* 1997;111:1061–1076.

Roach M III, Gandara DR, Yuo HS, et al. Radiation pneumonitis following combined modality therapy for lung cancer: analysis of prognostic factors. *J Clin Oncol* 1995;13:2606–2612.

Rodrigues G, Lock M, D'Souza D, et al. Prediction of radiation pneumonitis by dose-volume histogram parameters in lung cancer: a systematic review. *Radiother Oncol* 2004;71:127–138.

Section 7
RENAL AND METABOLIC DISORDERS

93 ACUTE RENAL FAILURE

Nina M. Patel

KEY POINTS

- Acute renal failure is common in the ICU and associated with substantial mortality.
- Dividing the causes among pre-renal azotemia, intrinsic renal failure, and post-renal failure is useful. Intravascular volume and renal perfusion should be judged and obstruction excluded, generally by assessing patency of a urinary catheter and performing renal ultrasound.
- Critical electrolyte disorders should be anticipated, sought, and corrected.
- No specific therapy has been shown to reduce the severity or duration of acute tubular necrosis. In particular, dopamine is clearly ineffective and should not be used for this purpose.
- Indications for renal replacement therapy include hyperkalemia, severe acidemia, fluid overload, and uremia.
- It is uncertain whether continuous renal replacement therapy is superior to intermittent dialysis.
- More than 50% of survivors will recover sufficient renal function to avoid long-term dialysis.

EPIDEMIOLOGY

- Acute renal failure (ARF) occurs in up to 20% of ICU patients.
- Mortality rates associated with ARF in the ICU are 50–70%.
- Survivors of ARF will recover renal function (no longer require dialysis) in 50–75% of cases.
- Approximately 30% of survivors will require lifelong hemodialysis.
- Acute tubular necrosis (ATN) and prerenal azotemia are the two most common causes of hospital-acquired ARF.
- Sepsis accounts for >50% of cases of ARF in the ICU.

PATHOPHYSIOLOGY

- Acute renal failure constitutes a sudden loss in renal function (decrease in glomerular filtration rate [GFR]) with consequent derangement of electrolytes, acid-base regulation, and extracellular fluid balance.
- ARF may also manifest with increasing blood urea nitrogen (BUN) and decreasing urine output (UO).
- The classification of ARF is stratified into prerenal, intrinsic renal, and postrenal azotemia.
- Prerenal azotemia results from decreased renal perfusion. Hospital-acquired prerenal azotemia is most often caused by systemic hypotension due to volume loss (hemorrhage, gastrointestinal [GI] bleed, or GI loss) or effective hypoperfusion (congestive heart failure [CHF], cirrhosis, sepsis).
- Nonsteroidal anti-inflammatory drugs (NSAIDs), angiotensin-converting enzyme (ACE) inhibitors, calcineurin inhibitors (tacrolimus, cyclosporine), amphotericin B, and radiocontrast media (RCM) can induce a decrease in glomerular perfusion and/or renal vasoconstriction.
- Intrinsic renal azotemia is subclassified into vascular, interstitial, glomerular, or tubular causes of disease.
  - Atheroemboli (recent intravascular procedure), malignant hypertension (HTN), vasculitis, hemolytic uremic syndrome/thrombotic thrombocytopenic purpura (TTP), and scleroderma are vascular etiologies of ARF.
  - A number of commonly administered medications precipitate acute interstitial nephritis (NSAIDs, penicillin, cephalosporins, sulfonamides, ciprofloxacin, furosemide, thiazides, phenytoin, allopurinol, rifampin, cimetidine).

- Glomerular diseases (nephrotic and nephritic syndromes) are often associated with systemic disease (connective tissue disease, vasculitis) and characteristically display an active urine sediment.
- Prolonged systemic hypotension, medications (e.g., aminoglycosides, RCM, and amphotericin), cast nephropathy due to myeloma light chains, uric acid nephropathy in tumor lysis syndrome, and myoglobinuria in rhabdomyolysis frequently cause ATN.

- Postrenal azotemia occurs when there is obstruction in urinary flow at any level between the renal pelvis and the urethra. Nephrolithiasis, prostate disease, retroperitoneal obstruction (e.g., lymph nodes or mass), and medication-induced crystalluria (protease inhibitors, methotrexate, acyclovir, sulfonamides) commonly lead to obstructive uropathy.

CLINICAL FEATURES

- Clinical history focuses on identification of volume loss, changes in color or quantity of urine, intake of nephrotoxic medications or illicit substances, presence of concurrent illnesses (e.g., HTN, diabetes mellitus [DM], CHF, and cirrhosis), and symptoms or signs of obstructive uropathy.
- Assessing intravascular volume status is valuable in distinguishing prerenal azotemia from other causes of ARF. Dry oral mucous membranes, tachycardia, and orthostatic hypotension are consistent with intravascular volume depletion. Inpatients should have daily weights checked to monitor for changes in volume status.
- Skin examination should center on presence of rash, purpura, livedo reticularis or stigmata of endocarditis or other systemic conditions associated with intrinsic renal disease.
- Nephrolithiasis may manifest as flank pain and costovertebral angle tenderness.
- UO is variable, but can be useful in determining etiology and prognosis in ARF.
- A severe vascular insult (bilateral renal artery or vein occlusion), complete urinary tract obstruction, bilateral cortical necrosis, severe ATN, or rapidly progressive glomerulonephritis may produce anuria (UO <50–100 mL/day).
- Nonoliguric ATN (UO >500 mL/day) often, but not always, has a lower rate of progression to dialysis than oliguric ATN (UO <500 mL/day).

DIFFERENTIAL AND DIAGNOSIS

- There are no standard criteria for the diagnosis of ARF, though it is often defined as a 50% decrease in GFR, a 0.5 mg/dL increase in plasma creatinine (Pcre), or a 25% decrease in creatinine clearance.
- Creatinine clearance is used as an estimate of GFR and is calculated based on a 24-hour urine collection (CREcl mL/min = [Ucre × (volume/Pcre)] × 1000/1440). Normal values: men = 120 ± 25 mL/min; women = 95 ± 20 mL/min.
- Limitations in use of CREcl are that tubular secretion of CRE increases with decreasing GFR, resulting in an overestimation of GFR and renal function. Also, some drugs [e.g., trimenthoprim (TMP) and cimetidine] compete with creatinine for secretion.
- When available, current Pcre should be compared to a baseline value to determine the acuity of presentation.
- An electrolyte panel, calcium, magnesium, phosphorus, uric acid level, creatine kinase (CK), and liver function panel should be checked in the initial assessment.
- Urinalysis (UA) may reveal muddy brown casts, granular casts, and epithelial cell casts in ATN. RBC casts and proteinuria occur in glomerular disease.
- A number of urine and serum examinations help differentiate ATN and prerenal azotemia:

	PRERENAL AZOTEMIA	ATN
Plasma BUN/Cre	>20:1	<10–15:1
Una	<20 meq/L	>40 meq/L
Uosm	>500 mOsm/kg	<400 mOsm/kg
FEna	<1%	>1%

(FEna; fractional excretion of Na = [Una × Pcre/Pna × Ucre] × 100)

- Patients with chronic renal failure or patients on diuretic therapy will have altered excretion of water and sodium. If prerenal azotemia is highly suspected, patients should undergo a trial of volume repletion for at least 24 hours. If unsuccessful, ATN is likely.
- Renal ultrasound (US) should be obtained and may reveal hydronephrosis in significant urinary obstruction. Doppler US may demonstrate renal vein thrombosis or renal artery stenosis.
- Plain films of the abdomen reveal radiopaque calculi (calcium, struvite, cystine).
- Non-contrast-enhanced computed tomography (CT) is the gold standard for suspected nephrolithiasis and can diagnose radiolucent as well as radiopaque stones. With IV contrast, CT can also diagnose renal cell cancer and renal vein thrombosis.
- Intravenous pyelogram (IVP), MRI, and radionuclide studies can be utilized for specific indications.
- Renal biopsy is indicated for suspected glomerulonephritis or vasculitis, or when noninvasive measures have failed to yield a diagnosis.

TREATMENT

- Initial management includes identifying the etiology and either discontinuing the nephrotoxic agent, relieving the obstruction, or treating the insult, and always, assuring adequate renal perfusion.
- Severe electrolyte derangements (e.g., hyperkalemia and hyperphosphatemia) should be corrected and enteral (when possible) nutritional support provided.
- Subsequent management of ARF is divided into nondialytic and dialytic therapy.
- Crystalloid infusion is an effective means of expanding intravascular volume. Indiscriminate use of crystalloids can lead to pulmonary edema. Fluid management should be titrated to markers of volume status and perfusion (fluid balance, daily weight, central venous pressure, central venous O_2%).
- Vasoactive agents are utilized to augment systemic blood pressure (BP), if intravenous fluids (IVFs) alone fail. Dobutamine, vasopressin, and norepinephrine have variable effects on UO and CREcl, and do not appear to compromise renal perfusion.
- "Renal dose" dopamine (0.5–2 μg/kg/min) does *not* improve outcomes (Pcre, mortality, length of stay, dialysis) and should not be used in patients with ARF.
- Fenoldopam (selective dopamine$_1$-receptor agonist) and *N*-acetylcysteine, in concert with hydration, have been shown to decrease rates of radiocontrast-mediated nephropathy. Sodium-bicarbonate therapy pre- and postradiocontrast exposure has also been shown to decrease the development of radiocontrast nephropathy.
- Indications for dialysis are hyperkalemia, severe metabolic acidosis, fluid overload, and uremia.
- Preliminary studies suggest that increased doses of dialysis (Kt/Vurea) and use of biocompatible membranes are improving survival in ARF and ATN.
- ICU patients who received daily hemodialysis versus intermittent hemodialysis were observed to have lower mortality rates.
- Data regarding continuous renal replacement therapy (CRRT) versus intermittent hemodialysis is controversial. At present, CRRT does not confer a survival benefit.

CONCLUSIONS

- Acute renal failure occurs frequently in the ICU, and is a major cause of ICU morbidity and mortality.
- Diagnosing the etiology of ARF can be challenging. Urine studies, renal US, rigorous attention to iatrogenic sources of renal failure (e.g., medications and contrast) and at times, renal biopsy are useful to discern the etiology of decreased renal function.
- Medical therapies for the prevention and treatment of ARF are targeted at the inciting insults. If metabolic derangements, fluid overload, or uremia ensue, renal replacement therapy is indicated.

BIBLIOGRAPHY

Liano F, Junco E, Pascual J, et al. Epidemiology of acute renal failure: a prospective, multicenter, community-based study. *Kidney Int* 1996;50(3):811–818.

Wan L, Bellomo R, Di Giantomasso D, et al. The pathogenesis of septic acute renal failure. *Curr Opin Crit Care* 2003;9: 496–502.

Albright RC. Acute renal failure: a practical update. *Mayo Clin Proc* 2001;76(1):67–74.

Esson ML, Schrier RW. Diagnosis and treatment of acute tubular necrosis. *Ann Intern Med* 2002;137(9):744–752.

Lameire NH, De Vriese AS, Vanholder R. Prevention and nondialytic treatment of acute renal failure. *Curr Opin Crit Care* 2003;9:481–490.

Birck R, Krzossok S, Markowetz F, et al. Acetylcysteine for prevention of contrast nephropathy: meta-analysis. *Lancet* 2003;362:598–603.

Merten GJ, Burgess WP, Gray LV, et al. Prevention of contrast-induced nephropathy with sodium bicarbonate: a randomized controlled trial. *JAMA* 2004;291:2328–2334.

Van Biesen W, Vanholder R, Lameire N. Dialysis strategies in critically ill acute renal failure patients. *Curr Opin Crit Care* 2003;9:491–495.

Schiffl H. Daily haemodialysis for acute renal failure. *Curr Opin Nephrol Hypertens* 2002;11:589–592.

For further reading, please refer to Hall, Schmidt & Wood, *Principles of Critical Care*, 3rd ed.

94 RENAL REPLACEMENT THERAPY IN THE ICU

Ignatius Y. Tang

KEY POINTS

- Primary indications for RRT include uremia, hyperkalemia, acidemia, volume overload, and drug intoxication.
- Continuous dialytic modalities are better tolerated in the setting of hemodynamic instability or hypoperfused states.
- Some form of anticoagulation is almost always required during dialytic therapy.

INDICATIONS

- Uremia
- Hyperkalemia refractory to medical therapy
- Volume overload refractory to diuretics
- Severe metabolic acidosis
- Some drug intoxications (e.g., lithium, ethylene glycol, methanol, salicylates, theophylline, and phenobarbital. Digoxin and tricyclic antidepressants are insignificantly removed by dialysis because of their large volumes of distribution. Phenytoin and warfarin are not significantly removed because of their high protein binding.)

TIMING OF INITIATION OF RENAL REPLACEMENT THERAPY

- There is no evidence that initiating renal replacement therapy (RRT) prophylactically would alter the outcomes of acute renal failure (ARF). However, one should not delay therapy until the patient has complete renal shutdown.

MODALITIES OF RENAL REPLACEMENT THERAPY

- Intermittent hemodialysis (IHD)
- Continuous venovenous hemofiltration (CVVH)
- Continuous venovenous hemodialysis (CVVHD)
- Continuous venovenous hemodiafiltration (CVVHDF)
- Continuous arteriovenous hemofiltration (CAVH)
- Continuous arteriovenous hemodialysis (CAVHD)
- Continuous arteriovenous hemodiafiltration (CAVHDF)
- Slow continuous ultrafiltration (SCUF)
- Slow low efficiency dialysis (SLED)
- Peritoneal dialysis (PD)

NOTES ON RENAL REPLACEMENT THERAPY MODALITIES

- All the modalities above except PD require a vascular access and an artificial membrane (dialyzer or filter). Biocompatible membranes which minimally activate complement are usually used.
- In PD, a catheter is placed in the peritoneal cavity. Dialysis solution is infused via the catheter into the peritoneal cavity. This is not commonly done for ARF.
- The continuous modalities are done continuously, 24 hours a day while the intermittent modalities are done 4–6 hours (IHD) or 8–16 hours (SLED) per session daily or every other day, depending on the patient's needs.
- PD is rarely used because of its inferior solute clearance compared to hemodialysis and hemofiltration.
- CVVH was shown to be more effective and improve survival in a population with infection and sepsis who developed ARF.
- Continuous arteriovenous renal replacement therapies are also rarely used because of the bleeding complications that occur with arterial cannulation.
- SCUF is used only for fluid removal; it does not provide significant solute clearance.

PRINCIPLES OF SOLUTE CLEARANCE DURING RENAL REPLACEMENT THERAPY

- *Diffusion*: solute removal based on concentration gradient; effective for small molecule removal.
- *Convection*: solute removal based on ultrafiltration; more effective for large molecule removal.
- *Hemodialysis*: diffusive clearance. Blood and dialysis solution flow in countercurrent directions while diffusion occurs across the membrane.
- *Hemofiltration*: convective clearance. No dialysis solution is used. Instead, replacement fluid is used to replete the solutes that are cleared.
- *Hemodiafiltration*: diffusive and convective clearance, that is, combination of hemodialysis and hemofiltration. Both replacement fluid and dialysis solution are used.
- *PD*: diffusive and convective clearance. PD solution is placed in the peritoneal cavity. Diffusion across the peritoneal membrane occurs during the dwell period.
- In hemodialysis, increasing either the blood or the dialysate flow rates, or both would increase solute clearance. In contrast to IHD in which blood flow rates of 300–450 mL/min and dialysate flow rates of 600–800 mL/min are employed, lower blood and dialysate flow rates for a prolonged period of time are used in SLED. In continuous hemodialysis or hemodiafiltration, typical blood and dialysate flow rates are 150–200 mL/min and 16–32 mL/min, respectively. Using a dialyzer with a large surface area also results in increased clearance.
- In hemofiltration, increasing the ultrafiltration (or effluent) flow rates would increase solute clearance. The blood flow rates are 150–200 mL/min.

PRINCIPLES OF FLUID REMOVAL DURING RENAL REPLACEMENT THERAPY

- Fluid removal is effected by ultrafiltration.
- In hemodialysis, hemofiltration, and hemodiafiltration, the driving force for ultrafiltration is the hydraulic

pressure gradient across the membrane. High ultrafiltration rates can be achieved with high flux membranes that have a high ultrafiltration coefficient.
- In PD, the driving force for ultrafiltration is the osmotic gradient generated by the high glucose contents of the peritoneal dialysate solutions.

ANTICOAGULATION

- Anticoagulation is usually required during RRT to prevent clotting of the dialyzer/filter and the RRT circuit because clotting of the dialyzer/filter would compromise the efficiency of solute clearance of RRT. Frequent clotting of the RRT circuit also results in increased blood loss.
- Heparin is the usual anticoagulant. Citrate, lepirudin, and argatroban are alternative choices in patients who cannot tolerate heparin, for example, those with heparin-induced thrombocytopenia.
- Lepirudin is rarely used because it is renally excreted and accumulates in renal failure. Citrate and argatroban may not be used in patients with severe liver dysfunction because both are hepatically metabolized.
- PD does not require anticoagulation.

COMPLICATIONS OF RENAL REPLACEMENT THERAPY

- Hypotension (excessive ultrafiltration)
- Bleeding (excessive anticoagulation)
- Clotting (inadequate anticoagulation)
- Infection (catheter-associated)
- Pneumothorax and hemothorax (catheter-associated)
- Increased intracranial pressure (rapid osmotic shifts in IHD)
- Anaphylactoid reaction with certain membranes (e.g., AN69 with angiotensin-converting enzyme [ACE] inhibitors)
- Citrate toxicity (arrhythmia, metabolic alkalosis, and hypocalcemia)
- Electrolyte imbalance (errors in replacement fluid or dialysate, parenteral nutrition, and other intravenous fluids)

DOSE ADJUSTMENT IN RENAL FAILURE AND DURING RENAL REPLACEMENT THERAPY

- The doses for all drugs and those with active metabolites that are mainly renally eliminated should be adjusted. Drugs may be removed by RRT.
- Rules of thumb: drugs with small molecular weights, small volumes of distribution, or low protein/tissue binding can be removed during RRT and may need supplementation. Lipophilic drugs are less likely to be removed. High flux membranes can remove large molecules such as vancomycin and vitamin B_{12}.

IMPACT OF RENAL REPLACEMENT THERAPY ON SURVIVAL

- There appears an association of improved outcome with increased dose of RRT.
- Daily IHD was associated with a lower mortality rate and a shorter duration of ARF when compared to alternate-day IHD.
- CVVH has been shown in a prospective randomized-controlled study to improve outcomes if the ultrafiltration rate is 35 mL/kg/h.
- RRT does not hasten renal recovery. It only supports the patient during ARF.

INTERMITTENT VERSUS CONTINUOUS TREATMENTS

- No difference in survival benefits is proven. Continuous RRT (CVVH, CVVHD, and CVVHDF) is usually indicated for hemodynamically unstable patients.
- Continuous RRT is useful in critically ill patients with multiorgan failure, requiring significant nutritional and fluid support.
- It may also be useful in liver failure patients with hepatic encephalopathy or stroke patients to avoid increase in intracranial pressure.

BIBLIOGRAPHY

Forni LG, Hilton PJ. Continuous hemofiltration in the treatment of acute renal failure. *N Engl J Med* 1997;336:1303–1309.

Johnson CA, Simmons WD. *2004 Dialysis of Drugs.* Nephrology Pharmacy Associates, Inc. Available at: http://www.nephrologypharmacy.com/downloads/us_dod_2004.pdf. Accessed July 17, 2006.

Pastan S, Bailey J. Dialysis therapy. *N Engl J Med* 1998;338:1428–1437.

Phu NH, Hien TT, Mai NTH, et al. Hemofiltration and peritoneal dialysis in infection-associated acute renal failure in Vietnam. *N Engl J Med* 2002;347:895–902.

Ronco C, Bellomo R, Homel P, et al. Effects of different doses of continuous veno-venous haemofiltration on outcomes of acute renal failure: a prospective randomized trial. *Lancet* 2000;356:26–30.

Schiffl H, Lang SM, Fischer B. Daily hemodialysis and the outcome of acute renal failure. *N Engl J Med* 2002;346:305–310.

95 SEVERE ELECTROLYTE DISORDERS

William Schweickert

KEY POINTS

- Disorders of sodium concentration are nearly always caused by excess free water (hyponatremia) or free water loss (hypernatremia).
- Severe or symptomatic acute hypernatremia should be corrected rapidly (2 mEq/L/h) but only partially, generally using hypertonic saline.
- Severe hypernatremia should be corrected only slowly, since rapid correction risks cerebral swelling.
- Mild hypokalemia (>2.5 mEq/L) is generally asymptomatic and does not benefit from urgent correction.
- Severe hyperkalemia risks life-threatening arrhythmias: treatment may include dialysis, diuretics, kayexalate, insulin with glucose, sodium bicarbonate, and calcium gluconate.
- Hypocalcemia is common in critical illness and generally does not benefit from treatment.

HYPONATREMIA

- Hyponatremia should be envisioned as a problem of free water excretion. In the event of a large free water intake, two processes prevent its occurrence: (1) kidney formation of a dilute filtrate in the Loop of Henle and (2) antidimone (ADH) is turned off. When these two steps are impaired, hyponatremia results.
- Symptoms are due to cerebral edema as the extra water enters the brain, causing headache, nausea, or lethargy; severe disease may culminate in seizures or coma.
- First step is to determine tonicity (to exclude pseudohyponatremia)—generally unnecessary, but can be proven by checking serum osmolality.
    - *Isotonic hyponatremia*: rare lab artifact due to hyperlipidemia or hyperproteinemia.
    - *Hypertonic hyponatremia* (high serum osmolality): presence of another effective osmole (glucose, mannitol) that moves free water into the extracellular volume. Recall that each 100 mg/dL increase in glucose >100 mg/dL, plasma Na will decrease by 1.6 meq/L.
    - *Hypotonic hyponatremia*: true excess of water relative to sodium. Almost entirely due to increased ADH secretion, but will need to determine if this is appropriate (decreased effective circulating volume) or inappropriate. *Note*: primary polydipsia is an exception.
        - *Hypovolemic* (primary Na loss with secondary water gain):
            - Urinary Na levels to determine source of loss.
            - Renal losses will have a U_{Na} >20 meq/L and FE_{Na} >1%. Etiologies include diuretics, hypoaldosteronism, and salt-wasting nephropathy.
            - Extrarenal losses produce a U_{Na} <10 meq/L, FE_{Na} <1%, frequently mediated by gastrointestinal (GI) losses, third spacing, and insensible losses.
        - *Euvolemic* (primary water gain): utilize U_{osm} to determine cause:
            - Syndrome of inappropriate antidiuretic hormone (SIADH): patients are euvolemic or mildly hypervolemic with an inappropriately high U_{osm} (>100). Seek etiology: endocrinopathies (hypothyroidism, adrenal insufficiency), pulmonary or intracranial pathology, malignancy, pain, nausea, drugs (neuroleptics).
            - Psychogenic polydipsia: usually requires intake of >12–20 L/day, U_{osm} <100, low uric acid.
            - Reset osmostat (ADH regulation reset to regulate a lower Na)—variable U_{osm}.
        - *Hypervolemic* (low *effective circulating* volume):
            - Etiologies include congestive heart failure (CHF), cirrhosis, nephrotic syndrome—all lead to decreased effective arterial volume = U_{Na} <10 meq/L, FE_{Na} <1%.
            - Advanced renal failure (U_{Na} >20 meq/L).
- Treatment:
    - Rate of correction:
        - *Chronic* hyponatremia, brain cells excrete osmoles to minimize intracellular swelling. Correcting too rapidly can increase serum osmolality relative to brain, create water shift from brain with resultant brain dehydration: cerebral pontine myelinolysis. Therefore, rate of increase of Na should not exceed 0.5 meq/L/h.
        - Patients with serious neurologic symptoms or a sodium concentration <100 meq/L need an initial rapid correction until symptoms resolve or a safer level is reached. The goal is to correct the serum Na at a rate of 1.5–2 meq/L/h. Consider the use of hypertonic saline.
    - Hypovolemic hyponatremia: calculate sodium deficit and replace with 0.9 normal saline:
        - (0.6 × ideal body weight × (140 – measured Na) × 0.85 (in women only)
    - Hypervolemic hyponatremia: sodium and water restriction (<1 L/day).
    - SIADH—free water restriction usually suffices. If chronic can use demeclocycline.

HYPERNATREMIA

- Hypernatremia is simply a deficit of water relative to sodium; this is almost always due to loss of hypotonic fluid and impaired access to free water. The body usually defends against this with the potent mechanism of thirst, but critically ill patients are often unable to drink.
- Symptoms are due to osmotic shrinkage of brain cells and include lethargy, seizures, and coma.
- First, check volume status and determine why the patient is not drinking.
  - If *hypovolemic*, determine source of loss (renal vs. nonrenal) via U_{Na} levels:
    - Renal losses (U_{Na} >20 meq/L, ↑ urine volume, U_{osm} = 300–600): diuretics, osmotic diuresis
    - Extrarenal losses (U_{Na} <10 meq/L, ↓ urine volume, U_{osm} >600): GI or insensible losses
  - If *euvolemic*, determine whether there is a lack of ADH activity:
    - Diabetes insipidus (DI): ADH is absent (central) or has no effect (nephrogenic):
      - Central: central nervous system (CNS) trauma, surgery, hemorrhage, tumor, idiopathic
      - Nephrogenic: drugs (lithium, amphotericin), metabolic (hypercalcemia, hypokalemia), sickle cell, sarcoid, amyloid
      - Tests: U_{osm} <300 in complete, 300–600 in partial OR water deprivation test
    - Reset osmostat
  - If *hypervolemic*, usual causes are exogenous NaCl infusion (high U_{osm} >600), or mineralocorticoid excess.
- Treatment:
  - Rate of correction: in *chronic hypernatremia*, brain cells generate osmoles to minimize intracellular dehydration. Too rapid correction prompts decrease serum osmolality relative to high brain osmolality, water passes into the brain with resultant swelling. Therefore, rate of increase of sodium should not exceed 0.5 meq/L/h
  - Hypovolemic hypernatremia: replace volume until clinically judged euvolemic and initiate free water replacement. Utilize free water deficit equation:
    - [Ideal body weight × 0.6 × (measured Na/140 − 1) (0.85 in women)]
  - Hypervolemic hypernatremia: loop diuretics + D_5W
  - Central DI: desmopressin (dDAVP)
  - Nephrogenic DI: treat underlying cause; salt restriction + thiazide diuretic

HYPOKALEMIA

- Potassium enters the body via oral intake or IV infusion and is largely stored in cells, and excreted in urine. Hypokalemia can ensue in the setting of decreased intake, increased translocation into cells, or (most commonly) increased losses in urine or the GI tract or sweat.
- Symptoms: Severe hypokalemia (<2.5 meq/L) can be accompanied by diffuse muscle weakness, mental status changes. Milder forms of hypokalemia are generally asymptomatic.
- ECG manifestations:
  - Mild hypokalemia: flat or inverted T waves, ST depression, prolonged Q_T interval
  - Severe hypokalemia: prominent U waves, ventricular tachycardia, or fibrillation
- Workup:
  - Evaluate for possible causes of transcellular shifts:
    - Insulin, albuterol, refeeding, periodic paralysis
  - Determine whether potassium depletion is due to GI or renal losses via U_K:
    - GI losses: U_K <25 meq/L; renal losses: U_K >30 meq/L
  - GI loss: vomiting, nasogastric (NG) drainage; diarrhea, villous adenoma
  - Renal loss: determine blood pressure and acid-base status:
    - Hypo- or normotensive:
      - Acidosis: diabetic ketoacidosis (DKA), renal tubular acidosis (RTA, types 1 and 2)
      - Alkalosis: diuretics, Bartter, or Gitelman syndrome, loss of gastric fluid
      - Either: magnesium deficiency
    - Hypertensive:
      - Hyperaldosteronism: primary or secondary
      - Pseudohyperaldosteronism: Cushing syndrome, licorice
- Treatment: Enteral or intravenous replacement of potassium combined with chloride or other anions.
  - Severe hypokalemia requires rapid intravenous infusion. If K is <2 meq/L, maximum 40 meq/h is necessary. Recheck values frequently.
  - When K is >2 meq/L and there are no ECG changed, 10 meq/h suffices.
  - Remember to treat any coexisting hypomagnesemia (avoid lethal arrhythmia)!

HYPERKALEMIA

- Urinary excretion is stimulated by a rise in plasma potassium, plasma aldosterone, or enhanced distal delivery of sodium and water. Hyperkalemia rarely occurs with isolated intake and release of intracellular potassium can cause a transient plasma elevation. Persistent hyperkalemia requires an impairment in urinary potassium excretion.
- Symptoms include weakness, irritability, paresthesias, and paralysis.

- ECG manifestations:
  - Mild hyperkalemia: peaked T waves, premature ventricular contractions (PVCs)
  - Severe hyperkalemia: widening of QRS, depressed ST, prolonged PR, sinus arrest, ventricular arrhythmia (tachycardia, fibrillation, or arrest)
- Workup:
  - Exclude pseudohyperkalemia (hemolyzed specimen, severe thrombocytosis/leukocytosis)
  - Evaluate for transcellular shifts:
    - Beta-blocker, insulin deficiency, digoxin intoxication, massive cellular necrosis, hyperkalemic periodic paralysis
  - Determine whether severely decreased or normal glomerular filtration rate (GFR):
    - Normal GFR: determine why there is decreased aldosterone function
      - Hyporeninemic: type 4 RTA (diabetic nephropathy, angiotensin-converting enzyme inhibitor [ACEI], nonsteroidal anti-inflammatory drugs [NSAIDs])
      - Primary adrenal: Addison disease, congenital adrenal hyperplasia, heparin
      - Renal tubular disorder: K-sparing diuretics, cyclosporine, systemic lupus erythematosus (SLE), multiple myeloma
    - Decreased GFR: any cause of acute oligo- or anuric renal failure or chronic disease
- Treatment:
  - Correct underlying disorder
  - Effectively decrease total body potassium
    - Kayexalate (oral or rectal), diuretics (furosemide), hemodialysis (definitive)
  - Transient effect: insulin (usually accompanied by glucose), consider bicarbonate
  - Stabilize membranes to avoid arrhythmia (with any ECG changes): calcium gluconate

HYPOCALCEMIA

- The free or ionized calcium is physiologically relevant. Total calcium levels must be interpreted relative to the plasma albumin concentration
  - Recall the approximation: for every 1.0 mg/dL that the albumin is below 4.0, the calcium is lowered by about 0.6 mg/dL. Alkalemia causes more calcium to bind to albumin and will drop ionized calcium further
- Symptoms, when severe: tetany, including laryngospasm, mental status changes, and seizures
- ECG changes: QT prolongation
- Causes:
  - Vitamin D deficiency
    - Malnutrition, poor sunlight exposure, malabsorption, drugs (e.g., phenytoin and phenobarbital), renal failure
  - Hypoparathyroidism (postsurgical or idiopathic)
    - Hypomagnesemia impairs parathyroid hormone (PTH) release
  - Uptake by necrotic tissue (severe pancreatitis, rhabdomyolysis)
  - Impaired action of PTH occurs in severe sepsis
- Diagnosis: measure PTH levels as well as concurrent phosphate level
- Treatment: correct underlying cause. Replace ONLY if the patient is symptomatic
  - Evidence that calcium administration in the critically ill may cause hypoxic cell damage
  - Remember to correct magnesium (to avoid arrhythmia)!

HYPERCALCEMIA

- Most common cause of severe disease is malignancy (bone involvement or ectopic PTH-like hormone). Others: hyperparathyroidism, vitamin D toxicity, or sarcoidosis.
- Manifestations: lethargy and mental status changes, vomiting, reversible nephrogenic DI, renal insufficiency, and ectopic calcifications.
- ECG changes: Q_T interval shortening, potentiation of digoxin toxicity.
- Treatment: increasing urine output with saline, followed by loop diuretics once euvolemic:
  - Slow effectors—pamidronate (or equivalent), calcitonin

HYPOPHOSPHATEMIA

- Causes include depleted stores, refeeding syndrome, malabsorption, phosphate-binding antacids, renal losses (RTA type 2, acute tubular necrosis [ATN], hyperparathyroidism), or transcellular shifts (insulin, DKA recovery, catecholamine infusion, alcohol withdrawal).
- Symptoms/adverse effects: muscular and diaphragmatic weakness, heart failure, arrhythmias, confusion, and rhabdomyolysis when severe.
- Treatment: oral supplementation, unless severe (below 1.0 mg/dL).

HYPERPHOSPHATEMIA

- Four main causes include excessive administration (laxatives), decreased renal excretion, transcellular

shift out of cells (respiratory acidosis, rhabdomyolysis, chemotherapy), and artifact from hemolysis.
- Usually requires some degree of renal failure, although it may result from severe tissue necrosis in normal renal function.
- Severe acute toxicity can result in ectopic calcification and hypocalcemia.
- Treatment: dietary restriction, phosphate binders when mild, dialysis if severe. Saline hydration or acetazolamide may help in those without renal failure.

HYPOMAGNESEMIA

- Results from malnutrition and chronically decreased body stores (alcoholism), diarrhea, or urinary wasting (diuretics, cisplatin, or amphotericin).
- Manifestations: tetany, laryngospasm, cardiac arrhythmias, hypocalcemia (and its effects).
- Correction may require large doses, critically ill patients require intravenous replacement (oral poorly tolerated).

HYPERMAGNESEMIA

- Causes: decreased renal excretion (renal failure, salt depletion), excessive intake (laxative or antacids), endocrinopathies, and tissue breakdown (rhabdomyolysis).
- Results in lethargy, weakness, and hyporeflexia. When severe, bradycardia, heart block, and hypotension may ensue.
- Treatment: hydration with loop or thiazide diuretic if patient urinates. Dialysis if anuric.
  - Intracardiac conduction abnormalities can be remedied with IV calcium gluconate.

BIBLIOGRAPHY

Kapoor M, Chan GZ. Fluid and electrolyte abnormalities. *Crit Care Clin* 2001;17(3):503–529.

Kraft MD, Btaiche IF, Sacks GS, et al. Treatment of electrolyte disorders in adult patients in the intensive care unit. *Am J Health Syst Pharm* 2005;62(16):1663–1682.

Topf JM, Rankin S, Murray P. Electrolyte disorders in critical care. In: Hall JB, Schmidt GA, Wood LDH, eds., *Principles of Critical Care*, 3rd ed. New York, NY: McGraw-Hill; 2005: 1161–1199.

96 ACID-BASE BALANCE

Meredith McCormack

KEY POINTS

- Acid-base homeostasis is important to maintain tissue and organ performance. Both acidosis and alkalosis can have harmful effects and when severe, can be life threatening.
- It is the nature of the condition responsible for the acid-base disturbance that largely determines the patient's prognosis.
- It is appropriate to focus on diagnosing and treating the underlying disorder, as most acid-base derangements do not benefit from specific correction of the abnormal pH.

INTRODUCTION

- The Henderson-Hasselbalch equation demonstrates the relationship between key components of the blood that determine acid-base balance. Here, the relationship among pH, HCO_3^-, and $PaCO_2$ can be readily seen.

$$pH = pK_a + \log([HCO_3^-]/(PCO_2 \times 0.03))$$

- The Henderson-Hasselbalch equation predicts that acidemia results from conditions that increase the PCO_2 or decrease the HCO_3^-. Conversely, alkalemia results from decreased PCO_2 or increased HCO_3.
- Compensatory responses tend to return the pH to normal.
- There are four primary acid-base disorders.
  - Metabolic acidosis
    - Characterized by a decrease in plasma $[HCO_3^-]$ through loss of HCO_3^- or accumulation of H^+
    - Accompanied by compensatory fall in $[PCO_2]$ through hyperventilation
  - Respiratory acidosis
    - Characterized by an increase in $[PCO_2]$ (hypoventilation)
    - Compensatory increase in $[HCO_3^-]$ via renal excretion of H^+ occurs slowly over days
  - Metabolic alkalosis
    - Characterized by increase in plasma $[HCO_3^-]$ through H^+ loss or HCO_3^- gain
    - Accompanied by compensatory rise in $[PCO_2]$ through hypoventilation

- Respiratory alkalosis
  - Characterized by decrease in [PCO_2] (hyperventilation)
  - Compensatory decrease in [HCO_3^-] via renal excretion of NH_4^+

METABOLIC ACIDOSIS

- Diagnostic evaluation
  - The presence of a low pH and a low [HCO_3^-] are the cardinal features of a metabolic acidosis.
  - Determination of the presence of an anion gap (AG) will aid in determining the underlying cause.
    - The formula is:
    - AG = [Na^+] – ([Cl^-] + [HCO_3^-]) and the expected value is between 8 and 10.
    - The AG is comprised largely of albumin and to a lesser extent, phosphate. Chronically, low albumin or phosphate will affect the value.
    - To correct for this, the expected value can be calculated as corrected AG = 2(albumin [g/dL]) + 0.5 (phosphate [mg/dL]).
  - Determination of the presence of an osmolar gap may also be helpful in determining the etiology of the metabolic acidosis.
    - Calculated serum osmolality = 2[Na^+] + glucose/18 + blood urea nitrogen (BUN)/2.8.
    - Osmolal gap = measured serum osmolality – calculated serum osmolality.
    - The presence of an elevated osmolal gap suggests the presence of an additional solute in the plasma.
  - To determine if there is appropriate respiratory compensation, one can use Winter formula.
  - $PCO_2 = 1.5[HCO_3^-] + 8 \pm 2$.
  - If this equation is not balanced by inserting the PCO_2 from the patient's arterial blood gas and the [HCO_3^-] from a blood chemistry drawn simultaneously, this suggests the presence of a secondary process.
  - Investigate the presence of a secondary process using the delta formula.
    - Here, the change in the AG is calculated (compared to predicted) and the change in [HCO_3^-] is calculated compared to the normal value of 24.
    - $\Delta AG > \Delta[HCO_3^-] \rightarrow$ concomitant metabolic alkalosis.
    - $\Delta AG = \Delta[HCO_3^-] \rightarrow$ no secondary metabolic disorder.
    - $\Delta AG < \Delta[HCO_3^-] \rightarrow$ concomitant nongap met acidosis.
- AG metabolic acidosis
  - Lactic acidosis
    - Lactic acidosis is the most important cause of metabolic acidosis in critical illness.
    - Lactic acid has been shown to correlate with outcome in hemorrhagic and septic shock.
    - Inadequate tissue oxygenation underlies the lactic acidosis in many patients.
    - Therapy should focus on restoring circulation and tissue oxygenation while diagnosing and treating the underling etiology (i.e., sepsis, hemorrhage, and bowel infarction).
    - Administration of sodium bicarbonate has not been shown to improve outcomes in patients with lactic acidosis.
  - Renal failure
    - Renal failure is often associated with a hyperchloremic metabolic acidosis that is partially associated with an elevated AG.
    - The AG reflects retained sulfates, phosphate, and other organic ions.
    - Hemodialysis will permit removal of these ions and will restore Na^+ and Cl^- balance.
  - Diabetic ketoacidosis
  - Poisoning/ingestion
    - Ethanol: alcoholic ketoacidosis is associated with both an elevated AG and an elevated osmolar gap.
    - Methanol and ethylene glycol are both associated with elevated anion and osmolal gaps.
    - Salicylate ingestion usually results in a mixed disturbance, a metabolic acidosis and a respiratory alkalosis.
      - Respiratory alkalosis is caused by the direct stimulation of the respiratory center by the salicylate and the metabolic acidosis is caused by lactate accumulation.
- Non-AG metabolic acidosis
  - Renal tubular acidosis (RTA)
    - The defect in all types of RTA is the inability to excrete Cl^- in proportion to Na^+.
    - Type I (classic distal) RTA can present with profound hypobicarbonatemia and hypokalemia and replacement with sodium bicarbonate and potassium infusion is usually required.
    - Type IV RTA is associated with aldosterone deficiency or resistance. Clinical features include high serum potassium and low urine pH (<5.5). Treatment is directed at the underlying cause.
  - Diarrhea
    - Loss of bicarbonate through the digestive tract is typically accompanied by losses of Na^+ that are out of proportion to the losses of Cl^-.
    - This results in a non-AG hyperchloremic metabolic acidosis.
    - Pancreatic diversion can have a similar effect.
  - Hyperalimentation
    - Parenteral nutrition with excess Cl^- can cause hyperchloremic acidosis.

- Weak anions such as acetate are often used in addition to Cl^- to allow adjustment for a patient's acid-base status.

RESPIRATORY ACIDOSIS

- Diagnostic evaluation
  - Diagnosis of respiratory acidosis involves recognizing the decrease in pH accompanied by an elevated PCO_2.
  - Assessment of the clinical situation and reviewing the serum bicarbonate concentration in relation to the PCO_2 can help determine the chronicity.
  - In an acute respiratory acidosis, $[HCO_3^-]$ should increase about 1 meq/L for every 10 mmHg rise in PCO_2.
  - In chronic respiratory acidosis, the $[HCO_3^-]$ should increase about 3–5 meq/L for every 10 mmHg rise in PCO_2.
- Differential diagnosis
  - Central nervous system (CNS) suppression
    - CNS disease
    - Drugs
  - Neuromuscular disease
    - Myasthenia gravis
    - Guillain-Barré syndrome
    - Hypophosphatemia
    - Hypokalemia
  - Pulmonary disease
    - Chronic obstructive pulmonary disease (COPD)
    - Obesity-hypoventilation
  - Mechanical derangement of the chest wall

METABOLIC ALKALOSIS

- Metabolic alkalosis occurs as either a loss of anions (Cl^- from the stomach) or an increase in cations, which is rare.
- Chloride responsive metabolic alkalosis
  - This is a consequence of temporary chloride loss.
  - Urine chloride is typically below 20 mmol/L.
  - Most common causes are vomiting, gastric drainage, volume contraction. Diuretic use is also chloride responsive but urine chloride may be >20 mmol/L.
  - Treatment is replacement of chloride and volume loss. Saline with potassium supplementation is often given.
- Chloride-resistant metabolic alkalosis
  - This is typically a consequence of a hormonal mechanism and is less easily corrected by the administration of chloride.
  - Urine chloride is typically elevated (>20 mmol/L).
  - Most common causes are processes involving excess mineralocorticoid activity. Examples include hypercortisolism, hyperaldosteronism, sodium bicarbonate therapy, and severe renal artery stenosis.
  - Treatment is directed at the underlying cause.
- Other causes
  - Rarely, metabolic alkalosis is a consequence of cation administration rather than anion depletion.
  - Examples include the milk-alkali syndrome and massive blood transfusions or plasma exchange. The latter occurs because Na^+ is paired with citrate (a weak anion) instead of Cl^-.

RESPIRATORY ALKALOSIS

- Respiratory alkalosis is the most common acid-base disorder. It occurs during normal pregnancy and at high altitudes. In critically ill patients, it often indicates poor prognosis.
- Diagnostic evaluation
  - Requires recognition of elevated pH and decreased PCO_2.
  - In an acute process, the compensatory response is an approximate decrease in $[HCO_3^-]$ of about 1–2 meq/L for every 10 mmHg decrease in PCO_2.
  - In a chronic process, the compensatory response is an approximate decrease in $[HCO_3^-]$ of about 5 meq/L for every 10 mmHg decrease in PCO_2.
- Differential diagnosis
  - Hypoxemia
    - High altitude
    - Pulmonary disease
    - Heart failure
    - Anemia
  - Respiratory center stimulation
    - Pregnancy
    - CNS disease
    - Liver disease
    - Sepsis
    - Drugs
  - Pulmonary disease
    - Pneumonia
    - Interstitial lung disease
    - Pulmonary emboli
- Treatment is directed at the underlying cause.

BIBLIOGRAPHY

Adrogue H, Madias NE. Management of life-threatening acid-base disorders. *N Engl J Med* 1998;338:26–34, 107–111.

Seifter JL. Acid-base disorders. In: Goldman L, Ausiello D, eds., *Cecil Textbook of Medicine*, 22nd ed. Philadelphia, PA: W.B. Saunders; 2004:688–699.

97 DIABETIC KETOACIDOSIS IN ADULTS

Steve Skjei

KEY POINTS

- Ketoacidosis is a common complication of DM and produces a host of metabolic disturbances.
- Common triggers include noncompliance, infection, or acute medical disorders.
- Dehydration with a requirement for large volume resuscitation is the rule.
- Management requires volume and electrolyte correction, insulin to clear acidemia, and a simultaneous search and treatment of precipitating disorders.
- Continuous insulin administration is essential in DKA.

DEFINITION

- Reduced circulating insulin action (due to insulin deficiency and/or resistance) and consequent elevation in hormones yielding hyperglycemia, hyperosmolality, and lipolysis leading to fatty acid oxidation and subsequent ketoacidosis. Serious and potentially lethal complication of type 1 or, less commonly, type 2 diabetes.

COMMON CAUSES OF DIABETIC KETOACIDOSIS

- Infection (pneumonia, urinary tract infection [UTI], gastroenteritis)
- New-onset type 1 diabetes mellitus (DM)
- Discontinuation of insulin therapy or inadequate insulin therapy in type 1
- Drugs (e.g., corticosteroids)
- Acute illness such as myocardial infarction (MI), pancreatitis, and cerebral vascular accident (CVA)
- Trauma

COMMON SYMPTOMS OF DIABETIC KETOACIDOSIS

- Usually begins with polyuria, polydipsia, polyphagia, and weight loss
- Dehydration
- Altered mental status
- Abdominal pain, nausea, and vomiting (can also be caused by pancreatitis or intra-abdominal infection, both potential causes of diabetic ketoacidosis [DKA])

FREQUENT PHYSICAL EXAMINATION FINDINGS IN DIABETIC KETOACIDOSIS

- Kussmaul (deep, rapid) respirations and a "fruity" odor to breath (from ketones)
- Tachycardia and/or hypotension (from volume depletion)
- Dry mucous membranes
- Altered mental status

FREQUENT METABOLIC DERANGEMENTS IN DIABETIC KETOACIDOSIS

- Hyperglycemia (blood sugar usually but not always >250 mg/dL)
- Hyperosmolality
- Ketonemia and secondary anion gap acidosis
- Volume depletion due to osmotic diuresis (due to glycosuria)
- Hyperkalemia or hypokalemia (due to potassium losses from osmotic diuresis leading to total body potassium depletion)
- Hyponatremia (due to volume depletion, hyperglycemia, or hypertriglyceridemia)
- Hypophosphatemia, hypomagnesemia

INITIAL MANAGEMENT

- After the initial basic assessment of the patients' airway, breathing, and cardiovascular status and vital signs, the following information is gathered:
  - Directed history including history of DM, treatment history, and any recent changes in treatment of DM, prior episodes of DKA, and evidence of infection or other precipitating cause.
  - Arterial blood gas (ABG), serum electrolytes, complete blood count (CBC), blood and urine cultures and possibly throat cultures, chest x-ray (CXR), ECG.
  - Urine and serum ketones. Beta-hydroxybutyrate (not detected by ketone assay) is converted to acetoacetate in the process of treating DKA. If ketones are frequently monitored, this may give the impression that ketonemia is worsening.
  - Head computed tomography (CT) and/or lumbar puncture (LP) if clinical suspicion warrants.
  - Evaluation for other causes of anion gap metabolic acidosis, if discovered on evaluation.

DIAGNOSIS

- Mild DKA: pH 7.25–7.30, urine/serum ketones (+), glucose >250, bicarb 15–18, anion gap >10, patient alert

- Moderate DKA: pH 7.00 to <7.24, urine/serum ketones (+), glucose >250, bicarb 10 to <15, anion gap >12, altered sensorium
- Severe DKA: pH <7.00, urine/serum ketones (+), glucose >250, bicarb <10, anion gap >12, stupor/coma

DIFFERENTIAL DIAGNOSIS

- Starvation ketosis (bicarb usually ≥ 18, pH usually normal)
- Alcoholic ketoacidosis (decreased caloric intake in alcoholic patients in whom alcohol has stimulated liver's ketogenic response; often normal blood sugar or hypoglycemic)
- Other causes of anion gap metabolic acidosis (MUDPALES—methanol, uremia, diabetic ketoacidosis, paraldehyde, alcoholic ketoacidosis, lactic acidosis, ethylene glycol, salicylates)

TREATMENT PRINCIPLES

- ICU monitoring
- ABCs
- Volume resuscitation, initially with isotonic fluids
- Correction of hyperglycemia, acidosis, and electrolyte imbalance
- Search for and treat underlying precipitant
- Uninterrupted insulin therapy

TREATMENT SPECIFICS

- Intravenous fluids (IVFs): Choice and rate guided by volume status to maintain adequate circulating volume. Also guided by corrected serum sodium (= measured sodium + (0.016 × [glucose − 100])) and osmolality to avoid overly rapid correction of hyperosmolality/ hyponatremia. Add 5% dextrose to infusion when glucose <250 to keep glucose 150–200.
- Insulin therapy: Often in adults treat initially with regular insulin 0.15 units/kg IV, followed by 0.1 units/kg/h gtt with infusion rate adjusted to decrease glucose by 50–70 mg/dL/h. Continue insulin gtt until acidosis resolved. Must treat with subcutaneous insulin before discontinuation of gtt to prevent redevelopment of DKA.
- Potassium: When potassium normalizes add potassium to IVFs to prevent development of hypokalemia and potentially severe arrhythmias, as long as the patient is not oliguric. Potassium management must be undertaken with patient's renal function in mind.
- Bicarbonate: Controversial due to lack of efficacy and concern for harm, especially in children. Complications may include intracellular acidosis, impaired tissue oxygen extraction, and hypokalemia.
- Phosphate and magnesium deficiencies should be repleted.

MONITORING

- Frequent vital signs
- ECG monitoring (for QRS duration, T-wave morphology)
- Monitor glucose q 1 h
- Monitor basic metabolic profile (BMP), magnesium, phosphorus q 2 h
- Beta-hydroxybutyrate (not detected by ketone assay) is converted to acetoacetate in the process of treating DKA. If ketones are frequently monitored, this may give the impression that ketonemia is worsening. Therefore, the anion gap is a better means of monitoring improvement in acid-base status
- Cerebral edema may be a serious, even fatal consequence of treatment of DKA. The best means of prevention is ensuring that osmolality is not corrected too rapidly and that sodium bicarbonate is not used.

BIBLIOGRAPHY

Buse JA, Polonsky KS. Diabetic ketoacidosis, hyperglycemic hyperosmolar nonketotic coma, and hypoglycemia. In: Hall JB, Schmidt GA, Wood LDH, eds., *Principles of Critical Care*, 2nd ed. New York, NY: McGraw-Hill; 2005:1209–1217.

Kitabchi AE, Umpierrez GE, Murphy MB, et al., for the American Diabetes Association. Hyperglycemic crises in diabetes. *Diabetes Care* 2004;27(Suppl 1):94–102.

98 INTENSIVE INSULIN THERAPY IN THE CRITICALLY ILL

Steve Skjei

KEY POINTS

- Hyperglycemia is common in acute illness in both diabetic and nondiabetic patients.
- Hyperglycemia in this setting is a risk factor for poor outcome that is potentially modifiable.

- Studies evaluating restoration of normoglycemia or near-normoglycemia have shown improvement in outcome in patients treated with IV insulin infusion with the goal of decreasing hyperglycemia and normalizing blood glucose concentrations.
- Hypoglycemic episodes are an almost inevitable consequence of protocols used to achieve "tight" glycemic controls and efforts must be expended to minimize this complication.

MECHANISMS OF HYPERGLYCEMIA IN THE CRITICALLY ILL

- Increased levels of "stress" hormones such as cortisol, epinephrine, and glucagon inhibit glycogen production and stimulate gluconeogenesis.
- Cytokine production in response to stress increases insulin resistance.
- Medications frequently used in critical illness such as corticosteroids and vasopressors may exacerbate insulin resistance.

INTENSIVE INSULIN THERAPY IN CRITICALLY ILL PATIENTS

- Patients in a surgical intensive care unit (ICU) were prospectively randomized to "conventional" or intensive insulin therapy.
    - Conventional treatment was an IV insulin drip if glucose exceeded 215 mg/dL, with target levels of 180–200 mg/dL.
    - Intensive treatment was an IV insulin drip if glucose exceeded 100 mg/dL, with target levels of 80–110 mg/dL.
    - Hypoglycemia (glucose <40 mg/dL) occurred more frequently in the intensive treatment group (5.2% vs. 0.8%) but did not cause hemodynamic disturbance.
    - Overall, mortality was significantly lowered in the intensively treated group (4.6% vs. 8.0%) with the greatest effect demonstrated in those patients with ICU stays >5 days and in those with multiorgan failure secondary to a septic focus. The study was stopped early due to this difference (Fig. 98-1).
    - Benefit was noted across the range of APACHE II scores.
    - Several markers of morbidity were improved, such as markers of inflammation (white blood cell count [WBC], C-reactive protein [CRP], fever).
- Additional studies in patients undergoing coronary artery bypass graft (CABG) and in patients with myocardial infarction (MI) have shown improvements in outcome with intravenous insulin infusion.
- A study of medical ICU patients treated with a similar goal of euglycemia did not reveal a difference in survival related to this intervention although post hoc subset analysis revealed that longer-term admissions

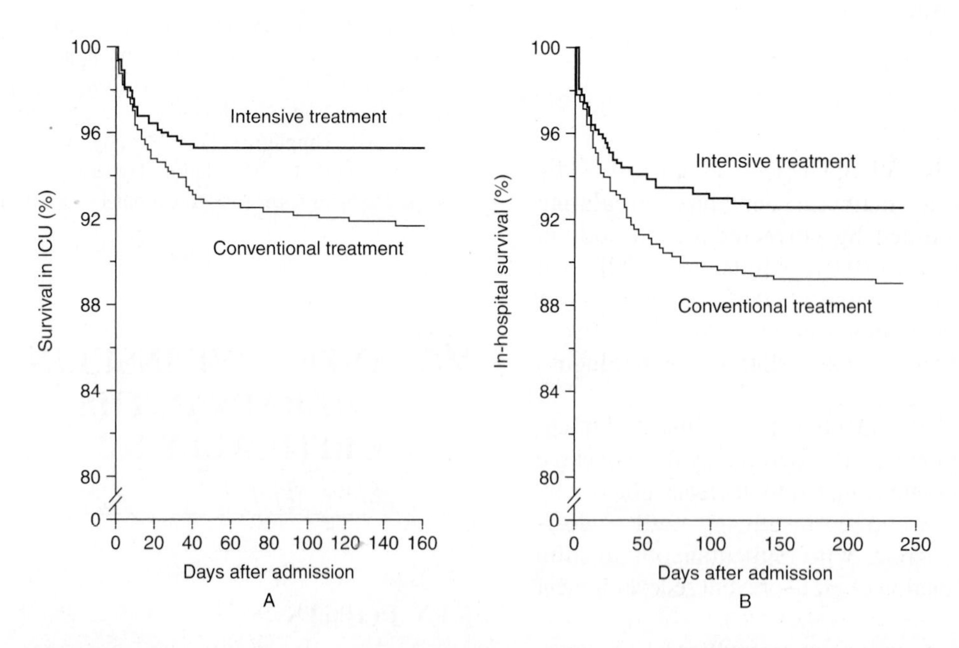

FIG. 98-1 Survival curves comparing intensive insulin therapy to conventional treatment in critically ill patients in a surgical ICU.
SOURCE: Adapted from Van den Berghe G, Wouters P, Weekers F, et al. Intensive insulin therapy in critically ill patients. *N Engl J Med* 2001;345:1359–1367.

to the ICU did exhibit a difference in outcome associated with tight glycemic control.

- Questions have arisen regarding the mechanism of benefit observed in these studies
  - Avoidance of hyperglycemia
    - Degree of hyperglycemia has been associated with increased risk of in-hospital mortality post-MI.
    - Osmotic diuresis from hyperglycemia may decrease cardiac output.
    - Hyperglycemia may decrease complement activation.
  - Insulin drug effect
    - Insulin may improve immune function.
    - Insulin may have anti-inflammatory properties.
    - Insulin inhibits lipolysis, thus reducing free fatty acids which may contribute to cardiac arrhythmias.
    - Insulin may have anabolic effects in critical illness.
- Whether antihyperglycemic strategies other than insulin may be effective in improving ICU outcome remains to be determined.
- At present, there is no consensus on a target glucose level or specific insulin infusion protocol.

BIBLIOGRAPHY

Chinsky K. The evolving paradigm of hyperglycemia and critical illness. *Chest* 2004;126:674–676.

Furnary A, Gao G, Grunkemeier GL, et al. Continuous insulin infusion reduces mortality in patients with diabetes undergoing coronary artery bypass grafting. *J Thorac Cardiovasc Surg* 2003;125:1007–1021.

Garber AJ, Moghissi ES, Bransome ED Jr, et al. American College of Endocrinology position statement on inpatient diabetes and metabolic control. *Endocr Pract* 2004;10(Suppl 2):5–9.

Krinsley JS. Effect of an intensive glucose management protocol on the mortality of critically ill adult patients. *Mayo Clin Proc* 2005;79:992–1000.

Malmberg K. Prospective randomized study of intensive insulin treatment on long term survival after acute myocardial infarction in patients with diabetes mellitus. *BMJ* 1997;314:1512–1515.

Umpierrez GE, Isaacs SD, Bazargan N, et al. Hyperglycemia: an independent marker of in-hospital mortality in patients with undiagnosed diabetes. *J Clin Endocrinol Metab* 2002;87:978–982.

Van den Berghe G, Wilmer A, Hermans G, et al. Intensive insulin therapy in the medical ICU. *N Engl J Med* 2006;354:449–461.

Van den Berghe G, Wouters P, Boullion R, et al. Outcome benefit of intensive insulin therapy in the critically ill: insulin dose versus glycemic control. *Crit Care Med* 2003;31:359–366.

Van den Berghe G, Wouters P, Weekers F, et al. Intensive insulin therapy in critically ill patients. *N Engl J Med* 2001;345:1359–1367.

99 THYROID DISEASE

Stephen Skjei, Shashi Kiran Bellam

KEY POINTS

- Most patients admitted to the ICU have low levels of T_3 and T_4 with normal to low levels of serum thyrotropin, a condition termed "euthyroid sick syndrome"; TFTs need to be interpreted on this background.
- T_3 is the logical replacement therapy for those patients who do need treatment of severe hypothyroidism.
- Management of myxedema coma (MC) should include glucocorticoids while the adrenal status is being assessed.
- Thyroid storm is often signaled by hyperthermia and altered mental status.
- Thyroid hormone secretion can be blocked by addition of iodine to an antithyroid drug; iopanoic acid is useful in life-threatening thyrotoxicosis.
- Beta-blockers are useful to ameliorate some cardiac effects of thyrotoxicosis and to offer perioperative protection, but need to be used with caution in the elderly and those with cardiomyopathy and airway disease.

THYROID BASICS

- Thyroid hormone production by the thyroid occurs under the control of thyroid-stimulating hormone (TSH), produced in the pituitary gland.
- Thyroid releases thyroid hormone 80% in form of T_4, 20% in form of T_3.
- T_3 is the primary active hormone.
- T_4 is metabolized to T_3 at the tissue level by tissue deiodinases, including type 1 deiodinase.
- Type 2 deiodinase is found primarily in brain/pituitary, metabolizes $T_4 \rightarrow T_3$.
- Type 3 deiodinase metabolizes $T_4 \rightarrow$ reverse T_3 (rT_3) which is hormonally inactive.
- Thyroid hormone participates in a negative feedback loop, inhibiting release of TSH by pituitary.
- Laboratory measurements of T_4 or T_3 usually measure total hormone, which is mixture of "free" and protein "bound" hormone. The free fraction is hormonally active. This is approximated by free thyroxine index (FTI) measurements or by nondialysis "free T_4" measurements. It can be directly measured by free T_4 by dialysis.

THYROID HORMONE AND THYROID FUNCTION TESTS IN ILLNESS

- Nonthyroidal illness (NTI) syndrome or euthyroid sick syndrome (ESS) frequently seen in acutely/chronically ill patients or in states of starvation.
  - Type 1 deiodinase inhibition with increase in type 3 deiodinase activity may produce low levels of T_3 with elevated levels of reverse T_3.
  - May also produce state of low T_4 and low T_3 with normal or slightly low TSH—these patients are often very sick and T_4 levels may correlate inversely with mortality.
  - Recovery from NTI syndrome frequently leads to elevated TSH.
  - Whether or not treatment is beneficial is still controversial—thyroid hormone may increase cardiac oxygen demand and/or precipitate arrhythmias; many studies evaluating T_4 or T_3 therapy in these patients with conflicting results.
- Other factors common in critical illness may lead to abnormal thyroid function tests (TFTs).
  - Hemodialysis
  - Corticosteroid treatment
  - Vasopressor treatment
  - Altered levels of binding proteins—thus, FTI or free T_4 are more informative tests
  - Total T_4 measurements
- Interpretation of TFTs in critical illness is often complicated and may require endocrine consultation.

HYPOTHYROIDISM IN THE INTENSIVE CARE UNIT

- Hypothyroidism is defined as an inadequate tissue delivery of thyroid hormone.
- Most cases of hypothyroidism in the United States are due to autoimmune thyroid (Hashimoto) disease. The second most common cause is postsurgical; medications such as amiodarone and lithium may cause hypothyroidism as well. Iodine deficiency is still common in parts of the world. History of thyroid disease, neck surgery, medication use and compliance, and pregnancy should be sought.
- Hypothyroidism must be differentiated from NTI syndrome mentioned as above.
- Symptoms/signs of hypothyroidism include cold intolerance, fatigue, dry skin, constipation, bradycardia, anemia.
- Consideration should always be given for pituitary cause of hypothyroidism.
- In the ICU, clinically significant hypothyroidism may develop in patients with primary hypothyroidism when challenged by an intercurrent illness.

MYXEDEMA COMA

- Myxedema coma (MC) typically occurs in a patient with long-standing hypothyroidism suffering some event (e.g., illness/infection, surgery, stroke, trauma, cold weather, and drug overdose such as tranquilizers, narcotics, and sedatives) that leads to decompensation.
- MC is characterized by hypothermia, hypoventilation, altered mental status, bradycardia, and hyponatremia. It carries a high risk of morbidity and mortality; endocrine consult should be obtained.
- Physical signs of severe hypothyroidism are present and include dry skin, thinning of eyebrows, delayed relaxation phase of deep tendon reflexes, and macroglossia.
- Laboratory evaluation reveals a markedly decreased serum T_4 level and elevation of TSH (except in the setting of central hypothyroidism).
- Pulmonary complications of MC include hypoventilation, aspiration pneumonia, and laryngeal obstruction.
- Cardiac complications of MC include pericardial effusion (common but rarely causing tamponade).
- Treatment includes supportive care and thyroid hormone replacement. One regimen would be to give an intravenous load of 400 μg T_4 followed by 50–100 μg T_4 IV qd until improvement occurs, then transition to a maintenance dose. Doses are given intravenously at first due to impaired absorption seen in hypothyroidism. Some thyroidologists recommend T_3 therapy instead, and others use a combination of T_4 and T_3. Doses may need to be decreased in the elderly and those with heart disease.
- There is a 5–10% incidence of concurrent hypoadrenalism, so a cosyntropin stimulation test should be administered if possible, and then empiric glucocorticoids should be given until adrenal status is known (routine doses of 50–100 mg hydrocortisone q 6 h). Glucocorticoids should be given prior to levothyroxine because of the risk of precipitating adrenal crisis if T_4 is given to a patient with hypoadrenalism, so a full stimulation test may not be always be possible.
- Supportive care may include intubation and mechanical ventilation. An underlying precipitant such as infection or ischemia should be sought and treated. Hyponatremia, if present, may be due to impaired free water clearance and may be managed with free water restriction.

HYPERTHYROIDISM IN THE INTENSIVE CARE UNIT

- Hyperthyroidism (thyrotoxicosis) is most commonly due to hypersecretion of thyroid hormone by an abnormal thyroid gland such as multinodular goiter, solitary adenoma, or Graves' disease. Occasionally, patients will develop a transient hyperthyroidism due to thyroid inflammation (thyroiditis) following an upper respiratory infection (URI). Hyperthyroxinemia due to exogenous overdose may also occur.

- Patients with preexisting multinodular goiter who are euthyroid or slightly hyperthyroid may develop hyperthyroidism if large doses of exogenous iodine are given, such as commonly occurs with IV contrast radiologic studies and amiodarone administration.
- Symptoms/signs of thyrotoxicosis include tremulousness, weight loss, irritability, palpitations, irregular menstrual periods, diarrhea, heat intolerance, and atrial fibrillation. Occasionally, patients present with cardiomyopathy and congestive heart failure (CHF). Symptoms may be muted in the elderly.
- Important elements of the history include prior history of thyroid disease and treatment, duration of symptoms, recent history of URI, history of ocular symptoms or pretibial myxedema to suggest Graves' disease, recent history of IV contrast or amiodarone administration, history of goiter, and any possibility of pregnancy.
- Physical examination and historical features should be used to attempt to differentiate the cause of hyperthyroidism, as treatment differs between causes. Endocrine consultation should usually be sought.
- The two principal antithyroid drugs used are propylthiouracil (PTU) and methimazole. Side effects of these medications include rash, agranulocytosis, hepatitis, cholestatic jaundice, and arthritis. Agranulocytosis and hepatotoxicity may be life threatening.
- Patients with hyperthyroidism may develop an extreme form of the condition if an intercurrent illness develops. This syndrome is called thyroid storm.

THYROID STORM

- Thyroid storm usually occurs in patients with poorly controlled thyrotoxicosis who develop a precipitating factor, such as surgery, infection, pulmonary embolism, or myocardial infarction.
- Symptoms and signs include fever, altered mental status, arrhythmias, tachycardia, CHF, and a widened pulse pressure.
- Consideration of this condition should prompt endocrine consultation.
- Treatment should be focused on four modalities: (1) decrease thyroid hormone levels, (2) decrease action of thyroid hormones on peripheral tissues, (3) prevent cardiovascular collapse, and (4) treat precipitating factors.

1. PTU or methimazole prevents further synthesis of thyroid hormone. PTU has theoretical advantage of blocking $T_4 \rightarrow T_3$ conversion in periphery. One regimen of PTU would be 250 mg PO q6.

   Once further synthesis is blocked, iodine (such as SSKI) may be administered to inhibit thyroid hormone release from the gland. Glucocorticoids may also be administered to further diminish $T_4 \rightarrow T_3$ conversion. Other treatments are available, but are beyond the scope of this discussion.

   Hyperthyroidism may be especially difficult to treat in those patients treated with amiodarone.
2. Beta-blockers decrease the action of thyroid hormones on peripheral tissues. Beta-blockade should be used cautiously and perhaps not in elderly patients, asthmatics, or patients with cardiomyopathies. Short-acting intravenous beta-blockade (esmolol) allows for rapid termination of therapy in the event of serious adverse effects.
3. External cooling and sedation can decrease heat generation and systemic oxygen consumption. Atrial fibrillation is commonly seen; ventricular response rate should be controlled with beta-blockers.
4. Precipitating factors should be sought and treated.

PREGNANCY AND THYROID DISEASE

- Cases of thyroid disease in pregnant women should prompt endocrine consultation as any potential diagnostic or therapeutic modalities will have implications for mother and fetus.
- In general, PTU is the favored thionamide in pregnancy. If hyperthyroid patients are unable to tolerate PTU, they may require thyroidectomy for treatment of hyperthyroidism.
- TFTs may be difficult to interpret in pregnancy due to estrogen-related changes in thyroid-binding globulin levels. Additionally, human chorionic gonadotropin (hCG) is a weak TSH receptor agonist. hCG peaks at the end of the first trimester, and thus these patients may have TFTs that seem to reflect hyperthyroidism (low TSH, elevated T_4). In this case, patients frequently do not require treatment as the effect is transient. However, patients with Graves' disease may present similarly. Endocrine consultation should be sought to distinguish between the two and to determine if treatment is necessary.

BIBLIOGRAPHY

Davies TF, Larsen PR. Thyrotoxicosis. In: Larsen PR, Kronenberg HM, Melmed S, eds., *Williams Textbook of Endocrinology*, 10th ed. Philadelphia, PA: W.B. Saunders; 2003: 374–421.

Greenspan FS. The thyroid gland. In: Greenspan FS, Gardner DG, eds., *Basic and Clinical Endocrinology*, 7th ed. New York, NY: McGraw-Hill; 2001:215–294.
Larsen PR, Davies TF. Hypothyroidism and thyroiditis. In: Larsen PR, Kronenberg HM, Melmed S, eds., *Williams Textbook of Endocrinology*, 10th ed. Philadelphia, PA: W.B. Saunders; 2003:423–455.
Weiss RE, Refetoff S. Thyroid disease. In: Hall JB, Schmidt GA, Wood LDH, eds., *Principles of Critical Care*, 3rd ed. New York, NY: McGraw-Hill; 2005:1231–1244.
Yamamoto T, Fukuyama J, Fujiyoshi A, et al. Factors associated with mortality of myxedema coma: report of eight cases and literature survey. *Thyroid* 1999;9(12):1167–1174.

100 ADRENAL INSUFFICIENCY

Shashi Kiran Bellam

KEY POINTS

- Traditional criteria for diagnosing adrenal insufficiency are based on the response of normal, nonstressed, healthy controls. These criteria are not appropriate for evaluating adrenal function in critically ill patients.
- Hypotensive ICU patients should have a random serum cortisol level assessed. If >25 μg/dL, they have sufficient adrenal function. If not, they may have relative adrenal insufficiency and should be considered for replacement corticosteroids.
- Nonhypotensive ICU patients should undergo a low-dose (1 μg) cosyntropin stimulation test. If any cortisol level is >25 μg/dL, they likely have sufficient adrenal function. If not, they have relative adrenal insufficiency and should receive replacement corticosteroids.
- The recommended replacement corticosteroid dose is either hydrocortisone 50 mg IV q 6 h or hydrocortisone 100 mg IV q 8 h.

PHYSIOLOGY OF ADRENAL FUNCTION

- Cortisol is the primary glucocorticoid hormone, secreted by the adrenal glands.
- In healthy, unstressed persons, cortisol is secreted in a diurnal pattern under the influence of corticotropin (adrenocorticotrophic hormone [ACTH]), which is released from the pituitary gland.
- Aldosterone is the primary mineralocorticoid hormone in the body. It is secreted by the adrenal gland.
- Aldosterone secretion is regulated primarily by the renin-angiotensin system and potassium levels.
- Cortisol binds to the glucocorticoid receptor (GR) present on all cells.

ACUTE STRESS RESPONSE

- Acute stress (including infection, surgery, trauma, burns, or illness) causes an increase in production of corticotropin-releasing hormone (CRH) and ACTH, which leads to increased cortisol production proportional to the severity of illness.
- Diurnal variation in cortisol secretion is lost.
- There is decreased production of the other adrenal hormones (aldosterone and androgens).
- GRs are increased in number in acute stress, thereby increasing the cellular response to secreted cortisol.
- The sum total of response to acute stress is a dramatic increase in cellular glucocorticoid activity which contributes to the maintenance of cellular and organ homeostasis.

PHYSIOLOGIC ACTIONS OF GLUCOCORTICOIDS IN ACUTE STRESS

- Glucocorticoids increase blood glucose levels by increasing hepatic gluconeogenesis and inhibiting adipose tissue glucose uptake.
- Glucocorticoids stimulate free fatty acid release from adipose tissue and amino acid release from body proteins.
- These responses facilitate delivery of energy and substrate to cells and organs to respond to stress and repair from injury.
- Glucocorticoids are required for the normal heart response to angiotensin II, epinephrine, and norepinephrine, contributing to the maintenance of cardiac contractility, vascular tone, and blood pressure.
- Glucocorticoids decrease the production of vasorelaxants such as nitric oxide and vasodilatory prostaglandins.
- Glucocorticoids attenuate both the accumulation at inflammatory sites and function of most cells involved in immune and inflammatory responses.

ASSESSMENT OF ADRENAL FUNCTION IN THE CRITICALLY ILL

- The diagnosis of adrenal insufficiency is based on the measurement of serum cortisol levels.
- The traditional criteria for diagnosing adrenal insufficiency are based on the response of normal, nonstressed, healthy controls. These criteria are not appropriate for evaluating adrenal function in critically ill patients.

- In addition, the high-dose cosyntropin stimulation test is probably not appropriate for critically ill patients.
- For hypotensive critically ill patients with an appropriate adrenal response to illness, the baseline cortisol level (at any time of the day) should be >25 μg/dL.
- For nonhypotensive critically ill patients, the normal adrenal response to a low-dose cosyntropin stimulation test (which consists of administering 1–2 μg of synthetic corticotropin and measuring cortisol levels at baseline, 30 minutes, and 60 minutes after that dose) should be a cortisol level >25 μg/dL.

ADRENAL INSUFFICIENCY IN THE CRITICALLY ILL

- The reported incidence is approximately 30% and can be as high as 60% for patients in septic shock.
- Acute adrenal insufficiency can present with hypotension, mild eosinophilia, unexplained fever, hyponatremia, and hyperkalemia.
- Chronic adrenal insufficiency presents with weakness, weight loss, anorexia, lethargy, slowed mentation, and general failure to thrive.
- Causes of acute adrenal insufficiency include hypothalamic and pituitary disorders (secondary adrenal insufficiency), and destruction of the adrenal glands (primary adrenal insufficiency).
- Synthetic glucocorticoids (orally or intravenously) may cause adrenal suppression if used for more than 5 days.
- Primary adrenal insufficiency in immunocompromised patients (e.g., HIV) is commonly due to adrenal gland infection with cytomegalovirus, tuberculosis, cryptococcus, and other organisms.
- Certain drugs (e.g., ketoconazole, megestrol acetate, and etomidate) can impair adrenal function.
- In sepsis, circulating suppressive factors released during systemic inflammation may cause adrenal insufficiency.
- Once the septic episode has resolved, adrenal function commonly returns to normal.
- Treatment with cortisol has been shown to improve shock reversal, decrease days on vasopressors, shorten ventilator time, and shorten ICU stay.
- The dosage of replacement corticosteroid is 100 mg hydrocortisone IV q 8 h or 50 mg IV q 6 h.

BIBLIOGRAPHY

Coursin DB, Wood WK. Corticosteroid supplementation for adrenal insufficiency. *JAMA* 2002;287:236–240.

Marik P, Zolaga G. Adrenocortical insufficiency. In: Hall JB, Schmidt GA, Wood LDH, eds., *Principles of Critical Care*, 3rd ed. New York, NY: McGraw-Hill; 2005:1219–1230.

101 RHABDOMYOLYSIS

Steven Q. Davis, Suneel M. Udani

KEY POINTS

- Rhabdomyolysis is caused by damage to skeletal muscle resulting in the release of myoglobin. It should be suspected in all patients with crush or burn injuries as well as renal failure of unclear etiology.
- Intravascular volume depletion as well as severe electrolyte and metabolic derangements can be profound requiring aggressive fluid resuscitation as well as frequent monitoring of electrolytes and volume status.
- Refractory electrolyte and metabolic derangement may necessitate renal replacement therapy to prevent life-threatening arrhythmias, seizures, or multisystem organ failure.

PATHOPHYSIOLOGY

- The final common pathway resulting in rhabdomyolysis is adenosine triphosphate (ATP) supply-demand mismatch. Therefore, any process causing inadequate ATP generation or inadequate ATP delivery to muscles may result in muscle injury and rhabdomyolysis.
  - Specifically, ATP is responsible for maintaining normal balance of intracellular and extracellular sodium and calcium. Increased metabolic activity or direct muscle injury (from burns, trauma, or direct toxin) causes influx of sodium and calcium into the cell. Massive influx overwhelms the ATP-dependent electrolyte balance resulting in pathologic concentrations of calcium inside the cell.
  - The high intracellular calcium concentrations trigger persistent muscle contraction depleting already diminished energy stores. Free intracellular calcium may also activate a variety of proteases and catalytic enzymes further causing cellular destruction. Finally, the resulting activation of the inflammatory cascade intensifies the destructive process ultimately leading to an active myolysis on top of cell necrosis.
- Once muscle death has occurred, myoglobin is released into the bloodstream and filtered into the renal tubules. Myoglobin accumulates in the renal tubules (exacerbated by the usual concomitant intravascular volume depletion) eventually precipitating and causing tubular obstruction, damage, and necrosis.
- Metabolic and electrolyte derangements result from initial cell death and are complicated further by renal insufficiency.

 - Cell death causes the release of organic and inorganic acids as well as electrolytes which are normally maintained at a low extracellular concentration but have high intracellular concentration (e.g., potassium and phosphate).
 - Hypocalcemia may occur in the early stages of rhabdomyolysis from accumulation in necrotic muscle as well as from the precipitation of calcium-phosphate complexes caused by increased extracellular phosphate concentration. Once perfusion is restored to muscle and the active lysis process completes, the sequestered calcium may be released into the bloodstream resulting in a late-stage hypercalcemia.
 - The accumulation of organic and inorganic acids into the bloodstream causes a metabolic acidosis. The acidosis and acidemia may lower urinary and intratubular pH, facilitating further myoglobin precipitation, tubular obstruction, and renal insufficiency. Worsening renal insufficiency can further exacerbate the ongoing metabolic acidosis.

ETIOLOGY

- Causes of rhabdomyolysis may be classified into four, broad categories: direct trauma or muscle injury, excessive muscle activity, inherited defects of enzyme muscle, and "other" medical causes.
  - Direct muscle injury causes rhabdomyolysis by injury to myocytes. The direct injury disrupts normal cellular membranes, initiating the cascade described above resulting in increased intracellular calcium. This etiology was the first recognized cause of rhabdomyolysis. While crush injury is the most apparent cause, direct muscle injury can also result from burns or electrical shock injuries.
  - Excessive muscle activity remains an important cause of rhabdomyolysis in the appropriate clinical setting. Many of these instances may initially go unrecognized, at least as regards the potential for skeletal muscle injury. However, in the setting of concomitant intravascular volume depletion and/or previous renal insufficiency, rhabdomyolysis, with its subsequent clinical sequelae can occur. Injury to muscle is directly related to the duration and intensity of muscle activity. Therefore, situations such as marathons or intensive military training in previously sedentary individuals have been identified as common clinical scenarios. Prolonged seizures with excessive muscle activity can also precipitate muscle injury.
  - Inherited diseases that result in decreased synthesis of ATP such as McArdle's can also lead to rhabdomyolysis. As outlined above, ATP supply-demand mismatch leads to muscle injury. When the degree of mismatch and resulting injury is severe, rhabdomyolysis may ensue. In individuals with unexplained muscle damage, a family history of rhabdomyolysis or multiple episodes, an inherited muscle enzyme defect should be suspected.
- The range of "other" medical causes of rhabdomyolysis is extensive. While the first three categories of etiology may be readily apparent, the "other" causes are more subtle and require a broad differential to identify. The medical causes of rhabdomyolysis may, themselves, be classified into four categories: drugs or toxins, infection, alterations in temperature, and metabolic derangements.
  - Drugs or toxins may be the most common etiology of rhabdomyolysis in the adult, Western world where crush and burn injuries are not routinely seen.
    - Alcohol remains the toxin most frequently encountered, likely, because of its widespread abuse and the multiple pathways by which it can cause muscle injury. Primarily, ethanol is directly myotoxic by inhibiting calcium accumulation by the sarcoplasmic reticulum, disturbing intra-extracellular electrolyte balance by inhibition of the Na-K-ATPase and disruption of cellular membranes. Asymptomatic elevations in creatinine kinase (CK) and histologic evidence of muscle injury have been seen in otherwise healthy individuals ingesting large amounts of alcohol. Alcohol may also indirectly lead to muscle injury by the concomitant electrolyte imbalance seen in individuals ingesting large amounts of alcohol. The malnutrition (as well as the vomiting and/or diarrhea) associated with chronic alcohol abuse leads to depleted potassium and phosphate stores. Potassium and phosphate stores are critically important in maintaining adequate energy supply for active muscles. Specifically, hypokalemia results in impaired glycogen metabolism and hypophosphatemia results in impaired ATP synthesis. Once again if muscle demand of ATP exceeds supply, muscle injury may ensue.
    - Drugs of abuse other than alcohol may also lead to rhabdomyolysis. Cocaine, phencyclidine (PCP), methylenedioxymethamphetamine (MDMA), and other sympathomimetic drugs or drug combinations lead to rhabdomyolysis primarily by the combination of excessive muscle activity and intravascular volume depletion.
    - Prescription medications, especially lipid-lowering agents, are an increasingly important etiology of rhabdomyolysis. Fibrates may be directly myotoxic, although the mechanism has not been elucidated. A large and ever-growing population of people is currently taking lipid-lowering agents in the "statin" class or hydroxymethylglutaryl coenzyme

A (HMG-CoA) reductase inhibitors. While the exact mechanism leading to muscle injury has not been determined, two theories predominate. The first is that statins inhibit not only cholesterol synthesis but also inhibit the formation of coenzyme Q, an important coenzyme in ATP synthesis. If ATP synthesis is significantly impaired and demand exceeds supply, muscle injury ensues. The second theory relates to the inhibition of cholesterol synthesis. Decreased cholesterol synthesis results in decreased lipid availability for cellular membrane synthesis. Membranes may lose their integrity predisposing them to injury and death. While the use of statins in most patients is very safe, the risk of adverse effects may be increased when medications affecting CYP 450 and, thereby, statin metabolism, such as antifungals and macrolide antibiotics, are used at the same time.

- ◦ Infections, both viral and bacterial may lead to rhabdomyolysis by either direct muscle invasion or toxin-mediated myocyte death. Viral infection leading to muscle injury is more common, the predominant viruses being influenza A and B and slightly less commonly coxsackie and HIV. While muscle biopsy has not been able to provide direct evidence, muscle invasion is the presumed mechanism of injury. A review of bacteria responsible for causing rhabdomyolysis identified *Legionella* species as the most common. Other infectious diseases associated with rhabdomyolysis include tularemia, pneumococcal pneumonia, salmonellosis, and staphylococcal sepsis (especially toxic shock syndrome). Both toxin-mediated and direct muscle invasion are thought to be responsible and histologic evidence of invasion by *Streptococcus*, *Salmonella*, and *Staphylococcus* species has been found.
- ◦ Extreme alterations in temperature may trigger muscle injury and rhabdomyolysis. While hyperthermia is a more common cause, muscle injury has also been seen with severe hypothermia. Hyperthermia resulting from neuroleptic malignant syndrome (NMS), heat stroke, and malignant hyperthermia are the most common pathways of injury. In NMS, the triad of excessive muscle rigidity, fever, and mental status changes after the administration of haloperidol or phenothiazines (sometime in combination with anti-Parkinsonian agents or tricyclic antidepressants) leads to muscle injury by a combination of excessive muscle activity and intravascular volume depletion. Malignant hyperthermia, an inherited (most commonly autosomal dominant) disorder of the calcium channel in the sarcoplasmic reticulum and heat stroke may lead to muscle injury and rhabdomyolysis by the same combination of effects.
- ◦ Electrolyte and metabolic derangements may be, as in the case of alcohol abuse, a secondary cause of muscle injury. However, they may also be the primary precipitant. Specifically, muscle hypoxia from generalized suffocation or inadequate local blood flow will precipitate muscle injury. Severe hypokalemia or hypophosphatemia, as previously outlined, can lead to rhabdomyolysis. Their role as a primary precipitant may be difficult to detect, however, because of the release of potassium and phosphate into the bloodstream after myocyte death. Therefore, after clinical presentation potassium and phosphate levels may be elevated, while they were initially extremely low.
- ◦ The above represent the common identified causes of rhabdomyolysis. More causes clearly exist and in one large review of causes of rhabdomyolysis a single etiology could not be identified in 3% of cases.

CLINICAL PRESENTATION, DIAGNOSTIC EVALUATION, AND CLINICAL CONSEQUENCES

- Rhabdomyolysis, clearly, does not always present "classically" with the triad of muscle pain, weakness, and "tea-colored" urine. While the symptoms may be elicited once the diagnosis is suspected, often rhabdomyolysis is asymptomatic until it is more advanced and metabolic derangements manifest. Ultimately, laboratory evaluation is necessary to make a diagnosis of rhabdomyolysis. Specifically, serum CK levels are useful to detect muscle injury. While the concentration of myoglobin in the blood and myoglobinuria is more important in the actual process of injury, hepatic metabolism and myoglobin's relatively small molecular weight allows its rapid clearance from the bloodstream into the urine. Therefore, serum myoglobin assays are unreliable for predicting clinical consequences. While no established value of CK is diagnostic of rhabdomyolysis, levels in the 10,000–100,000s are not uncommon. Myocardial injury as a cause of elevated CK level must always be excluded and a CK level less than five times the upper limit of normal in the setting of renal failure must make one suspect other potential etiologies of renal failure. Urine myoglobin assay may be helpful to confirm myoglobinuria and clinical suspicion.
- Once rhabdomyolysis has occurred, the metabolic and electrolyte abnormalities previously outlined may manifest. The clinician should specifically monitor for:
  - ◦ Hyperkalemia
  - ◦ Hyperphosphatemia
  - ◦ Hypocalcemia early, hypercalcemia late

  - Anion gap metabolic acidosis
  - Acute renal failure (incidence varies but may complicate approximately 30% of cases of rhabdomyolysis)
- The most devastating consequences of rhabdomyolysis are usually a result of these metabolic derangements and the subsequent renal failure. These include, but are not limited to, seizures and tetany from severe hypocalcemia, life-threatening cardiac arrhythmias from hyperkalemia, and severe acidosis and, in extreme cases, multisystem organ failure. Respiratory failure from fluid overload and/or direct lung injury may be a late-stage manifestation. Disseminated intravascular coagulation (DIC) may occur as a result of activation of the coagulation cascade by muscle breakdown products. When it does occur, DIC has its peak incidence on days 3–5. In these instances supportive care remains the treatment.
- In the absence of obvious causes from history and physical examination, any of the above medical causes may be responsible. Toxicology assays and the previously mentioned viral and bacterial serologies should be sent as part of the diagnostic evaluation.

TREATMENT

- If any reversible cause or ongoing muscle injury is present, it must be treated aggressively and as quickly as possible.
- Once muscle injury has occurred, the mainstay of treatment for rhabdomyolysis is aggressive volume resuscitation to prevent renal failure and correction of electrolyte imbalances. In patients whose muscles are compressed as a result of trauma, initiating fluid resuscitation prior to extrication of the injured limb may prevent exacerbation of ongoing intravascular volume depletion from sequestration of blood flow to the injured limb as part of the reperfusion process.
- While the type of fluid to be used for resuscitation is debated, the amount of fluid needed and goals of diuresis is not. To restore adequate intravascular volume, intravenous fluids in the 10 L range may be necessary and goal diuresis should be approximately 200 cc/h to continuously flush the renal tubules of myoglobin in an attempt to prevent precipitation and tubular obstruction.
- The type of fluid administered has been debated and, while no absolute recommendation exists, the general recommendation is large amounts of iso- or slightly hypertonic crystalloid. Sodium bicarbonate (in the form of 0.45 normal saline [NS] with 2 amps of $NaHCO_3$) may be preferable to NS in attempt to alkalinize the urine and help prevent further myoglobin precipitation. No randomized trial, however, has confirmed its benefit. The administration of mannitol has been used as a standard in traumatic causes of rhabdomyolysis and some nontraumatic cases. In theory, mannitol, as an osmotic diuretic, helps to flush myoglobin out of the renal tubules. Randomized trials of adequate methodology have not been carried out to confirm its benefit and a recent retrospective review in a series of trauma patients did not find a benefit to administering mannitol to posttrauma patients with rhabdomyolysis.
- Once aggressive fluid resuscitation has been initiated, frequent monitoring is of the utmost importance, with attention to electrolytes, acid-base balance, and intravascular volume.
- The indications for dialysis in rhabdomyolysis patients remain the same as general indications for dialysis—profound acidosis, pulmonary edema leading to impending respiratory failure, electrolyte imbalances refractory to conservative measures, that is, hyperkalemia causing electrocardiographic changes that are not responsive to intestinal potassium binders (sodium polystyrene sulfate or Kayexalate).
- Hypocalcemia, while often seen in the early stages of rhabdomyolysis, rarely needs treatment as the deficit does not represent a total body deficit and the initial calcium sequestered in injured muscle may redistribute into the bloodstream.

BIBLIOGRAPHY

Allison RC, Bedsole L. The other medical causes of rhabdomyolysis. *Am J Med Sci* 2003;326:79–88.

Brown CVR, Rhee P, Chan L, et al. Preventing renal failure in patients with rhabdomyolysis: do bicarbonate and mannitol make a difference? *J Trauma* 2004;56:1191–1196.

deMeijer AR, Fikkers BG, deKeijzer MH, et al. Serum creatine kinase as predictor of clinical course in rhabdomyolysis: a 5 year intensive care study. *Intensive Care Med* 2003;29: 1121–1125.

Singh D, Chander V, Chopra K. Rhabdomyolysis. *Methods Find Exp Clin Pharmacol* 2005;27:39–48.

Section 8
GASTROINTESTINAL DISORDERS

102 UPPER GASTROINTESTINAL HEMORRHAGE

Maria Dowell

KEY POINTS

- The majority of GI bleeding encountered in the ICU is from an UGI source.
- Large-bore intravenous access and proactive resuscitation with crystalloids and blood products are essential.
- Massive bleeding typically engenders a coagulopathy that requires factor and platelet replacement.
- Early intervention with endoscopy, angiography, or surgery may be needed, and critical care management of these patients should coordinate these various subspecialties as resuscitation is ongoing.

EPIDEMIOLOGY

- Upper gastrointestinal (UGI) bleeding is defined as bleeding located proximal to the ligament of Treitz.
- Approximately 75% of all GI bleeding comes from an UGI source. The mortality from UGI bleeding requiring intensive care unit (ICU) admission may be as high as 10%.

PRESENTATION AND EVALUATION

- Upper gastrointestinal bleeding commonly presents with hematemesis and/or melena. A nasogastric lavage often, but not always, yields blood or coffee-ground material.
- Initial management is directed at maintaining hemodynamic stability. Intravenous access with two large-bore catheters should be maintained at all times. Evidence of hypotension or shock requires prompt resuscitation with crystalloid and packed red blood cells. Pay close attention to end-organ perfusion and in particular, coronary and renal perfusion. If variceal hemorrhage is suspected, central venous pressure (CVP) monitoring may be useful.
- Hematocrit should be maintained >30% in order to ensure adequate oxygen-carrying capacity and to prevent end-organ ischemia. The initial hematocrit with an acute bleed may be misleading as both loss of erythrocytes and plasma are equivalent. Platelets should be maintained >50,000/mm^3 and any coagulopathy should be corrected with fresh frozen plasma.
- With active hematemesis, a nasogastric tube should be placed to reduce the risk of aspiration. Endotracheal intubation is indicated with hematemesis and decreased mental status, prior to endoscopy for active hematemesis, prior to insertion of esophageal tamponade tube, and in the setting of shock.
- Radiology and surgery should be consulted early in the course of management. When endoscopic evaluation is unable to identify the etiology of bleeding, angiography and radionuclide studies may be of help. Angiography can visualize acute arterial hemorrhage in 75% of UGI bleed patients but it must be bleeding at a brisk rate of 0.5–1 mL/min. Radionuclide using ^{99m}Tc-pertechnetate-labeled red blood cells can detect bleeding <0.5 mL/min using intermittent scan over 1–2 days. This scan, however, can only localize the bleeding to an area and cannot precisely determine the mucosal location.
- Continuous hemodynamic monitoring should be performed as rebleeding is a definite risk.

VARICEAL HEMORRHAGE

- Presents as symptom of decompensated cirrhosis in up to 50% of patients and accounts for 30% of all deaths related to cirrhosis. Overall mortality is 50%.

The first phase of bleeding is the initial episode of hemorrhage in which 50% stop spontaneously. The initial bleed is followed by the second phase lasting about 6 weeks and is defined by a high risk of recurrent bleeding especially within 48–72 hours.

INITIAL MANAGEMENT

- Cardiopulmonary management includes intubation for airway protection, especially in the setting of encephalopathy, active hematemesis, or emergent endoscopy. Hypotension refractory to fluid resuscitation should be treated with the vasoconstrictor; norepinephrine is a reasonable first choice agent (avoid dopamine as it can cause splanchnic vasodilatation and worsen the bleeding).
- Respiratory, ascitic fluid, and urinary tract infections are common and prophylactic antibiotics have been shown to reduce these and improve short-term mortality. In addition to fresh frozen plasma, recombinant factor VIIa is emerging as a procoagulant that can rapidly correct severe coagulopathy associated with decompensated liver disease and promote hemostasis. If decreased mental status is present, hepatic encephalopathy should be considered as a potential cause and empiric lactulose therapy should be initiated.

PHARMACOTHERAPY

- Selective splanchnic vasoconstrictors have the added advantage of diverting blood flow from the splanchnic circulation to the systemic circulation, thereby improving blood pressure and renal perfusion. The agent of choice is octreotide at a recommended dose of 50 μg IV bolus followed by an infusion of 50 μg/h for 5 days. Terlipressin, a long-acting vasopressin analogue, has recently been shown to reduce mortality but is awaiting larger prospective trials for confirmation of this early observation.

ENDOSCOPIC THERAPY

- Endoscopy may be performed under stable conditions within the first 24 hours. Emergent endoscopy with therapeutic hemostatic intent is recommended for patients with GI hemorrhage who have been initially stabilized with fluid and blood product resuscitation and continue to bleed. Determining the source of bleeding is important since esophageal varices are amenable to endoscopic therapy, whereas gastric varices may require more aggressive salvage measures.
- Endoscopy for esophageal varices is based on interrupting blood flow using either endoscopic sclerotherapy (EST) or endoscopic variceal band ligation (EVL). EVL has been shown to be superior to EST as the initial therapy unless the endoscopic field of view is too poor.
- Absolute contraindication to endoscopy includes suspected GI perforation, uncontrolled unstable angina, severe coagulopathy, untreated respiratory decompensation, and severe agitation. Complications include ulceration, dysmotility and stricture formation, esophageal perforation, mediastinitis, and portal hypertensive gastropathy. With massive exsanguinations, emergent surgical intervention should be considered instead of endoscopy.
- Gastric varices may initially be controlled with EVL; however, this is not always effective. Other interventions include nonendoscopic esophageal tamponade tubes (e.g., Sengstaken Blakemore tube) once an endotracheal tube is secured. This should be done by skilled personnel as esophageal ulceration and perforation may occur. Following temporary stabilization, creation of an artificial vascular shunt between the systemic and portal circulation to decompress the varices can be performed. This may be accomplished by a transjugular intrahepatic portosystemic shunt (TIPS) with a radiologically guided metallic stent. Since the advent of TIPS, there has been a reduction in surgical decompression.
- Once hemodynamically stable, nonspecific beta-blockade should be initiated (nadolol 20–40 mg daily) to decrease portal hypertension.

NONVARICEAL HEMORRHAGE

- These lesions have a more favorable prognosis compared to variceal bleeding. Peptic ulcer disease (PUD) accounts for the majority of nonvariceal bleeds.

PEPTIC ULCER DISEASE

- Thermal therapy and injection therapy with epinephrine are the most commonly used hemostatic endoscopic methods. Thermal therapy produces coagulation and dehydration at the ulcer base resulting in constriction and destruction of the submucosal feeding vessels. Injection therapy causes vasoconstriction and necrosis of the bleeding vessel and surrounding tissue. Combination therapy with injection and thermal coagulation is superior to either monotherapy in active bleeding although thermal therapy may be used alone with nonbleeding ulcers.

- Acid suppression with proton pump inhibitors is used as an adjunct to endoscopic hemostasis. Octreotide may be considered as a pharmacologic adjunct as well.
- In a minority of patients, endoscopy may not visualize the lesion and angiography may be required. Angiography with the option of hemostatic therapy using the vasoconstrictor, epinephrine, or embolization is reserved for poor surgical candidates or unstable patients awaiting surgery.
- Surgical therapy should be considered for life-threatening hemorrhage that is refractory to medical and endoscopic intervention and for the patient in whom medical management has failed to heal or prevent recurrence of the ulcer.
- Once hemodynamically stable, long-term acid suppressive therapy with either oral H_2-receptor blockers or proton pump inhibitors should be started. If evaluation for *Helicobacter pylori* is positive, treatment should be initiated.

MALLORY-WEISS TEAR

- Generally a self-limiting cause of bleeding and rarely requires more than supportive measures. Patients with portal hypertension, however, are at increased risk of massive bleeding and EVL or EST should be performed. In the rare instance, a Mallory-Weiss tears continues to bleed in patients without portal hypertension; endoscopic therapy with either thermal or injection therapy should be attempted prior to surgical oversewing. Acid suppression therapy is given as adjunctive therapy to accelerate healing.

DIEULAFOY LESION

- This lesion results from a dilated submucosal vessel which erodes the overlying epithelium in the absence of a primary ulcer. Massive bleeding can occur if the eroding vessel is an artery. The endoscopic treatment of choice is combination epinephrine injection and thermal coagulation. EVL has also reportedly been successful; however, the risk of bleeding after any endoscopic therapy is up to 40%. If rebleeding occurs, surgical wedge resection should be performed.

STRESS-RELATED MUCOSAL DAMAGE

- This is the result of multiorgan system failure in critically ill patients. Mortality is >30% when bleeding is substantial, likely a reflection of the underlying disease(s). Two major risk factors are coagulopathy and mechanical ventilation >48 hours. Other suggested risk factors include sepsis, shock, acidosis, peritonitis, extensive burns, hepatic failure, and renal failure.
- Endoscopically, stress-related mucosal damage (SRMD) appears as multiple shallow erosions or submucosal hemorrhage that progress to deeper ulcerations which may erode into the submucosa.
- Therapy is supportive with an attempt to correct precipitating factors. Acid suppression is used as an adjunct to endoscopic or angiographic interventions. Surgery should be avoided, since near-total gastrectomy is required, and mortality exceeds 50%.
- Prophylactically, acid suppression and adequate nutritional support, preferably enteral, have been shown to decrease the incidence of SRMD.

BIBLIOGRAPHY

Subramanian RM, McCashland TM. Gastrointestinal hemorrhage. In: Hall JB, Schmidt GA, Wood LDH, eds., *Principles of Critical Care*, 3rd ed. New York, NY: McGraw-Hill; 2005: 1261–1278.

103 LOWER GASTROINTESTINAL HEMORRHAGE

Maria Dowell

KEY POINTS

- Massive bleeding from the upper GI tract (UGIH) may mimic bleeding from the lower GI tract (LGIH) and must be considered in the patient passing frank blood per rectum.
- The two most common causes of LGIH are diverticulosis and angiodysplasia.
- When the rate of bleeding precludes direct visualization by colonoscopy, imaging by tagged red cell scanning or angiography should be considered.

EPIDEMIOLOGY

- Lower gastrointestinal (LGI) bleeding is defined as bleeding from a source distal to the ligament of Treitz.
- 10% of patients thought to have LGI bleed are found to have an upper source.

PRESENTATION AND EVALUATION

- Hematochezia is the most common presenting sign. In patients with hematochezia and hemodynamic compromise, however, a brisk upper GI (UGI) bleed should be included on the differential diagnosis.
- The two most frequent LGI bleeding sources are diverticulosis and angiodysplasia.
- Initially, concentrate evaluation on resuscitation and correction of coagulopathy. Nasogastric tube aspiration is then performed and if positive, an urgent esophagogastroduodenoscopy (EGD) is warranted. If the aspiration is negative or patient has low risk for upper bleed, an urgent colonoscopy should be done after rapid oral purge.

COLONOSCOPY

- Emergent colonoscopy after rapid oral purge (4 L of Golytely orally or via nasogastric tube over 2 hours) is the initial approach. Metoclopramide (10 mg) is given at the start of the cleansing to facilitate intestinal transit time and minimize emesis.
- Following colonic cleansing, colonoscopy has higher diagnostic yield and lower complication rate compared to angiography.
- Overall diagnostic yield of emergent colonoscopy is 69–80%.
- Aside from diverticular bleeding and angiodysplasia, the most common findings are colitis, neoplasia, and anorectal disease.
- If the source is not determined on colonoscopy and an upper endoscopy is negative, a small bowel etiology should be considered. Small bowel evaluation with push enteroscopy, capsule endoscopy, or enteroclysis may be done once hemostasis is achieved.

ENDOSCOPIC THERAPY

- As with UGI bleeding, both thermal coagulation and injection therapy with epinephrine have been used to obtain hemostasis in acute LGI bleeding.
- Thermal coagulation and injection therapy with epinephrine can achieve hemostasis and may prevent recurrent diverticular bleeding and the need for hemicolectomy. Unfortunately, massive diverticular bleed may not be amenable to endoscopic therapy due to poor visualization thereby necessitating angiographic or surgical therapy.
- Angiodysplastic lesions are often located in the cecum and right colon and are frequently responsive to endoscopic therapy. Additional lesions responsive to endoscopic therapy include postpolypectomy sites, radiation colitis, and anorectal sources. Argon-plasma coagulation has been used effectively in radiation colitis and postpolypectomy bleeding. Band ligation similar to esophageal variceal band ligation can also be used to treat bleeding from internal hemorrhoids.

RADIONUCLIDE STUDIES

- Radionuclide scanning using ^{99m}Tc-pertechnetate-labeled red blood cells is often used to localize LGI bleeding. Nuclear scan can detect bleeding rates as low as 0.1 mL/min and repeat imaging may be performed within the 48-hour stability of the tagged red blood cell.
- Nuclear scanning has a high sensitivity but low specificity for precise localization compared to positive endoscopy or angiography.
- A positive scan localizes the bleeding only to an area of the abdomen and should be used to direct attention to specific sites to be examined by angiography or repeat endoscopy. Surgical intervention should not be based on nuclear scan alone.

ANGIOGRAPHIC THERAPY

- Angiography with therapeutic intent is the preferred treatment in the setting of massive bleeding that precludes colonoscopy or after a nondiagnostic colonoscopy.
- Overall diagnostic yield ranges from 40 to 78% with diverticular disease and angiodysplasia being the most common findings. Initial hemostasis using intra-arterial vasopressin or embolization ranges from 60 to 100% although recurrent bleeding can be as high as 50% following vasopressin therapy.
- Intra-arterial vasoconstrictive therapy is associated with a major complication rate of 10–20% and includes arrhythmias, ischemia, and pulmonary edema. Transcatheter embolization with gelatin sponges and microcoils is a more definitive means of controlling bleeding but carries up to a 20% risk of intestinal infarction.
- In the absence of localization via nuclear imaging, the superior mesenteric artery is examined first followed by the inferior mesenteric and celiac vessels.
- If therapeutic angiography does not achieve permanent homeostasis, emergent surgical therapy is indicated. Angiography can also be used to temporarily control bleeding and allow surgical intervention in a controlled setting with improved operative mortality.

SURGICAL THERAPY

- Surgical therapy should be reserved for hemorrhage that is refractory to nonsurgical interventions. The patient who is exsanguinating from LGI bleed, however, should undergo emergent subtotal colectomy.
- Preoperative localization by angiography or colonoscopy is crucial to avoid extensive surgical resection and ensure that the bleeding is truly arising from a lower source. Exploratory laparotomy with intraoperative endoscopy can be used to localize the source, especially in the small intestine.
- Once the source is identified, segmental colectomy can be performed. A subtotal colectomy is indicated for the exsanguinating patient or patient with persistent hemorrhage without a source and involves resection from the cecum to proximal rectum with an ileoproctostomy.

OBSCURE BLEEDING AND SMALL BOWEL EVALUATION

- Occasionally, patients undergo nondiagnostic evaluations for GI bleeding but clinically stabilize. Emergent surgical exploration and intraoperative endoscopy may not be indicated and they should undergo further evaluation directed at the small bowel.
- Novel endoscopic modalities exist that can visualize more distal portions of the small bowel. Push enteroscopy uses a pediatric endoscope passed beyond the ligament of Treitz to visualize the proximal 60 cm of jejunum and allows biopsy or therapy of visualized lesions. Diagnostic yield is 50% with angiodysplasia being the most common lesion. Sonde enteroscopy should be considered if push enteroscopy is negative. It is performed by passing a long flexible enteroscope passively by intestinal peristalsis but does not allow biopsy or therapy of the lesions. Wireless capsule endoscopy provides a noninvasive method of examining the entire small bowel via peristaltic propulsion of an endoscopic capsule. Approximately 50,000 images are taken as it traverses the small bowel over 12–15 hours but biopsy and therapeutic interventions cannot be performed. Enteroclysis radiology is a double contrast study performed by injecting barium, methylcellulose, and air via a tube in the proximal small bowel. It has a yield of only about 10% but is considered superior to standard small bowel follow through studies.
- Small intestinal angiodysplasia accounts for the majority of lesions associated with obscure bleeding. End-stage renal disease, von Willebrand disease, and Osler-Weber-Rendu are all associated with increased incidence of small bowel angiodysplasia.
- Hemobilia is bleeding from the liver, bile ducts, or pancreas and usually results from blunt or sharp trauma to the liver. Hemobilia should be considered when melena occurs in conjunction with jaundice, after blunt trauma or acute pancreatitis. Angiographic therapy may allow temporary control of hemobilia but generally definitive surgery is required.
- Aortoenteric fistula occurs rarely following abdominal vascular surgery with synthetic graft placement. The fistula arises from the proximal anastomosis of the graft and communicates with the fourth portion of the duodenum. Evaluation should begin with endoscopy and if this fails to identify the source, angiography should be performed.
- Meckel diverticulum should be considered in younger patients with massive bleeding. ^{99m}Tc-pertechnetate scan has a diagnostic sensitivity of 75% and surgical resection provides definitive therapy.

BIBLIOGRAPHY

Subramanian RM, McCashland TM. Gastrointestinal hemorrhage. In: Hall JB, Schmidt GA, Wood LDH, eds., *Principles of Critical Care*, 3rd ed. New York, NY: McGraw-Hill; 2005: 1261–1278.

104 ACUTE HEPATIC FAILURE

D. Kyle Hogarth

KEY POINTS

- Fulminant hepatic failure (FHF) is defined as the onset of hepatic oncephalopathy (HE) within 8 weeks of the onset of liver-related symptoms.
- Common complications in patients with FHF include encephalopathy, cerebral edema, cardiovascular instability, renal failure, and infection.
- Supportive management of FHF consists of (1) airway protection, (2) ICP monitoring in the sickest patients, and (3) treatment of complications and monitoring for infection.
- Patient survival is inversely related to the number and extent of extrahepatic organ dysfunction, so early recognition and management of organ system deterioration is mandatory.
- All FHF patients should be assumed to have an unpredictable clinical course, which may require liver transplantation.

- Orthotopic liver transplantation (OLT) is the only definitive therapy for FHF. Among severe FHF patients, expected recovery with medical management is only 10–40%. Liver transplantation has survival rates of 60–80% for FHF.

DEFINITIONS

- There are multiple ways to classify fulminant hepatic failure (FHF), which are useful from a research and retrospective analysis point of view. However, the classification systems do not provide prospective guidelines for initial management of FHF.
- FHF is defined as the onset of hepatic encephalopathy (HE) within 8 weeks of the onset of liver-related symptoms.
- HE is graded using the following scale:
  - Grade 1: confused or has an altered mood
  - Grade 2: somnolent or displays inappropriate behavior
  - Grade 3: stuporous but arousable or displays moderately confused behavior
  - Grade 4: the patient is unresponsive or comatose

ETIOLOGIES

- Careful history taking from the patient, family, and significant others is mandatory and may provide valuable information in identifying the etiology of FHF.
- In the United States, acetaminophen toxicity has replaced acute viral hepatitis as the most common cause of FHF.
- Of the viral causes of FHF, hepatitis A and B are the most common with hepatitis C rarely causing FHF. Other viral causes include herpes simplex virus and Epstein-Barr virus.
- Drugs other than acetaminophen causing FHF include halothane, ampicillin-clavulanate, ciprofloxacin, erythromycin, isoniazid, nitrofurantoin, tetracycline, sodium valproate, phenytoin, lovastatin, tricyclic antidepressants, gold, flutamide, dipyridium, Antabuse, cyclophosphamide, methyldioxymethamphetamine (ecstasy), loratadine, propylthiouracil, and troglitazone.
- FHF results from toxins including Amanita phalloides, organic solvents, herbal medicines, and bacterial toxins (*Bacillus cereus* and *Cyanobacteria*).
- Miscellaneous rare causes of FHF include acute Budd-Chiari syndrome (hepatic vein thrombosis), hepatic ischemia from shock, Wilson disease, Reye syndrome, acute fatty liver of pregnancy, heatstroke, extensive hepatectomy, and autoimmune hepatitis.

INITIAL EVALUATION AND MANAGEMENT

- Patients suspected of having FHF should be managed in a critical care unit associated with an active liver transplant program.
- A history of preexisting liver disease, toxin exposure (e.g., alcohol, acetaminophen, and nonsteroidal anti-inflammatory drugs [NSAIDs]), acute viral illness, or predisposing medical condition should increase suspicion of FHF in a patient presenting with altered mental status, transaminase elevation, and synthetic dysfunction.
- Synthetic function of the liver is best followed by the international normalization ratio (INR) or prothrombin time. A rising INR coincident with falling liver transaminases is an ominous sign suggestive of nonrecoverable ongoing hepatic necrosis.
- Progression of FHF may lead to significant hemodynamic instability. Often, the hemodynamic changes resemble those associated with septic shock, and include a hyperdynamic circulation and a decreased systemic vascular resistance.
- Episodes of hypotension require aggressive evaluation and correction to prevent cerebral hypoperfusion, worsening injury to the blood-brain barrier, and multisystem organ failure.
- When the intracranial pressure (ICP) is being measured, cerebral perfusion pressure (CPP) serves as the major parameter for titration of fluid and vasoactive therapy (goal >60 mmHg), rather than the mean arterial pressure (MAP).

MONITORING

- Among patients with grade 3 or 4 encephalopathy, endotracheal intubation is necessary for airway protection, oxygenation, and control of respiratory acidosis.
- ICP monitoring is strongly recommended for direct measurement of ICP in patients with grade 3 or 4 HE. Extradural catheter monitoring is preferred in this setting for its safety and ease in placement.

WORKUP FOR ETIOLOGY AND POSSIBLE TRANSPLANT

- The initial laboratory evaluation should try to determine the potential causes of FHF as well as evaluate other organ system function in the patient.
- A complete blood count, platelet count, chemistries, albumin, bilirubin, alkaline phosphatase, aspartate

aminotransferase (AST), alanine aminotransferase (ALT), prothrombin time (INR), arterial blood gas, factor V level, blood glucose, and ammonia level are required for initial evaluation and management.
- Possible causes of FHF are sought through serologic assays for hepatitis A (anti-HAV IgM) and hepatitis B (anti-HBV IgM, HBsAg, HBcAb) and serum assays for ceruloplasmin, iron binding capacity, toxic substances, and acetaminophen. HIV testing should also be performed.
- A right upper quadrant ultrasound is useful in providing information regarding the patency of hepatic vessels, liver size, presence of ascites, and degree of compression of the porta hepatitis by intra-abdominal masses.
- The role for liver biopsy is controversial.

COMPLICATIONS

ENCEPHALOPATHY AND CEREBRAL EDEMA

- Dysfunction of cerebral blood flow autoregulation, cerebral vasodilation, and a disrupted blood-brain barrier all contribute to the accumulation of interstitial cerebral fluid, resulting in increased ICP in the FHF patient.
- In the acute setting, cerebral edema is clearly evident in patients with grade 3 and 4 encephalopathy.
- Computed tomography (CT) has limited sensitivity in detecting cerebral edema, therefore, repeated clinical evaluation and grading of encephalopathy is required, preferably by the same senior staff member.
- Other external variables that may contribute to worsening encephalopathy include hypoglycemia, hypoxia, electrolyte abnormalities, gastrointestinal bleeding, and sepsis.
- Treatments normally effective in the encephalopathy of decompensated chronic liver disease, such as selective gut decontamination, lactulose, and dietary nitrogen restriction, do not help in FHF.
- Initial management of cerebral edema in FHF should include avoidance of unnecessary stimulation, including respiratory suctioning in intubated patients, which may cause acute elevations in ICPs.
- The head of the patient's bed should be elevated to 30° and the patient's head should be maintained in a neutral position.
- Brain blood flow is determined largely by the CPP, a function of MAP and ICP: CPP = MAP − ICP. The optimal CPP is between 60 and 80 mmHg.
- Mannitol can be used as medical therapy of cerebral edema in FHF. Careful monitoring of the serum osmolality should occur. When osmolality exceeds 320 mOsm/L, the mannitol should be held.

RENAL FAILURE

- Acute renal failure is a frequent occurrence in the patients with FHF and is associated with a poor prognosis.
- The incidence of renal insufficieny approaches 75% among patients with acetaminophen-induced FHF and 30–50% among patients with FHF from other causes. Prerenal azotemia, acute tubular necrosis, hepatorenal syndrome, and nephrotoxic drugs may contribute to renal dysfunction and should be investigated and treated.
- Continuous renal replacement therapies are the preferred modality for dialysis as significant fluctuations in hemodynamic and ICP have been demonstrated with intermittent hemodialysis.

RESPIRATORY FAILURE

- The onset of hypoxic respiratory failure is usually associated with development of multisystem organ failure and predicts an overall poor prognosis.
- Diagnostic and therapeutic bronchoscopy should generally be avoided in these patients because of the potential to raise ICP dramatically.
- The presence of hypoxemia requiring >60% FiO_2 is likely to present difficulties with posttransplant management and survivability.

INFECTIONS

- Patients with FHF have a high incidence of bacterial and fungal infections. Eighteen percent of all patients with FHF ultimately die of infectious-related complications.
- Central venous catheters should be inserted using full barrier precautions and maintained with sterile technique. When line sepsis is suspected, all lines must be removed and replaced at alternative sites. Before a new line is inserted, reassess if the patient truly needs the central access.
- Urinary catheters can be removed from anuric patients to limit the risk of an ascending urinary tract infection.
- Systemic infection usually contraindicates transplantation because of the high level of immunosuppression subsequently required. However, this contraindication is not absolute.

LIVER TRANSPLANTATION

- Liver transplantation for the treatment of FHF has dramatically improved survival and should be considered the primary mode of therapy.

- The only factor consistently associated with poor outcome was level of encephalopathy at the time of admission.
- No consistent patient characteristic could be correlated with survivability without liver transplantation.

OTHER THERAPEUTIC INTERVENTIONS

- Many other treatment options have been investigated, and many showed early promise. However, none have proven benefit. Potential treatment options in a research setting include high volume plasma exchange, steroids, prostaglandin E, auxiliary liver transplantation, and extracorporeal liver support.

BIBLIOGRAPHY

Barr, WG and Robin JA. Rheumatology in the ICU. In: Hall JB, Schmidt GA, Wood LDH, eds., *Principles of Critical Care,* 3rd ed. New York, NY: McGraw-Hill; 2005:1573–1592.

105 CHRONIC LIVER DISEASE

Josh Levitsky

KEY POINTS

- Decompensation in patients with chronic liver disease and cirrhosis often results from infection, bleeding, and/or encephalopathy.
- Clinicians should have a low threshold for paracentesis in patients with chronic ascites and even modest evidence of infection to clarify the potential diagnosis of SBP.
- Massive ascites may compromise respiratory function and lead to an abdominal compartment syndrome.

EPIDEMIOLOGY

- In 2000–2001, over 360,000 hospital discharges and 27,000 deaths in the United States resulted from complications of chronic liver disease.
- Complications are related to the development of portal hypertension.
- Most common diagnoses on ICU admission are: sepsis, spontaneous bacterial peritonitis (SBP), variceal hemorrhage, hepatic encephalopathy (HE), massive ascites, and renal failure.

PATHOPHYSIOLOGY

- Portal hypertension = portal pressure gradient (pressure difference between the portal vein and inferior vena cava [IVC]) >5 mmHg; clinically significant >10 mmHg (formation of gastrointestinal varices) or >12 mmHg (risk of variceal hemorrhage).
- Portal hypertension leads to cirrhotic circulatory dysfunction, characterized by splanchnic vasodilation, activation of the renin-angiotensin and sympathetic nervous systems, and subsequent systemic vasoconstriction.
- Renal failure due to portal hypertension (e.g., hepatorenal syndrome) is caused by systemic and intrarenal vasoconstriction.
- Ascites develops with avid fluid and sodium retention by the kidneys, excessive lymph formation, and increased intrahepatic resistance.
- HE may be caused by portosystemic shunting of neurotoxins (e.g., ammonia, endogenous benzodiazepines, manganese, and gamma-aminobutyric acid [GABA]).

CLINICAL FEATURES

- Relative hypotension is important to confirm as hypotension (systolic blood pressure [SBP] ~80–90 mmHg) is common at baseline.
- Tachypnea may be due to intrapulmonary (hepatic hydrothorax, pulmonary edema, pneumonia) or extrapulmonary (tense ascites, metabolic acidosis due to sepsis, cirrhotic cardiomyopathy, encephalopathy) causes.
- Fetor hepaticus: sweet breath odor caused by increased dimethylsulphide concentrations (portosystemic shunting).
- Neurologic: stage I HE: anxiety, short attention span, sleep-wake reversal; stage II HE: lethargy, inappropriate behavior, slurred speech, asterixis; stage III HE: severe confusion, somnolent but arousable, hyperreflexia; stage IV HE: obtundation, loss of reflexes.
- Cardiovascular: hypotension, tachycardia, bounding pulses.
- Pulmonary: tachypnea, small lung volumes from ascites, decreased breath sounds, and dullness to percussion from associated pleural effusions.
- Gastrointestinal: flank or shifting dullness, splenomegaly, caput medusa, abdominal tenderness or rebound (SBP). Hepatomegaly suggests posthepatic cause or infiltrative disorder.
- Genital: testicular atrophy.
- Extremity: edema or anasarca, clubbing (often in primary biliary cirrhosis or hepatopulmonary syndrome), Dupuytren contracture (often in alcoholics), Muehrcke (white bands separated by normal color) or

Terry (proximal two-thirds of nail plate appears white) nails.
- Dermatologic: jaundice, spider angiomata, palmar erythema.
- Miscellaneous: gynecomastia, parotid hypertrophy (often in alcoholics).

LABORATORY FEATURES

- Leukopenia: often due to hypersplenism.
- Thrombocytopenia: hypersplenism, decreased thrombopoietin levels from liver disease, alcoholism.
- Anemia: hypersplenism, anemia of chronic disease, acute blood loss (bleeding or hemolysis), vitamin deficiency, alcoholism, renal failure.
- Coagulopathy: elevated international normalized ratio (INR), correlates with severity of liver disease, less common disseminated intravascular coagulation (DIC), fibrinolysis, dysfibrinogenemia.
- Liver tests: hypoalbuminemia (not specific for liver disease), hyperbilirubinemia, aspartate aminotransferase (AST)/alanine aminotransferase (ALT) >1 often seen in cirrhosis, >2 suggestive of alcohol-related liver disease, elevated alkaline phosphatase and gamma-glutamyltransferase in cholestatic disorders (primary biliary cirrhosis, primary sclerosing cholangitis).
- Chemistry: hyponatremia, hyperkalemia (use of potassium-sparing diuretics, renal failure), metabolic alkalosis.

PRINCIPLES OF DIAGNOSIS AND MANAGEMENT

- Infection (general): Pan-culture (blood, urine, peritoneal fluid if ascites present), chest x-ray (CXR). If no obvious initial source, consider broad-spectrum antibiotics until further data (culture or imaging results) direct management.
- SBP: Diagnostic paracentesis for culture, Gram's stain, and cell count. Diagnosis made with a polymorphonuclear (PMN) count ≥250/μL. Organism isolated in only 50–60% of cases. Start cefotaxime (2 g IV every 6–8 hours) or ceftriaxone (2 g IV every 24 hours). Albumin infusion at the time of diagnosis (1.5 g/kg) and day 3 (1 g/kg) to reduce risk of renal dysfunction. Repeat diagnostic paracentesis in 48–72 hours: if no improvement in cell count, culture is polymicrobial, or ascites glucose <50 mg/dL or ascites lactate dehydrogenase (LDH) >serum LDH, consider secondary peritonitis.
- HE: Often precipitated by progression of liver disease, missed scheduled medications, infection, gastrointestinal blood loss, hypovolemia, sedative use, electrolyte imbalances (hyponatremia, hypokalemia, hypoglycemia, alkalosis, renal failure), protein load, hepatocellular carcinoma. Treat underlying cause + lactulose (goal: 2–3 soft stools per day). If no resolution, consider other causes of encephalopathy.
- Variceal hemorrhage: Initial management—protect airway (consider endotracheal intubation), consider central venous catheter; resuscitate with fresh frozen plasma, red blood cells, platelets, and/or saline. Avoid excessive transfusions. Start octreotide (initial IV bolus 25–50 μg followed by 25–50 μg/h infusion) and broad-spectrum antibiotic prophylaxis. Urgent upper endoscopy for variceal sclerotherapy or banding. If unsuccessful, balloon tamponade tube or urgent portosystemic shunt (transjugular intrahepatic portosystemic shunt [TIPS]).
- Ascites: Exclude infectious peritonitis. Low sodium diet and diuretics. Avoid >10 L paracentesis and give 8 g albumin/1 L ascites, $^1/_2$ after paracentesis, and $^1/_2$ 6 hours later. Consider TIPS in refractory cases if no contraindications (encephalopathy, severe hepatic dysfunction).
- Renal failure: Evaluate for prerenal, intrarenal, and postrenal causes. Assess volume status and evidence of infection. Discontinue nephrotoxic drugs. Trial of 1.5 L of normal saline or equivalent. Order urinalysis, urine sodium, renal ultrasound. If no etiology or improvement in 24–48 hours, likely hepatorenal syndrome: avoid overzealous paracentesis, maintain volume status, consider systemic vasoconstrictors (terlipressin, octreotide + midodrine). TIPS is considered experimental.

BIBLIOGRAPHY

Angeli P, Volpin R, Gerunda G, et al. Reversal of type 1 hepatorenal syndrome with the administration of midodrine and octreotide. *Hepatology* 1999;29:1690–1697.

Arias E, Anderson RN, Kung HC, et al. Deaths: final Data for 2001. *Nat Vital Stat Rep* 2003;52:1–116.

Kozak LJ, Hall MJ, Owings MF. National Hospital Discharge Survey: 2000 annual summary with detailed diagnosis and procedure data. National Center for Health Statistics. *Vital Health Stat* 2002;13–199.

Ortega R, Gines P, Uriz J, et al. Terlipressin therapy with and without albumin for patients with hepatorenal syndrome: results of a prospective, nonrandomized study. *Hepatology* 2002;36:941–948.

Sort P, Navasa M, Arroyo V, et al. Effect of intravenous albumin on renal impairment and mortality in patients with cirrhosis and spontaneous bacterial peritonitis. *N Engl J Med* 1999;5:403–409.

106 BLEEDING ESOPHAGEAL VARICES AND TIPS

Sunana Sohi

KEY POINTS

- A large fraction of patients with cirrhosis will experience at least one episode of variceal bleeding.
- Without treatment, variceal bleeding has a high rate of recurrence.
- Initial stabilization can be challenging given the propensity for massive and rapid blood loss.
- In advance of diagnostic procedures, large-bore access should be established, blood product and fluid resuscitation initiated, coagulopathy addressed, and in many patients, intubation performed to protect the airway.

EPIDEMIOLOGY

- Liver cirrhosis affects approximately 3.6 out of 1000 adults in the United States.
- In the United States, alcohol abuse is the most common cause of cirrhosis.
- Approximately 10% of upper gastrointestinal bleeds are variceal in nature, and 25–40% of patients with cirrhosis will develop a variceal bleed.
- One-third of all cirrhosis-related deaths are secondary to variceal bleeds.
- A single variceal bleeding episode is associated with a 30% mortality rate.
- Whereas approximately 90% of nonvariceal upper gastrointestinal bleeds resolve spontaneously, less than half of variceal bleeds resolve without treatment.

ETIOLOGY

- Varices develop as a result of portal hypertension, which is caused by resistance to outflow from the portal vein. This can happen at several levels:
  - *Presinusoidal* (e.g., portal vein thrombosis and splenic vein thrombosis)
  - *Sinusoidal* (alcoholic cirrhosis being the most common, but other causes include schistosomiasis, the various hepatitides, Wilson disease, hemochromatosis, and alpha$_1$-antitrypsin deficiency)
  - *Postsinusoidal* (including Budd-Chiari syndrome and inferior vena cava thrombosis)
- In cirrhosis, portal hypertension develops secondary to sinusoidal obstruction and is associated with splanchnic vasodilation, which increases portal inflow.
- Varices form as portosystemic collaterals to divert obstructed blood flow back to the systemic vasculature, thus decompressing the portal system. This happens when the pressure gradient between the two systems exceeds 12 mmHg. The most significant collaterals are the gastroesophageal varices, which drain blood from the portal system into the azygous vein.
- Increased expression of the vasoconstrictor endothelin-1 has been related to the pathogenesis of varices; endothelin-1 is produced by the hepatic sinusoids and its vasoconstrictor effects serve to increase portal pressure. Additionally, the cirrhotic liver sinusoids have been shown to downregulate production of the vasodilator nitric oxide. Together, these mechanisms increase hepatic vascular resistance.
- Factors predicting variceal progression are similar to those predicting bleed (see "Factors Predicting a Variceal Bleed," below). Varices are more likely to progress if the patient has a higher Child-Pugh score (Table 106-1), if they are a large size, and if they have red wale signs (long erythematous streaks on the varices) seen on endoscopy.

FACTORS PREDICTING A VARICEAL BLEED

- *A previous bleed*: Almost 75% of patients will rebleed.
- *Size and appearance*: Varices that are more likely to bleed are larger and have endoscopic red signs: red wale markings, cherry red spots (clearly demarcated

TABLE 106-1 Child-Pugh Score*

	1 POINT	2 POINTS	3 POINTS
Total bilirubin	<2 mg/dL	2–3 mg/dL	>3 mg/dL
Serum albumin	>3.5 g/dL	2.8–3.5 g/dL	<2.8 g/dL
International normalized ratio (INR)	<1.7	1.7–2.2	>2.2
Ascites	None	Mild	Moderate/severe
Encephalopathy	None	Mild	Moderate/severe

*Class A: 5–6 points; class B: 7–9 points; class C: 10–15 points.

flat spots), hemato cystic spots (clearly demarcated raised spots), or simply diffuse erythema.
- *Child-Pugh score*: As a marker of liver dysfunction, those patients with Child class B or C are more likely to bleed than those with Child class A.
- *Alcohol intake*: Patients still actively consuming alcohol are more likely to have a variceal bleed than those who abstain.
- *High variceal pressure*: Variceal pressure can be measured using an endoscopic gauge, and the higher the pressure within the varices, the more likely they are to bleed.

PROPHYLAXIS AGAINST A FIRST VARICEAL BLEED

- Therapies are aimed at either decreasing portal pressure or locally minimizing the varices.
- *Nonselective beta-blockers*: Nonselective beta-blockers, such as propranolol, nadolol, and timolol, are commonly used as prophylaxis against variceal bleeds. They increase splanchnic vascular tone by blocking beta-adrenergic-mediated vasodilation, and they therefore decrease blood flow to the portal system. Their use is associated with an approximately 50% risk reduction of hemorrhage, but they have not yet been consistently proven to decrease mortality. Nadolol is used most commonly as it is dosed once per day. The typical starting doses are: nadolol 20–40 mg PO qd. Alternative beta-blockers include propranolol 10 mg PO tid, and timolol 10–20 mg PO bid. Doses are adjusted based on heart rate, with the aim being a relative bradycardia.
- *Nitrates*: Long-acting nitrates, such as isosorbide mononitrate, decrease portal pressure, but they have not been demonstrated to decrease mortality when used as a single agent, nor have they been shown conclusively to prevent bleeding, even when used in conjunction with a beta-blocker. Therefore, they are not used routinely.
- *Sclerotherapy*: Endoscopic sclerotherapy is an effective treatment of bleeding esophageal varices, but as there are many risks to the procedure (see "Endoscopic Sclerotherapy or Band Ligation," below), is not currently recommended as prophylaxis against a first variceal bleed.
- *Band ligation*: A meta-analysis of endoscopic band ligation has shown the procedure to decrease the risk of a first variceal hemorrhage and bleeding-related mortality; however, it has not been shown to decrease mortality overall. Additionally, as with sclerotherapy, band ligation has risks, and does not permanently remove varices. Currently, its use is limited to patients with a high risk of hemorrhage who are unable to tolerate beta-blocker prophylaxis.
- *Surgical portal decompression and TIPS (Transjugular Intrahepatic Portosystemic Shunts):* These treatments are very effective at preventing variceal hemorrhage, but their complications (see individual sections) preclude their use as a prophylactic measure against a first variceal bleed.

TREATMENT OF A VARICEAL BLEED

- Supportive measures are key in the treatment of a variceal bleed, as patients can exsanguinate quickly. Obtaining large-bore venous access is a first priority.
- The preferred first direct therapy for variceal bleeding includes pharmacologic treatment with octreotide or somatostatin, quickly followed by endoscopic sclerotherapy or band ligation.
- Treatment of a variceal hemorrhage is aimed at addressing the bleed site directly, via sclerotherapy, band ligation, or balloon tamponade, and decreasing portal pressure, via pharmacotherapy, TIPS, or surgical shunt creation (Table 106-2).

SUPPORTIVE TREATMENT

- *Hemodynamic support*: Volume resuscitation with normal saline should be initiated via two large-bore peripheral IVs or a central line. Additionally packed red blood cells may be transfused to replace blood loss, and fresh frozen plasma may be needed to replace clotting factors that may be deficient due to the cirrhotic liver.
- *Nasogastric (NG) tube placement*: A NG tube should be placed for decompression and to lavage the stomach for greater visibility during endoscopy.
- *Intubation*: NG tube decompression may reduce aspiration risk, but if there is a concern for aspiration, the patient may require intubation for airway protection.

TABLE 106-2 Treatment Modalities

Site-specific
Endoscopic sclerotherapy
Endoscopic band ligation
Balloon tamponade
Portal pressure reduction
Somatostatin
Octreotide
Vasopressin (rarely used)
Terlipressin (not available in the United States)
TIPS
Surgical shunt

PHARMACOTHERAPY

- *Somatostatin and octreotide*: Somatostatin and octreotide, is long-acting synthetic analog, inhibit glucagon and thus constrict the mesenteric vasculature, which decreases portal pressure. Their effects on the portal system are similar to that of vasopressin but with fewer systemic side effects (see below). This makes somatostatin and octreotide first-line pharmacotherapy for an acute variceal bleed, though they have not been shown to decrease mortality.
- *Vasopressin*: Vasopressin constricts the splanchnic bed, thereby decreasing portal inflow and thus portal pressures. It may be beneficial in the initiation of hemostasis, but as its vasoconstrictor effects are not limited to the mesenteric system, it can increase mortality by causing organ ischemia. In the past, it was used with nitroglycerin in an attempt to counteract systemic vasoconstriction, but with the development of somatostatin and octreotide, its use has fallen out of favor.
- *Terlipressin*: Although not available in the United States, terlipressin is a synthetic vasopressin analog used commonly in Europe. It has a longer half-life and can be given in IV boluses instead of continuous infusion. It is the only pharmacologic agent associated with decreased mortality.

ENDOSCOPIC SCLEROTHERAPY OR BAND LIGATION

- Endoscopic treatment is diagnostic as well as therapeutic and has been shown to achieve hemostasis 80–90% of the time.
- *Sclerotherapy*: Sclerotherapy involves the injection of a "sclerosant" (usually sodium tetradecyl sulfate or sodium morrhuate) into the varices on visualization during endoscopy. The procedure is associated with a 2% mortality rate. Complications include mucosal ulceration, esophageal perforation, mediastinitis, and, in the long term, approximately 15% of patients will develop esophageal stricture.
- *Band ligation*: This involves the deployment of small elastic bands around the varices, causing subsequent strangulation and then fibrosis of the vessels. Its major limitation is impaired visibility caused by the banding attachment device, although this has improved with the development of clear devices. Local complications, such as esophageal stricture, are less common, but band ligation is associated with rebleeding during the procedure.
- Both have fairly equivalent rates of hemostasis; utility of one over the other is based on operator preference.
- If endoscopic treatment fails, balloon tamponade, surgical treatment, or TIPS are second-line therapies.

BALLOON TAMPONADE

- Balloon tamponade, via the Sengstaken-Blakemore tube, Minnesota tube, or Linton-Nachlas tube, is used for short-term hemostasis if endoscopic treatment fails. It is less likely to be successful if the patient has failed pharmacotherapy or has developed early rebleeding.
- Generally, the tube is advanced through the oropharynx, and placement is confirmed via endoscopy or a radiograph or ultrasound. The balloon is then inflated in the stomach and pulled up against the gastroesophageal junction, compressing the varices. Tension is held until hemostasis is achieved.
- Complications associated with balloon tamponade include a high risk of rebleeding after the balloon is deflated and a risk of esophageal rupture if the balloon is overinflated. The procedure is associated with a risk of aspiration pneumonia and thus the patient is commonly intubated for airway protection. Because of these complications, tamponade is used primarily to stabilize the patient briefly prior to a more definitive treatment, such as TIPS or surgical shunt creation.

TRANSJUGULAR INTRAHEPATIC PORTOSYSTEMIC SHUNTS

- Transjugular intrahepatic portosystemic shunts involve the use of a metal stent to create a connection between the hepatic vein and the intrahepatic portion of the portal vein, thus decompressing the portal system. It has the added benefit of decompressing the hepatic sinusoids, thereby also decreasing ascites.
- TIPS is not first line in the treatment of acute variceal bleeds. Endoscopic treatment is first line; however, 10–20% of patients may rebleed after endoscopic therapy. Sclerotherapy or band ligation may be attempted again, but if this fails again, TIPS may be attempted. It is indicated in patients who rebleed and are poor surgical candidates.
- TIPS has been associated with a lower rebleeding rate compared with endoscopy, however, it is also associated with higher rates of hepatic encephalopathy and liver failure, as well as a higher mortality rate.

MAJOR COMPLICATIONS ASSOCIATED WITH TIPS

- *Rebleeding*: The main causes of rebleeding after TIPS include a recurrence of portal hypertension due to stent thrombosis, kinking, or stenosis, and the development of right heart failure.
- *Stent stenosis*: This is the most common complication after TIPS and is caused by pseudointimal hyperplasia, or growth of the liver tissue into and around the lumen of the stent. Almost 50% of patients will occlude their

shunts within 1 year of the procedure, thus surveillance Dopplers or angiograms are standard.
- *Stent thrombosis*: Anticoagulation carries with it such a high risk of bleeding in this patient population that it is not used as a prophylactic measure. Approximately 8% of patients will develop stent, portal vein, or splenic vein thrombosis, usually within 1–2 months of the procedure. If this develops, thrombolytics, anticoagulation, or suction thrombectomy are used; liver transplant is the definitive treatment.
- *Procedural complications*: Patients must be monitored for cardiac arrhythmias as the catheter is passed through the heart. There is also a risk of fatal hemoperitoneum if the liver capsule is punctured, if a TIPS-biliary fistula is created, or if the portal vein is punctured in the extrahepatic region.
- *Complications of shunt creation*: These complications also apply to the creation of surgical shunts. Twenty-five percent of patients develop portosystemic encephalopathy within 2–3 weeks of the procedure. They present with altered sleep, confusion, or hepatic coma. Portosystemic encephalopathy is also associated with a high ammonia level, although the level is not correlated with the severity of the encephalopathy. Patients should be treated with lactulose while other causes for encephalopathy, such as infection, subclinical bleed, metabolic and acid-base disturbances, are ruled out.

SURGICAL PORTAL DECOMPRESSION

- There are three types of surgical shunts. The side-to-side portocaval shunts decompress the entire portal tree and are thus nonselective; the selective distal splenorenal shunt decompresses the varices while keeping pressure in the superior mesenteric artery high; and the partial shunts only partially decompress the portal tree while maintaining some amount of liver perfusion.
- Surgical shunts are very successful at creating hemostasis but they interfere with the potential for future liver transplant. As with TIPS, they are associated with about a 50% encephalopathy rate.
- They may be used in patients who are good surgical candidates and fail emergent endoscopic treatment.

RECURRENT BLEEDING EPISODES

- The greatest likelihood of rebleeding occurs within the first 2–3 days after stabilization, but the patient is still considered high risk for approximately 6 weeks after treatment.
- Survivors of an acute variceal bleed have a 70% risk of recurrent hemorrhage within 1 year. Up to one-third of these events are fatal.
- Risk factors for a rebleeding episode include age >60, the presence of renal failure, large variceal size, and a severe initial bleed (hemoglobin <8 when admitted).

PREVENTION OF RECURRENCE

- Data regarding a first-line treatment for the prevention of recurrence of variceal bleeds has not been consistent. Currently, the American College of Gastroenterology recommends endoscopic band ligation as a primary treatment.
- Surveillance endoscopy should be performed every 6 months for the first year after the bleeding episode, and then every year thereafter, to monitor for recurrent varices.
- Many of the medications used for the prevention of variceal bleeding are also used in the prevention of recurrence. Nonselective beta-blockers, with or without the addition of a long-acting nitrate, are commonly administered.
- Treatment choices are based on Child-Pugh class. Clinicians are more likely to attempt medical management on patients with Child's score A, while patients with Child's score C would benefit from repeat endoscopic sclerotherapy or band ligation, with consideration for TIPS or surgical shunt creation as salvage therapy if patients continue to rebleed. Additionally, Child's score C patients should be listed for liver transplant.
- Liver transplantation is the only long-term treatment that reliably prevents against rebleeding, with survival rates of 80–90% at 1 year posttransplant and 60% at 5 years after transplant.

BIBLIOGRAPHY

De Franchis R, Prigmani M. Why do varices bleed? *Gastroenterol Clin North Am* 1992;21:85–96.

Imperiale T, Chalasani N. A meta-analysis of endoscopic variceal ligation for primary prophylaxis of esophageal variceal bleeding. *Hepatology* 2001;33:802–807.

Merli M, Giorgia N, Stefania A, et al. Incidence and natural history of small esophageal varices in cirrhotic patients. *J Hepatol* 2003;38:266–272.

Sanyal A, et al. Transjugular intrahepatic portosystemic shunts compared with endoscopic sclerotherapy for the prevention of recurrent variceal hemorrhage: a randomized, controlled trial. *Ann Intern Med* 1997;126:849–857.

Williams S, Westaby D. Management of variceal hemorrhage. *BMJ* 1994;308:1213–1217.

107 ACUTE PANCREATITIS

Maria Dowell

KEY POINTS

- The most common causes of pancreatitis causing admission to the ICU include alcohol and biliary obstruction; the most common causes of pancreatitis arising during other critical illness include direct surgical trauma, hypoperfusion, and drugs.
- Severe pancreatitis causes a generalized Systemic Inflamatory Response Syndrome (SIRS) with a high risk of evolution of other organ failures.
- Fluid requirements may be large early in the course, with risks of low pressure pulmonary edema and large intra-abdominal fluid collections.
- Carefully timed imaging of the abdomen is crucial to assess for anatomic complications of pancreatic inflammation.

BACKGROUND AND ETIOLOGY

- Often a self-limiting disease but 10% can develop severe form that carries a 30–40% mortality rate.
- Many causes with the most common being alcohol and gallstones. Other causes include postcardiopulmonary bypass, abdominal aortic aneurysm repair, posttransplantation of organs including the heart, kidney, and liver.
- Regardless of initiating cause, common pathogenetic mechanisms involve an intense systemic inflammatory response syndrome (SIRS) and hypoperfusion injury. The exact mechanism of injury is not known and is likely multifactorial.

DIAGNOSIS

- Clinical signs and symptoms are notoriously variable and may include abdominal pain, nausea, vomiting, leukocytosis, fever, and hemodynamic instability. Serum lipase may be more reliable and specific than amylase.
- Abdominal and chest radiographs should be used to rule out perforation and intestinal obstruction. X-rays may suggest pancreatitis by demonstrating pleural effusions, local ileus, widened duodenal loop, gallstones, absent psoas shadow, free intraperitoneal fluid, or pancreatic calcifications.
- *Computed tomography (CT) scan (IV contrast if possible)*: The gold standard for assessing retroperitoneal morphology and recommended in the presence of diagnostic uncertainty at the time of initial presentation. Can be useful to have a baseline scan but critical value is in detection and follow-up of pancreatitis complications. It is recommended that CT for detection of local complications be delayed for 48–72 hours when possible, as necrosis may not be visible earlier.
- *Ultrasound*: The most available and convenient bedside test for edematous pancreatitis that responds rapidly to supportive therapy and monitoring resolution of pseudocysts. Results may be hampered by obesity and ileus.

SEVERITY OF DISEASE

- Ranson criteria were used extensively in the past but several scoring systems employing clinical, biochemical, and radiologic features are currently available. These models should not replace frequent serial clinical assessments. Many centers use the Atlanta classification, based on the patient's presentation, Ranson score, APACHE (Acute Physiology and Chronic Health Evaluation) II score, and organ dysfunction. The Balthazar score is based on CT findings.

TREATMENT

- The mainstay of initial treatment is fluid resuscitation, respiratory and nutritional support, as well as attention to the primary disease state. Current sepsis guidelines should be initiated once the presence of infection is suspected and sepsis physiology is present.
- *Metabolic and hemodynamic effects*: Close clinical observation is required as patients usually require early and aggressive fluid resuscitation (may be up to 10 L isotonic fluid). Monitoring should focus on intravascular volume assessment (examination, urine output, acid-base status, central venous pressure) and pulmonary function. Use of pulmonary artery catheters remains controversial.
- *Respiratory and renal support*: Increased capillary permeability related to serotonin release, breakdown of surfactant by pancreatic phospholipase A, or activation of complement cascade are all mechanisms implicated in development of acute respiratory distress syndrome (ARDS) in acute pancreatitis. Ventilatory support is often required. Acute tubular necrosis and resulting renal insufficiency or failure usually results from hypoperfusion injury.
- *Nutrition*: Enteral nutrition via nasojejunal or percutaneous jejunal tube is recommended in preference to

parenteral nutrition. Infusion into the proximal jejunum bypasses stimulatory effects of feeding on pancreatic secretion, has fewer complications, is less costly than total parenteral nutrition (TPN), helps maintain mucosal function, and limits absorption of endotoxins and cytokines from the gut. TPN should only be used after 5–7 days' trial if enteral nutrition has failed.

- *Control of pancreatic enzyme secretion*: Numerous strategies attest to the failure of most of them to alter the course of the inflammatory process.

LOCAL COMPLICATIONS OF NECROTIZING PANCREATITIS

- Uncommon but potentially lethal intra-abdominal hemorrhage may occur. Necrosis, abscess, pseudocyst, perforation, and abdominal compartment syndrome may occur due to further hypoperfusion injury to the pancreas.
- *Pancreatic and peripancreatic necrosis*: Patients who die from necrotizing pancreatitis usually do not die in the early resuscitation phase. The patchy devitalization of the pancreas develops days to weeks after the onset of inflammation and may occur with or without infection of this tissue. Abdominal pain, persistent fever, leukocytosis, and radiologic evidence are useful in making the diagnosis. Ultrasound or CT-guided fine needle aspiration (FNA) with Gram's stain should be done to discern sterile from infected necrosis. Debridement and/or drainage are not recommended for sterile necrosis.
- *Infected necrosis and pancreatic abscess*: Debridement or drainage should be performed with infected necrosis or abscess confirmed by radiologic gas or FNA culture to avoid the sequelae of systemic infection.
- *Antibiotic therapy*: Although the latest consensus recommends against routine prophylactic systemic antimicrobial or antifungal agents or selective decontamination of the gastrointestinal (GI) tract in patients with necrotizing pancreatitis, it remains common practice. There may be a subset of patients (posttransplant, immunocompromised) identified by future investigations who may benefit from use of these agents.
- *Surgical debridement*: The gold standard is open operative debridement. Whenever possible, necrosectomy and/or drainage should be delayed 2–3 weeks to allow for demarcation of the necrotic pancreas; however, the clinical picture should be the primary determinant of when the patient needs to proceed to the operating room.
- *Gallstone pancreatitis*: In the setting of obstructive jaundice, urgent endoscopic retrograde cholangiopancreatography (ERCP) should be performed within 72 hours of onset of symptoms or, if ERCP unavailable, alternative methods of biliary drainage must be considered.
- *Pseudocysts*: Persistence of lesser sac fluid implies communication with pancreatic duct system. Cysts do not mandate immediate treatment unless they become symptomatic, infected, rupture, or grow quickly. Percutaneous decompression or endoscopic drainage is often employed. Surgery is required for bleeding or free rupture.

BIBLIOGRAPHY

American Thoracic Society. Executive Summary: management of the critically ill patient with severe acute pancreatitis. *Proc Am Thorac Soc* 2004;1:289–290.

Dervenis C, Smailis D, Hatzitheoklitos E. Bacterial translocation and its prevention in acute pancreatitis. *J Hepatobiliary Pancreat Surg* 2003;10:415–418.

Swaroop VS, Chari ST, Clain JE. Severe acute pancreatitis. *JAMA* 2004;292:23.

Taylor BR. Acute pancreatitis in the critically ill. In: Hall JB, Schmidt GA, Wood LDH, eds., *Principles of Critical Care*, 3rd ed. New York, NY: McGraw-Hill; 2005:1299–1308.

108 MESENTERIC ISCHEMIA

Joseph Levitt

KEY POINTS

- Acute mesenteric ischemia is rare but often fatal when diagnosis is delayed and thus a high index of suspicion is necessary in at-risk patients.
- Presentation can vary from a dramatic acute abdomen and shock in acute embolic events to vague nonspecific abdominal pain and changed bowel habits with chronic ischemia or venous thrombosis.
- Mesenteric angiography is the investigation of choice and may offer therapeutic options. CT angiography is commonly used and widely available and allows insight into status of the bowel.
- Treatment is generally surgical with restoration of blood flow via endarterectomy or bypass and resection of nonviable bowel.

- Prognosis remains poor even at specialist centers with diagnostic delay being the greatest hurdle to improved outcomes.

ANATOMY AND PATHOGENESIS

- The bowel is supplied by three branches of the aorta. The celiac artery supplies the foregut and hepatic and splenic circulations. The superior mesenteric artery (SMA) supplies the midgut and the inferior mesenteric artery (IMA) supplies the hindgut. With chronic ischemia significant collateral circulation can develop.
- At baseline, the intestine receives 20–30% of cardiac output, which can increase to 50% after meals.
- Acute drops in cardiac output cause intense vasoconstriction of the mesenteric circulation that can be out of proportion to the fall in cardiac output.
- Decreases in blood supply to the mesentery lead to an increased O_2 extraction by the bowel, thus lowering the O_2 content of the portal circulation and increasing the risk of hepatic ischemia.
- The mucosal layer receives 70% of intestinal blood supply and is the most sensitive to ischemia. Twenty minutes of ischemia can lead to injury and loss of mucosal villi. Prolonged ischemia will progress to mucosal sloughing (which presents as bloody diarrhea) and eventually transmural infarction with perforation and septic peritonitis.
- Reperfusion after prolonged ischemia can release a host of metabolic byproducts into systemic circulation causing an intense systemic inflammatory response syndrome (SIRS) or promote translocation of intestinal bacteria and sepsis.

PRESENTATION

- It is important to be able to recognize the signs and symptoms of both acute and chronic mesenteric ischemia as they can have very different presentations and therapies but the same catastrophic result if not recognized early.
- Chronic ischemia may be subtle and presents with the classic triad of weight loss, intestinal angina (pain after eating and food phobia), and a change in bowel habits.
- Acute ischemia has a range of presentations depending on its cause:
  - *Embolic* (usually to SMA)—severe abdominal pain (often out of proportion to the physical examination because of poor localization of pain to palpation) with nausea, vomiting, and diarrhea. Patients may choose a "chin to knee" position and be restless from the pain. As ischemia progresses to perforation, patients may develop peritonitis and a more acute abdominal examination. History should focus on predisposing factors such as atrial fibrillation, dilated cardiomyopathy, or recent aortic instrumentation.
  - *Thrombotic*—usually presents in the setting of acute-on-chronic ischemia where collateral circulation allows for a more subtle onset of vague pain and a change in bowel habits. However, due to diffuse disease of all three major circulations, it may progress to massive infarction. History should focus on occult symptoms of chronic ischemia and other sites of atherosclerosis (i.e., stroke, coronary, or peripheral vascular disease).
  - *Nonocclusive mesenteric ischemia (NOMI)*—occurs in setting of shock and use of vasopressors with a nonspecific presentation of persistent ileus, abdominal distention, melena or hematochezia, and occult sepsis.
  - *Mesenteric vein thrombosis*—onset may be acute or delayed with several weeks' history of vague pain and changed bowel habits. Risk factors include prior abdominal surgery, thrombophilia, history of mesenteric or deep venous thrombosis, malignancy, and cirrhosis.
  - *Miscellaneous causes*—include aortic surgery or dissection, trauma, aneurysms, arteritis or extrinsic compression (low pressure veins are more susceptible and may be seen with severe intestinal distention, volvulus or intussusception, or by tumor).

DIAGNOSIS

- Early diagnosis requires a high index of suspicion and early utilization of appropriate diagnostic testing.
- Clinical presentation can vary from vague abdominal discomfort with a benign examination to overt shock. Laboratory studies are generally not helpful. Leukocytosis is nearly universal but nonspecific while lactate has poor sensitivity and should not delay more definitive diagnostic testing.
- Mesenteric angiography remains the definitive diagnostic test and may provide therapeutic options but is invasive and not always readily available.
  - Emboli are seen as rounded filling defects at arterial branch points.
  - Thrombosis appears as abrupt cutoffs usually near the ostia of larger vessels in the setting of extensive collaterals.
  - NOMI shows diffuse narrowing with a "sausage string" appearance and should have an acute response to papaverine infusion.
  - Venous thrombosis shows decreased portal vein filling in the late phase of infusion.

- Computed tomography (CT) angiography is often the first test of choice in the algorithm of abdominal pain and has the advantage of wide availability and high diagnostic yield but may not be as sensitive or specific as invasive angiography. CT also has the added benefit of evaluating to the condition of the bowel, which has important treatment implications and is not provided by angiography.
- Ultrasound with duplex is the test of choice in chronic ischemia with diagnostic criteria being based on velocity of flow in SMA and celiac artery. In acute ischemia, potential findings of ileus and bowel wall thickening are nonspecific.
- MRI has gained acceptance in diagnosing chronic ischemia but currently is not indicated in the acute setting.
- Abdominal x-ray is insensitive and nonspecific. Supportive information may include ileus, luminal distention, or diffuse calcification of mesenteric vasculature. Classic findings of intestinal wall thickening ("thumbprinting"), pneumatosis intestinalis, and free air are very late findings.

TREATMENT

- First-line therapy is supportive and should always start with the ABCs (airway, breathing, circulation) of resuscitation. Correction of electrolyte abnormalities, placement of a nasogastric tube to decompress the bowel, broad-spectrum antibiotics, and full-dose heparin are also recommended. Analgesia should not be withheld while workup proceeds.
- If no evidence of infarct exists, then angiography may have therapeutic implications. In NOMI, papaverine infusion into the SMA for 24 hours is the treatment of choice. For occlusive etiologies, surgery is still the standard of care but percutaneous procedures including clot suctioning, angioplasty, and stenting and thrombolysis are gaining ground at specialized centers.
- When concern for bowel infarction exists, urgent laparotomy should be performed to evaluate intestinal viability. This can be confirmed with good sensitivity by the character of pulsation of the mesenteric arcade vessels (either manually or with sterile Doppler probe), bleeding, color, and peristalsis.
- Revascularization should be attempted by endarterectomy or, if not successful, bypass. If >6 ft of small bowel is clearly viable then liberal excision of suspect portions may be performed with primary anastomosis. With more extensive involvement, bowel-sparing procedures with delayed reanastomosis may be necessary to prevent long-term dependence on parenteral nutrition. A second exploration within 48 hours will often be necessary to confirm viability of all remaining bowel segments.
- Postoperative care should always be in an intensive care unit. Reperfusion may cause severe SIRS or overt sepsis requiring aggressive fluid resuscitation and vasoactive drugs. Attention should be paid to the risk of developing abdominal compartment syndrome due to bowel edema and massive third spacing of fluid. Parental nutrition may be necessary for prolonged periods. Heparin should be continued and transitioned to warfarin when enteral feeding resumes.
- Further diagnostic testing may include transthoracic or transesophageal echocardiography to look for an embolic source or laboratory testing to rule out a thrombophilia.

PROGNOSIS

- Prognosis is generally poor, with perioperative mortality ranging from 22 to 96% in different case series and is related to the etiology of the ischemia. Venous thrombosis and arterial embolism have better prognosis (postsurgical mortality of 32% and 54%, respectively) compared to arterial thrombosis and NOMI (postsurgical mortality 77% and 73%, respectively).
- These differences are likely related to greater comorbidities associated with the latter two etiologies as well as a more subtle presentation leading to delayed diagnosis and greater bowel involvement at time of intervention.
- For those who survive the perioperative period, they are generally able to return to preoperative levels of function but significant late mortality persists, related to underlying comorbidities.
- Poor prognosis should dissuade pursuit of heroic measures in the elderly: presence of significant comorbidities, advanced shock, or extensive tumor involvement.

BIBLIOGRAPHY

Harkin DW, Lindsay TF. Mesenteric ischemia. In: Hall JB, Schmidt GA, Wood LDH, eds., *Principles of Critical Care*, 3rd ed. New York, NY: McGraw-Hill; 2005:1309–1319.

Schoots IG, Koffeman GI, Legemate DA, et al. Systematic review of survival after acute mesenteric ischaemia according to disease aetiology. *Br J Surg* 2004;91:17–27.

109 ABDOMINAL COMPARTMENT SYNDROME

Michael Moore

KEY POINTS

- Increases in abdominal pressure to a point compromising local and systemic perfusion and impairing pulmonary function can occur in a number of medical and surgical contexts, a circumstance termed as abdominal compartment syndrome.
- Clinicians must have a high index of suspicion for this condition and if clarification is required, bladder pressure can be measured at the bedside as a surrogate for IAP.
- Surgical decompression may be required in the most severely affected patients.

INTRODUCTION AND DEFINITION

- Abdominal compartment syndrome (ACS) can be defined as symptomatic organ dysfunction resulting from increased intra-abdominal pressure (IAP). ACS has been described in patients with multiple medical and surgical conditions.
- ACS is often hard to diagnose because patients are often critically ill and progressive organ dysfunction may be attributed to other causes. Prompt recognition of increased IAP before ACS develops may prevent progressive tissue hypoperfusion, multiple organ dysfunction, and death.
- The reported mortality has been between 42 and 100%.

PATHOPHYSIOLOGY

- Intra-abdominal pressure is normally 0 mmHg.
- IAP is slightly positive in patients on positive pressure ventilation and increases in direct relationship to body mass index.
- As volume of the peritoneal cavity increases, the IAP rises in proportion to the pressure-volume relationship of the abdominal cavity.
- Once a "critical IAP" is reached, abdominal wall compliance decreases and results in a rapid increase in IAP.
- The increased IAP has two important physiologic consequences:
  - Decreased perfusion to the intra-abdominal vascular beds (hepatic, splanchnic, and renal)
  - Increased intrathoracic pressures via mechanical coupling of the intra-abdominal and thoracic cavities through the diaphragm
- Compression of the intra-abdominal vascular beds and increased juxtacardiac and pleural pressures lead to decreased organ perfusion, interfere with cardiac and respiratory function, and lead to clinical ACS.
- The compliance of the abdominal wall tends to limit the rise of IAP and states that are associated with increased compliance may protect against ACS (pregnancy, cirrhosis, morbid obesity).

RISK FACTORS

MEDICAL

- Massive volume resuscitation
- Bowel obstruction
- Pancreatitis
- Massive ascites
- Peritonitis
- Peritoneal dialysis
- Gastric over distention following endoscopy
- Pneumothorax (rare)
- Any condition that results in tissue edema, intraperitoneal or retroperitoneal bleeding, bowel distention, or third spacing of fluids

SURGICAL

- Trauma patients who require massive volume resuscitation
- Laparoscopy
- Postoperative edema
- Liver transplantation
- Abdominal wall restriction (abdominal burns with fascial scaring, MAST [medical antishock trousers] garments)
- Tight surgical closure following laparotomy
- Pneumoperitoneum

CLINICAL MANIFESTATIONS

- Abdominal compartment syndrome can compromise the function of every organ system and organ dysfunction is further exacerbated by the presence of hypotension and shock.

CARDIOVASCULAR

- Direct compression the heart resulting in decreased ventricular compliance and contractility resulting in a decreased cardiac output.
- Elevated IAP decreases venous return by compressing the inferior vena cava (IVC) resulting in peripheral edema, increased risk of venous thrombosis, and decreased cardiac output from the lower venous return.

PULMONARY

- Hypoxemia and hypercarbia are common.
- Extrinsic compression of the pulmonary parenchyma results in atelectasis, decreased oxygen transport, increased intrapulmonary shunt fraction, and increased alveolar dead space.
- Increased peak and mean airway pressure in mechanically ventilated patients.
- Decreased chest wall compliance and tidal volumes result in V/Q mismatching and increased work of breathing.
- Increased risk of pneumonia.

RENAL

- Progressive decline in glomerular filtration rate (GFR) and urine output directly related to IAP.
- Oliguria develops at IAP of 15 mmHg.
- Anuria develops at IAP of 30 mmHg.
- Results in "prerenal" picture with FE_{Na} (fractional excretion of sodium) <1%.
- Mediated via increased venous resistance and arterial vasoconstriction mediated by sympathetic and renin-aldosterone systems.

GASTROINTESTINAL

- Gastrointestinal (GI) system is the most sensitive to changes in IAP.
- Mesenteric blood flow is compromised at relatively low levels of IAP and results in intestinal mucosal ischemia.
- IAP causes compression of mesenteric veins promoting venous hypertension and edema.
- Intestinal edema further increases IAP and can result in a vicious cycle of worsening hypoperfusion and ischemia.
- Gut hypoperfusion results in loss of mucosal barrier which may contribute to bacterial translocation, sepsis, and multisystem organ failure.

HEPATIC

- Decreased hepatic perfusion
- Decreased lactate clearance

CENTRAL NERVOUS SYSTEM

- Increased IAP increases central venous pressure (CVP) and will increase intracranial pressure.
- High CVP in setting of hypotension may result in decreased cerebral perfusion pressure and progressive cerebral edema.

DIAGNOSIS

- Suspect diagnosis with clinical syndrome of tense abdominal distention with the signs and symptoms of splanchnic hypoperfusion, systemic hypoperfusion, or increased work of breathing.
- Physical examination findings have sensitivity of only 40%.
- Chest x-ray (CXR) findings of small lung volumes, atelectasis, and elevated hemidiaphragms are suggestive.
- Computed tomography (CT) findings include tense infiltration of the retroperitoneum out of proportion to peritoneal disease, extrinsic compression of the IVC, massive abdominal distention, direct real compression or displacement, bowel wall thickening, and bilateral inguinal herniation.
- Neither physical examination nor imaging studies are adequate for diagnosis.
- The gold standard is to indirectly measure the IAP by transducing the intra-abdominal bladder pressure (IAPB).

INTRA-ABDOMINAL BLADDER PRESSURE MEASUREMENT

- Bladder acts as a passive reservoir that can transmit IAP using the bladder wall as a transducing membrane.
- IABP is well correlated with directly measured IAP (Fig. 109-1).
- Technique:
  - Instill 50 mL of sterile water into the bladder via a Foley catheter with the drainage tube clamped.
  - Insert an 18-gauge needle connected to a pressure transducer into the aspiration port of the catheter.
  - Measure the pressure with the transducer zeroed at the level of the pubic symphysis.

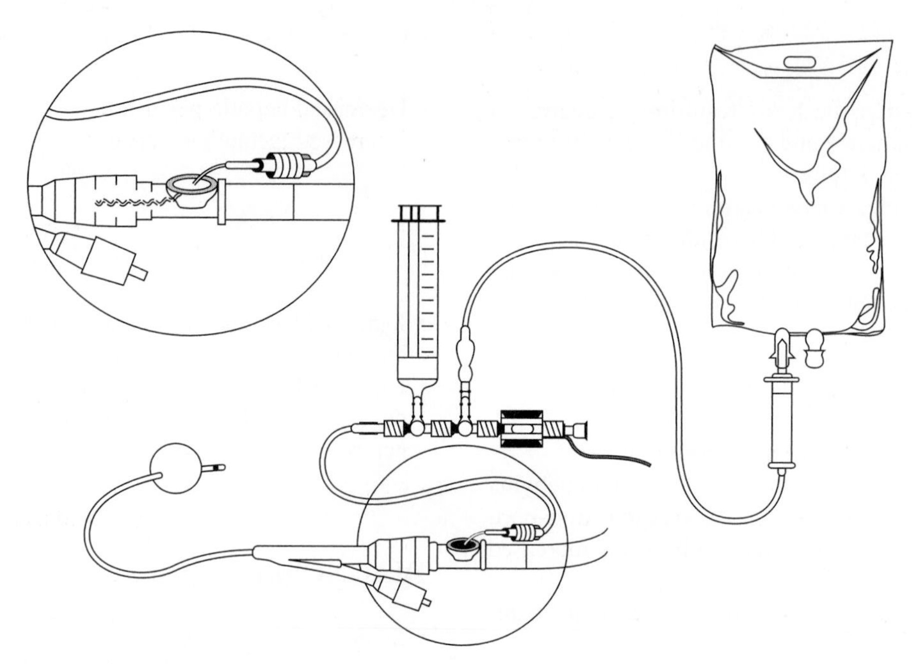

FIG. 109-1 Bladder transduction system. Using a patient Foley catheter with clamped drainage tube, 50–100 mL sterile water is infused into the bladder via a three-way stopcock system. The bladder pressure measured with a transducer correlates well with directly measured IAP.

- Certain clinical states may interfere with accurate measurements:
  - Intraperitoneal adhesions
  - Pelvic hematomas
  - Pelvic fractures
  - Abdominal packing
  - Neurogenic bladder
- Certain clinical states associated with chronic intra-abdominal hypertension (IAH) (pregnancy, morbid obesity, and ascites) complicate the diagnosis of ACS while small increases in IAP in this setting may be tolerated less well.
- The critical IAP varies from patient to patient and within patients based on severity of illness so no single value in individual patients can accurately diagnose ACS.
- In general, an IABP ≤10 mmHg rules out ACS and >25 mmHg rules in ACS.

TREATMENT

- Successful management requires attention to prevention, maintaining a high index of suspicion, and early recognition with prompt decompression.
- Preventative techniques include temporary abdominal closure following laparotomy in surgical patients and avoiding supranormal resuscitation of critically ill medical patients.
- Low threshold for checking bladder pressures in patients at risk for or suspected of having ACS.
- Follow patients with elevated IAP with serial measurements.
- ACS secondary to tense ascites may be managed with serial or large volume paracentesis.
- Supportive care including endotracheal intubation and mechanical ventilation.
- When positive end-expiratory pressure (PEEP) is required to maintain adequate oxygenation, use the least PEEP associated with a nontoxic Fio_2.
- Volume resuscitation will, at least temporarily, improve cardiac output, pulmonary function, renal function, and visceral perfusion but may also be associated with worse outcome.
- Definitive management for ACS is surgical decompression and maintenance of an open abdomen with temporary wall closure.
- The critical IAP that identifies the need for decompressive laparotomy, the timing, and procedure of choice are not well defined.

BIBLIOGRAPHY

Balogh Z, McKinley BA, Cocanour CS, et al. Patients with impending abdominal compartment syndrome do not respond to early volume loading. *Am J Surg* 2003;186:602–607.

Cullen DJ, Coyle JP, Teplick R, et al. Cardiovascular, pulmonary and renal effects of massively increased intra-abdominal pressure in critically ill patients. *Crit Care Med* 1989;17:118–121.
Hall JB, Schmidt, GA, Wood LDH. *Principles of Critical Care*, 3rd ed. New York, NY: McGraw-Hill; 2005:1123–1136.
Hong JJ, Cohn SM, Perez JM, et al. Prospective study of the incidence and outcome of the abdominal compartment syndrome. *Br J Surg* 2002;89:591–596.
Kirkpatrick AW, Brenneman FD, McLean RF, et al. Is clinical examination an accurate indicator of raised intra-abdominal pressure in critically injured patients? *Can J Surg* 2000;43:207–211.
Malbrain ML. Different techniques to measure intra-abdominal pressure (IAP): time for a critical re-appraisal. *Intensive Care Med* 2004;30:357–371.
Pickhardt PJ, Shimony JS, Heiken JP, et al. The abdominal compartment syndrome: CT findings. *AJR Am J Roentgenol* 1999;173:575–579.
Sanchez NC, Tenofsky PL, Dort JM, et al. What is normal intra-abdominal pressure? *Am Surg* 2001;67:243–248.

110 INFLAMMATORY BOWEL DISEASE

Timothy L. Zisman

KEY POINTS

- Inflammatory bowel disease consists of two separate but related diseases of the bowel, Ulcerative Colitis (UC) and Crohn's Disease (CD).
- IBD can have serious complications associated both with the underlying disease process as well as the disease treatments.
- Complications of the GI tract include massive hemorrhage, toxic megacolon, bowel obstruction, fistula formation, intra-abdominal abscess, and bowel perforation.
- Immunosuppressive and cytotoxic medications used to treat IBD can predispose patients to a variety of infectious complications.
- Extraintestinal manifestations of IBD include peripheral and axial arthritis, ocular disease, aphthous ulcers, erythema nodosum, pyoderma gangrenosum, PSC, venous thrombosis, and pulmonary fibrosis.

EPIDEMIOLOGY AND GENETICS

- Crohn disease (CD) has an annual incidence of approximately 3–8 per 100,000 persons, with a prevalence of 1 in 1–2000. Ulcerative colitis (UC) has an annual incidence of 2–12 per 100,000 persons, with a prevalence of 1 in 1–2000.
- Disease onset occurs in a bimodal distribution, with the largest peak at age 15–25 and a second smaller peak later in life at age 50–80.
- The incidence of inflammatory bowel disease (IBD) is much higher in developed countries than in the developing world. Within a given country the incidence appears to be higher in the northern regions.
- IBD is more common in Jewish than non-Jewish populations. Prevalence amongst whites and blacks is higher than among Asians, Hispanics, and Native Americans.
- CD is slightly more common in women, whereas UC is slightly more common in men.
- Familial aggregation of IBD has been well established. Approximately 20% of IBD patients are able to identify another family member with IBD. Amongst monozygotic twins, the concordance rate is 58% for CD and 6–18% for UC.
- Interestingly, tobacco use appears to offer a symptomatic protective effect for patients with UC. Disease onset is often associated with smoking cessation, in many cases as far as a few years after stopping smoking.
- Investigations into the genetics of IBD have identified mutations in the NOD2 gene on chromosome 16 which appear to confer susceptibility to ileal and stricturing CD.

CLINICAL FEATURES

ULCERATIVE COLITIS

- The inflammation in UC invariably involves the rectum, with extension of disease proximally in a contiguous distribution. Approximately 50% of patients have disease limited to the rectum and sigmoid colon, 30% have involvement of the descending colon as well, and 20% have extensive involvement of the entire colon.
- Bowel inflammation outside the colon does not occur in UC, with the exception of "backwash ileitis," an inflammation of the distal terminal ileum seen in some patients with extensive colitis.
- Patients with UC often report hematochezia, diarrhea associated with urgency and nocturnal awakenings, abdominal cramping, bloating, poor appetite, and weight loss.
- Physical examination may reveal fever, tachycardia, dehydration, and signs of anemia. A tender and distended abdomen with absent bowel sounds may suggest toxic dilatation of the colon.
- Serologic studies may demonstrate anemia, an elevated erythrocyte sedimentation rate, and hypoalbuminemia.
- Stool analysis will reveal gross blood with presence of fecal leukocytes. Stool culture and examination for ova and parasites will be negative.

TABLE 110-1 Clinical Features of CD and UC

	CD	UC
Pattern of distribution	Patchy, discontinuous areas of inflammation	Contiguous from rectum, extending proximally
Involved bowel	Anywhere from mouth to anus, most commonly in terminal ileum	Large intestine only
Thickness	Transmural	Mucosa only
Endoscopic findings	Ulcers in otherwise normal mucosa, cobblestoning	Friable mucosa, ulcers only in inflamed mucosa
Biopsy	Granulomatous inflammation	Neutrophilic infiltrate, crypt abscesses
Major complications	Fistulas, strictures, abscesses, bowel obstruction	Massive hemorrhage, toxic megacolon, bowel perforation

- Endoscopic findings may show edematous, granular, erythematous, and friable mucosa with areas of gross ulceration. Dysplasia in UC often appears as flat lesions and may be difficult to identify. Although not done routinely, colonoscopy can be safely performed in patients with acute severe colitis.
- Biopsy of the colon demonstrates superficial inflammation involving only the mucosa. Common findings include alteration of crypt architecture with neutrophilic infiltrate and crypt abscesses (Table 110-1).

CROHN'S DISEASE

- Crohn disease is an inflammatory condition of the bowel that can occur anywhere along the gastrointestinal (GI) tract from mouth to anus. Thirty percent of patients have disease confined to the small bowel, 25% have only colonic involvement, and 40% have both small and large bowel inflammation.
- Patients frequently report abdominal pain and cramping, diarrhea, low-grade fever, poor appetite, and weight loss. Hematochezia is less common than with UC.
- Physical examination may be significant for weight loss, dehydration, abdominal tenderness, and a right lower quadrant mass. Perianal examination may show skin tags, fissures, enterocutaneous fistula tracts, or perirectal abscesses.
- High-grade fever and a tender abdominal mass may represent intra-abdominal abscess and should prompt further investigation.
- Laboratory studies may show leukocytosis, anemia (from iron deficiency, chronic disease, or vitamin B_{12} deficiency), hypoalbuminemia, and elevated acute phase reactants.
- Patients with extensive small bowel involvement may have steatorrhea with consequent vitamin deficiencies. Laboratory findings in these patients may reveal hypocalcemia, prolongation of the prothrombin time, and hyperoxaluria with nephrolithiasis.
- Endoscopic features characteristically include discrete ulcers in normal mucosa, linear ulcerations, discontinuous areas of involvement, rectal sparing, strictures, and "cobblestoning."
- Classic histologic findings include aphthoid ulcers overlying lymphoid follicles, lymphoid aggregates and fibrosis of the bowel wall, and granuloma formation.
- Radiologic studies may aid in diagnosis or in assessment of extent and severity of disease. Computed tomography (CT) often reveals bowel wall thickening with adjacent fat stranding, and is superior to ultrasound for identifying intra-abdominal abscesses. Small bowel series may be useful in identifying areas of stricture or fistula tracts (Table 110-1).

DIAGNOSIS

- Both UC and CD are diagnosed clinically, taking into consideration the sum of available evidence, including the patient's signs and symptoms, as well as endoscopic, histologic, and radiologic features.
- Anti-*Saccharomyces cerevisiae* antibodies (ASCA) and perinuclear antineutrophil cytoplasmic antibodies (p-ANCA) have been proposed as serologic tests for CD and UC, respectively. However, due to inadequate sensitivity and specificity these tests are not currently recommended for routine use as either a screening or diagnostic tool.

EXTRAINTESTINAL MANIFESTATIONS

- Ocular findings include uveitis and iritis, which tend to occur independent of bowel disease activity, and episcleritis, which is more coincident with active bowel symptoms.
- Cutaneous manifestations include oral aphthous ulcers, erythema nodosum, and pyoderma gangrenosum.
- Peripheral arthritis is a common feature of IBD that occurs in approximately 20% of patients, and the severity of joint inflammation correlates with the activity of bowel disease. Typically, the large joints are involved, especially knees ankles, hips, and shoulders.

IBD patients are also at increased risk for an axial arthritis akin to ankylosing spondylitis, which occurs in 3–5% of patients and is independent of bowel disease activity.

- Bronchopulmonary disease is uncommon in IBD but is becoming increasingly recognized. Inflammations of the airways, pulmonary parenchyma, and pleura have all been reported and are attributed both to the disease itself as well as the medications used to treat IBD.
- Hepatobiliary manifestations in patients with UC include primary sclerosing cholangitis (PSC) which may progress to liver failure or be complicated by cholangiocarcinoma. Crohn patients are predisposed to develop cholelithiasis which results from depletion of bile salts in patients with inflammation or surgical resection of the terminal ileum.
- Anemia is quite common in IBD patients and may be multifactorial in etiology. Chronic blood loss can lead to iron deficiency, whereas chronic inflammation can result in anemia of chronic disease. CD patients may also have vitamin B_{12} deficiency with consequent megaloblastic anemia.
- Hypercoagulability associated with IBD predisposes to venous, and occasionally arterial, thromboembolism.
- Osteopenia and osteoporosis are common in IBD and are related both to calcium malabsorption and chronic steroid use. Low body weight may exacerbate problems with decreased bone mineral density.
- Nephrolithiasis, particularly with calcium oxalate stones, may complicate CD. Impaired reabsorption of bile salts may result in intraluminal chelation of calcium, with consequent increased absorption of oxalate.
- Immunosuppression is a common side effect of many of the medications used to treat IBD, particularly glucocorticoids, azathioprine (AZA), 6-mercaptopurine (6-MP), infliximab, and cyclosporine. Consequently, patients are at increased risk for a variety of infections with ordinary pathogens and opportunistic organisms.

BOWEL COMPLICATIONS

FULMINANT COLITIS AND TOXIC MEGACOLON

- Approximately 10–15% of UC patients develop fulminant colitis, characterized by severe diarrhea (>10 bowel movements daily), hemorrhage requiring transfusion, high fever, tachycardia, dehydration, marked abdominal tenderness, and leukocytosis.
- A severely dilated colon of more than 6 cm on abdominal x-ray, associated with absent peristalsis, an acute abdomen, and signs of systemic toxicity are worrisome findings suggestive of toxic megacolon.
- Development of toxic megacolon may be precipitated by hypokalemia or by the use of narcotic, antidiarrheal, or anticholinergic medications in patients with fulminant colitis.
- Abdominal radiograph may show "thumbprinting" from bowel wall edema or pneumatosis.
- In addition to supportive care with fluids, electrolytes, and blood products, initial management should include serial abdominal examinations and radiographs, and decompression of the bowel with nasogastric suction.
- Intravenous corticosteroids should be continued and may mask signs of systemic toxicity.
- Broad-spectrum antibiotics with sensitivity against gram negatives and anaerobes should be administered in anticipation of possible peritonitis or perforation.
- Signs of decreasing peristalsis or worsening bowel dilatation may indicate impending perforation that should prompt urgent surgical evaluation. Likewise, failure to improve within 48–72 hours despite aggressive medical therapy is an indication for surgical intervention. Free air under the diaphragm on upright chest radiography indicates perforation and requires urgent surgical intervention.
- With prompt recognition, close monitoring, and aggressive medical and surgical therapy, the mortality rate associated with fulminant colitis and toxic megacolon has been reduced to 6%.

COLON CANCER

- Colorectal carcinoma is a well-established long-term complication of UC. The association between CD and cancer has been increasingly reported and is now accepted as well.
- The risk of cancer in UC increases with the duration of disease and is estimated to be 2% at 10 years of disease, 8% at 20 years, and 18% at 30 years.
- Factors associated with an increased risk of colon cancer include longer duration of disease, younger age at diagnosis, greater extent of disease, family history of colorectal cancer (independent of a history of IBD), and the presence of PSC.
- Evidence from observational studies suggests that regular use of 5-aminosalycylate medications and folate may provide chemoprotection against colon cancer.
- Unlike in sporadic colorectal carcinoma, malignant lesions in IBD do not arise from polyps, but rather from areas of dysplasia in flat mucosa.
- Patients with IBD should undergo periodic surveillance colonoscopies beginning 8–10 years after disease onset with the goal of identifying potentially malignant lesions at a precancerous stage when surgical cure is still feasible.

- Patients with low-grade or high-grade dysplasia on colonoscopy should be referred for surgery because of the high rate of progression to frank carcinoma.

FISTULAS/ABSCESSES

- The transmural inflammation in CD can lead to fistula tracts between the bowel and adjacent anatomic structures. Fistulas and abscesses are not part of the clinical picture in UC.
- Enterovesical or enterovaginal fistulas can lead to recurrent infections.
- Enteroenteric or enterocolic fistulas may result in bacterial overgrowth with consequent diarrhea, malabsorption, and weight loss.
- Fistulas to the mesentery may cause intra-abdominal abscesses that typically manifest as fever and a tender abdominal mass.
- Computed tomography is more sensitive than ultrasound for identifying abscesses.
- Abscesses, if present, require percutaneous or surgical drainage as well as antibiotic therapy.

BOWEL OBSTRUCTION

- Obstruction may complicate stricturing CD, especially of the small bowel.
- Patients often present with postprandial crampy abdominal pain, bloating, and distention.
- Nasogastric tube insertion with low intermittent suction is advised to decompress the bowel.
- Although medical therapy may be attempted, most patients will require surgery to alleviate their obstruction.

HEMORRHAGE

- Severe hemorrhage requiring transfusion can be seen in 10–15% of UC patients. The incidence in CD is much lower.
- Initial management of massive hemorrhage is similar to non-IBD patients, and involves immediate resuscitation and correction of coagulopathy with intravenous fluids and blood products.

MALABSORPTION

- Loss of bile salts may occur in Crohn patients with active inflammation or prior resection of the terminal ileum, leading to malabsorption and steatorrhea.
- Patients may develop nutritional deficiencies, especially from poor absorption of fat-soluble vitamins.
- Loss of fluids can result in profound dehydration and electrolyte disturbances, especially hypokalemia.
- Surgical resection of the small bowel decreases the absorptive area of the gut and, if extensive, can result in the short gut syndrome with consequent malnutrition and weight loss. Total parenteral nutrition may be necessary to meet metabolic requirements.

COMPLICATIONS OF EXTRAINTESTINAL DISEASE

PULMONARY DISEASE

- Involvement of the respiratory system in IBD is relatively uncommon, but is being increasingly recognized, especially in association with UC.
- Pulmonary involvement may manifest as airway inflammation, lung parenchymal disease, or pleuritis.
- Airway inflammation can occur in the large or small airways, and often presents as cough with or without sputum production and wheezing.
- Bronchiolitis obliterans with organizing pneumonia (BOOP) presents as fever, cough, shortness of breath, and pleuritic chest pain.
- Interstitial lung disease may manifest as dyspnea. Chest CT may show interstitial opacities.
- Sulfasalazine, one of the mainstays of pharmacotherapy for IBD, has been associated with eosinophilic pulmonary infiltrates.

PRIMARY SCLEROSING CHOLANGITIS

- Primary sclerosing cholangitis is an idiopathic inflammatory condition of the biliary tree that leads to fibrosis and stricturing of the intra- and extrahepatic bile ducts.
- PSC occurs in only 1–4% of UC patients. However, 70% of patients with PSC have IBD, predominantly UC.
- Patients may present with signs or symptoms of obstructive jaundice, or they may have asymptomatic elevation of alkaline phosphatase on routine labs.
- Serious long-term complications of PSC include progression to biliary cirrhosis, and development of cholangiocarcinoma in up to 15% of patients.
- Medical therapy with ursodeoxycholic acid may provide symptomatic benefit but does not alter the progression of disease.
- Biliary stricturing may be managed with endoscopic dilatation and stent placement initially. However, liver transplantation is the procedure of choice once cirrhosis develops.

IMMUNOSUPPRESSION

- Many of the medications used to treat IBD can cause serious immunosuppression that places patients at risk for infections with typical and opportunistic pathogens.
- The differential diagnosis and empiric antibiotic coverage should remain broad for IBD patients on immunosuppressive medications who appear infected.

MEDICAL THERAPY

5-AMINOSALICYLATES

- Mesalamine, sulfasalazine, olsalazine, and balsalazide are all derivatives of 5-aminosalicylic acid (5-ASA), and are considered the mainstay of therapy for patients with IBD.
- 5-ASA medications are first-line agents for both induction of remission and maintenance in mild to moderately active UC and CD.
- Regular use of 5-ASA products may reduce the risk colorectal carcinoma in patients with IBD, suggesting an additional role for these medications as chemopreventive agents.
- While the sulfapyridine moiety in sulfasalazine is associated with a fair amount of adverse effects, the other 5-ASA medications are generally well tolerated with only minor side effects.

CORTICOSTEROIDS

- Corticosteroids are highly effective in inducing remission for both UC and CD, however, the side effects associated with chronic therapy preclude their use as maintenance medications.
- Ideally, steroids should be initiated for disease flares and then be tapered after 2–3 weeks. Many patients, however, are unable to withdraw completely from steroids. In these patients, it is appropriate to initiate steroid-sparing agents such as AZA or 6-MP.
- Budesonide is an oral steroid that acts topically in the gut, and subsequently undergoes significant first-pass metabolism in the liver, thereby limiting systemic effects. It is effective for inducing remission in ileal CD, but should not be used as maintenance therapy.
- Intravenous corticosteroids should be reserved for patients with severe disease requiring admission to the hospital. After symptomatic improvement, patients can transition to oral steroids and begin a taper.

IMMUNOMODULATORS

- Azathioprine is a prodrug that is metabolically converted to 6-MP. Both AZA and 6-MP therapy have a role as steroid-sparing agents in the long-term management of patients who are unable to taper completely off of oral corticosteroids.
- These medicines take 3–6 months for peak effect and should therefore be started well before steroid tapering is undertaken.
- Approximately 1 in 10 patients will have to discontinue these medications due to significant side effects including bone marrow suppression, hepatitis, pancreatitis, rash, or infections.
- Deficiency of thiopurine-*S*-methyltransferase (TPMT), the enzyme that metabolizes AZA and 6-MP, is present in 1 in 300 people and can predispose to life-threatening bone marrow suppression.
- Methotrexate has also been shown to be effective in inducing remission, but its use is mainly limited by side effects and the greater convenience of other immunomodulatory drugs.

CYCLOSPORINE

- Cyclosporine should be reserved for patients with severe or fulminant colitis who fail to respond to an appropriate course of intravenous steroids.
- Although initial clinical response to cyclosporine is good, many of these patients will go on to have relapse of colitis that ultimately requires colectomy.

ANTIBIOTICS

- Antibiotics may be helpful as adjuvant therapy in the management of CD patients with active colonic involvement or with fistulizing disease.
- Ciprofloxacin and metronidazole are the best-studied antibiotics, although rifaximin is being increasingly studied with encouraging results.

TUMOR NECROSIS FACTOR-ALPHA INHIBITORS

- Infliximab is a chimeric monoclonal antibody directed against human tumor necrosis factor-alpha (TNF-alpha).
- TNF-alpha has been implicated as a key mediator in the inflammatory cascade of CD, and inhibition of TNF-alpha with infliximab has been shown to improve endoscopic and histologic inflammation in CD patients.

TABLE 110-2 Major Side Effects of Medications Used to Treat IBD

MEDICATION	MAJOR SIDE EFFECT
Sulfasalazine	Nausea, headache, fever, rash, male infertility, hypersensitivity reaction (in sulfa-allergic patients), pancreatitis, agranulocytosis, pericarditis, pneumonitis
5-Aminosalicylates	Fever, rash, pancreatitis, pneumonitis
Corticosteroids	Lymphopenia, osteopenia, avascular necrosis, impaired wound healing, gastritis, hyperglycemia, hypertension (HTN), accelerated atherosclerosis
AZA and 6-MP	Fever/rash, pancreatitis, nausea, bone marrow suppression, hepatitis, infections
Methotrexate	Nausea, abdominal pain, joint pain, myelosuppression, hepatotoxicity
Cyclosporine	Nephrotoxicity, HTN, hyperglycemia, infections, neurotoxicity
Infliximab	Infusion reactions, immunosuppression, life-threatening infections, hepatotoxicity, possible lymphoproliferative disorder

- Infliximab is currently recommended for both induction and maintenance of remission in CD patients with moderate to severe disease activity, or with fistulizing disease, who fail to respond to conventional therapy.
- Common side effects include acute infusion reactions (shortness of breath, hypotension, urticaria, fever), delayed hypersensitivity reactions, drug-induced autoantibodies, arthralgias, rash, GI upset, and minor infections.
- Serious adverse effects include severe or life-threatening infections (4%), bone marrow suppression, hepatotoxicity, and a possible association with lymphoma (Table 110-2).

SURGICAL MANAGEMENT

ULCERATIVE COLITIS

- Surgical removal of the colon should be considered for patients with disease refractory to medical treatment or for those who develop massive hemorrhage, perforation, toxic megacolon, dysplasia, or frank adenocarcinoma of the colon.
- Approximately one in four patients with UC will eventually require surgery.
- Surgery, if undertaken, should consist of total abdominal colectomy, and is considered curative.
- In the majority of cases, patients are able to maintain intestinal continuity with the construction of an ileal J-pouch that is anastomosed to the anal canal. These patients typically will have 4–6 soft bowel movements daily with normal bowel continence.
- Approximately 50% of these patients will develop an inflammatory condition of the ileal pouch called "pouchitis" that symptomatically mimics their UC and is usually responsive to antibiotic therapy with either ciprofloxacin or metronidazole.
- In patients who are unable to have ileal pouch anal anastomosis, an ileostomy is created. The major complication of ileostomy formation is local skin breakdown.

CROHN DISEASE

- Surgery should be considered in patients with intractable symptoms despite medical therapy, strictures with obstruction, enterovesical or enterovaginal fistula formation, intra-abdominal abscesses, massive hemorrhage, or colorectal carcinoma.
- Approximately three of four patients with CD will eventually require surgical intervention.
- Surgery is not curative for CD, and every effort should be made to spare as much bowel as possible from resection. Techniques such as stricturoplasty can be employed to limit the need for resection.
- Surgical anastomoses are often sites of disease recurrence.
- Complications of surgery include short gut syndrome with consequent nutritional deficiency.
- Following surgical resection of diseased bowel, patients should be placed on medication for maintenance of remission.

BIBLIOGRAPHY

Bamias G, Nyce MR, De La Rue SA, et al. New concepts in the pathophysiology of inflammatory bowel disease. *Ann Intern Med* 2005;143:895–904.

Domenech E. Inflammatory bowel disease: current therapeutic options. *Digestion* 2006;73:67–76.

Hanauer SB. Inflammatory bowel disease: epidemiology, pathogenesis, and therapeutic opportunities. *Inflamm Bowel Dis* 2006;12:S3–S9.

Section 9

THE SURGICAL PATIENT

111 ACUTE ABDOMEN

Nina M. Patel

KEY POINTS

- Intra-abdominal crises may present in subtle ways in patients in the ICU.
- Early diagnosis is essential to optimize outcome.
- A low threshold for imaging the abdomen with ultrasonographic or CT techniques should exist.
- A patient with signs and symptoms of sepsis and who does not have a plausible source identified outside of the abdomen should be evaluated for the possibility of an intra-abdominal source.

DEFINITION

- The "acute abdomen" is defined as the sudden onset of severe abdominal pain.

CLINICAL FEATURES

- Patients in the ICU are often unable to verbally express pain due to endotracheal intubation, sedation, and/or compromised mental status. Consequently, the clinical presentation of the acute abdomen in an ICU patient is vastly different than that in an outpatient.
- Nonspecific findings, including fever, hemodynamic instability, abdominal distention, and unexplained sepsis may be surrogate markers of an acute abdomen.
- If clinical suspicion for an abdominal emergency is present, prompt diagnostic evaluation should be effected with radiologic imaging (generally abdominal computed tomography [CT] or ultrasound [US]) and/or gastroenterologic and surgical consultation.

DIFFERENTIAL DIAGNOSIS

- Traditional causes of the acute abdomen can be classified into categories based on the etiology and quality of the pain: inflammatory (e.g., appendicitis and diverticulitis), colicky (e.g., biliary or renal), vascular (e.g., mesenteric ischemia), urologic/gynecologic, or related to systemic disease (e.g., sickle cell crisis).
- This chapter will focus on a number of causes of intra-abdominal sepsis (IAS) that are specific to the ICU setting:
    - Primary peritonitis
    - Secondary peritonitis
    - Biliary sepsis
    - Intra-abdominal abscess—intravisceral or extravisceral
    - Occult IAS

PATHOPHYIOLOGY, DIAGNOSIS, AND THERAPY

- Primary peritonitis is a spontaneous phenomenon that occurs most frequently in patients with ascites due to congestive heart failure, cirrhosis, or renal failure. It can also occur consequent to more esoteric causes (e.g., tuberculosis [TB] peritonitis).
    - It is speculated that infection results from a hematogenous source or from bacterial translocation across the intestinal wall.
    - Diagnosis is based on clinical suspicion and paracentesis. Ascites fluid reveals a neutrophil count of >250 and/or a positive culture. Aerobic, enteric organisms are the most commonly isolated infectious agents.
    - Empiric antibiotic therapy should be initiated while awaiting culture results, with either an aminoglycoside, a third-generation cephalosporin, or ciprofloxacin + enterococcal coverage (e.g., ampicillin). A response to therapy is marked by a decline in the ascitic neutrophil count.

- Secondary peritonitis results from inflammation of the peritoneal lining secondary to polymicrobial infection and/or chemical irritation of the peritoneal lining (e.g., bile). Visceral inflammation and/or perforation (e.g., bowel infarction and gallbladder perforation), retroperitoneal pathology (e.g., infected pancreatic pseudocyst), and postoperative complications (e.g., wound dehiscence) are frequent causes of secondary peritonitis.
  - Patients may experience substantial fluid shifts into the abdomen with subsequent hypovolemia.
  - A plain film of the abdomen should be performed in the initial evaluation, as a rapid means of assessing for the presence of free air under the diaphragm.
  - Rapid intervention with surgical treatment, however, is frequently the only way to diagnose and/or correct the primary process. As such, patients often proceed to laparoscopy prior to obtaining imaging studies.
  - Although few patients will respond to medical therapy alone, broad-spectrum antibiotic coverage (gram-negative, gram-positive, and anaerobic organisms) is necessary as adjunctive therapy pre-, peri-, and postoperatively to treat IAS and/or systemic bacteremia.
  - Aggressive supportive care with antibiotic therapy, intravenous fluid (IVF) hydration and hemodynamic support, enteral feeding (as tolerated), and renal replacement therapy (if necessary) are essential components of the intensivist's care.
  - If fever, bandemia, or ileus fail to regress with appropriate surgical and medical therapy, postoperative complications (e.g., wound dehiscence, abscess, and enterocutaneous fistula) or the possibility of extraperitoneal infection should be considered.
  - Prior to postoperative days 5–7, repeat surgical exploration is necessary if clinical symptoms and abdominal examination are not regressing. Abdominal CT may be helpful in delineating complications after this time point.
  - Risk of wound dehiscence is greatest at postoperative days 4–8.
- Biliary sepsis is a consequence of (a) acute calculous cholecystitis, (b) ascending cholangitis, and (c) acalculous cholecystitis.
  - Diagnosis of biliary sepsis may first be inferred by the presence of jaundice and hyperbilirubinemia. Appropriate initial triage includes liver function testing (LFT) and right upper quadrant (RUQ) US. Acute calculous cholecystitis seldom necessitates ICU intervention.
  - Acute cholangitis, characterized by fever, RUQ pain, and jaundice, is an infection within the biliary ductal system due to biliary obstruction and stasis. If RUQ US does not demonstrate biliary ductal dilatation in the appropriate clinical setting, patients may require endoscopic retrograde cholangiopancreatography (ERCP) or percutaneous transhepatic cholangiography (PTC) for diagnosis. Biliary decompression is the definitive therapy and should be pursued emergently with sphincterotomy, stent placement, or T-tube placement. Patients should be concurrently treated with broad-spectrum antibiotic coverage (gram negatives, *Enterococcus* species).
  - Acalculous cholecystitis is an indolent process that occurs in 0.5–1.5% of patients who are hospitalized in the ICU for >1 week.
  - It is characterized by gallbladder wall inflammation and infection with enteric organisms as well as cystic duct edema and functional occlusion due to increased viscosity of bile.
    - Preventive measures are limited as the pathophysiology of this process is not well understood.
    - The utility of most diagnostic tests is limited in acalculous cholecystitis. LFTs do not aid in diagnosis, and US or CT may show a thickened gallbladder wall, pericholecystic fluid, or intramural gas. Hydroxy iminodiacetic acid (HIDA) scan can be helpful by ascertaining patency of the cystic duct.
    - Unrecognized acalculous cholecystitis will proceed to complete gallbladder necrosis. Therefore, if clinical suspicion is high, patients should proceed rapidly to the operating room (OR) for cholecystectomy. If deemed too ill for the OR, percutaneous drainage can be performed as a temporizing measure.
- Intra-abdominal abscesses may be visceral or extravisceral.
  - Visceral abscesses (e.g., hepatic or splenic) may result from hematogenous seeding or direct extension of an infectious process.
  - Extravisceral abscesses are most often due to postoperative complications, though they also can develop from direct extension.
  - Presentation tends to be nonspecific, with fever, ileus, and occasionally abdominal pain or peritoneal signs.
  - Abdominal CT or US are the diagnostic tests of choice, and US the preferred test to visualize pelvic fluid collections.
  - Therapy consists of broad-spectrum antibiotic coverage with percutaneous or surgical drainage/resection of the fluid collection.
- Occult IAS
  - Microabscesses, short segments of infarcted bowel, or bacterial translocation from the gastrointestinal (GI) tract are all postulated etiologies of IAS of unknown cause.

  - Radiologic imaging is likely to be unhelpful in making a diagnosis of occult IAS. Similarly, blind laparoscopy to seek out a cause of IAS is also unlikely to improve patient outcome.

CONCLUSIONS

- Intensivists must maintain a high level of suspicion to diagnose an acute abdomen in the ICU.
- Diagnosis is often challenging and necessitates a low threshold to proceed to radiologic imaging and/or surgical consultation.
- Treatment consists of supportive medical therapy and broad-spectrum antibiotic coverage, often in concert with percutaneous drainage and/or surgical intervention.
- If a patient's clinical course is not improving following "definitive" therapy, the intensivist should pursue evaluation of postoperative complications.
- If no intra-abdominal source of sepsis is found and extra-abdominal sepsis has been effectively ruled out, occult sources of IAS should be considered.

BIBLIOGRAPHY

Achkar E. Abdominal pain. In: Andreoli TE, Carpenter CJ, Griggs RC, et al., eds., *Cecil Essentials of Medicine*, 5th ed. Philadelphia, PA: W.B. Saunders; 2000:303–305.

Marincek B. Nontraumatic abdominal emergencies: acute abdominal pain: diagnostic strategies. *Eur Radiol* 2002;12:2136–2150.

Mustard RA, Bohnen JMA, Schouten BD. The acute abdomen and intra-abdominal sepsis. In: Hall JB, Schmidt GA, Wood LDH, eds., *Principles of Critical Care*, 3rd ed. New York, NY: McGraw-Hill; 2005: 1345–1353.

112 COMPLICATIONS OF SOLID ORGAN TRANSPLANTATION

Nathan Sandbo

KEY POINTS

- The immunosuppressive regimens used for solid organ transplantation result in a high incidence of infectious complications in certain patient groups, and the time from transplant is useful to consider potential infecting organisms.
- Each transplanted organ has a characteristic pattern of rejection, which is generally characterized as acute or chronic, with adjustment of immunosuppression determined in part by the time course.

GENERAL ASPECTS

- Over 25,000 solid organ transplants (kidney, liver, heart, lung, pancreas, small intestine) were performed in 2003, with 1 year survival at ~90% for most recipients, with the exception of lung (~70%).
- Immunosuppressive agents usually fall into four main categories, each with unique toxicities.
  - Corticosteroids, which are commonly used in high doses in the initial posttransplant period, and then are slowly tapered. They are also commonly used in pulse doses to treat episodes of acute rejection. The most common side effects include insulin resistance, impaired wound healing, and adrenal insufficiency.
  - Calcineurin inhibitors, which are commonly part of the initial immunosuppression regimen. Cyclosporine is the founding member of this class, but tacrolimus is a more recent agent, which is often employed to treat acute rejection. The most common side effects of each of these agents include nephrotoxicity, hypertension, neurotoxicity, and tremors.
  - Antiproliferative agents, such as azathioprine, and more recently, mycophenolate mofetil (MMF). Usually one of these agents is initially included in the induction and maintenance of immunosuppression, with MMF often reserved for the treatment of rejection. The most common toxicities are bone marrow suppression and hepatotoxicity.
  - Antilymphocyte antibodies, such as OKT3, antilymphocyte globulin (ALG), and antithymocyte antibody (ATG). Most often these agents are employed only for therapy-resistant acute rejection, as their toxicity is high. OKT3, for instance, can result in lymphokine-mediated toxicity, anaphylaxis, pulmonary edema, and fevers.
- Induction therapy is generally based on cyclosporine and corticosteroids, with addition of one antiproliferative agent, most typically, azathioprine. Dosing is generally high in the perioperative period, with subsequent tapering to maintenance doses after allograft implantation.

PERIOPERATIVE CONSIDERATIONS

- Perioperative complications are similar to those found with any large intra-abdominal or intrathoracic surgery, but also includes pulmonary edema from fluid overload, electrolyte abnormalities, engraftment syndrome, and hypotension secondary to hypovolemia, and graft dysfunction due to surgical technique or primary graft failure of any transplanted organ. The risk of primary graft failure increases with cold ischemic time.

SPECIFIC ORGAN CONSIDERATIONS

- *Renal*: Initial organ function is characterized by urine output in the immediate postoperative period, and adequate circulating intravascular volume is imperative. Special attention is needed to identify and treat hyperkalemia, acidosis, and fluid overload.
- *Liver*: The monitoring of organ function and detection of abdominal hemorrhage are paramount in the posttransplant period, as both can lead to rapid deterioration and death in the organ recipient.
- *Heart*: Denervated heart lacks the ability to manifest reflex tachycardia in response to hypovolemia, thus maintenance of euvolemia is important. Similarly, normal neuroendocrine responses are not present in the immediate posttransplant period, such that systemic hypertension is a common finding.
- *Lung*: Pulmonary edema from volume expansion, or ischemia-reperfusion injury is a common finding. Lung protective ventilator strategies and moderation in volume repletion are important considerations during this time.

REJECTION

HYPERACUTE REJECTION

- Rarely seen—results from ABO incompatibility of donor organ. Within hours of transplant, there is rapid onset of complete dysfunction in the transplanted organ and the presence of a systemic inflammatory response syndrome, progressing to shock and death.

ACUTE CELLULAR REJECTION

- A T-cell-mediated phenomenon occurring between 1 week and 1 year. Often characterized by fever, leukocytosis, or organ dysfunction and requires lab studies of physiologic function of grafted organ and tissue biopsy to ascertain diagnosis. Treatment usually consists of increased immunosuppression, often with pulsed corticosteroids, the administration of second-line immunosuppressives (such as tacrolimus), or the initiation of salvage immunosuppression with antilymphocyte antibodies (OKT3, ALG).

CHRONIC REJECTION

- Characterized by a slowly progressive, angiocentric fibroproliferative response that is generally resistant to treatment with immunosuppressive agents, and is characterized by a slow deterioration of organ function. Early posttransplant infections (especially viral) may be a risk factor for the early development of clinically significant chronic rejection.

INFECTIOUS COMPLICATIONS

THE FIRST MONTH (PERIOPERATIVE PERIOD, ASSOCIATED WITH HIGH LEVELS OF IMMUNOSUPPRESSION)

- Approximately 90% of infections during this period are bacterial infections related to surgery. Common sites include intravascular catheter-related sepsis, wound infections, and hospital-acquired pneumonias. The overall risk is dependent on the integrity of mucocutaneous barrier (presence of indwelling devices), degree of immunosuppression, and coexistent morbidities.
- Viral infections may begin to present late in this period. Reactivation of herpes simplex virus (HSV) is the most common etiology, however the prophylactic use of acyclovir may decrease its incidence. Exacerbation of chronic hepatitis B or C (in liver transplant patients) may also present during this period.
- Fungal infections usually do not present during this early period, with the exception of candidal infections related to hospitalization (indwelling catheters). In addition, pulmonary aspergillosis may occasionally present during this early period.

1–6 MONTHS (EMERGENCE OF OPPORTUNISTIC INFECTIONS)

- This period is characterized by the onset of the "classic" post-transplant-related viral infections.
  - Cytomegalovirus (CMV) is the most common viral illness encountered during this period.
    - Occurs either by reactivation or through de novo acquisition from the graft, with de novo infections tending to be most severe. Antilymphocyte globulin (ALG) treatment increases the risk and severity of infection.

    - Symptoms classically include a mononucleosis-like syndrome of fever, malaise, and leukopenia, as well as concurrent end-organ involvement (pneumonitis, hepatitis, chorioretinitis, gastroenteritis).
    - Active CMV infection is thought to result in further systemic immunosuppression, and often heralds subsequent infectious complications later in the posttransplant period.
    - CMV infection also is associated with an increased risk for the development of Epstein-Barr virus (EBV)-related posttransplant lymphoproliferative disorder (PTLD) and chronic rejection.
  - Other viral illness include EBV (usually only seen in seronegative recipients receiving a seropositive graft), varicella-zoster virus (VZV) reactivation (shingles), respiratory syncytial virus (RSV, associated with risk of chronic rejection, bronchiolitis obliterans syndrome [BOS], in lung transplant recipients), adenovirus, and influenza.
- Opportunistic bacterial infections
  - Nocardia, most often presenting as pulmonary infiltrates. However, this is less common in the era of pneumocystis pneumonia (PCP) prophylaxis with trimethoprim/sulfamethoxazole.
  - Listeria—frequent cause of central nervous system (CNS) infection.
  - Mycobacterial disease
    - Tuberculosis (TB) usually is due to reactivation rather than primary infection. Presenting symptoms typically include fever, with other constitutional symptoms. Half of patients have lung involvement alone, one-third dissemination with lung involvement, and one-sixth extrapulmonary TB alone. Mortality is 25–40%, even in modern treatment era.
    - Nontuberculous infection is also a cause of pulmonary infiltrates in the posttransplant period (especially in lung transplant). Mycobacterium-avium complex accounts for the majority of infections.
- Opportunistic fungal infections
  - *Aspergillus*
    - Incidence is as high as 5% in heart, lung, and liver transplants, but lower in kidney. Usually presents as invasive disease in the lung, with fever, cough, chest pain, and hemoptysis.
    - Radiographically presents with one or more nodular opacities, which often cavitate.
    - Diagnosis can be difficult to obtain, empiric therapy with either liposomal amphotericin B or voriconazole is the current standard of care.
  - *Cryptococcus*—also a frequent cause of meningitis and brain abscess
  - PCP
    - Incidence is now decreasing due to effective prophylactic therapy with trimethoprim/sulfamethoxazole.
  - Endemic fungi should be considered in any transplant patient who has lived in an appropriate geographic area:
    - Histoplasmosis (Ohio and Mississippi river valleys), coccidioidomycosis (Southwestern United States), and blastomycosis (Midwest).
    - Disease most often is due to reactivation and is more likely to present with dissemination in solid organ transplant patients.
- Opportunistic parasitic infections
  - Toxoplasma accounts for the majority of parasitic infections, with CNS infection (abscess, meningitis) the most common site.

>6 MONTHS POSTTRANSPLANT (MAINTENANCE IMMUNOSUPPRESSION)

- This period is characterized by tapering to maintenance immunosuppression, and, consequently, a shift in the epidemiology of infections to community-acquired pathogens.
- Indolent viral infections can become apparent, such as BK virus in renal transplants and reactivation of varicella virus (herpes zoster).
- Chronic rejection may become apparent, especially in patients with previous viral infections or acute rejection.
- Vascular insufficiency due to stenosis of anastomoses can lead to progressive deterioration of organ function.

POSTTRANSPLANT LYMPHOPROLIFERATIVE DISORDER

- Comprises several EBV-driven disorders including uncomplicated EBV posttransplant infection (mononucleosis), to true malignancy with clonal chromosomal abnormalities. Historically, mortality ranges between 50 and 80% in patients with the monoclonal-derived malignancy.
- Risk factors include EBV infection in the early post-transplant period, CMV disease, type and intensity of immunosuppression, and type of solid organ transplant (lung, heart; due to degree of immunosuppression). Importantly, EBV seronegative recipients have a 10–76% greater likelihood of developing PTLD early in the transplant period.
- Diagnosis is based on histologic criteria, with a gold standard of pathologic examination of either surgical or needle biopsies.

- Therapy consists of reduction of immunosuppressive therapy, consideration of local resection for isolated lesions, consideration for use of anti-CD20 antibodies (rituximab), and consideration of antiviral agents or interferon-α for selected patients.

BIBLIOGRAPHY

Christie JD, Sager JS, Kimmel SE, et al. Primary graft failure following lung transplantation. *Chest* 1998;114:51–60.

Fishman JA, Rubin RH. Infection in organ-transplant recipients. *N Engl J Med* 1998;338:1741–1751.

Kotloff RM, Ahya VN, Crawford SW. Pulmonary complications of solid organ and hematopoietic stem cell transplantation. *Am J Respir Crit Care Med* 2004;170:22–48.

Preiksaitis JK, Keay S. Diagnosis and management of posttransplant lymphoproliferative disorder in solid-organ transplant recipients. *Clin Infect Dis* 2001;33(Suppl 1):S38–S46.

Scales DC, Granton JT. The transplant patient. In: Hall JB, Schmidt GA, Wood LDH, eds., *Principles of Critical Care*, 3rd ed. New York, NY: McGraw-Hill; 2005:1355–1374.

Snydman DR. Epidemiology of infections after solid-organ transplantation. *Clin Infect Dis* 2001;33(Suppl 1):S5–S8.

Speich R, van der Bij W. Epidemiology and management of infections after lung transplantation. *Clin Infect Dis* 2001;33(Suppl 1):S58–S65.

113 CARE OF THE MULTISYSTEM TRAUMA PATIENT

William Schweickert

KEY POINTS

- Mortality from trauma has a trimodal distribution—a first peak (seconds to minutes after the traumatic event) produced by essentially lethal injuries; a second peak (minute to hours after the traumatic event) produced by injuries of potentially lethal nature (usually neurologic injury and hemorrhage); and a third peak (days or weeks) due to sepsis and multiple system organ failure. The intensivist can help to intervene in the latter instances, especially the third peak, utilizing medical knowledge, resources, persistence, and attention to detail to reduce the impact.
- On admission to the ICU, patients usually have been previously evaluated (emergency physician, trauma/general surgeon); however, patients remain at risk for deterioration due to unrecognized injuries, iatrogenic complications of initial diagnostic studies and therapy, and general complications of critical care.

STEP 1: REASSESSMENT OF THE PRIMARY SURVEY

AIRWAY (A)

- If the patient is intubated, the patency and position of the endotracheal tube should be assessed, especially given risk of dislodgement during transport.
- If the patient is spontaneously breathing, verify that the oral cavity is clear without evidence of airway obstruction from the loss of tone of the musculature supporting the tongue or foreign material.
- In the multisystem trauma patient, particularly with blunt injuries above the clavicle, a cervical spine injury should be assumed and immobilization must be maintained until proven otherwise.

BREATHING (B)

- Inspect patient for asymmetric/paradoxical chest wall movement and/or tracheal deviation.
- Auscultate and percuss the chest for hyperresonance or dullness suggesting pneumo- or hemothorax.
- Hypoxemia should be rapidly addressed with either supplemental FiO_2 via face mask or in concert with positive end-expiratory pressure (PEEP) via a ventilator to ensure an oxygen saturation goal of >95%.

CIRCULATION (C) AND HEMORRHAGE CONTROL

- Verify adequate resuscitation, seeking weak pulses, cool/clammy skin, and delayed capillary refill to indicate further needs. Tachycardia with cool extremities suggests hypoperfusion until proven otherwise. This is usually as a result of hemorrhage, although other causes of hypoperfusion (tension pneumothorax, cardiac tamponade, myocardial contusion, open pneumothorax, flail chest, and limb vascular injury) must be considered.
- Intravascular access should be reviewed. Such traumas require at least two large-bore (14- to 16-gauge) intravenous catheters; central venous catheters should be directed to large bore, number 8 French introducers (over a multilumen catheter) for the ability to achieve high flow rates. All catheters should have confirmed

patency and appropriate placement. Replace any unsterile lines once stabilized.
- Review the total volume of intravenous (IV) fluids administered since presentation. If normalization of blood pressure is not accomplished after ~50 mL/kg of crystalloid, blood should be administered (uncrossmatched group O if necessary). All blood products and IV fluids must be prewarmed when administered in massive quantities or at rapid infusion rates to prevent or correct hypothermia.

NEUROLOGIC DISABILITY (D)

- A full neurologic evaluation, including level of consciousness, mentation, and pupillary size and reaction must be performed on arrival and compared to previous examination results.
- Any significant deterioration mandates a more detailed examination, including oxygenation, ventilation, and perfusion, and investigation of intracranial pathology with immediate brain computed tomography (CT) scan without contrast.

EXPOSURE (E)

- The patient MUST be completely (RE)exposed to evaluate external injuries.

STEP 2: REVIEW THE TRAUMA EVENT'S HISTORY AND MEDICAL HISTORY CLOSELY

- Trauma details: mechanism of injury, event, and environment related to the accident, details of the prehospital course. Think about the possible intentional drug overdose prior to injury.
- Medical history (often obtained from family/friends): medications, allergies, and especially any history of drug or alcohol use. Ongoing drug or alcohol dependence is present in over 30% of patients admitted for complications of trauma. These patients have higher risks of complications, including withdrawal.

STEP 3: EXCLUDE UNDIAGNOSED INJURIES

- The incidence of missed injuries despite complete primary and secondary surveys has been estimated to be as high as 10% in patients with blunt injury. Reasons for injuries to be missed: altered mental status due to head injury or alcohol intoxication, severe multiple injuries, instability requiring immediate operation, lack of symptoms on admission, and low index of suspicion.
- Potentially life-threatening injuries that may have been missed include head injury (especially intracranial hemorrhage), aortic injury, intra-abdominal injury, and rhabdomyolysis. These require careful initial radiographic interpretations and serial neurologic examinations. Intra-abdominal injury should be considered in all patients with blunt or penetrating trauma and evidence of ongoing unexplained blood loss. Rhabdomyolysis is evidenced by the clinical history, elevated creatine kinase, and should be managed with fluids, maintenance of high urine output, and consideration for intravenous bicarbonate-containing fluids.

STEP 4: AVOIDANCE OF IATROGENIC AND GENERAL COMPLICATIONS OF CRITICAL ILLNESS

- Transfusion-related complications. Avoid hypothermia by warming blood, dilutional coagulopathy by following coagulation studies and replacing platelets and/or fresh frozen plasma, monitor and treat hypocalcemia. Recognize that massive transfusion may lead to acute lung injury independently.
- Venous thromboembolic disease (due to prolonged immobilization, pelvic and lower extremity injuries, and direct vascular injuries). Utilize antiembolism stockings, sequential compression devices. Anticoagulation or inferior vena cava filter placement may be necessary in high-risk situations.
- Stress ulcers. Recommend prophylaxis via acid inhibition (either antihistamine or proton pump inhibitors).
- Contrast nephropathy. Maintenance of renal perfusion, euvolemia, and urinary flow are necessary. Adjunctive *N*-acetylcysteine or intravenous sodium bicarbonate has been shown to improve outcomes in selected populations.

BIBLIOGRAPHY

Birck R, Krzossok S, Markowetz F, et al. Acetylcysteine for prevention of contrast nephropathy: meta-analysis. *Lancet* 2003;362:598–603.

Merten GJ, Burgess WP, Gray LV, et al. Prevention of contrast-induced nephropathy with sodium bicarbonate: a randomized controlled trial. *JAMA* 2004;291:2328–2334.

Soderstrom CA, Dischinger PC, Smith GS, et al. Psychoactive substance dependence among trauma center patients. *JAMA* 1992;267:2756–2759.

114 SPINE INJURIES

D. Kyle Hogarth

KEY POINTS

- In any trauma setting, spinal injury should always be assumed to be present until appropriate assessment has ruled it out.
- All spinal injuries must be considered unstable until they are thoroughly evaluated.
- Spinal cord injury can be minimized by limiting the secondary ischemic phase and maintaining appropriate spinal immobilization.
- Complete spinal cord injuries have no potential for functional recovery.
- Incomplete injuries have recovery potential, which must be maximized.
- Rehabilitation must be initiated at the beginning of the hospitalization.

GENERAL THOUGHTS

- Life-threatening injuries from trauma requiring ICU admission can potentially delay the diagnosis and management of spinal injury as the team focuses on the immediate obvious injuries.
- It is estimated that approximately 20% of patients sustaining multiple injuries have associated spinal column injury.
- The possibility of cervical spine injury must be considered in anyone who has suffered significant injuries to the face or head, especially those unconscious from trauma.
- Furthermore, patients with preexisting conditions that put them at risk for spinal injury, such as ankylosing spondylitis, may suffer serious neck injury from apparently "minor" traumatic events.

NEUROLOGIC INJURY

- Physical disruption of the spinal cord results in complete, irreversible loss of function.
- The effect and extent of injury is directly related to the magnitude of the force applied and the length of time it was applied.
- The management goal for a spine injury is to prevent further force being applied to the injured area. This is accomplished via immobilization and then relief of the compression on the spine from displaced bony fragments and discs.

SPINAL CORD SYNDROMES

ANTERIOR CORD SYNDROME

- Complete motor loss below the level of injury.
- Loss of light touch sensation below the level of injury.
- Preservation of position, vibration, and deep touch sensation.

CENTRAL CORD SYNDROME

- Motor loss in the extremities: the upper extremities experience greater loss than the lower extremities.
- Sensation is variably altered.
- Caused by central hemorrhage in the cord.

BROWN-SÉQUARD SYNDROME

- Motor is lost on the ipsilateral side of injury.
- Pain and temperature are lost on the contralateral side, one or two segments below the level of the injury.

CAUDA EQUINA SYNDROME

- The degree of neurologic loss with this syndrome varies greatly, depending on the extent of nerve root damage.
- The motor and sensory loss is symmetrical.
- May have loss of bladder and bowel control.

SPINAL SHOCK

- There can be a physiologic block to conduction from any force applied to the spine. This is clinically manifested as complete cessation of all neurologic function—motor, sensory, and autonomic—below the level of the injury.
- Spinal shock and complete block to conduction can last from minutes to weeks.

INITIAL CLINICAL ASSESSMENT

- A history of the mechanism of injury is helpful in predicting the type of neurologic injury.
- Any evidence of head or facial trauma (i.e., bruises, lacerations, or abrasions) can suggest the direction from which the force was applied and can help predict injury.
- Evaluate for asymmetry of the head position and tenderness along the sternomastoids.

- Examine the chest for the presence of a paradoxical pattern of respiration.
- A detailed neurologic examination should be performed and recorded on a flow sheet to allow for serial examination.
- The patient who is stabilized in a cervical collar and is manually secured in traction may be slowly log-rolled to allow examination of the back for the following: tenderness, malalignment of the spinous processes, a boggy gap in the supraspinous ligament, sensation in the perianal area, rectal examination, and testing of the bulbocavernosus reflex.

RADIOLOGY

- The initial films that should be done are lateral cervical spine films and an anteroposterior view of the chest and pelvis.
- Other x-ray views, such as oblique and swimmer's may help visualize the spine.
- Computed tomography (CT) allows for routine, coronal, sagittal, and three-dimensional reconstructions of the spine. CT requires only a single transfer of the patient: this is done with a spine board.
- Myelography should only be done in three different clinical scenarios:
  - The extent of the injury cannot be explained by the plain films or CT.
  - Increasing neurologic loss without severe encroachment on the neural canal.
  - When demonstration of defects or avulsed nerve roots needs to occur.
- Magnetic resonance imaging (MRI) can be used to assess soft tissue and ligamentous injury in the spine, but surprisingly the results have not shown much advantage compared to conventional films and CT.
- MRI has a very high negative predictive value for significant soft-tissue injury.

IMMEDIATE GENERAL MANAGEMENT

- Patients with spinal injuries should be taken directly to a level 1 tertiary care center.
- The advanced cardiac life support (ACLS) requirements for management of airway, breathing, and circulation do not change even in the presence of a spinal injury.
- Spinal immobilization should continue until the patient has either been cleared or appropriate management of the injury has occurred.
- The arterial PaO_2 should be at least 100 mmHg. Supplemental oxygen should be delivered to ensure this.
- The blood pressure should be at least 100 mmHg systolic.

MANAGEMENT OF NEUROGENIC SHOCK

- Patients with neurogenic shock will be hypotensive and bradycardic secondary to increased vagal tone and peripheral vasodilation. This is treated with crystalloid infusion.
- Placement of a central line for monitoring of the central venous pressure should occur.
- Small doses of vasopressors can be used.

OTHER MANAGEMENT ISSUES

- Respiratory complications after cervical spinal cord injury occur in 60% of patients.
- Loss of phrenic nerve function occurs in spinal lesions above C5.
- Acute spinal cord injury may be associated with pulmonary edema.
- Almost all spine injury patients develop a transient ileus.
- 50% of patients with spinal cord injuries develop deep vein thrombosis and prophylaxis with low-dose heparin appears ineffective. Calf compression and low-molecular weight heparin seem to be more effective.
- Care should be taken to avoid decubitus ulceration of the skin.
- Spinal injury patients become catabolic. As soon as the ileus resolves, eating should resume.

SURGICAL MANAGEMENT

- Indications for surgical decompression of spinal cord are:
  - Progressive neurologic loss
  - Failure or anticipated failure of nonoperative decompression (owing to retained bone or disc fragments)
  - Incomplete cord and/or cauda equina lesions with residual compression
- Contraindications for surgical decompression as it will not benefit or may even harm:
  - A complete spinal cord lesion in a patient out of spinal shock
  - Progressive neurologic loss due to ischemia, with no blockage or significant residual compression as seen on myelography

STEROIDS

- Glucocorticoids (e.g., dexamethasone) are presumed to help in spine injury by decreasing modulating catecholamines, stabilization of cell membranes, and prevention of immune cell release of lysosomal enzymes and prevention of complement activation.
- Controversy exists regarding the effectiveness of steroids.

COMPLICATIONS OF SPINAL CORD INJURY

- Hypothermia secondary to lack of vasoconstriction due to loss of thoracic sympathetic outflow as well as being unable to shiver to maintain core temperature can lead to hypotension and bradycardia.
- Autonomic dysreflexia can occur in patients with injuries above T6 at any time after the stage of spinal shock. Symptoms include hyperhidrosis, headache, and vasodilation above the level of the neurologic loss with nasal stuffiness. The cardinal sign of autonomic dysreflexia is paroxysmal hypertension. Typical precipitating events are distention or manipulation of the bladder or rectum or intra-abdominal pathology.

BIBLIOGRAPHY

Bagley LJ. Imaging of spinal trauma. *Radiol Clin North Am* 2006;44(1):1–12.

Johnson GE. Spine injuries. In: Hall JB, Schmidt GA, Wood LDH, eds., *Principles of Critical Care*, 3rd ed. New York, NY: McGraw-Hill; 2005: 1409–1420.

115 TORSO TRAUMA

Kaveeta P. Vasisht

KEY POINTS

- Torso trauma can occur due to blunt or penetrating trauma.
- The critical care physician needs to be prepared for any injury to a thoracic or abdominal organ when treating a patient who has trauma to the torso.
- Careful history and examination of a torso trauma patient can allow quick identification of a life-threatening injury.

OVERVIEW

- Generally, torso trauma is classified as blunt versus penetrating. Clinically, it is useful to differentiate injuries that are immediately life threatening versus injuries in a hemodynamically stable person. This chapter will focus on the potentially life-threatening injuries where lifesaving skills are within the realm of practicing intensivists.

TENSION PNEUMOTHORAX

- *Pathophysiology*: Injury to the lung results in gas accumulation in the pleural space which is normally apposed by the parietal and visceral pleura. A one-way valve mechanism is created by which air enters the pleural space with each respiratory cycle but cannot escape. Eventually, the intrathoracic pressure becomes increased such that the ipsilateral lung is compressed and displaced to the opposite side. This rise in intrathoracic pressure will cause impedance of venous return. In addition, mediastinal shifting occurs, which may cause occlusion of the major vessels resulting in worsening venous return.
- *Diagnosis*: The diagnosis is made clinically. Patients may present with severe dyspnea, tachypnea, hyperresonance, and absent or decreased breath sounds on the affected side. The trachea may be shifted away from the side of the tension pneumothorax.
- *Treatment:* Immediate needle decompression with a large-bore needle in the second intercostal space, midclavicular line. This action is then followed by tube thoracostomy placement.

OPEN PNEUMOTHORAX

- *Pathophysiology*: Free communication between the pleural space and the atmosphere through a chest wall wound. This results in collapse of the ipsilateral lung.
- *Diagnosis*: Generally, there is a visible wound and audible noise from atmospheric air entry into the pleural space.
- *Treatment*: Occlusion of the open wound, which can usually be accomplished by occlusive gauze dressings. This should be followed by tube thoracostomy placement.

MASSIVE PNEUMOTHORAX

- *Pathophysiology*: Persistent pneumothorax despite an adequately functioning chest tube with respiratory instability is a sign of a large pulmonary defect. The air is leaving the pulmonary system faster than the chest tube can remove it from the thorax.

- *Diagnosis*: This is a clinical assessment. A massive pneumothorax suggests a large airway laceration.
- *Treatment*: 100% oxygen and immediate surgical intervention.

MASSIVE HEMOTHORAX

- *Pathophysiology*: Blunt or penetrating trauma results in injury to a major central vascular structure or laceration of a systemic artery.
- *Diagnosis*: Severe hypotension from blood loss followed by hypoxemia from lung collapse secondary to mass effect of blood in the thoracic cavity. Dullness to percussion on affected side. Diagnosis is confirmed if after chest tube placement a large volume of blood is drained.
- *Treatment*: Volume resuscitation, chest tube placement. If blood continues to drain at 100 cc/h the patient needs surgical intervention.

FLAIL CHEST

- *Pathophysiology*: Chest trauma results in rib fractures, which result in a segment of the chest wall moving paradoxically. During inspiration the flail segment moves inward with negative pleural pressure and outward with expiration.
- *Diagnosis*: The diagnosis is often difficult to make clinically. On chest x-ray (CXR), the presence of multiple adjacent rib fractures involving the same rib in different segments of the CXR would suggest flail chest.
- *Treatment:* A hemodynamically unstable patient requires positive pressure ventilation (PPV) and chest tube placement on the involved side to prevent tension pneumothorax on institution of PPV. Liberation from mechanical ventilation can occur once the gas exchange abnormality is corrected. However, if there is no hemodynamic compromise, not all flail chest patients need to be mechanically ventilated.

CARDIAC TAMPONADE

- *Pathophysiology*: Blood accumulation in the pericardial sac secondary to trauma resulting in impaired cardiac filling and reduced stroke volume and cardiac output.
- *Diagnosis*: Requires a high index of clinical suspicion in anyone who has had blunt or penetrating trauma to the chest and is hypotensive without obvious signs of blood loss.
  - Beck triad includes hypotension, decreased heart sounds, and jugular venous distention. However, this is not always present.
  - Pulsus paradoxus (the difference between systolic blood pressure during inspiration and expiration) above 10 mmHg may also be evident.
  - One should note that distended neck veins and hypotension are present in both tension pneumothorax and cardiac tamponade. If there is a doubt to the diagnosis always treat tension pneumothorax first.
- *Treatment*: If available in the emergency setting ultrasound probe placement is helpful in the diagnosis of hemopericardium. The initial treatment involves IV fluid administration and prompt pericardiocentesis.

TRAUMATIC AIR EMBOLISM

- *Pathophysiology*: Systemic air embolism occurs when a direct communication exists between the air passages and the blood vessels. In chest trauma, scattered loss of integrity of the pulmonary blood vessels, air passages, and alveoli creates such a pathway.
- *Diagnosis*: High index of clinical suspicion in anyone that suffers sudden cardiovascular collapse after chest trauma who demonstrates a neurologic deficit, especially after PPV. May see bubbles in arterial puncture (need to make sure the syringe connector is not loose and giving bubbles via this mechanism).
- *Treatment*: Left lateral decubitus positioning of the patient. Maintenance of high systemic pressures (with alpha agonists if needed) may limit gradient for air entry at some vascular sites.

BIBLIOGRAPHY

Ali J. Torso trauma. In: Hall JB, Schmidt GA, Wood LDH, eds., *Principles of Critical Care*, 3rd ed. New York, NY: McGraw-Hill; 2005:1421–1442.

116 PELVIC AND EXTREMITY TRAUMA

Shashi Kiran Bellam

KEY POINTS

- Pelvic and extremity trauma require a careful evaluation for neurologic and vascular injury.
- Serial examination of the traumatic area, and areas distal to the injury, should be performed after initial

stabilization with careful attention to the neurovascular examination.
- Early consultation with surgical colleagues should be sought for trauma patients.
- Long-bone injuries can lead to local complications, such as compartment syndrome, bleeding, and neurologic injury.
- Long-bone injuries can also lead to distant complications, such as fat embolism.

EXTREMITY INJURIES

COMPARTMENT SYNDROME

- Compartment syndrome is defined as an elevation of the interstitial pressure in a closed osseofascial compartment, resulting in microvascular compromise, and occurs after prolonged external pressure, direct trauma, and vascular injury, commonly in the forearm or leg, less commonly in the hand, foot, or thigh.
- Physiologically, compartment syndrome involves the accumulation of fluid in a nondistensible compartment leading to increased absolute compartment pressure, decreased venous blood exit, decreased capillary flow, tissue hypoperfusion, and eventually, anaerobic metabolism. Muscle and nerve necrosis may occur while distal pulses are still maintained.
- Clinical signs and symptoms in a conscious patient include: pain disproportionate to the known cause of pain; swelling and tenderness over the involved compartment; hypesthesia in the cutaneous nervous distribution for nerves within the compartment; and severe weakness of involved muscles. In an unconscious patient, a greater degree of physician awareness for a possible compartment syndrome is required.
- Measurement of the intracompartmental pressures can be helpful. The pressure should be below 30 mmHg, but the degree of injury is related to both the absolute pressure and the duration of increased pressure. Compartment syndrome may occur at lower intracompartmental pressures in the face of hypotension due to decreased tissue perfusion pressures.
- Nonoperative management of compartment syndrome is only appropriate in the earliest stages and consists of removal of all external sources of pressure, elevating the limb to the level of the heart to maintain perfusion but limit edemagenesis. If nonoperative management is successful, there should be complete resolution of signs and symptoms within 1 hour.
- Surgical management involves an open release of the entire compartment involved, stabilization of underlying fractures, fasciotomy incisions packed to allow secondary suturing, or skin grafting within 4–7 days. Immediate skin grafting of the incision site is also acceptable.
- Secondary complications of compartment syndrome include myoglobinuria and acute renal failure, infection of the fasciotomy wound, loss of range of motion of affected joints, and muscular weakness and contracture.

PERIPHERAL NERVE INJURY

- A detailed neurologic examination with attention to extremities with known injury should be done by identifying the nerve to be tested, examining sensation in the distribution of cutaneous innervation of that nerve, and examining motor activity in a muscle that is most distal, least cross-innervated, and not inhibited by pain.
- Once peripheral nerve injury is documented, expected recovery is 1 mm/day after a 1-month delay at the site of injury, followed by monitoring Tinel sign (pain or paresthesia in the distribution of the nerve elicited by tapping over the course of the nerve distal to the injury). If serial examination shows that Tinel sign is progressing distally, nerve regeneration is occurring. If serial examination does not show that Tinel sign is progressing distally, then structural disruption of the nerve is likely present and nerve repair should be considered.

VASCULAR INJURIES

BLUNT

- If an open vascular injury due to penetrating or blunt trauma occurs, operative repair is essential and postoperative management for shock or reperfusion injury in the ICU may be required.
- Multiple trauma patients may be initially evaluated in the ICU for assessment and management.
- Arterial occlusion with hypotension will lead to ischemic injury to muscles and nerves in the affected region. Muscle cell death occurs after 6 hours of ischemia. Revascularization must be accomplished within this time frame to preserve the function of the limb.
- Traction injuries to the shoulder girdle may be associated with brachial plexus palsy and innominate, subclavian, or axillary artery injury.
- Injuries above the knee may be associated with popliteal artery occlusion.
- Clinical signs of extremity ischemia should be suspected in the traumatized extremity and are summarized by the 5 P's: pain, pallor, paresthesias, paralysis, and pulselessness. Pulselessness with hemodynamic stability should be presumed to be due to arterial occlusion and an arteriogram should be performed. Angiographic documentation of patent circulation allows continued management by observation alone.

- Compromised arterial circulation should be repaired operatively. Supportive therapies include protection from additional trauma, occlusive dressings on wounds, and stabilization of fractures. Concomitant venous repair is usually performed. In the absence of multiple injuries, systemic heparinization should be instituted preoperatively if the limb is ischemic. Concomitant fasciotomy should be performed if ischemia has lasted more than 6 hours or if there is evidence of compartment syndrome before or after revascularization.

PENETRATING

- Penetrating vascular injuries may or may not present with the 5 P's (see above). Some arterial injuries do not cause ischemia. Venous injuries do not cause ischemia. Evidence of massive blood loss is sufficient to warrant either exploration or angiography. Arterial injuries may present with a pulsating or expanding hematoma. Antibiotic and tetanus prophylaxis should be given perioperatively.

FRACTURES

- Fractures and joint injuries may pose a life-threatening problem via sepsis, hemorrhage, or fat embolism.
- Definitive management of fractures involves reduction, maintenance, and rehabilitation.
- Immediate operative management of fractures in multisystem trauma can reduce the incidence of many complications that can occur with more conservative management (fat embolism, pulmonary failure, sepsis).
- Early nutrition is also likely to improve outcomes.
- Compound fractures are frequently complicated by infection and patients should receive prophylactic antibiotics to cover common skin pathogens as well as any specific pathogens related to the injury (e.g., *Clostridium* in farmyard injuries).
- Early cleaning and debridement of compound fractures is a surgical emergency and failure to perform it within 8 hours will turn a contaminated wound into an infected one.

PELVIC FRACTURES

- The mortality rate from major pelvic injury is approximately 10%.
- Pelvic instability is implied when there is obvious pelvic displacement, a compound wound, injury to neurovascular structures, or marked tenderness or bruising posteriorly.
- Palpation and manipulation of the pelvis may also demonstrate instability.
- Bleeding at the urethral meatus indicates a urethral tear.
- Standard radiologic assessment includes a routine anteroposterior view; an inlet view may show posterior displacement; an outlet view shows superior migration or rotation. Computed tomography (CT) may be the most helpful study.
- Initial management includes massive fluid replacement, type and screen for packed red blood cell (RBC) transfusion, and stabilization of the fracture via application of an external frame or clamp.
- Bleeding or hemodynamic instability may warrant angiography. Diagnostic peritoneal lavage is frequently positive due to transperitoneal leakage of a pelvic hematoma.
- Definitive stabilization may be delayed up to 1 week after the injury to allow for the patient's generalized condition to be stabilized.
- Major complications include: massive hemorrhage, visceral and soft-tissue injuries, and deep venous thrombosis.

FAT EMBOLISM

- Criteria for the diagnosis of fat embolism syndrome (FES) include respiratory insufficiency, cerebral involvement, and a petechial rash. Minor features include fever, tachycardia, anemia, thrombocytopenia, and lipiduria.
- FES usually occurs 48–72 hours following injury and initially can present with disorientation, lethargy, or irritability. Petechiae are present in 60% of cases, usually in the upper trunk, axillary folds, conjunctiva, or fundi.
- There is usually a fall in hemoglobin of 3–4 g/dL. There is usually thrombocytopenia and increased fibrin degradation products, but rarely clinical bleeding.
- Chest x-ray (CXR) may show a diffuse infiltrate.
- Management is primarily preventive (early fracture stabilization and splinting) and supportive (mechanical ventilation as needed).
- There is no proven role for corticosteroids.

BIBLIOGRAPHY

Liew ASL. Pelvic ring injuries and extremity trauma. In: Hall JB, Schmidt GA, Wood LDH, eds., *Principles of Critical Care*, 3rd ed. New York, NY: McGraw-Hill; 2005:1443–1450.

117 ELECTRICAL TRAUMA

Steven Q. Davis, Chris E. Keh

KEY POINTS

- The extent of electrical injury is dependent on duration, voltage, resistance, type of current, and distribution.
- Initial examination may be normal, but this does not rule out serious complications as delayed and subtle injuries can occur.
- The extent of injuries can include most organ systems, including cardiac, neurologic, and musculoskeletal injuries.

PHYSICS OF ELECTRICAL INJURY

- Ohm's law ($I = V/R$) describes the relationship of current (I), voltage (V), and resistance (R).
- The duration of contact with the power source, the type of current, the voltage/resistance, and the distribution of current throughout the body determine the extent of injury. Prediction of the amount of heat produced from current flow can be calculated from Joule's law, energy = $(V^2 \times \text{time})/R$.
- Alternating current (ac) is found in household current and is defined by a current that changes the direction of electron flow in a cyclical manner. Direct current (dc), in which the direction of electron flow is constant, is found in batteries, electronics, and lightning.
- Current density is usually greatest at the contact points with the power source.
- Nerve and blood vessels have the least electrical resistance (good conductor of electricity), while bone has the highest resistance (poor conductor of electricity). Muscle has resistance that is intermediate between the two.

CLASSIFICATION OF INJURY

- *Low-voltage injuries*: Most often domestic electricity, in which there is often an entry and exit point. Cutaneous burns are often minor or absent, although ac has the potential to interfere with cardiac cycle leading to ventricular fibrillation.
- *High-voltage injuries*: Found in power lines and lightning. Minimal contact results in severe cutaneous burns.
  - *True high tension*: Occurs at voltage ≥1000 V. This type of injury is associated with massive tissue damage and aggressive monitoring and resuscitation is often needed.
  - *Flash (arc)*: Occurs when an arc of current strikes or affects the skin, but does not pass through the body.
  - *Lightning*: The arc temperature of a lightning strike is approximately 3000°C. A direct lightning strike is most often fatal. Survivors of lightning strike were most likely in the vicinity of a surface strike and experience surface burns and arc effects.

CELLULAR RESPONSE TO ELECTRICAL TRAUMA

- Tissue destruction occurs both by thermal injury and nonthermal electroporation (production of holes in cell membranes).
- If the victim is holding the power source, muscles will initially have involuntary spasms, then tetanic contraction. This leads to the "no-let-go" phenomenon, when the victim is unable to let go of the power source when held in the hand because of strong contractions of the hand and forearm flexor muscles.
- If the victim is close to but not touching the power source, muscle contractions generally push the victim away from the source. High-voltage contacts will also tend to throw the victim from the source, due to a single strong muscle contraction.

CLINICAL PRESENTATION

- *Cardiac*: Ventricular arrhythmias account for a significant portion of the initial morbidity and mortality from electrical injury.
  - Low-voltage ac often produces ventricular fibrillation, while high-voltage ac and dc can produce asystole and other cardiac arrhythmias.
  - Approximately half of victims have electrocardiographic (ECG) or rhythm disturbances. Most commonly these are nonspecific ST-T-wave changes and sinus tachycardia, both of which usually resolve over time.
  - Because of the extensive muscular damage in an electrical injury, determination of cardiac damage by biochemical markers can be difficult. Because ECG changes usually revert to normal, these are also unreliable for the diagnosis of ischemia.
  - Generally, as typical victims tend to normally be active and healthy, preexisting cardiac disease is usually not present and treatment (including surgery) may proceed. Any history of cardiac disease

should raise concern for myocardial damage during the electrical injury and may warrant more dedicated investigation.

- *Renal*: Roughly 10% of victims will develop renal dysfunction, which is most commonly due to hypovolemia secondary to extravascular extravasation of fluid. Creatine phosphokinase (CPK) isoenzymes and urine myoglobin should be measured frequently. If myoglobin fails to clear or enzymes continue to rise, an occult focus of muscle injury should be sought.
- *Musculoskeletal*: Soft-tissue injuries should always be assumed to be worse than is superficially apparent. Compartment syndromes are common and lead to significant morbidity if not addressed rapidly. Pain with passive movement is an early finding of compartment syndrome. A fluid pressure >30 mmHg in a compartment indicates the need for fasciotomy. All nonviable tissue should be debrided.
- *Skin*: Injury can range from first-, second-, or third-degree burns. The amount of cutaneous injury can severely underestimate the amount of internal injury. Lightning injury can present with characteristic cutaneous markings.
- *Neurologic*: Effects may be transient or permanent, immediate or delayed.
  - Up to 65% of patients lose consciousness secondary to neuronal depolarization in the brain.
  - Ischemic brain damage can occur if respiratory movement is compromised.
  - Acute deficits of the spinal cord tend to resolve relatively quickly; delayed onset spinal cord injuries are much less likely to resolve.
  - Median nerve damage is the most common manifestation of peripheral nerve injuries. Immediate decompression of the compartments of the arm may prevent significant functional decline and permanent injury.
  - Long-term sequelae include headache, dizziness, vertigo, seizure activity, mood or personality changes, and impotence. Cognitive decline has also been documented. Sensorimotor neuropathies, paresthesias, dysesthesias, reflex sympathetic dystrophy, and cold intolerance may manifest long after the injury is sustained and may last several years or remain permanent. Paraplegia and quadriplegia have occurred years after the injury.
- *Pulmonary*: Pulmonary dysfunction is usually related to central nervous system (CNS) damage or injury to the chest wall. If the current path traverses the upper airway, particular attention should be paid to the potential for life-threatening airway edema. Furthermore, inhalation injuries from chemical toxins (ozone) or carbon monoxide can occur in arc injuries, explosions, or fires.

MANAGEMENT

- As with any major trauma, attention must first be paid to the airway, breathing, and circulation (ABCs). Advanced trauma life support (ATLS) guidelines should also be followed, with special attention to cervical spine immobilization and possible airway burns or smoke inhalation.
- A careful examination should be performed to look for contact points. Obvious cutaneous injury often represents a small fragment of the total injury.
- If cardiopulmonary arrest occurs, resuscitation attempts should be aggressive and prolonged if necessary. Anecdotal evidence reports survival after several hours of resuscitation. All patients should have close hemodynamic and cardiac monitoring with ECG on presentation.
- Laboratory evaluation with complete blood count, serum electrolytes including creatinine, and urine analysis in patients with more than minor injury.
- Assess the amount of muscle necrosis by obtaining CPK or urine/serum myoglobin. Suspicion for compartment syndrome should be high and consultation with surgeons for possible fasciotomy or escharotomy should occur early.
- Large volumes of isotonic fluid should be used during resuscitation.
  - The goal for urine output is 0.5–1 mL/kg/h, which increases to 1.5–2 mL/kg/h if myoglobin or free hemoglobin is found in the urine. Alternatively, initial intravenous fluid rate can be started at 20–40 mL/kg/h with reassessment after the first hour.
  - Mannitol (12.5 mg IV) may be necessary to achieve the large amounts of diuresis. If myoglobinuria persists, a continuous infusion of 12.5 g/h may be used or alkalinization of the urine may be considered.
- Any change in the level of consciousness requires a thorough evaluation given the high coincidence of head trauma. Tests to be considered include electroencephalogram, arterial blood gas, and toxicology screen. Only after other causes have been ruled out can a change in the level of consciousness be attributed to the electrical injury itself.
- Imaging with chest radiographs, bone radiographs to rule out fractures (due to tetanic muscle contractions and falls), or computed tomography may be initiated according to risk for secondary injuries.
- Prophylaxis against streptococcal and clostridial organisms should be considered, along with administration of tetanus vaccine.
- Those with lightning injury should have evaluation for cataract formation and otoscopic abnormalities.

BIBLIOGRAPHY

Cawley JC, Homce GT. Occupational electrical injuries in the United States, 1992–1998, and recommendations for safety research. *J Safety Res* 2003;34:241–248.

Gottlieb LJ, Lee RC. Electrical trauma. In: Hall JB, Schmidt GA, Wood LDH, eds., *Principles of Critical Care*, 3rd ed. New York, NY: McGraw-Hill; 2005:1451–1456.

Hettiaratchy S, Dziewulski P. Pathophysiology and types of burns. *BMJ* 2004;328:1427–1429.

Martin TA, Salvatore NF, Johnstone B. Cognitive decline over time following electrical injury. *Brain Inj* 2003;17:817–823.

118 BURNS

Maria Dowell

KEY POINTS

- The morbidity and mortality of burns is determined by the wound surface area, wound depth, age, and associated injuries.
- Early resuscitation of the burn victim involves aggressive fluid administration and attention to respiratory compromise if present.
- The intermediate phase of burn management is characterized by a hypermetabolic state, need for nutritional support, and a growing risk of infectious complications.
- The late phase of burn management, extending through the period of wound closure, is marked by continued risk of infection as well as other general complications of critical illness.

PATHOPHYSIOLOGY

- Burn patients are trauma patients and their condition changes significantly over the course of the injury.
- First-degree burns involve only the thin outer epidermis, appear as erythema, produce mild discomfort, and heal rapidly. Second-degree burns are defined as injury to the entire epidermis and variable portions of the dermis. Third-degree burns destroy the entire epidermis and dermis leaving no residual epidermal cells to repopulate the area. Skin grafting is often required.
- Estimating the size of the burn is guided by the *rule of nines*. The head and each arm are 9% while the chest/abdomen, back, each lower extremity are 18% of the total body surface (TBS). The Lund and Browder chart is more accurate and should be used for precise calculation.
- The morbidity/mortality is based on the wound size and depth, patient's age, and associated injuries.
- Physiologic and metabolic parameters substantially change due to the cardiopulmonary instability, onset of intense wound inflammation, immunosuppression, and infection.
- Treatment is based on clear understanding of differences in the postburn phases.

INITIAL RESUSCITATION PERIOD (0–36 HOURS)

- This phase is characterized by cardiopulmonary instability including life-threatening airway and breathing problems and hypovolemia due to plasma volume loss.
- Pulmonary insufficiency caused by heat and smoke is the major cause of mortality and accounts for >50% of fire-related deaths.
- Carbon monoxide (CO) toxicity symptoms usually appear when the CO concentration exceeds 15% and are manifested as neurologic changes and metabolic acidosis. Hydrogen cyanide exposure is a well-recognized byproduct of burning synthetics such as polyurethane and presents in a similar fashion. Persistent metabolic acidosis despite adequate volume resuscitation suggests CO or cyanide inhalation even though the PaO_2 remains normal. Toxicology screen is warranted as ethyl alcohol (EtOH) and drugs can cause similar neurologic dysfunction. CO toxicity requires early administration of 90–100% O_2 to displace CO from hemoglobin. Hyperbaric O_2 is best reserved for severe neurologic compromise with high CO level. Cyanide toxicity treatment involves administration of sodium nitrite followed by sodium thiosulfate to help clear the cyanide.
- Upper airway obstruction from airway edema after heat exposure may not occur for 12–18 hours. The external burn edema and airway edema have a parallel time course and local edema can resolve in 4–5 days. Inspection of the oropharynx for soot or heat injury should be routine. Intubation should occur if there is significant inhalation injury, deep facial burns, respiratory distress, hemodynamic instability, impaired consciousness, or indecision. Use the largest endotracheal tube (ETT) possible as very thick secretions develop.
- Chemical burns of the upper and lower airway from toxic gases may become evident only after 24–48 hours.

Breath-holding and laryngospasm are protective measures in the conscious patient, however, the unconscious patient loses this protection and sustains more injury to the lower airway. Early bronchospasm and edema from the irritant gases result in decreased dynamic lung compliance and ventilation-perfusion mismatching. Initial treatment consists of maintenance of small airway patency (with positive end-expiratory pressure [PEEP]) as well as removal of secretions. Increased airway resistance >18–24 hours after the injury is due to bronchiolar edema and plugging more than bronchospasm.

- Hemodynamic instability and impaired O_2 delivery can occur with massive fluid shifts during resuscitation. Increased vascular permeability, increased osmotic forces in burned tissue, and cellular swelling contribute to intravascular volume loss into burned and nonburned tissues. The fluid and protein shifts are the greatest in the first several hours. The quantity of edema depends on the adequacy of fluid resuscitation. Major protein losses in the first 6–8 hours can result in severe hypoproteinemia. Edema may take days to weeks to resolve depending on the restoration of lymphatic patency. Cardiac output is depressed primarily due to hypovolemia but myocardial edema can be seen with third-degree burns >40% of the TBS. Afterload is increased due to increased systemic vascular resistance (SVR) from catecholamines.
  - Intravenous access should be through peripheral vein catheters in nonburned tissue to avoid line sepsis (older patients with massive burns or inhalation injury are typically monitored with a central catheter).
  - Parameters of perfusion to monitor include a mean arterial pressure >85 mmHg, heart rate <130, urine output 0.5–1 mL/kg/h, trends in base deficit as indicator of adequacy of restoration of perfusion, and avoidance of hypothermia.
  - Use crystalloid without glucose (except in small children) initially and colloid about 8–12 hours later for protein restoration. The total 24-hour volume is calculated as (4 mL)(% burn)(body weight in kg) and 50% of this is generally given in the first 8 hours.
  - This general guideline should be modified by serial clinical assessments of the intravascular volume.
- Hematologic disorders to look for after major burns include hemolysis due to red cell fragility, early leukocytosis, thrombocytopenia, and hypercoagulability from consumption of clotting factors.
- Pain and anxiety management should begin soon after the injury to avoid excessive stress response. A continuous background of narcotics and low doses of benzodiazepines are commonly used.
- The burn itself is a low priority for initial care.

POSTRESUSCITATION PHASE (2–6 DAYS)

- This phase is a period of transition from the shock phase to the hypermetabolic phase.
- Five major pulmonary abnormalities impair pulmonary function during this period.
  - Upper airway and facial edema from heat-induced damage begins to resolve between days 2 and 4.
  - Impaired chest wall compliance may occur, especially in circumferential third-degree burns and is improved, but not eliminated, by escharotomy.
  - Mucosal irritation and ciliary dysfunction from a chemical burn to the airways cause bronchorrhea, cough, increased mucus production, and may progress to bacterial tracheobronchitis and diffuse bronchopneumonia.
  - If infection can be controlled, the acute process will resolve over 7–10 days.
  - Pulmonary edema and surgical anesthesia-related pulmonary dysfunction may also be present.
- Maintaining hemodynamic stability can be challenging. Fluid losses from surface evaporation, increases in intravascular fluid from absorption of edema and decreases in hematocrit from red cell membrane damage, and low production all contribute.
- Persistently elevated catecholamines from the hypermetabolic state give tachycardia.
- O_2 consumption peaks around 5–7 days postburn.
- Release of pyrogens from the wound increases body temperature by 1–2°F.
- Rate of protein loss is massive as a result of increased catecholamines and cortisol as well as inflammatory cytokines that stimulate gluconeogenesis and protein breakdown. Muscle loss of 1 kg/day is common with large burns. All of this contributes to reduced wound healing and immune dysfunction.
- A common error is continued infusion of isotonic crystalloid in the absence of major sodium losses. A 5% glucose-containing solution with low sodium and increased potassium is the primary replacement fluid for evaporative and urinary losses during this phase. Initiation of nutrition, preferably enteral, is essential.
- Care of the burn wound becomes increasingly important. Burn wounds are never sterile. Many of the early colonizing bacteria originate from the heat-injured skin, nares, oropharynx, perineum, and stool. Silver sulfadiazine is the most common and least toxic topical antibiotic used. Mafenide (carbonic anhydrase inhibitor) is more potent but reserved for deep infections. Infection of the wound indicates invasion of viable tissue and may lead to sepsis. Diagnosis

is difficult and may require biopsy. *Staphylococcus aureus* is common in the first week with gram-negative organisms more evident after the first week. *Enterococcus* and *Candida albicans* are present in 50% of wounds.
- Surgical excisions should begin as soon as the patient is hemodynamically stable, to avoid having extensive burns still in place when the infection-inflammation phase begins.

INFLAMMATION-INFECTION PHASE (DAY 7 TO WOUND CLOSURE)

- This is the most complicated phase of management evidenced by marked catabolism with loss of body protein, increased metabolic rate, bacterial colonization of the wound, and concern for wound sepsis. Intense inflammation is seen at 7–10 days in deep burns.
- Sepsis is the leading cause of morbidity/mortality during this period with the most common sites being the lungs, burn wound, and vascular catheters. Respiratory failure and pneumonia surpass burn wound sepsis as causes of mortality. Approximately 50% of burn patients with both inhalation injury and major body burn develop pneumonia. Both the immunocompromised state and high incidence of virulent organisms in the ICU contribute to the risk. Prevention of pneumonia is important as eradication of established pneumonia is difficult.
- The antimicrobial doses required to obtain adequate tissue levels are much higher in hypermetabolic burn patients.
- Consider tracheostomy early if there is a persistent need for intubation.
- Evaporative water and protein losses from the wound remain increased until wound closure. The hypermetabolic-catabolic state persists with elevated catecholamine levels, increased O_2 consumption, hepatic gluconeogenesis requiring rapid body protein breakdown, suboptimal nutrition, growth hormone decrease, and reduced antioxidants.
- It is important to control the source of the stress response and increase the process of anabolism through nutrition, nutritional adjuvants, and increased muscle activity. Liberal use of analgesics, anxiolytics, and other methods to control stress are required. Relative adrenal insufficiency has also been reported.
- Parenteral nutritional support is preferred and 30–35 cal/kg/day are required for burns >30% TBS. Increasing carbohydrate intake reduces gluconeogenesis and proteolysis. Protein requirements are two to three times the recommended daily allowance and supplements are often necessary. Glutamine replacement as well as vitamin and mineral replacement are essential. Occasionally, growth hormone and the testosterone analog, oxandrolone, are used to increase anabolic activity.

BIBLIOGRAPHY

Demling RH, Desanti L. Burns: inflammation-infection phase (day 7 to wound closure). In: Hall JB, Schmidt GA, Wood LDH, eds., *Principles of Critical Care*, 3rd ed. New York, NY: McGraw-Hill; 2005:1473–1478.

Demling RH, Desanti L. Burns: postresuscitation phase (days 2 to 6). In: Hall JB, Schmidt GA, Wood LDH, eds., *Principles of Critical Care*, 3rd ed. New York, NY: McGraw-Hill; 2005: 1467–1472.

Demling RH, Desanti L. Burns: resuscitation phase (0 to 36 hours). In: Hall JB, Schmidt GA, Wood LDH, eds., *Principles of Critical Care*, 3rd ed. New York, NY: McGraw-Hill;2005: 1457–1466.

119 CARE OF THE POSTCARDIAC SURGERY PATIENT

J. Matthew Brennan

KEY POINTS

- Hypotension following cardiac surgery has a broad differential diagnosis that is informed by chest radiography, measurement of central venous pressure, monitoring of chest drains, and echocardiography.
- Respiratory dysfunction may be caused by pulmonary edema, consequences of cardiopulmonary bypass, transfusion (transfusion-related acute lung injury, TRALI), and phrenic nerve injury.
- Renal dysfunction complicates 30% of patients following bypass grafting and, when nonoliguric, generally resolves quickly.
- Operative complications (tamponade, hemorrhage, acute graft failure) are uncommon but require prompt diagnosis and treatment.
- Atrial fibrillation is common: rate or rhythm control are equally effective.

GENERAL MANAGEMENT ISSUES

HYPOTENSION

- See Table 119-1 for details.

RISK FACTORS
- Decreased left ventricular (LV) function
- Diastolic dysfunction
- Increased cardiopulmonary bypass (CPB) duration
- Periop acute myocardial infarction (AMI)/graft failure
- Coronary artery air embolism

MECHANICAL SUPPORT
- Intra-aortic balloon pump (IABP): most placed in the operating room if blood pressure (BP) unstable following CPB. A survival benefit has been noted with IABP use.

TABLE 119-1 Hypotension—Diagnosis and Treatment

CVP	DDX	CLINICAL FEATURE	TREATMENT (IN ORDER OF PREFERENCE)	COMMENT
High	LV failure	Decreased EF with pulmonary edema	Dobutamine 1–20 μg/kg/min	Increased contractility with decreased SVR Need central IV access for doses above 5–10 μg/kg/min
			Milrinone Loading dose: 50 μg/kg Maintenance: 0.4–0.5 μg/kg/min	Increased contractility with decreased SVR Need central IV access
			IABP	Decreased afterload with increased coronary perfusion See below for details
			Epinephrine 0.05–0.25 μg/kg/min	Increased contractility and SVR Need central IV access
			Norepinephrine 0.05–0.25 μg/kg/min	Vasoconstrictor Need central IV access
			Dopamine 2.5–20 μg/kg/min	Vasoconstrictor >6 μg/kg/min increases SVR Need central IV access
			VAD	See text for details
	Diastolic dysfunction	Normal EF with pulmonary edema	IVF (goal: MAP 15–20 mmHg)	Secondary to long-standing HTN or myocardial stunning postinfarction
	RV failure	Dilated/hypocontractile RV with dry lungs	Sildenafil (Viagra) if increased pulmonary vascular resistance Dobutamine Vasopressin 0.02–0.04 units/min Norepinephrine Epinephrine VAD	PE vs. pulmonary vasoconstriction
	Tamponade	See Chap. 135	Surgical correction	TTE often shows RV/RA dimpling Elevated and equalized RAP, RVEDP, PA diastolic pressure and PCWP
	Tension PTX	Decreased breath sounds; mediastinal shift away from PTX	Chest tube or Angiocath (2nd intercostal space, midclavicular line)	Diagnosed by physical examination and CXR
	Mechanical dysfunction	New, loud systolic murmur	Surgical repair	Papillary muscle rupture, VSD
	Arrhythmia	Bradycardia	Atrial, AV, or ventricular pacing, atropine	Determine if cause is sinus node or AV nodal dysfunction by ECG
		Tachyarrhythmias	See appropriate sections for management	
Low	Hypovolemia	Cold skin	IVF and blood products, as needed	Vigorous LV function on TTE
	Vasodilatory	Warm skin	Vasopressin 0.04 units/min Norepinephrine	CPB effect with cytokine release, sepsis or adrenal insufficiency

ABBREVIATIONS: CVP, central venous pressure; dDx, differential diagnosis; EF, ejection fraction; PTX, pneumothorax; IVF, intravenous fluid; MAP, mean arterial pressure; SVR, systemic vascular resistance; HTN, hypertension; PE, pulmonary embolism; RV, right ventricle; RA, right atrium; RAP, right atrial pressure; RVEDP, right ventricular end-diastolic pressure; PA, pulmonary artery; PCWP, pulmonary capillary wedge pressure; CXR, chest x-ray; VSD, ventricular septal defect.

- Mechanism of Action (MOA): increase coronary perfusion and decrease afterload
- Indications:
  - Decreased cardiac output with optimization of preload/afterload/heart rate
  - Moderate dose dopamine (10 μg/kg/min) or equivalent dobutamine/epinephrine with hemodynamic (HD) instability
- Initially 1:1 ratio (60–100 cycles/min); then, titrated to 1:3 as cardiac output improves

- Ventricular assist devices (VADs): placed in the operating room if BP unstable following CPB despite IABP use
  - Indications:
    - Decreased cardiac index (<1.5 L/min/m^2) despite IABP and moderate dose inotropic support following discontinuation of CPB, and
    - If myocardial dysfunction expected to resolve in course of a few days, or if patient <65–70 years old (y/o) and transplant candidate
  - Short- and long-term devices are available

PULMONARY DYSFUNCTION

Risk Factors

- Age: <2 y/o or >60 y/o
- Chronic obstructive pulmonary disease (COPD)
- Preop use of amiodarone
- Oxygenators other than membrane type
- Increased CPB duration
- Increased left atrial pressure
- If reintubation is necessary, consider tracheostomy at 7 days postop

Cardiopulmonary Bypass Effects

Treatment

- Noninvasive positive pressure ventilation (NIPPV)
- Judicious use of diuretics
- Oxygen
- Chest physiotherapy (PT)
- Steroids

Phrenic Nerve Palsy

Epidemiology

- 11% of patients with left lower lobe atelectasis in the postop period suffer from phrenic nerve palsies.

Risk Factors

- The major risk factor is use of ice slush rather than cold saline for cardioplegia.

Treatment

- Spontaneous recovery occurs within 6 months in the majority of patients.

RENAL FAILURE

Epidemiology

- *Renal dysfunction* is defined as an increase in serum creatinine by >50% above the baseline, and *renal failure* is an acute increase in serum creatinine ≥2 times the baseline value.
- Renal dysfunction is present in ~30% of patients post-coronary artery bypass graft (post-CABG).
- In adults with normal preop renal function, there is a 1% incidence of renal failure with rare progression to HD. However, in patients with abnormal preop renal function the incidence may be as high as 16–20% with nearly 1 in 5 progressing to acute dialysis.
- Oliguric acute renal insufficiency (ARI) often occurs within 12–18 hours postop, is recalcitrant to dopamine and diuretics, but resolves completely in the majority of patients. In contrast, nonoliguric ARI may occur as late as 3–4 days with a blood urea nitrogen (BUN) and creatine peak around days 7–10, and is only associated with a 75% rate of resolution.
- Nonoliguric ARI is associated with a 90% survival rate; however, among patients with acute renal failure progressing to end-stage renal disease (ESRD), there is a 50% in-hospital mortality rate.
- Aprotinin causes renal artery stenosis and oliguric azotemia resolving in 1–2 days.
- The possible utility of nesiritide in the treatment of hypervolemia is controversial due to its association with renal dysfunction.

Risk Factors

- Preop chronic kidney disease (CKD)
- Diabetes
- Renal artery stenosis
- Emergent operations
- Re-exploration for bleeding
- Advanced atherosclerosis
- Class III/IV heart failure
- Cyanotic heart disease
- Old age (>70 y/o)
- Increased time of CPB
- CPB prime with whole blood (instead of hemodilution)
- Increased plasma hemoglobin (>40) during and following CPB
- Acute postop decrease in cardiac output
- Preop use of radiocontrast dye
- Use of certain antibiotics (especially gentamicin)

PATHOPHYSIOLOGY AND DIAGNOSIS
- See Chap. 79 for details.

Prerenal
- Most frequently an issue of volume status or cardiac output.
- If not receiving loop diuretics (i.e., furosemide): check serum and urine sodium and creatinine; FeNa <1% indicates prerenal etiology, >2% indicates intrinsic renal dysfunction.
- If receiving loop diuretics: check serum BUN and creatinine and urine urea and creatinine; FeUrea <35% indicates prerenal etiology, >35% indicates intrinsic renal dysfunction.

Renal

- Most often due to acute tubular necrosis (ATN), acute interstitial nephritis (AIN), or pyelonephritis.
- Check urine for eosinophils (AIN), casts (ATN), or bacteria and WBCs (pyelonephritis).

Postrenal

- Most often due to Foley catheter dysfunction.
- Flush and/or replace Foley catheter if high suspicion.

PREVENTION AND TREATMENT
- The cornerstone of prevention involves appropriate fluid management and maintenance of a good cardiac output.
- Treatment initially involves optimizing preload and afterload.
- Dopamine 2.5 μg/kg/min may increase glomerular filtration rate (GFR), but is controversial.
- Fenoldopam 0.01 μg/kg/min may increase GFR, but is controversial.
- Some centers use furosemide q 6-12 h × 3 days in escalating doses with or without albumin to increase tubular flow and help manage fluid status. This does not aid recovery of kidney function.
- "Renal Cocktail" infusion (400 mg furosemide + 100 mL 20% mannitol) at 1 mg/kg/h furosemide rate, alternating 4 hours "on" and 4 hours "off" has also been used by some. Serum osmolarity must be monitored frequently and the infusion is stopped if >310 mOsm/L.
- Early HD/continuous venovenous hemodialysis (CVVHD)/slow continuous ultrafiltration (SCUF); CVVHD associated with decreased ventilator days, decreased ICU stay, and increased renal recovery rate.

CARDIOVASCULAR ACCIDENT

EPIDEMIOLOGY
- Rates of postop cardiovascular accidents (CVAs) leading to hemiplegias or hemiparesis are age dependent: 5% in patients >65 y/o, 8% in those >75 y/o. They occur in up to 16% of all patients undergoing combined CABG and intracardiac procedures.
- Approximately 12% of patients with periop CVAs die.

RISK FACTORS
- Increased age
- Prior CVA/transient ischemic attack (TIA)
- Severe ascending aortic atherosclerosis
- Increased CPB duration
- Decreased postop cardiac output

DIAGNOSIS AND TREATMENT
- Head computed tomography (CT) with and without IV contrast
- Maintain systolic blood pressure (SBP) between 130 and 160 mmHg to prevent extension of infarct

PANCREATITIS

EPIDEMIOLOGY
- Postop increases in serum amylase are noted in 25–30% of patients; however, most is thought to be secondary to salivary amylase production. An increase in lipase is seen in only 10% of patients. Clinical signs of pancreatitis are far less common (0.04–1%).

PREVENTION
- Administration of calcium chloride is associated with an increased risk of postop erative pancreatitis.

TREATMENT
- Symptomatic pancreatitis is treated with bowel rest (often with intermittent nasogastric [NG] tube suction) and opioid analgesics. Enteral nutrition improves outcome in severe pancreatitis.

HYPERTHERMIA

- Postcardiac surgery patients frequently experience noninfectious fevers for 4–5 days after surgery persisting for up to 2 weeks without active infection. Some have attributed this phenomenon to the release of interleukins associated with the damaging effects of CPB.

HYPERGLYCEMIA

- Post-CABG blood glucose levels >175 mg/dL lead to increased mortality, deep sternal wound infections, length of hospital stay, and cost of hospitalization.
- Blood glucose levels >110 mg/dL in a general ICU population leads to increased mortality rates.

TREATMENT
- Goal: 80–175 mg/dL (80–110 mg/dL is likely most beneficial)
- IV insulin drips are most effective means to tight glycemic control

SPECIFIC POSTOP COMPLICATIONS

POSTOP HEMORRHAGE

CLINICAL FEATURES
- Excessive bleeding:
  - There is no accepted standard.
  - 500 mL/h in 1st hour; 400 mL/h in first 2 hours; 300 mL/h in first 3 hours; 200 mL/h in first 6 hours; or increasing bleeding rate at any postop time.
  - Others use 200 cc/h over first 3 hours or >1 L over 24 hours.

EPIDEMIOLOGY
- 30% of patients require postop transfusions; however, only 3–5% have severe bleeding (>10 U packed red blood cells [PRBC]).

RISK FACTORS
- Low preop hemoglobin
- Low weight
- Older age
- Female gender
- Emergency operation
- Open heart procedure
- Aortic operation

DIAGNOSIS AND DIFFERENTIAL DIAGNOSIS
- Increased partial thromboplastin time (PTT) and activated clotting time (ACT): heparin effect
- Increased prothrombin time (PT)/international normalized ratio (INR): shock liver
- Decreased platelet count: hemodilution or disseminated intravascular coagulation (DIC)
- Decreased factor VIII level: DIC
- Normal coagulation profile, platelet count, factor VIII levels: mechanical vascular dysfunction (i.e., anastomotic failure)
- High-risk anatomic sites:
  - Graft anastomosis or side branch
  - Cannulation sites
  - Aortotomies/cardiotomies
  - LV aneurysm resection lines
  - Pericardial edges
  - Coronary sinus
  - Sternal wire sites
  - Pleural/pericardial fat pad
- CPB effect:
  - Fibrinolysis—risk increases with increased CPB times
- Meds:
  - Aspirin and Clopidogrel lead to platelet dysfunction
  - Heparin
- Hemodilution of clotting factors and platelets
- Hypothermia and CPB effects lead to platelet dysfunction

TREATMENT
- Fibrinolysis:
  - Transexemic acid
  - Epsilon-aminocaproic acid
- Reverse heparin with protamine (amount is based on ACT level).
- Replace fibrin with fresh frozen plasma (FFP, 500 mg/U) or cryoprecipitate (150 mg/U) if fibrinogen level <100 mg/dL.
- NovoSeven can be used if factor VIII or IX levels are decreased due to hemophilia, DIC, or hemodilution or if inhibitors to factors VIII or IX are present.
- Some centers suggest increasing positive end-expiration pressure (PEEP) to 10–15 cmH_2O to tamponade hemorrhage.
- If continued hemorrhage despite correction of coagulation cascade, consider a mechanical dysfunction (i.e., anastomotic failure) and return patient to OR.

PERICARDIAL TAMPONADE

CLINICAL FEATURES
- See Chap. 135 for details.

EPIDEMIOLOGY
- 84% of postop patients have pericardial effusions on transthoracic echocardiography (TTE).
- 30% have large effusions by postop days 4–10, mostly found in cardiac transplant patients and those with excessive postop hemorrhage. Most effusions regress starting on day 10.
- Clinical tamponade is present in only 1% of patients, but can develop up to 4 months after cardiac surgery.

DIAGNOSIS AND DIFFERENTIAL DIAGNOSIS
- See Chaps. 13 and 135 for details.

TREATMENT
- Reentry into the chest

ACUTE GRAFT FAILURE/PERIOP MYOCARDIAL INFARCTIONS

EPIDEMIOLOGY
- Seen in 2–5% of post-CABG patients
- Associated with increased inpatient mortality (9.7% vs. 1.0%)

RISK FACTORS
- Cardiomegaly
- Increased CPB time
- Repeat CABG
- CABG plus other open heart surgery (OHS)

PATHOGENESIS
- Acute graft failure may occur as a result of graft thrombosis (32%), poor distal run-off (17%), graft stenosis (7%), and anastomotic stenosis (5%).

DIAGNOSIS
- Periop AMI is defined by the presence of new Q waves on a postop ECG or CK-MB increasing to >5 times the upper limits of normal 8–16 hours postop.
- Troponin elevation is considered the most reliable marker by some.

TREATMENT
- The mainstay of treatment involves postop coronary catheterization with rescue percutaneous coronary intervention (PCI) or reoperation (see Chap. 18).

POSTOP ATRIAL FIBRILLATION

EPIDEMIOLOGY
- The risk of postop atrial fibrillation (AF) depends on the surgical procedure performed; 15–40% incidence following CABG; 37–50% postvalve surgery; 60% with combined valvular and CABG surgery; 11–24% following cardiac transplant.
- Peak risk occurs at 2–3 days postop.
- Most postop AF is transient, and converts to normal sinus rhythm (NSR) within 2–3 days with treatment (unless chronic preop AF). If no prior history, 15–30% convert to NSR within 2 hours, 80% within 24 hours; however, 43% of patients experience recurrent episodes.
- New-onset postop AF leads to increased morbidity, length of stay, and cumulative cost.

RISK FACTORS
- Prior AF
- Discontinuation of periop beta-blockers
- Age: 4% <40 y/o, 18% <60 y/o, 30% >70 y/o, 52% >80 y/o
- COPD
- CKD
- Mitral valvular disease (esp. stenosis)
- Left atrial enlargement (LAE), cardiomegaly
- Increased CPB
- Prior OHS
- Elevated preop brain natriuretic peptide (BNP)
- Right coronary artery (RCA) stenosis
- Risk prediction models have been developed

PREVENTION AND TREATMENT
- The cornerstone of prevention involves the use of periop beta-blockers beginning on the morning following surgery. Angiotensin-converting enzyme (ACE) inhibitors have also been shown to decrease the risk of recurrent postop AF. Postop beta-blockers should be continued at least until 1st postop clinic visit.
- Postop biatrial pacing is the most effective form of prevention.
- Treatment strategies consist of either rate or rhythm control. No difference in time to NSR, AF relapse, proportion of patients in NSR at 2 months has been shown between the two strategies.
  - Hemodynamic instability:
    - Rhythm control:
      - Pacing via biatrial pacing wires
      - External defibrillation
      - Amiodarone 5 mg/kg IV bolus; then 0.25–0.5 mg/min infusion with conversion to PO when stable
  - Hemodynamically stable:
    - Rate control:
      - IV beta-blocker with conversion to PO meds when clinically stable
    - Anticoagulate with warfarin is only necessary if AF >48 hours and acceptable bleeding risk with target INR = 2–3

MEDIASTINITIS

CLINICAL FEATURES
- Characterized by sternal instability, retrosternal fluid collections identified on CT scan, and retrosternal purulent drainage.

EPIDEMIOLOGY
- Mediastinitis develops in 0.8–1.5% of post-CABG patients and 2.5–7.5% of posttransplant patients.
- There is an increased risk with VADs, and in patients not given periop prophylactic antibiotics (50% infection rate).
- 83% of sternal wound infections are monomicrobial.
- 57% are associated with bacteremia.
- The median time to onset is 7 days with two-thirds of cases occurring within 2 weeks.
- They are associated with an increased length of stay by 38–51 days extra with 2–3 times increased cost of care.
- A wide range of mortality rates has been reported from 6 to 70%, but current series support a likely rate of 5–10% with early treatment.
- Favorable outcomes are typical with appropriate antibiotic therapy.

Risk Factors

- Retrosternal hematoma
- Increased operative time
- Incomplete sternal closure
- New York Heart Association (NYHA) class IV congestive heart failure (CHF)
- Prior OHS
- Obesity
- Smoking
- Diabetes
- COPD
- Male sex (possibly secondary to practice of chest shaving on day prior to surgery)
- Prolonged postop ventilation
- Steroid use
- Pre- and periop hyperglycemia
- Bilateral IMA use (secondary to decreased sternal blood supply)
- Of note, reoperation has not been shown to be an independent risk factor for mediastinitis

Pathophysiology

- Organism isolates <30 days postop:
  - Methicillin-susceptible *Staphylococcus aureus* (MSSA) 45%
  - Methicillin-resistant *S. aureus* (MRSA) 16%
  - Gram-negative bacilli 17%
  - Coagulase-Negative Staphylococcus species (CoNS) 13%
  - Streptococci 5%
  - *Candida albicans* also cultured

Diagnosis

- Computed tomography scan is the best diagnostic modality, but its sensitivity and specificity vary according to the timing of the scan (100% sensitive, 33% specific if performed before 14 days; 100% sensitivity and specificity if performed >14 days). Overall sensitivity and specificity have been reported as 67% and 83%, respectively.

Prevention and Treatment

- Prophylactic antibiotics with one dose prior to anesthesia, one prior to CPB, and one post-CPB; continuing until postop day 2 or until last IV/ET tube is removed. Longer durations have not been shown to decrease rates of infection. Recommended regimens:
  - Cefazolin 1 g if <80 kg or 2 g if >80 kg
  - Cefuroxime 1.5 g
  - If penicillin (PCN) allergy: vancomycin 10–15 mg/kg or clindamycin 600–900 mg
- Tight glycemic control

Therapy

- Surgical management

POSTCARDIOTOMY SYNDROME

Clinical Features

- Pleuritic and pericardial chest pain occurring usually >2 weeks following surgery with a peak incidence at 4 weeks postop. Pericardial and pleural friction rubs are often present, and it is occasionally associated with tamponade.
- Fever, pleural/pericardial pain with associated eosinophilia and atypical lymphocytosis.

Epidemiology

- Median duration is 22 days (range 2–100 days), and there is a 21% recurrence rate by 30 days.

Pathophysiology

- It is thought to be secondary to heart-reactive antibodies.

Treatment

- Treatment is with high-dose aspirin or nonsteroidal anti-inflammatory drugs (NSAIDs) unless the patient is taking diuretics. If pain persists and infection has been ruled out or if patient is on diuretics, prednisone (40 mg daily with a 4–8 weeks taper) has been advocated.

BIBLIOGRAPHY

Aranki S, Aroesty JM. Early complications of coronary artery bypass graft surgery. 2005. Available at: http://www.uptodateonline.com/application/topic.asp?file=chd/27202&type=A&selectedTitle=1~95. Accessed September 1, 2005.

Bharucha DB, Marinchak RA. Arrhythmias after cardiac surgery: atrial fibrillation and atrial flutter. 2005. Available at: http://www.uptodateonline.com/application/topic.asp?file=carrhyth/43828&type=A&selectedTitle=16~95. Accessed September 1, 2005.

Postoperative care. In: Kouchoukos NT, Blackstone EH, Doty DB, et al., eds., *Kirklin/Barratt-Boyes Cardiac Surgery: Morphology, Diagnostic Criteria, Natural History, Techniques, Results, and Indications*, 3rd ed. Philadelphia, PA: Elsevier; 2003:195–253.

Rasmussen C, Thiis JJ, Clemmensen P, et al. Significance and management of early graft failure after coronary artery bypass grafting: feasibility and results of acute angiography and re-revascularization. *Eur J Cardiothorac Surg* 1997;12:847–852.

Salenger R, Gammie JS, Vander Salm TJ. Postoperative care of cardiac surgical patients. In: Cohn LH, Edmunds LH Jr, eds., *Cardiac Surgery in the Adult*, 2nd ed. New York, NY: McGraw-Hill; 2003:439–469.

Sexton DJ. Postoperative mediastinitis. 2005. Available at: http://www.uptodateonline.com/application/topic.asp?file=pulm_inf/2544&type=A&selectedTitle=10~95. Accessed September 1, 2005.

Silvestry FE Overview of the postoperative management of patients undergoing cardiac surgery. 2005. Available at: http://www.uptodateonline.com/application/topic.asp?file=cc_medi/22438&type=A&selectedTitle=3~95. Accessed September 1, 2005.

Thielmann M, Massoudy P, Marggraf G, et al. Role of troponin I, myoglobin, and creatine kinase for the detection of early graft failure following coronary artery bypass grafting. *Eur J Cardiothorac Surg* 2004;26:102–109.

Vijay V, Gold JP. Late complications of cardiac surgery. In: Cohn LH, Edmunds LH Jr, eds., *Cardiac Surgery in the Adult*, 2nd ed. New York, NY: McGraw-Hill; 2003:521–537.

Section 10
SPECIAL PROBLEMS IN THE ICU

120 PREGNANCY IN THE ICU

D. Kyle Hogarth

KEY POINTS

- The most common causes of ICU admission in pregnancy are complications of cesarean section, preeclampsia or eclampsia, and postpartum hemorrhage.
- The most common risk factors associated with ICU mortality include pulmonary complications, shock, cerebrovascular events, and drug dependence.
- A multidisciplinary team consisting of intensivists, high-risk obstetricians, anesthesiologists, and neonatologists should manage the gravid patient in the ICU.

PHYSIOLOGY OF PREGNANCY

- Blood volume increases with a decrease in albumin and hematocrit and hemoglobin.
- Heart rate, stroke volume, and cardiac output all increase while blood pressure decreases. Overall, the systemic and pulmonary vascular resistances decrease.
- Minute ventilation increases, as does oxygen consumption. Overall, the pregnant patient will have diminished PCO_2 with a decrease in HCO_3, giving the patient a compensated respiratory alkalosis. Understanding that a pregnant patient at baseline has a respiratory alkalosis with a compensatory metabolic acidosis is very important when interpreting the acid-base status of the patient during acute illness.
- A majority of pregnant patients will have a physiologic third heart sound, and this finding on examination cannot be interpreted as indicating ventricular failure with certainty.

THE FETO-PLACENTAL UNIT

- The fetus is very sensitive to changes in oxygen delivery, and pathologic changes in maternal physiology can quickly lead to diminished oxygen delivery.
- At baseline, the uterine artery is maximally dilated, so increased flow from local autoregulation cannot occur.
- Any condition leading to maternal general vasoconstriction will diminish oxygen delivery to the fetus. Worsening maternal alkalemia will also lead to vasoconstriction.
- The delivery of oxygen to the fetus is dependent on maternal cardiac output, as the oxygen-carrying capacity of the mother is diminished secondary to the lower level of hemoglobin.
- Monitoring fetal well-being through fetal heart rate is nonspecific, and fetal pH requires rupture of membranes. In general, the maternal acid-base status and parameters of oxygen delivery are adequate surrogates for fetal well-being.
- Maternal anemia sometimes needs to be corrected if oxygen delivery is compromised.

SHOCK IN PREGNANCY

- The approach to the hypoperfused pregnant patient is essentially the same for the nonpregnant patient. The initial management includes distinguishing between low flow and high flow states and assessing the volume status of the patient, keeping in mind the normal changes in physiology.
- If a right heart catheter must be placed, then the femoral position is relatively contraindicated secondary to vena caval obstruction by the gravid uterus and the possible need for emergent delivery of the fetus.

HYPOVOLEMIC SHOCK IN PREGNANCY

- The management of the pregnant patient with hypovolemic shock is essentially the same as the nongravid patient. While delivering the necessary volume to ensure adequate perfusion, a careful assessment of the cause of hypovolemia is undertaken.
- While assessing for causes of hemorrhage related to the gravid state, care must be taken to evaluate for nongravid causes of blood loss (i.e., gastrointestinal blood loss and hemolysis). Furthermore, critically ill gravid patients can frequently develop disseminated intravascular coagulation (DIC), so any massive bleeding should prompt a coagulopathy workup.
- Management of hemorrhage in pregnancy requires immediate intravenous access with two large-bore (16-gauge or larger) catheters. Resuscitation with crystalloid or colloid should be instituted until blood can be administered. The patient should be placed in the left lateral decubitus position. In patients receiving massive transfusions, a survey for resultant DIC should be undertaken. Patients should also be monitored for a secondary thrombocytopenia resulting from consumption.

SEPTIC SHOCK IN PREGNANCY

- Sepsis in an important cause of hypoperfusion in pregnancy, as it accounts for up to 15% of all maternal deaths.
- Normal pregnant circulatory physiology somewhat resembles early sepsis (high cardiac output, low vascular resistance), and sepsis can be difficult to diagnose in the febrile gravid patient.
- Chorioamnionitis or intra-amniotic infection occur in 1–4% of pregnancies and most commonly occur after prolonged rupture of membranes, prolonged labor, or postinvasive procedures such as amniocentesis or cervical cerclage. Patients typically have fever, tachycardia, uterine tenderness, and foul smelling amniotic fluid.
- The management of the septic gravid patient is similar to the nongravid patient.
- Cultures of blood, urine, and pelvic sites should be obtained. Empiric coverage with broad-spectrum antibiotics for polymicrobial infection should be initiated. If possible, aminoglycosides should be avoided in the gravid patient secondary to the risk of fetal nephrotoxicity and ototoxicity.
- The principles of assuring adequate venous return, cardiac filling pressures, and mixed venous oxygen saturation guide the ICU physician during the management of the gravid patient in a manner similar to the nongravid patient.
- Septic shock should be managed with early goal-directed therapy for a central venous pressure (CVP) of 10 mmHg and a mixed venous oxygen saturation of at least 70%. Inotropes to ensure adequate cardiac output and adequate mixed venous saturation are preferred over vasoconstrictors that may alter placental blood flow. However, if there is refractory hypotension after ensuring adequate filling pressures and mixed venous saturation, then vasoactive drugs should be employed.
- The role of drotrecogin alpha (activated) has not been defined in the pregnant population with sepsis. These patients were excluded in the original study. Pregnancy should be considered a relative contraindication for the use of activated protein C.

CARDIOGENIC SHOCK IN PREGNANCY

- Hypoperfusion secondary to cardiac dysfunction during pregnancy is often from preexisting conditions, such as valvular abnormalities, that emerge during the increased physiologic demands of pregnancy.
- Peripartum cardiomyopathy is an acquired cause of cardiac dysfunction that occurs with an incidence of 1/1300 to 1/4000 deliveries. Maternal mortality of patients with class III or IV heart failure is around 7%.
- This acquired heart failure of pregnancy usually occurs during the last month of pregnancy or during the first 6 months postpartum. Risk factors include African American race, older age, twin gestation, preeclampsia, and postpartum hypertension.
- Pregnant patients also have an increased risk for aortic dissection, possibly secondary to the increased shear stress from the elevated cardiac output. Dissection tends to present in the last trimester as a tearing sensation around the scapula.
- Risk factors for dissection include hypertension, increased age, multiparity, trauma, Marfan syndrome, Ehlers-Danlos syndrome, coarctation of the aorta, and bicuspid aortic valve. History and a widened mediastinum on chest x-ray should raise the suspicion for dissection. The diagnosis can be made with infused chest computed tomography (CT) or with transesophageal echocardiogram.
- Adequate preload needs to be ensured, and having the patient in the left lateral decubitus position is extremely important. If shock persists despite adequate preload, then management options include inotropic support and maximizing reduction in afterload.
- Dobutamine is the drug of choice for inotropic support, but it should be reserved for life-threatening situations because it has been shown in animal models to decrease placental blood flow.

- Afterload reduction with nitroprusside or nitroglycerin can be initiated if inotropic support does not correct the shock state. Nitroprusside can only be used for extremely brief periods of time because of the risk of cyanide and/or thiocyanate toxicity to the fetus. The dose and duration should be minimized, and the patient converted to oral hydralazine as soon as possible.
- Angiotensin-converting enzyme (ACE) inhibitors are absolutely contraindicated as they cause oligohydramnios and anuric renal failure in the fetus exposed in utero.
- When the patient with cardiogenic shock delivers, this should be an assisted vaginal delivery in the left lateral decubitus position with epidural anesthesia to minimize the tachycardic and hypertensive response to pain.

PREECLAMPSIA

- Preeclampsia is a circulatory disorder unique to pregnancy that occurs in 5–10% of pregnancies. It occurs usually after the 20th week of pregnancy, but may happen postpartum.
- It is characterized by the triad of hypertension, edema, and proteinuria. However, all three characteristics need not be present, and in some cases the manifestations may be mild.
- Risk factors for the development of preeclampsia include chronic hypertension, preexisting renal disease, diabetes, multiple gestations, hydatidiform mole, and the antiphospholipid antibody syndrome.
- Management of preeclampsia includes early diagnosis, close medical observation, and timely delivery. In most cases of preeclampsia, delivery is curative. In cases of severe preeclampsia, impending eclampsia, multiorgan involvement, or gestational age >34 weeks, immediate delivery is recommended.
- Conservative management involves close blood pressure control. A diastolic blood pressure of 110 mmHg or greater should be treated with the goal of maintaining a mean arterial pressure between 105 and 126 mmHg, with the diastolic between 90 and 105 mmHg. The goal of blood pressure management is to prevent the development of encephalopathy and lower the risk of cerebral hemorrhage.

ECLAMPSIA

- Eclampsia is a syndrome characterized by convulsions and increased risk for death in the setting of preeclampsia.
- The seizures of eclampsia can be controlled with magnesium, benzodiazepines, or phenytoin. Meta-analysis has suggested that magnesium is superior for control and prevention of further eclamptic seizures.
- No study has convincingly demonstrated prophylactic magnesium to be superior to blood pressure control in preventing eclampsia. However, magnesium and blood pressure control are superior to phenytoin in preventing eclampsia.
- Magnesium should be given for a minimum of 24 hours postdelivery in any woman with eclampsia.

HELLP SYNDROME

- An extremely fulminant complication of preeclampsia is the HELLP syndrome (Hemolytic anemia, Elevated Liver enzymes, Low Platelets), which occurs in 0.3% of deliveries.
- The HELLP syndrome is characterized by multiorgan system dysfunction arising from an unclear endothelial abnormality that results in secondary fibrin deposition and organ hypoperfusion.
- In up to 30% of patients who develop HELLP, the disease manifests 48 hours postpartum. Maternal mortality ranges from 0 to 24%, with fetal mortality ranging from 8 to 60%.
- The diagnosis is made based on laboratory values that demonstrate dropping platelets and elevated liver transaminases in the setting of a consumptive microangiopathic hemolytic anemia. Management is supportive and requires delivery of the fetus.

RESPIRATORY DISORDERS OF PREGNANCY

- The lower functional residual capacity of the lungs during pregnancy secondary to the enlarging abdomen can complicate chronic respiratory disorders such as asthma, cystic fibrosis, or chest wall restrictive lung disease (scoliosis).
- Tocolytic-induced pulmonary edema, amniotic fluid embolus, air embolus, aspiration, or pneumonia can complicate pregnancy.
- Management of many of these problems is supportive, and similar to the nonpregnant patient.

MECHANICAL VENTILATION OF PREGNANT PATIENTS

- The indications for intubation of a pregnant patient are no different than the nonpregnant patient. Noninvasive ventilation has not been studied extensively in this population.

- The guiding principle of ventilating the pregnant patient is ensuring adequate oxygen delivery. The goal is a PaO_2 of >90 mmHg.
- Positive end-expiratory pressure (PEEP) should be applied to keep the FiO_2 <60%, but the patient should be kept in the left lateral decubitus position to minimize the effect of PEEP on venous return. Ensuring adequate preload with intravenous fluids can also minimize the hemodynamic effects of PEEP and mechanical ventilation.
- Pregnant patients with ventilatory failure (e.g., from drug overdose and neuromuscular weakness) and without diffuse lung injury should have a target $PaCO_2$ of 27–30 mmHg, a eucapnic level during pregnancy.
- Pregnant patients with acute lung injury have not been well studied. Permissive hypercapnia, a strategy used in acute lung injury, may lead to fetal distress. If higher $PaCO_2$ levels are being sustained in the pregnant patient, then continuous fetal monitoring is required.
- In patients requiring neuromuscular blockade, short-term use of nondepolarizing agents such as pancuronium, vecuronium, and atracurium are safe for the fetus.
- Sedation with propofol and opioid drugs are safe, though the fetus may need to be intubated on delivery as these drugs cross the placenta.
- Benzodiazepines should be avoided as they have been shown to increase the incidence of cleft palate.
- Higher than normal peak and plateau airway pressures can be expected on the ventilator: compression of the diaphragm by the gravid uterus will increase respiratory system elastance.
- Fetal viability can be maintained while a patient is on mechanical ventilation, even during maternal brain death. Delivery or termination of pregnancy does not seem to improve the respiratory status of the mother, and therefore is not recommended.

CARDIOPULMONARY ARREST

- A pregnant patient requiring chest compressions should have a Cardiff Wedge or other device achieving approximately a 30° tilt placed under her back. This allows the patient to have adequate support of the torso for cardiopulmonary resuscitation (CPR) but also minimizes compression of the inferior vena cava (IVC). A backboard with rolled up towels or pillows under one side can substitute.
- The pregnant patient can safely undergo direct current cardioversion, both synchronized and unsynchronized. Drugs such as lidocaine, procainamide, adenosine, and quinidine can be safely used in the gravid patient. Amiodarone is contraindicated secondary to the possible effects on fetal thyroid development.
- It is possible for an emergent cesarean section to be performed during CPR.

BIBLIOGRAPHY

Afessa B, Green B, Delke I, et al. Systemic inflammatory response syndrome, organ failure, and outcome in critically ill obstetric patients treated in an ICU. *Chest* 2001;120:1271–1277.

Afessa B, Morales I, Cury JD. Clinical course and outcome of patients admitted to an ICU for status asthmaticus. *Chest* 2001;120:1616–1621.

Joglar JA, Page RL. Antiarrhythmic drugs in pregnancy. *Curr Opin Cardiol* 2001;16:40–45.

Lewin SB, Cheek TG, Deutschman CS. Airway management in the obstetric patient. *Crit Care Clin* 2000;16:505–553.

Ramsey PS, Ramin KD, Ramin SM. Cardiac disease in pregnancy. *Am J Perinatol* 2001;18:245–266.

Strek ME, O'Connor MF, Hall JB. Critical illness in pregnancy. In: Hall JB, Schmidt GA, Wood LDH, eds., *Principles of Critical Care*, 3rd ed. New York, NY: McGraw-Hill; 2005: 1583–1614.

121 RHEUMATOLOGY IN THE ICU

Janelle Laughlin

KEY POINTS

- Rheumatology patients are at increased risk for infection.
- Hypotension may be caused by adrenal insufficiency related to prior corticosteroid use without adequate stress dosing.
- Many rheumatologic diseases will present with pulmonary complications.
- Rheumatoid arthritis and lupus patients are at increased risk for coronary artery disease.
- Rheumatoid arthritis patients may have cervical neck instability.

EPIDEMIOLOGY

- Approximately one-third of patients admitted to the hospital with rheumatic disease require intensive care.

- 50% of intensive care unit (ICU) admissions are related to infection, and 25–35% are related to exacerbation of the rheumatic disease.
- Of the rheumatic diseases, rheumatoid arthritis (RA), systemic sclerosis (SSc), and systemic lupus erythematosus (SLE) account for more than 75% of admissions to the ICU.

IMMUNE STATUS OF THE RHEUMATIC PATIENT AND RISK FOR INFECTION

- Patients with rheumatic disease are often immunocompromised either due to the disease itself or therapies employed.
- For example, patients with SLE have impaired cellular immunity, altered phagocytic function, low complements, decreased production of immunoglobulin, and an impaired reticuloendothelial system necessary for organism elimination.
- Corticosteroids decrease phagocytic function as well as impair cell-mediated immunity.
- The incidence of infectious complications with corticosteroids increases with dose and duration over 4 weeks.
- Other immunosuppressives used can result in neutropenia, lymphopenia, T-cell signaling abnormalities, and other defects in immune response.
- Newer biologic therapies play a role in immunosuppression. These include monoclonal antibodies to tumor necrosis factor-alpha (TNF-α) (e.g., infliximab, etanercept, and adalimumab) and CD20 (e.g., rituximab).
- The TNF-α agents have been associated with infections with *Mycobacterium tuberculosis*, histoplasmosis, *Pneumocystis carinii*, coccidioidomycosis, and cryptococcus.
- Anti-CD20 therapies result in B-cell depletion and decrease production of immunoglobulins.

SYSTEMIC LUPUS ERYTHEMATOSUS

- Systemic lupus erythematosus is a systemic inflammatory disease, which can present in a variety of ways to the ICU.
- Pulmonary disease was the most common cause of admission in a series of 48 patients, occurring in 18 patients (37.5%). Other manifestations include neurologic and hematologic phenomena.
- Pulmonary manifestations of SLE include the following:
  - Pulmonary embolism
  - Pneumonia
  - Pneumonitis
  - Pulmonary hemorrhage
    - The mortality rates for lupus pneumonitis and pulmonary hemorrhage are high (up to 50%).
    - Patients may present with fever, tachypnea, and chest pain.
    - Hemoptysis does not need to be present.
    - Workup includes bronchoscopy or lung biopsy and markers of disease activity including complement levels, double stranded DNA antibodies, and markers of inflammation.
    - Infection must be ruled out.
    - Treatment should be aggressive although no consensus exists. Therapy includes pulse methylprednisolone 500–1000 mg intravenously for 3–5 days and/or intravenous cyclophosphamide. Plasmapheresis has been used as a temporizing measure although there are no controlled trials of its efficacy.
- Central nervous system (CNS) lupus ranges from cognitive dysfunction or peripheral neuropathy to seizures, psychosis, septic and aseptic meningitis, mononeuritis, and rarely transverse myelitis.
- Anemia and thrombocytopenia are common in SLE and can be refractory to therapy.
- It can be difficult to differentiate active SLE from thrombotic thrombocytopenic purpura (TTP) as these have been reported to coexist.

ANTIPHOSPHOLIPID SYNDROME

- Antiphospholipid syndrome (APS) is characterized by venous or arterial thrombosis and/or pregnancy morbidity in the setting of positive lupus anticoagulant, anticardiolipin antibodies, or anti-β_2-glycoprotein I antibodies.
- APS can present independently or along with other connective tissue disease.
- Less than 1% of APS patients present with life-threatening multiple-organ thrombosis and failure defined as catastrophic APS (CAPS).
  - CAPS is characterized by rapid diffuse small vessel ischemia and thrombosis affecting parenchymal organs.
  - Conditions associated with CAPS include malignant hypertension, acute respiratory distress syndrome, disseminated intravascular coagulation, microangiopathic hemolytic anemia, schistocytes, and thrombocytopenia.
  - "Trigger factors" such as recent surgical procedures or medications such as oral contraceptives have been described.
  - CAPS is fatal in approximately half of all patients despite treatment.

- First-line treatment consists of immediate anticoagulation with unfractionated or low-molecular weight heparin and high-dose corticosteroids.
- Corticosteroids are used to inhibit the excessive cytokine response but does not prevent further thrombotic events.
- Intravenous pulse methylprednisolone (1000 mg/day) for 3–5 days followed by high-dose methylprednisolone (1–2 mg/kg) is most commonly used. Second-line therapies include IVIg (in patients who are not IgA deficient) and plasma exchange with or with out fresh frozen plasma.

SCLERODERMA

- Life-threatening complications of SSc include renal crisis, undiagnosed or decompensated pulmonary artery hypertension (PAH), aspiration, alveolar hemorrhage, cardiac or gastrointestinal involvement.
- Scleroderma renal crisis presents with malignant hypertension and can progress to renal failure if treatment is not initiated.
  - There is an association with antecedent high-dose corticosteroids.
  - Laboratory data may show proteinuria, increased serum creatinine, and elevated plasma renin activity.
  - A microangiopathic hemolytic anemia may also be present.
  - Treatment includes the early use of angiotensin-converting enzyme (ACE) inhibitors and hemodialysis.
- SSc patients with PAH may present with symptoms of right ventricular failure.
  - Causes for decompensation should be investigated including but not limited to infection, thromboembolic disease, acute myocardial infarction, and cardiac tamponade.
  - Initial management should include administration of oxygen, use of pulmonary vasodilators, cardiac inotropes, and diuretics.
  - Diuresis can improve symptoms, however patients should be monitored carefully because of preload dependence.
  - Nitric oxide can be used to decrease pulmonary artery pressure without the risk of systemic hypotension.
  - Epoprostenol will reduce right ventricular afterload, however patients must be monitored for systemic hypotension. This should be administered in the ICU with the guidance of a pulmonary artery catheter.

RHEUMATOID ARTHRITIS

- Acute infection is the predominant reason for admission to the ICU in patients with RA.
- Standard evaluation for infectious source should include a thorough joint examination as RA patients are at increased risk for septic arthritis.
- Joint aspiration and culture should be performed especially if there is asymmetric swelling, redness, and warmth. The most common pathogen is *Staphylococcus aureus*.
- Patients with RA may present with respiratory failure.
  - Causes for respiratory failure are similar to those in the general population, but also include interstitial lung disease associated with RA, acute laryngeal stridor, and cricoarytenoid arthritis.
  - Airway management in these patients poses a special challenge. Obstacles in airway management include temporomandibular joint involvement, hypoplasia of the mandible, laryngeal or cricoarytenoid arthritis, as well as cervical spine disease including instability at the atlantoaxial joint.
  - For these reasons caution must be maintained for endotracheal intubation. It is important to avoid flexion of the neck. The cervical spine should be stabilized prior to intubation and intubation should occur under fiberoptic visualization. Continued neurologic monitoring for spinal cord dysfunction should be performed while patient remains intubated.

INFLAMMATORY MYOPATHY

- Dermatomyositis and polymyositis are idiopathic inflammatory muscle diseases presenting with proximal muscle weakness, which may include respiratory muscles and/or bulbar muscles.
- Severe disease may result in respiratory failure and/or aspiration.
- Patients who cannot protect their airway or who have difficulty adequately ventilating may require endotracheal intubation.
- Patients with dysphagia may require an enteral feeding tube to lessen aspiration risk.
- Electromyogram (EMG) and muscle biopsy are helpful in the diagnosis as well as laboratories for muscle enzymes and pulmonary function tests to diagnose respiratory muscle weakness.
- Respiratory muscle strength can be assessed at bedside via measurement of the negative inspiratory force.

BIBLIOGRAPHY

Alzeer AH, Al-Arfaj A, Basha SJ, et al. Outcome of patients with systemic lupus erythematosus in intensive care unit. *Lupus* 2004;13:537–542.

Coissio M, Menon Y, Wilson W, et al. Life threatening complications of systemic sclerosis. *Crit Care Clin* 2002;18:819–839.
Dedhia HV, DiBartolomeo A. Rheumatoid arthritis. *Crit Care Clin* 2002;18:841–854.
Erkan D, Cervera R, Asherson RA. Catastrophic antiphospholipid syndrome: where do we stand? *Arthritis Rheum* 2003;48:3320–3327.
Greenberg SB. Infections in the immunocompromised rheumatologic patient. *Crit Care Clin* 2002;18:931–956.
Janssen NM, Karnad DR, Guntupalli KK. Rheumatologic diseases in the intensive care unit: epidemiology, clinical approach, management, and outcome. *Crit Care Clin* 2002;18:729–748.
Wattenmaker I, Concepcion M, Hibberd P, et al. Upper-airway obstruction and perioperative management of the airway in patients managed with posterior operations on the cervical spine for rheumatoid arthritis. *J Bone Joint Surg Am* 1994;76:360–365.

122 DERMATOLOGY IN THE ICU

Joseph Levitt

KEY POINTS

- Observation and description of the lesions (morphology, distribution, feel) are important in developing a differential diagnosis.
- Mucous membranes (oral, ocular, nasal, genital, and perianal) should be examined in all patients.
- The skin may provide clues to an underlying, life-threatening condition, such as endocarditis, GVHD, bacterial sepsis, TSS, systemic vasculitis, or complications of HIV infection.
- Drug-related dermatoses are prevalent in the intensive care unit. Clues include a rapidly developing eruption; generalized, symmetrical, predominantly truncal distribution; maculopapular, urticarial, or acneiform morphology; and accompanying pruritus.
- Extensive skin disease can cause important fluid, electrolyte, and protein losses and predisposes the patient to life-threatening infection.

CHARACTERIZING THE LESION

- In approaching a patient with skin disease, careful observation, palpation, and description are critical in developing a differential diagnosis.
- Morphology may be flat (macule), elevated (papule, nodule, plaque, cyst, vesicle, bulla, pustule, hyperkeratosis), or depressed (ulcer, atrophy).
- Shape, margination (well or poorly defined borders), and arrangement of the lesions are important.
- Color may be white (leukoderma, hypomelanosis); red (erythematic); pink; violaceous (purple); brown (hypermelanosis, hemosiderin); black; blue; gray; yellow.
- Particular attention should be given to the distribution of the eruption (e.g., localized, systemic, truncal, acral, unilateral, or intertriginous).
- Palpation will help determine consistency, temperature, mobility, tenderness, and depth of lesion.
- When various lesions are present, one should attempt to identify the primary lesion.

INITIAL APPROACH

- Clinical history is an important part of any diagnosis. Symptoms (fever, malaise, arthralgias, myalgias, and so forth) should be questioned with particular attention paid to cutaneous symptoms (pruritus, pain, tenderness, burning, stinging). Careful medication history, including alternative and herbal remedies, is essential.
- Time course of the skin lesions should be determined and correlated with recent illness and medications.
- Common diagnostic aids include: skin biopsy for hematoxylin and eosin (H&E) or other special staining, direct immunofluorescence (DIF), or culture; potassium hydroxide (KOH) preparation (for dermatophytic infections); mineral oil mounts (for scabies); Gram's stain (for bacterial infections); fluid cultures; and Tzanck smears (for herpes simplex and varicella zoster virus infections).

DRUG REACTIONS

- Cutaneous drug reactions are the most common type of adverse drug reaction, and occur in 2–3% of hospitalized patients with 1 out of 1000 patients having a serious reaction.
- Multiple medications and delayed onset can make determination of the offending agent difficult in the ICU setting. Commonly identified agents include antiepileptics (e.g., phenytoin and carbamazepine), antibiotics (e.g., amoxicillin, penicillin, fluoroquinolones, sulfonamides, and cephalosporins), nonsteroidal anti-inflammatory agents (NSAIDs), and other analgesics.
- Morphology may be maculopapular, morbilliform, urticarial, fixed drug, or acneiform.
- Eruptions generally develop very rapidly and may be accompanied by pruritus.

- Onset is usually 1 week after exposure but may be significantly delayed, particularly with antibiotics.
- While usually benign, adverse reactions can progress to toxic epithelial necrolysis (TEN) or the Stevens-Johnson syndrome. Signs indicative of serious skin problems include mucosal involvement, blistering lesions, and a positive Nikolsky sign (sheering of epidermis when lateral pressure is applied to the skin).
- Systemic manifestations include hepatitis, fever, eosinophilia, glomerulonephritis, anaphylaxis, and angioedema.

SERIOUS CUTANEOUS DRUG REACTIONS

Chemotherapeutic Agents

- Stomatitis occurs in 40% of patients and can lead to significant discomfort and even difficulties with oral nutrition. Treatment consists of oral hygiene and topical regimens consisting of magnesium/aluminum hydroxide, diphenhydramine elixir, and viscous lidocaine/benzocaine solutions.
- Care should be taken to distinguish stomatitis from candidiasis (white adherent velvety plaques) and varicella and herpes zoster (lip and intraoral ulcers) infection. KOH preparations and Tzanck staining should be diagnostic in ambiguous situations.
- Extravasation of peripherally infused agents start as painful erythema and can lead to significant local tissue necrosis. Treatment consists of elevation of the effected limb, hot or cold packs, and if necessary surgical debridement. Specific antidotes to some agents exist and should be used early to prevent progression.
- Acral erythema occurs in 6–24% of patients and consists of painful erythema and edema of the palms and soles. Symptoms usually resolve within 4 weeks of discontinuation of offending agent.

Anticoagulant Agents

- Subcutaneous heparin on rare occassion is associated with local delayed type reaction at the injection site manifested by erythema and vesicular pruritic plaques (2–5 days) and local skin necrosis (5–10 days). Reactions are associated with increased risk of heparin-induced thrombocytopenia. Reports of cross-reactivity with low-molecular weight heparins and heparinoids have been reported and thus these agents should be avoided.
- Warfarin necrosis occurs on rare occasions on initiation of therapy as protein C and S levels decline prior to fall in procoagulant factors. Lesions, involving the breast, abdomen, and thighs, start as blue/black plaques with hemorrhagic bullae that necrose and form a central eschar. Predisposing factors include protein C deficiency and factor V Leiden mutations. Surgical debridement is often necessary but significant morbidity and mortality (15%) persists.

Vasopressor Agents

- Extravasation of peripherally infused α_1-agonists and vasopressin can cause severe local ischemic tissue necrosis. Even with when centrally delivered, high doses in low flow states (shock) can lead to necrosis of distal digits and diffuse ischemic skin lesions.

Stevens-Johnson Syndrome and Toxic Epithelial Necrolysis

- Histologically identical lesions, these syndromes are distinguished by amount of body surface area involved (SJS <10% and TEN >30%). Erythema multiforme shares similar histology but is limited to annular erythematous plaques with central areas of blistering and necrosis (target lesions) involving mucosal and extremity extensor surfaces.
- Fever, sore throat, and burning eyes may precede eruption of a painful erythematous maculopapular rash. Early stages may be indistinguishable from benign drug reactions, but lesions rapidly coalesce, progress to blisters and epidermal detachment in hours to days. Mucosal surfaces are involved in 85–95% of cases and, when present early, suggest a more serious reaction. Ocular and airway and gastrointestinal epithelial involvement are associated with increased morbidity.
- Anticonvulsants (phenytoin, valproic acid, phenobarbital, carbamazepine), antibiotics (sulfonamides, aminopenicillins), NSAIDs, chlormezanone, allopurinol and, paradoxically, corticosteroids are the most commonly implicated medications. Reactions occur more commonly in patients with HIV.
- Treatment is largely supportive and consists of nonadherent wrapping of affected areas to limit fluid losses. Silver or antibiotic (except sulfonamides) impregnated wraps may help to reduce infection. Airway involvement may require endotracheal intubation and aggressive fluid and electrolyte replacement may be necessary. Case reports have suggested benefit with early use of corticosteroids but multiple retrospective series imply a worse outcome and they are generally considered contraindicated. IVIg and plasmapheresis may be beneficial but no consensus exists on their utility.

MEDICAL DERMATOSES

ERYTHRODERMA

- Erythroderma or exfoliative dermatitis is a descriptive term for a clinical condition characterized by total body diffuse erythema and scaling, often accompanied by fever, chills, and lymphadenopathy.

- Loss of the percutaneous absorption barrier increases blood flow to the skin and may lead to hypoalbuminemia, peripheral edema, loss of muscle mass. High output cardiac failure may result with as much as 8% of cardiac output directed to the inflamed cutaneous vasculature.
- Risk factors for erythroderma include inflammatory conditions (psoriasis, atopic dermatitis, contact dermatitis, and pityriasis rubra pilaris), drug eruptions, cutaneous T-cell lymphoma, and systemic neoplasms.
- Treatment consists of careful attention to fluid and electrolyte balance, temperature regulation, and nutritional status. Topical therapies include medium potency steroid ointments covered with a bland ointment, such as zinc oxide ointment and wrapped with clean cloths, or topical steroids applied directly under a plastic sauna suit. Topical irritant agents, such as tar containing ointments, should be avoided. Wet dressings may help weeping or crusted areas. Pruritus and anxiety typically respond to the sedating antihistamines.

PURPURA

- Purpura results from the extravasation of blood into surrounding tissues and is associated with many conditions. Lesions are placed into two main categories, palpable or nonpalpable. Assessment of purpura includes evaluation of the patient's underlying conditions; potential precipitating events, current and past laboratory values, and medication history are analyzed.
- Nonpalpable (macular), nonblanching purpura arises from simple hemorrhage into tissue. Petechiae are lesions <0.2 cm in diameter that result from superficial vascular hemorrhage. Larger areas are termed ecchymoses. Nonpalpable purpura is most commonly attributed to fragility of the vascular tissue or defects in hemostasis. Examples include platelet disorders (thrombocytopenia, thrombocytopathia, and thrombocytosis), disseminated intravascular coagulation (DIC), and warfarin-associated necrosis. Skin biopsy may be helpful in diagnosis, especially in neutropenic patients who are unable to mount the immune response to cause dermal inflammation.
- Palpable purpura indicates underlying vasculitis (also called cutaneous necrotizing venulitis or leukocytoclastic vasculitis) resulting from segmental vascular inflammation, swelling, and necrosis of endothelial cells, and neutrophilic infiltration of vessel walls. For the first 24–48 hours, the lesions are a deep erythematous color that eventually becomes violaceous. Precipitating factors include infections, drugs, autoimmune diseases, and immunoglobulin-mediated complement activation. Common infectious agents include *Staphylococcus aureus*, hepatitis B, and hepatitis C. Drugs commonly associated with vasculitis include ampicillins, thiazides, phenytoin, sulfa-containing compounds, allopurinol, hydralazine, and propylthiouracil.
- Workup includes identification of a potential primary cause and evaluation for systemic involvement. In addition to a biopsy, a complete blood count, chemistry panel, liver function tests, urinalysis, stool guaiac, hepatitis B and C viral serologies, cryoglobulins, and complement levels are evaluated. Antinuclear antibody (ANA) titers are evaluated in patients with suspected connective tissue diseases. In patients with a fever and heart murmur, blood cultures and echocardiography should be performed.

GRAFT-VERSUS-HOST DISEASE

- Graft-versus-host disease (GVHD) is a complex syndrome following allogeneic bone marrow transplantation. The skin is often the first and is the most frequent organ involved in GVHD. Biopsy may help distinguish GVHD from other causes of erythema such as drug eruptions or viral exanthems. Acute GVHD usually occurs between days 10 and 30 after transplantation, but may appear anytime up to day 100.
- Skin changes consist of a generalized morbilliform eruption progressing to extensive redness, blistering, or skin necrosis. The earliest sign is pruritus and tenderness of the palms and soles with reddening of the dorsal aspects of the fingers followed by diffuse erythema of the hands and feet. Blisters (with a positive Nikolsky sign) and generalized desquamation portend a poor prognosis.
- Factors associated with developing GVHD include recipient cytomegalovirus seropositivity, pretransplant seropositivity for three to four different herpes viruses in the donor, early engraftment (<15 days), increased tumor necrosis factor (TNF) during conditioning, and prophylactic monotherapy.
- Treatment for acute GVHD includes continuing the original immunosuppressive prophylactic regimen (cyclosporine, tacrolimus, mycophenolate mofetil) and adding methylprednisolone at 2 mg/kg. Treatment protocols differ and may include antithymocyte globulin and monoclonal antibodies. Topical treatment is mainly supportive with emollients and topical steroids.

INFECTIONS

BACTERIAL INFECTIONS

NECROTIZING FASCIITIS

- This results from a suppurative bacterial infection of the superficial and soft tissues. Proximal spread along deep fascial planes can lead to rapid progression to gangrene, sepsis, and death. Although classically described with group A streptococcus alone or in combination with anaerobes, numerous organisms can be implicated depending on the clinical setting.

- Risk factors include any break in the skin (superficial infections, surgical procedures, cuts, burns, indwelling catheters, child birth), obesity, diabetes, cirrhosis, and immunosuppression (steroids, NSAIDs, TNF-alpha inhibitors).
- Patients present with erythema, edema, warmth, and severe tenderness often limited to one limb which may rapidly progress to a bluish hue with bullae formation. The diagnosis is primarily clinical. Necrotizing fasciitis (NF) is distinguished from cellulitis by rapid progression and the severity of pain on presentation. Computed tomography (CT) scans may help identify the extent of involvement, but should not delay or discourage definitive surgical exploration. Plain radiographs may show air in the soft tissues with concomitant anaerobic infections. Measurement of compartment pressures may help confirm the diagnosis. Superficial biopsies and cultures are not useful.
- Treatment consists of antibiotics and emergent fasciotomy and surgical debridement. Antibiotics alone are ineffective due to the vascular occlusion in effected areas. There is theoretical support for adding clindamycin for its disruption or protein synthesis since much of the intense inflammation is toxin mediated.

Toxic Shock Syndrome

- Toxic shock syndrome (TSS) is characterized by fever, shock, desquamating rash, and multiorgan system failure in association with toxins mediated from both group A streptococcal and *S. aureus* infections.
- Streptococcal TSS usually occurs in association with soft tissue infections, but less apparent portals can occur via the vagina or pharynx. Toxins may function as superantigens, binding directly to major histocompatibility complex (MHC) II cells and inducing a massive T-cell reaction.
- In Staph TSS diagnostic criteria include the presence of a normal to high normal WBC with extreme left shift, acute renal failure, hypotension, hypoalbuminemia, hypocalcemia, thrombocytopenia, hematuria, and elevated creatine kinases (CKs). Interestingly, renal failure often precedes the onset of hypotension.
- Staph TSS occurs in association with overgrowth of occluded mucosal surfaces (superabsorbent tampons and nasal packing) and presents with a scarlatiniform eruption with flexural accentuation. Erythema and edema of the palms and soles, hyperemia of conjunctiva and mucous membranes, and a strawberry tongue may also be present.
- Treatment is supportive and consists of penicillin and clindamycin and vasoactive drugs. IVIg may be of benefit when hypotension is present. Plasmapheresis and hyperbaric oxygen have also been used in Strep TSS.

Staphylococcal Scalded Skin Syndrome

- A desquamative exanthem that occurs in conjunction with infection by toxin producing *S. aureus*. The majority of patients are under age 5 and adults are only rarely affected. The major risk factors for developing staphylococcal scalded skin syndrome (SSSS) in adults are renal failure (owing to decreased filtration of toxin), hematologic malignancies, and immunosuppression. The concurrent use of NSAIDs may predispose to SSSS.
- Patients may have a preceding upper respiratory infection with rhinorrhea, pharyngitis, and conjunctivitis. The exanthem begins abruptly with diffuse tender erythema and subsequent superficial desquamation. Intact bullae are rarely seen but when present, may have a positive Nikolsky sign. Biopsy of the blister border may be necessary to distinguish from TEN.
- Treatment consists of appropriate antibiotics (nafcillin, methicillin, dicloxacillin, or a first-generation cephalosporin) and vigilant monitoring of fluids and electrolytes. Monotherapy is usually adequate, since multiresistant strains of *S. aureus* are rarely encountered among the toxigenic strains. Healing generally occurs in 7–10 days.

Pseudomonas Bacteremia

- A variety of skin manifestations of *Pseudomonas* bacteremia have been described. Ecthyma gangrenosum, usually found in the anogenital region, buttocks, or axilla, occurs in 5% of patients and is characterized by a localized, erythematous, tender plaque or bulla which subsequently develops central necrosis leaving a gangrenous eschar with an erythematous annular border.
- Vesicles or bullae may occur anywhere either singly or in clusters. Lesions frequently become hemorrhagic and may resemble ecthyma gangrenosum lesions when ruptured.
- Cellulitis, which in contrast to that caused by staphylococcal or streptococcal infections, tends to have sharply demarcated borders.
- Cellulitis may also form as small pink, round plaques or subcutaneous nodules concentrated on the trunk and proximal extremities which when incised and drained, grow *Pseudomonas aeruginosa* in culture.

Meningococcemia

- Acute infection with the gram-negative diplococcus *Neisseria meningitidis* is associated with petechiae,

ecchymoses, or palpable purpura, which may herald a rapidly progressive fatal disease. Petechiae may be preceded by an urticarial, rubella-like, papular or generalized scarlatiniform eruption for 2 days.
- Lesions may result from thrombosis precipitated directly by meningococcus, fibrin, and leukocytes with a corresponding leukocytoclastic vasculitis or DIC precipitated by meningococcal endotoxin resulting in microvascular fibrin thrombi.
- Differential diagnosis includes gonococcemia, Rickettsial infection, allergic vasculitis, and bacterial endocarditis. Gonococcemia is usually associated with arthritis and tenosynovitis. Petechiae of the palms and soles suggest Rocky Mountain spotted fever (infection with *Rickettsia rickettsii*).
- Rapid recognition and prompt antibiotic treatment is essential to reduce mortality which may be as high as 70% when progressing to shock.

Infective Endocarditis

- Petechiae, secondary to microemboli, are found in approximately 30% of patients. Roth spots may appear on conjunctiva, buccal mucosa, palate, and retina. Petechiae on fingers or proximal nail beds manifest as red to brown streaks termed splinter hemorrhages.
- Petechiae occurring on the palms and soles with a nodular character are termed Janeway lesions. Lesions are characteristically nontender and result from septic emboli consisting of bacteria, neutrophilic infiltration, and subcutaneous hemorrhage.
- Osler nodes are small 2–15 mm, painful nodules commonly found on the pads of the fingers, toes, or thenar eminences. Osler nodes are seen in 5–15% of patients with streptococcal-induced infective endocarditis but may also be seen in systemic lupus erythematosus, endocarditis due to fungal or gram-negative bacilli, typhoid fever, gonococcemia, and in the arms of patients with cannulated radial arteries.

VIRAL INFECTIONS

Herpes Simplex

- Cutaneous herpes infection, associated with herpes simplex virus (HSV) types 1 and 2 appear as clusters of vesicles or shallow erosions, usually over the lips, genitals, and lumbosacral region but can occur on any cutaneous area. When vesicles to go undetected, the patient may present with punched-out erosions or shallow ulcerations. Chronic perianal HSV ulcers are easily mistaken for decubitus ulcers. Scalloped borders and small circular ulcerations at the periphery of the ulcer may be helpful distinguishing signs.
- Rapid diagnosis may be done by DIF on cells smeared on a glass slide, or by direct fluorescent antibody (DFA) testing with monoclonal antibodies on cultured specimens. Bedside diagnosis can be made with a Tzanck smear by scraping the base of an unroofed vesicle with a blade or glass slide revealing multinucleated giant and/or balloon cells.
- All infections encountered in the ICU should be treated promptly with an antiviral agent such as acyclovir, famciclovir, or valacyclovir usually intravenously although the medications are effective orally.

Varicella Zoster

- Classic cutaneous findings consist of a generalized eruption of discrete vesicles on an erythematous base ("dewdrop on a rose petal") associated with prodromal symptoms of fever and malaise.
- Lesions, which first appear on the trunk and spread to the extremities, progress from an erythematous papule to a vesicle to a hemorrhagic crust and may be at various stages of development at any one time (in contrast to small pox in which lesions start centripedally and all are in the same stage of development).
- Patients are contagious from 2 days prior to the eruption until all lesions have crusted.
- While usually self-limited, infections in adults and the immunosuppressed can be life threatening. Encephalitis may be seen in patients with a persistent viremia. An immune complex vasculitis may lead to pancreatitis, myocarditis, arthritis, and palpable purpura.
- Zoster (shingles), a recrudescence of latent infection lying dormant in nerve roots, presents with a prodrome of intense pain followed by eruption of lesions in dermatomal pattern (thoracic 55% and trigeminal nerves 15–20%).
- Involvement of the eye, caused by infection of the ophthalmic branch of the trigeminal nerve, may lead to conjunctivitis, keratitis, and iridocyclitis. Ophthalmologic consultation is mandatory.
- In immunosuppressed patients, disseminated herpes zoster may occur and should be treated with full doses of intravenous antiviral therapy.

SUPERFICIAL FUNGAL INFECTIONS

- Primary cutaneous infection with *Candida albicans* is the most common fungal infection in the ICU. Lesions consist of bright red, moist plaques with satellite pustules occurring in moist, warm environments such as intertriginous areas. Associated skin breakdown may predispose to secondary bacterial infections.

- Candidemia, once rare, is a growing concern in ICUs. Usually associated with central venous lines, neutropenia, or multiorgan failure, candidemia is associated with a 30% mortality rate despite antifungal therapy.
- The diagnosis is supported by the typical pseudohyphae on KOH mount or culture of scales but visual inspection is often sufficient to begin topical therapy.

PRESSURE ULCERS

- Continuous pressure over a bony site obstructs microcirculation, leading to tissue ischemia and necrosis. Pressure ulcers constitute a major problem in the ICU, with reported prevalences as high as 40% (two- to threefold higher than other hospitalized patients).
- Risk factors include the duration of previous surgeries and number of operations, preoperative protein and albumin concentrations, skin moisture, use of inotropic drugs, fecal incontinence or diarrhea, altered circulatory status, diabetes mellitus, decreased mobility, and high Acute Physiology and Chronic Health Evaluation II (APACHE II).
- Ulcers are classified in four grades:
  - *Stage I*: An observable pressure-related alteration (redness, skin temperature, tissue consistency, and/or sensation) of intact skin.
  - *Stage II*: Partial thickness skin loss involving epidermis, dermis, or both. The ulcer is superficial and presents clinically as an abrasion, blister, or shallow crater.
  - *Stage III*: Full thickness skin loss involving damage to, or necrosis of, subcutaneous tissue that may extend down to, but not through, underlying fascia. The ulcer presents clinically as a deep crater with or without undermining of adjacent tissue.
  - *Stage IV*: Full thickness skin loss with extensive destruction, tissue necrosis, or damage to muscle, bone, or supporting structures (e.g., tendon and joint capsule). Undermining and sinus tracts also may be associated with stage IV pressure ulcers.
- Pressure ulcers lead to increased mortality rates, costs, and lengths of hospital stays and preventive strategies (risk assessment scales, repositioning the patient every 2 hours, the provision of dynamic or static support surfaces that redistribute pressure, and proper nutrition) should be implemented from the moment of entry into the ICU.
- Topical treatment consists of maintenance of a moist environment via one of many different dressings (transparent films, hydrocolloids, alginates, foams, hydrogels, or hydrofibers). These dressings require few changes and result in less need for nursing care, faster healing, and decreased infection. Gauze dressings, particularly wet to dry dressings, should be avoided. Surgery may be required for recalcitrant, full-thickness ulcers, however, recurrence rates are high.

BIBLIOGRAPHY

Cotran RS. The skin. In: Cotran RS, Kumar V, Collins T, et al., eds., *Robbins Pathologic Basis of Disease*, 6th ed. Philadelphia, PA: W.B. Saunders; 1999: 1170–1214.

Lacouture ME, Welsch MJ, Laumaun AE. Dermatologic conditions. In: Hall JB, Schmidt GA, Wood LDH, eds., *Principles of Critical Care*, 3rd ed. New York, NY: McGraw-Hill; 2005:1627–1654.

Roujeau JC, Stern RS. Severe adverse cutaneous reactions to drugs. *N Engl J Med* 1994;331:1272–1285.

123 TOXICOLOGY IN ADULTS

Michael Moore

KEY POINTS

- Supportive management is the most important aspect of treating most intoxications, although specific antidotes should be considered when indicated.
- Patients with depressed mental status should all receive empiric therapy with oxygen, dextrose, thiamine, and naloxone while evaluation is ongoing.
- Identification of toxidromes, guided largely by vital signs, pupillary findings, and aspects of autonomic function often helps to identify the class of agents that may be part of the poisoned patient.
- Poison control center consultation is an extremely useful source of information.
- An osmolal gap of large magnitude coupled to an anion gap acidosis suggests methanol or ethylene glycol poisoning.

EPIDEMIOLOGY

- In 2001, >2 million toxic exposure cases were reported to poison control centers in the United States.
- 85% were unintentional and 92% involved a single substance.
- Toxic exposures account for 5–10% of emergency department (ED) visits and >5% of all adult ICU admissions.
- Most common exposures: analgesics (10.6%), cleaning substances (9.5%), cosmetics (9.2%), foreign bodies (5.1%), plants (4.7%), sedative-hypnotics (4.4%), and cough/cold preparations (4.3%).

- Substances most associated with fatalities: carbon monoxide (CO), analgesics, sedative-hypnotics, antipsychotics, antidepressants, street drugs, cardiovascular drugs, or alcohols.

GENERAL APPROACH

DIAGNOSIS

- Suspect the diagnosis in patients with the clinical features found in Table 123-1.
- The history is paramount but may be missing or incomplete.
- Look for specific "toxidromes" (see Table 123-2).
- Physical examination:
  - Vital signs: tachycardia, bradycardia, hypo/hyperthermia
  - Ocular findings: mydriasis versus miosis, horizontal versus other nystagmus
  - Mental status/behavior: depressed mentation, agitation, delirium/confusion
  - Muscle tone: dystonias, dyskinesias, rigidity
- Urine toxicology screen can help confirm or refute exposure but is unlikely to alter early management.

TABLE 123-1 Clinical Features Mandating Consideration of Toxic Ingestion

History of drug overdose or substance abuse
Suicidal ideation or prior suicide attempts
History of other psychiatric illness
Agitation and hallucinations
Stupor and coma
Rotary nystagmus
Delirium or confusion
Seizures
Muscle rigidity
Dystonia
Cardiopulmonary arrest
Unexplained cardiac arrhythmias
Hyper/hypotension
Ventilatory failure
Aspiration
Bronchospasm
Liver failure
Renal failure
Hyper/hypothermia
Rhabdomyolysis
Osmolal gap
Anion gap acidosis
Hyper/hypoglycemia
Hyper/hyponatremia
Hyper/hypokalemia
Polypharmacy

SOURCE: Adapted from Corbridge TC, Murry P, Mokhlesi B. Toxicology in adults. In: Hall JB, Schmidt GA, Wood LDH, eds., *Principles of Critical Care*, 3rd ed. New York, NY: McGraw-Hill; 2005: 1506.

- Measure the anion gap, osmolal gap, and oxygen saturation gap.
- Contact local poison control center for additional help in suspected poison cases and to help guide initial management.

MANAGEMENT

- Initial support measures require attention to the "ABCs" (airway, breathing, circulation).

ELIXIR OF CONSCIOUSNESS

- Administer a combination of thiamine 100 mg IV, dextrose 50 g IV, and naloxone (initial dose of 0.2–04 mg IV) to patients who present with change in mental status.
- Consider administration of flumazenil for suspected cases of benzodiazepine overdose.

DECONTAMINATION

GENERAL

- Decontaminate skin by removal of toxin with soap and water. Remove contaminated clothing and store in adequate container to limit ongoing exposure to patient and health care providers.
- Ocular decontamination may require prolonged irrigation with normal saline solution.

EMESIS

- Can be considered for fully awake patient but rarely used since these patients usually have not ingested highly toxic substances or quantities.
- Contraindicated in patient at high risk for seizures, or poisoning with corrosives, petrolatum products, or antiemetics. Avoid in patients who are at risk for seizures.
- Dose 30 mL followed by 16 oz of water. Can be repeated in 30 minutes if no effect.

GASTRIC EMPTYING

- Large-bore (Ewald) tubes 37–40 F may be needed to remove gastric debris.
- Technique: Inspect mouth and clear off foreign material. Have suctioning equipment ready. Insert tube and confirm placement. Immediately withdraw as much of the gastric contents as possible. Instill 200 mL bolus of warmed water and aspirate gastric contents. Repeat until gastric aspirate is clear. This method of tube placement should not be used in patients with

TABLE 123-2 Common Toxidromes

TOXIDROME	FEATURE	DRUG/TOXIN	DRUG TREATMENT
Anticholinergic "Hot as a hare, dry as a beet, mad as a hatter"	Mydriasis Blurred vision Fever Dry skin Flushing Ileus Urinary retention Tachycardia Hypertension Psychosis Coma Seizures Myoclonus	Antihistamines Atropine Baclofen Benztropine Cyclic antidepressants Phenothiazines Propantheline Scopolamine	Physostigmine (do not use in cyclic antidepressant overdose) Sodium bicarbonate in cyclic antidepressant overdose
Cholinergic "SLUDGE"	Salivation Urination Diarrhea GI cramps Emesis Wheezing Diaphoresis Bronchorrhea Bradycardia Miosis	Carbamate Organophosphates Physostigmine Pilocarpine	Atropine Pralidoxime for organophosphates
Beta-adrenergic	Tachycardia Hypotension Tremor	Albuterol Caffeine Terbutaline Theophylline	Beta-blockade (caution in asthmatics)
Alpha-adrenergic	Hypertension Bradycardia Mydriasis	Phenylephrine Phenylpropanolamine	Treat hypertension with phentolamine or nitroprusside; not with beta-blockers alone
Beta- and alpha-adrenergic	Hypertension Tachycardia Mydriasis Diaphoresis Dry mucus membranes	Amphetamines Cocaine Ephedrine Phencyclidine Pseudoephedrine	Benzodiazepines
Sedative/hypnotic	Stupor and coma Confusion Slurred speech Apnea	Anticonvulsants Antipsychotics Barbiturates Benzodiazepines Ethanol Meprobamate Opiates	Naloxone for opiates Flumazenil for benzodiazepines Urinary alkalinization for phenobarbital
Hallucinogenic	Hallucinations Psychosis Panic Fever Mydriasis Hyperthermia	Amphetamines Cannabinoids Cocaine LSD Pneumocystis pneumonia (PCP)	Benzodiazepines Haloperidol
Extrapyramidal	Rigidity/tremor Opisthotonos Trismus Hyperreflexia Choreoathetosis	Haloperidol Phenothiazines	Diphenhydramine Benztropine
Narcotic	Altered mental status Slow respirations Miosis Bradycardia Hypotension Hypothermia Decreased bowel sounds	Dextromethorphan Opioids Pentazocine Propoxyphene	Naloxone

(Continued)

TABLE 123-2 Common Toxidromes *(Continued)*

TOXIDROME	FEATURE	DRUG/TOXIN	DRUG TREATMENT
Serotonin syndrome agents	Irritability Hyperreflexia Flushing Diarrhea Diaphoresis Fever Trismus Tremor Myoclonus	Fluoxetine Meperidine Paroxetine Sertraline Trazodone	Benzodiazepines

SOURCE: Corbridge TC, Murry P, Mokhlesi B. Toxicology in adults. In: Hall JB, Schmidt GA, Wood LDH, eds., *Principles of Critical Care*, 3rd ed. New York, NY: McGraw-Hill; 2005: 1507.

depressed level of consciousness unless intubation has been performed, since retching and vomiting is common.
- Indications: American Academy of Clinical Toxicology does not recommend routine use of gastric lavage (GL) unless the patient has ingested a potentially life-threatening amount of a poison and the procedure can be performed within 60 minutes of ingestion. The time to perform GL may be increased if the toxin is known to delay gastric emptying.
- Contraindications: Obtunded, comatose, or convulsing patients. Also ingestion of sustained-release or enteric-coated tablets and probably caustic liquids to avoid aspiration-induced lung injury.

ACTIVATED CHARCOAL

- Activated charcoal is a nontoxic, inert, nonspecific adsorbent that binds intraluminal drugs and decreases systemic absorption.
- Very effective for high molecular weight substances.
- Indications: As sole decontaminate or used after GL or ipecac-induced emesis.
- Contraindications: Patients unable to protect airway or during seizures.
- Complications: pneumonia, bronchiolitis obliterans, acute respiratory distress syndrome (ARDS), death.
- Dosing: If quantity of toxin known, give 10:1 charcoal: toxin ratio; can dose by weight 1 g/kg.

WHOLE-BOWEL IRRIGATION

- Polyethylene glycol (Colyte®) or potassium chloride (Golytely®) can be used to clear gastrointestinal (GI) tract of tablets or packages.
- Usual dose is 1–2 L/h.
- May be particularly effective in cases of ingestion of sustained-release tablets, drugs where activated charcoal is not effective (iron, lithium), or in cases of "body packing."
- Contraindications: ileus, GI hemorrhage, bowel perforation.

ENHANCEMENT OF ELIMINATION

MULTIPLE-DOSE ACTIVATED CHARCOAL

- Can enhance elimination of drugs that have already been absorbed.
- Interrupts enterohepatic/enterogastric circulation or binds drugs that can diffuse from circulation into gut lumen.
- Dose: initial 1 g/kg followed by 0.5 g/kg every 2–4 hours for at least 3 doses.
- Contraindications: inability to protect airway.
- Avoid cathartics to avoid hypernatremia, hypokalemia, and hypermagnesemia.
- Not studied in clinical trials; not shown to decrease morbidity or mortality.
- Should be reserved for life-threatening ingestion of carbamazepine, dapsone, phenobarbital, quinine, or theophylline.

HEMODIALYSIS

- Effective for removal of certain toxins and drugs (low molecular weight, water soluble, low protein binding, and small volume of distribution).
- Consider in cases where clearance is expected to be delayed or insufficient secondary to renal or hepatic insufficiency, toxin produced toxic metabolites, or when delayed toxicity is characteristic.
- Early use of hemodialysis (HD) is recommended for intoxication with methanol, ethylene glycol, boric acid, salicylates, and lithium.
- Effective for use in heavy metal intoxication in patients with renal failure.

HEMOPERFUSION

- Blood is pumped through an adsorbent system (usually a charcoal canister).
- Has been effectively used for intoxications with theophylline, phenobarbital, phenytoin, carbamazepine, paraquat, and glutethimide.
- Less effective for lithium, ethanol, methanol, CO, cocaine, and phencyclidine.
- Complications: cartridge saturation, thrombocytopenia, hypoglycemia, hypocalcemia, hypothermia, charcoal embolization.

HEMOFILTRATION

- Utilizes a highly porous membrane to remove drugs and toxins by convection.
- Potentially useful for removal of toxins that have a large volume of distribution, slow intracompartmental transfer, or extensive tissue binding.
- Specific hemofiltration cartridges can be used to effectively remove digoxin-Fab complexes, deferoxamine-iron complexes, and aluminum.

INDICATIONS FOR ADMISSION TO INTENSIVE CARE UNIT

- Based on observed and predicted severity of toxicity.
- Patients with mild toxicity or low predicted severity can be observed in the ED until asymptomatic. Patients with observed or predicted moderate toxicity should be admitted to an appropriate observation unit.
- One study retrospectively identified eight clinical risk factors in poisoned patients who are likely to require ICU interventions: $PaCO_2$ >45 mmHg, need for endotracheal intubation, toxin-induced seizures, cardiac arrhythmias, QRS duration ≥0.012 seconds, systolic blood pressure (BP) <80 mmHg, second- or third-degree AV block, unresponsiveness to verbal stimuli.
- See Table 123-3 for list of ICU admission criteria.

TABLE 123-3 Indications for Admission to ICU

Respiratory depression ($PaCO_2$ >45 mmHg)
Seizures
High-degree AV block
Systolic BP <80 mmHg
Glasgow Coma Scale <12
Need for emergent HD, hemoperfusion, or extracorporeal membrane oxygenation (ECMO)
Increasing metabolic acidosis
Hypo- or hyperthermia
Tricyclic or phenothiazine overdose with anticholinergic signs, neurologic abnormalities, or prolonged QRS/QT
Body packers
Drug bezoars
Need for naloxone by continuous infusion
Digitalis overdose and hypokalemia
Antivenom for envenomations

SOURCE: Adapted from Mokhlesi B, Leiken JB, Murry P. Adult toxicology in critical care. Part I. General approach to the intoxicated patient. *Chest* 2003;123:589.

SELECTED SPECIFIC INTOXICATIONS (LISTED ALPHABETICALLY)

ACETAMINOPHEN

- Most common overdose reported to poison control centers.
- Rapid oral absorption with peak levels in <1 hour.
- The toxic threshold is 150 mg/kg or 7.5–10 g in adults.
- There are four phases of toxicity:
  - *Phase 1*: first 24 hours: malaise, pallor, diaphoresis, nausea, and vomiting
  - *Phase 2*: 24–48 hours: onset of right upper quadrant (RUQ) pain and liver function test abnormalities. Initial symptoms may improve
  - *Phase 3*: 48–96 hours: encephalopathy, hypoglycemia, and coagulopathy. Aspartate transaminase (AST)/alanine transaminase (ALT) levels usually peak (≥10,000 IU/L) with severely abnormal prothrombin time and total bilirubin levels. Rare phase 3 complications include acute renal failure, hemorrhagic pancreatitis, and myocardial necrosis
  - *Phase 4*: >96 hours: full recovery or death
- The modified Rumack-Matthew nomogram allows stratification of risk based on acetaminophen level and time since ingestion (see Fig. 123-1).
- Successful use of the Rumack-Matthew nomogram requires attention to its limitations:
  - Less useful when patients present early (<4 hours) or late (>24 hours)
  - Chronic ingestion or ingestion with extended-release products
  - Nomogram does not take into account patients at high risk of toxicity (chronic alcohol users or patients with induced cytochrome P-450 system)
- Activated charcoal is the treatment of choice for gastric decontamination. GL is reasonable if administered within 1 hour of ingestion.

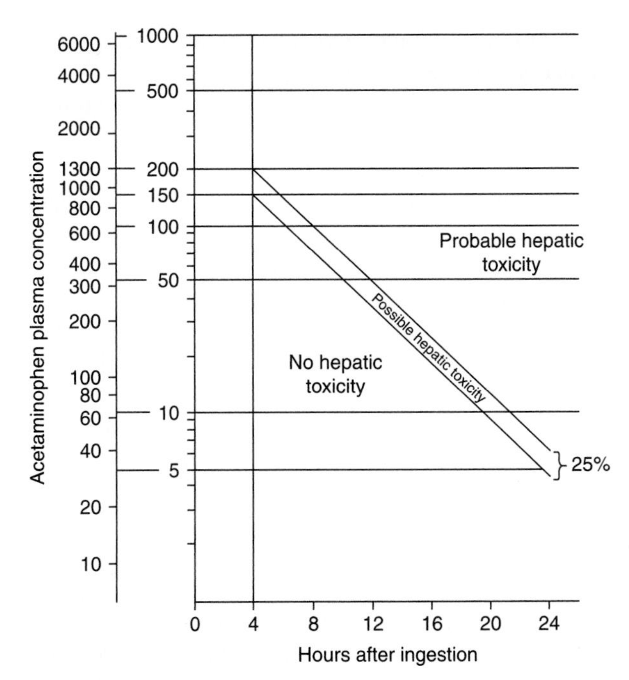

FIG. 123-1 Rumack-Matthew Nomogram.
SOURCE: Reproduced with permission (pending) from Rumack BH. Acetaminophen overdose in children and adolescents. *Pediatr Clin North Am* 1986;33:691.

- Indications for *N*-acetylcysteine (NAC) include:
  - Possible or probable risk of hepatic toxicity based on Rumack-Matthew nomogram
  - Acetaminophen level >5 μg/mL if time since ingestion unknown
  - Evidence of hepatotoxicity
  - Serum acetaminophen levels unavailable
- NAC is given as a 5% solution in juice with oral loading dose of 140 mg/kg followed by maintenance dose of 70 mg/kg q 4 h for 17 doses. Antiemetics can be given with repeat doses if patient vomits.
- IV dosing is now Food and Drug Administration (FDA) approved.
- Poor outcomes are seen in patients who present late or whose course is complicated by grade 3 or 4 encephalopathy, prolonged prothrombin time (PT), renal dysfunction, sepsis, or cerebral edema.

ALCOHOLS

- Ethylene glycol, methanol, and isopropanol are the most commonly ingested nonethanol alcohols. Intoxication suggested by signs and symptoms of inebriation with low or undetectable ethanol levels. Elevated anion gap and/or elevated osmolal gap are cardinal features of methanol and ethylene glycol intoxication. All are relatively weak toxins but all have toxic metabolites.

ETHYLENE GLYCOL

- Odorless and sweet tasting.
- Contained in antifreeze, deicers, and industrial solvents.
- Has a positive urinary fluorescence under a Wood lamp because of added dye.
- Metabolized eventually to oxalic acid.
- Precipitation of oxalic acid to calcium oxalate in the renal tubules produces calcium oxalate crystals. This contributes to development of acute tubular necrosis.
- Other complications include hypocalcemia and myocardial dysfunction.
- Ingestion of 100 mL can be lethal with significant toxicity at serum levels of >50 mg/dL.
- Clinical course:
  - *Stage I*: 30 minutes to 12 hours postingestion: inebriation, ataxia, seizures, variable levels of elevated anion gap metabolic acidosis with Kussmaul breathing, elevated osmolal gap, crystalluria, hypocalcemia; death or coma can occur from cerebral edema
  - *Stage II*: 12–24 hours postingestion: myocardial dysfunction, high or low pressure pulmonary edema; death can occur from myocardial dysfunction or aspiration pneumonia
  - *Stage III*: 2–3 days postingestion: acute renal failure
  - *Late*: 6–18 days postingestion: neurologic sequelae
- Treatment:
  - Inhibition if alcohol dehydrogenase and dialytic removal is cornerstone of therapy.
  - Supportive therapy includes GL in the first hour postingestion, thiamine, folate, and pyridoxine. Correct hypoglycemia and hypocalcemia.
  - Inhibition of formation of toxic metabolites:
    - Fomepizole: does not require blood monitoring; 15 mg/kg loading dose followed by a 10 mg/kg IV bolus q 12 h; after 48 hours, increase bolus dose to 15 mg/kg q 12 h. Continue therapy until levels <20 mg/dL.
    - Ethanol: can be given PO or IV to maintain serum levels between 100 and 200 mg/dL. Exacerbates inebriated state and requires monitoring of levels.
  - Indications for HD include ethylene glycol level >50 mg/dL, significant and refractory metabolic acidosis, or evidence of end-organ damage.

METHANOL

- Colorless, odorless, bitter tasting, and highly volatile.
- Commonly found in paint removers, duplicator fluid, gas-line antifreeze, windshield washing fluid, and canned solid fuel.
- Lethal doses can be as little as 150–240 mL of a 49% solution.
- Intoxication can occur via ingesting, inhalation, or dermal absorption.

- Metabolized by alcohol dehydrogenase to formaldehyde which is subsequently converted to formic acid by aldehyde dehydrogenase. Formic acid is primarily responsible for metabolic and ocular toxicity.
- Clinical course:
  - Initially: headache, inebriation, dizziness, ataxia, and confusion.
  - Formic acid accumulates over 6–12 hours, the anion gap increases, visual symptoms become more prominent; other complications include pancreatitis.
- Treatment:
  - Similar to ethylene glycol intoxication.
  - HD is indicated for serum levels >50 mg/dL, suspected ingestion of lethal dose, significant and refractory metabolic acidosis, or evidence of end-organ damage.
  - Continue HD until acidosis resolves and level is <25 mg/dL.

ISOPROPANOL

- Colorless, bitter tasting, with smell of acetone or alcohol.
- Commonly found in rubbing alcohol, skin lotions, hair tonics, aftershave, deicers, and glass cleaners.
- Isopropanol is metabolized by alcohol dehydrogenase to acetone. Acetone is eliminated via the kidneys and lungs.
- Diagnosis of isopropanol exposure is suggested by the combination of ketonemia, ketonuria, sweet-smelling breath, and absence of anion gap or metabolic acidosis along with hemorrhagic gastritis and an elevated osmolal gap. Diagnosis is confirmed by measuring serum levels.
- Treatment:
  - Supportive measures; GL in first hour postingestion.
  - HD is indicated when lethal doses have been ingested (150–240 mL of a 40–70% solution), lethal level detected in serum (>400 mg/dL), refractory shock, or prolonged coma.

AMPHETAMINES

- Includes illicit drugs like methamphetamine ("crank"), 3,4-methylenedioxy-methamphetamine ("ecstasy"), prescription stimulants: methylphenidate, dextroamphetamine, pemoline, and prescription anorexiants: diethylpropion and phentermine.
- Toxicity occurs via central nervous system (CNS) stimulation, peripheral release of catecholamines, inhibition of reuptake of catecholamines, or inhibition of monoamine oxidase.
- Low therapeutic index.
- Signs and symptoms of overdose: confusion, irritability, tremor, anxiety, agitation, mydriasis, tachyarrhythmias, myocardial ischemia, hypertension, hyperreflexia, hyperthermia, rhabdomyolysis, renal failure, coagulopathy, seizures.
- Death can result from hyperthermia, arrhythmias, status epilepticus, intracranial hemorrhage, fulminant liver failure, or aspiration pneumonia.
- Treatment is supportive with attention to specific signs and symptoms:
  - Hypertension: phentolamine or nitroprusside
  - Tachyarrhythmias: esmolol or propranolol
  - Agitation/violent behavior/psychosis: haloperidol, droperidol, benzodiazepines, or phenothiazines
  - Hyperthermia: cooling measures if temperature >40°C
- GL is effective if performed within 1 hour of ingestion.
- HD and hemoperfusion are not effective.

BARBITURATES

- Phenobarbital is prototypical agent.
- Mild-to-moderate overdose is characterized by decreased level of consciousness, slurred speech, and ataxia.
- Higher doses cause hypothermia, hypotension, bradycardia, flaccidity, hyporeflexia, coma, and apnea.
- Severe overdose can result in the appearance of brain death with absent electroencephalogram (EEG) activity.
- Cardiovascular and respiratory depression result in a hypotensive, hypercapnic, and hypoxemic state.
- Diagnosis is made clinically with confirmation of barbiturate exposure by routine toxicology screen. Serum levels correlate with severity but usually do not change management.
- Treatment:
  - Supportive
  - No antidote available
  - GL is useful for acute massive overdose within the first hour
  - Multiple-dose activated charcoal, charcoal hemoperfusion, and urinary alkalinization (phenobarbital only) enhances elimination
- If CNS depression persists, other etiologies should be considered.

BENZODIAZEPINES

- Common therapeutic agents used as hypnotics, anxiolytics, muscle relaxants, and sedatives.
- Frequently involved in single and multiple drug overdoses.
- Symptoms range from slurred speech and lethargy to respiratory arrest and coma.
- Benzodiazepines increase the inhibitory effects of gamma-aminobutyric acid (GABA) and cause general CNS depression.

- Diagnosis is clinical with confirmation of exposure by routine urine toxicology.
- Benzodiazepine coma patients present with hyporeflexia and small-to-midsize pupils.
- Treatment:
  - Supportive measures initially
  - Gastric emptying if performed within the first hour postingestion
  - Activated charcoal
  - No role for forced diuresis, dialysis, or hemoperfusion
  - Consider antidote flumazenil
- Flumazenil is a specific benzodiazepine antagonist:
  - Helpful as diagnostic challenge as it does not antagonize the effects of other CNS depressants.
  - May precipitate seizures in patients with mixed benzodiazepine and tricyclic antidepressant overdose or unmask seizure from any cause.
  - Avoid in patients taking benzodiazepines for control of seizures or increased intracranial pressure.
  - Can precipitate acute withdrawal in patients chronically exposed to these agents.
  - Initial dose is 0.2 mg IV over 30 seconds, repeat with 0.3 mg if no effect seen in 30 seconds. Additional doses can be given at 1-minute interval to a total loading dose of 3 mg.
  - Monitor for resedation which may occur 1–2 hours after administration.

BETA-BLOCKERS

- Competitive antagonists of beta-receptors found in the heart (β_1) and bronchial tree (β_2).
- Clinical features are variable but toxicity is increased in patients exposed to other cardioactive drugs and beta-blockers with membrane stabilizing effects (acebutolol, betaxolol, pindolol, propranolol).
- Diagnosis is clinical. Serum levels are available but do not correlate well with toxicity.
- Cardiovascular toxicity is usually seen within 4 hours postingestion. Asymptomatic patients with normal ECGs after 6 hours do not require ICU monitoring.
- Signs and symptoms of toxicity include hypotension, bradycardia, atrioventricular blocks, and congestive heart failure (CHF) with or without pulmonary edema. Other effects include bronchospasm, hypoglycemia, hyperkalemia, lethargy, stupor, coma, and seizures. There is an increased risk of seizures and cardiac arrest with propranolol.
- Treatment:
  - Supportive measures are indicated initially.
  - Induced emesis is contraindicated.
  - GL and activated charcoal if performed within 1 hour of ingestion.
  - Cardiovascular manifestations can be treated with IV fluids, vasopressor therapy, transvenous pacing, and glucagon.
- Glucagon as antidote:
  - Positive inotropic and chronotropic effects mediated via increases in cyclic adenosine monophosphate (cAMP).
  - Bolus dose of 5–10 mg IV over 1 minute followed by maintenance infusion of 1–10 mg/h.
  - Dilute in normal saline of dextrose solution to prevent phenol toxicity.

CALCIUM CHANNEL BLOCKERS

- Selectively inhibit calcium flux in cardiac and vascular smooth muscle.
- Cardiovascular effects are dependent on class effects. Dihydropyridine causes peripheral vasodilatation. Verapamil and diltiazem have negative inotropic effects, depress the sinus node, and slow conduction through the AV node.
- Signs and symptoms of toxicity including hypotension (most common) generally occur within 6 hours with immediate release and 12 hours with sustained-released formulations. Other effects may include hyperglycemia, lethargy, confusion, and coma.
- Treatment:
  - Poisoning with sustained-release products may be treated with GL up to 8 hours postingestion and whole-bowel irrigation.
  - Multiple-dose activated charcoal and HD are not usually helpful.
  - In hepatic dysfunction, verapamil overdose has been treated with charcoal hemoperfusion.
  - Hypotension is managed with IV fluid.
  - Refractory hypotension can be treated with calcium gluconate and/or glucagon.

CARBON MONOXIDE

- Nonirritating, colorless, tasteless, and odorless gas produced by incomplete combustion of carbon fuels.
- Toxicity is usually seen in setting of smoke inhalation, attempted suicide from automobile exhaust, and poorly ventilated charcoal or gas stoves.
- Most common cause of death by poisoning in the United States.
- Mechanism of CO toxicity:
  - Has 240 times greater affinity for hemoglobin versus oxygen.

- Decreases oxyhemoglobin and oxygen-carrying capacity.
- Results in tissue hypoxia and directly inhibits cellular respiration via cytochrome oxidase blockade.

- Diagnosis:
  - Have a high level of suspicion especially during cold months.
  - Historical clues include symptomatic coinhabitants, suspect heating devices, and problems with forced-air heating systems.
  - Carboxyhemoglobin (COHb) levels are determined by co-oximetry.
  - Pulse oximetry does not differentiate between COHb and oxyhemoglobin and overestimates oxyhemoglobin levels.
- Clinical features:
  - COHb levels up to 5% are generally well tolerated.
  - Mild toxicity (COHb 5–10%): headache, mild dyspnea. These levels can be seen in heavy smokers and commuters on polluted roads.
  - Moderate (COHb 10–30%): headache, dizziness, weakness, dyspnea, irritability, nausea, and vomiting.
  - Severe (COHb 10–30%): coma, seizures, cardiovascular collapse, and death.
  - COHb levels do not always correlate well with clinical severity.
  - Delayed neuropsychiatric sequelae (DNS):
    - 10–30% of survivors of CO intoxication.
    - Symptoms include persistent vegetative state, short-term memory loss, behavioral change, hearing loss, incontinence, and psychosis.
    - Most patients (50–70%) will have full recovery at 1 year.
- Treatment:
  - Administration of 100% oxygen decreases the half-life of COHb from 5 to 6 hours in ambient air to 40–90 minutes.
  - Hyperbaric oxygen therapy can additionally decrease the half-life to 15–30 minutes.

COCAINE

- Can be snorted nasally, orally ingested, smoked (crack cocaine), or injected IV.
- Toxicity stems from excessive CNS stimulation and inhibition of neural uptake of catecholamines.
- Onset of effects depends on route of administration, dose, and patient tolerance.
- Coingestion is common with heroin, phencyclidine, and alcohol.
- Toxicity:
  - CNS: euphoria, anxiety, agitation, psychosis, delirium, seizures
  - Cardiovascular: chest pain, myocardial ischemia, infarction, sudden death, arrhythmias, CHF, pulmonary hypertension, endocarditis, aortic dissection
  - Respiratory:
    - Status asthmaticus, upper airway obstruction, barotrauma, pulmonary edema, alveolar hemorrhage
    - Acute pulmonary syndrome associated with crack cocaine and characterized by dyspnea, diffuse infiltrates, and hemoptysis
  - Renal: acute rhabdomyolysis
  - Other: hyperthermia, muscle rigidity, disseminated intravascular coagulation (DIC), multiple system organ failure (MSOF)
- Treatment:
  - ABCs with immediate treatment of seizures, hyperthermia, or agitation
  - Decontamination with activated charcoal for oral ingestion
  - Enhanced elimination: HD and hemoperfusion ineffective
  - Avoid unopposed beta-blockade
  - Symptom-based:
    - Hyperthermia: active and passive cooling
    - Agitation: benzodiazepines
    - Chest pain: nitrates and calcium channel blockers
    - Bronchospasm: bronchodilators and corticosteroids

CYANIDE

- Found in a variety of materials including plastics, glue removers, wool, silks, various seeds, and plants.
- Poisoning usually occurs through inhalation of hydrogen cyanide gas when cyanide-containing products are burned. May also occur with nitroprusside infusion or when absorbed through skin from cyanide-containing solutions.
- Mechanism: inhibits cellular cytochrome oxidase and interferes with aerobic oxygen consumption.
- Toxicity:
  - Early signs include anxiety, headache, confusion, tachycardia, and hypertension.
  - Rapidly progresses to include stupor, coma, seizures, fixed and dilated pupils, hypoventilation, bradycardia, heart block, ventricular arrhythmias, and cardiovascular collapse.
- Diagnosis:
  - Usually made clinically based on history of smoke inhalation.
  - Rapid onset of coma, seizures, cardiovascular dysfunction in setting of severe lactic acidosis.
  - Blood level >0.5 mg/L is toxic.
  - Other hints include "arterialization" of venous blood seen on ophthalmoscopic examination or bitter almond smell of hydrogen cyanide gas.

- Treatment:
  - Most efficacious if started early.
  - Gastric emptying followed by activated charcoal appropriate for acute ingestions.
  - Immediate 100% oxygen therapy via mask or endotracheal tube (ETT).
  - Induce methemoglobinemia to scavenge unbound cyanide with amyl or sodium nitrite:
    - Amyl nitrite: inhaled by crushable pearls for 15–30 seconds with 30 seconds breaks in between inhalations
    - Sodium nitrite: 300 mg over 3 minutes IV
    - Induced methemoglobin levels usually <20%
    - Avoid methylene blue to treat methemoglobinemia
  - Sodium thiosulfate enhances conversion of cyanide to thiocyanate:
    - 12.5 mg IV over 10 minutes
    - May repeat 1/2 dose after 2 hours
    - HD is effective for possible thiocyanate toxicity

CYCLIC ANTIDEPRESSANTS

- Tricyclic antidepressants responsible for majority of antidepressant-related fatalities.
- Mechanism of toxicity is related to anticholinergic effects, inhibition of neurotransmitter reuptake, peripheral alpha-blockade, and cardiac membrane depressant effects.
- Clinical presentation:
  - Anticholinergic effects: mydriasis, blurred vision, fever, dry skin/mucus membranes, lethargy, delirium, coma, tachycardia, ileus, myoclonus, urinary retention
  - Cardiovascular:
    - Sinus tachycardia with prolongation of QRS, QTc, PR intervals
    - Ventricular tachycardia
    - QRS interval (limb lead) >0.10 seconds predicts seizures
    - QRS duration >0.16 seconds associated with ventricular arrhythmias
    - Atrioventricular block
    - Hypotension
  - Neurologic: seizures, mental status changes
- Diagnosis:
  - Can be made when there is a compatible history and consistent clinical features.
  - Suspect in all patients with a prolonged QRS duration.
  - Confirm exposure with urine toxicology screening.
  - Blood levels are available but not necessary as ECG findings adequately predict severity.
- Treatment:
  - Supportive while identifying potentially life-threatening complications
  - Immediate serum alkalinization if QRS prolonged:
    - Sodium bicarbonate 1–2 meq/kg IV
    - Continue until QRS interval normalizes or pH >7.55
    - Hyperventilation in intubated patients
  - Decontamination:
    - GL (within 2 hours postingestion)
    - Single-dose activated charcoal
    - Induced emesis contraindicated
    - Dialysis and hemoperfusion not effective
  - Specific complications:
    - Refractory ventricular arrhythmias: lidocaine drug of choice
    - High-grade AV block: temporary ventricular pacing
    - Hypotension: fluids, vasopressors
    - Seizures: benzodiazepines, phenobarbital
    - Refractory seizures: phenytoin, paralysis, or deep sedation
  - ICU monitoring for mental status changes, seizures, hypotension, metabolic acidosis, or cardiac arrhythmias

γ-HYDROXYBUTYRATE

- Drug of abuse also known as liquid ecstasy, liquid G, date-rape drug, fantasy.
- Mechanism: derived from GABA and may act as an inhibitory neurotransmitter through γ-hydroxybutyrate (GHB) receptors or via GABA receptors.
- Not used clinically; banned by FDA outside of clinical trials.
- Toxicity:
  - Tolerance and dependence has been reported
  - Delirium and psychosis after abrupt withdrawal
  - Low doses result in euphoria, emesis, hypothermia, symptomatic bradycardia, hypotension, respiratory acidosis
  - High doses can result in deep coma and death
- Treatment:
  - Supportive
  - Expect coingestions
  - Decontamination: not reported
  - Antidotes: no role for naloxone
  - Patients usually will regain consciousness spontaneously after 5 hours
- Diagnosis:
  - No readily available diagnostic tests
  - Can be detected in blood and urine by specialized laboratories

LITHIUM

- Monovalent cation used in the treatment of bipolar affective disorders.
- Low therapeutic index.

- Poisoning most often accidental in patients on chronic therapy or deliberate overdose with suicidal intent.
- Risk factors for toxicity in chronic users:
  - Elderly
  - Long-term therapy increases half-life of lithium
  - Volume depletion
  - Renal insufficiency
- Toxicity:
  - Mild:
    - <2.5 meq/L
    - Tremor, ataxia, nystagmus, choreoathetosis, photophobia, lethargy
  - Moderate:
    - 2.5–3.5 meq/L
    - Agitation, fascicular twitching, confusion, nausea, vomiting, diarrhea, signs of cerebellar dysfunction
  - Severe:
    - >3.5 meq/L
    - Seizures, coma, sinus bradycardia, hypotension
  - Levels do not correlate well with symptoms in acute toxicity
  - Chronic or acute-on-chronic toxicity:
    - Levels better correlated with symptoms
    - Severe symptoms may occur at lower serum levels
    - Associated with diabetes insipidus, renal insufficiency, hypothyroidism, and leukocytosis
- Treatment:
  - Supportive including treatment of seizures and hypotension with vasopressors
  - Decontamination:
    - GL
    - Activated charcoal not indicated
    - Sodium polystyrene: monitor for hypokalemia
    - Whole-bowel irrigation for sustained-release tablets
  - Enhanced elimination:
    - HD
      - Prototypical dialyzable intoxicant
      - Indications:
        - Acute intoxication serum level >3.5 meq/L
        - Chronic intoxication, renal insufficiency, or symptomatic patients with level >2.5 meq/L
        - Any serum level after large ingestion
      - May need to repeat HD secondary to drug redistribution
    - Multidose sodium polystyrene may result in GI dialysis
    - Saline and forced alkaline diuresis are not indicated

METHEMOGLOBINEMIA

- Formed by oxidation of reduced hemoglobin (Fe^{2+}) to methemoglobin (Fe^{3+}).
- Pathophysiology:
  - Cannot bind and transport oxygen
  - Shifts oxyhemoglobin dissociation curve to left
- Etiology:
  - Includes hereditary, dietary, drug-induced, idiopathic
  - Acquired methemoglobinemia is usually oxidant drug or toxin exposure induced
  - Many drugs are associated:
    - Antibiotics: dapsone, chloroquine, primaquine, sulfonamides
    - Anesthetics: lidocaine, benzocaine, bupivacaine
    - Nitrates: isosorbide dinitrate, nitric oxide, nitroglycerine, nitroprusside
- Clinical features:
  - Mild:
    - MetHb $<15\%$
    - May see cyanosis but usually asymptomatic
    - May be significant in setting of critical coronary artery stenosis
  - Moderate:
    - MetHb 15–60%
    - Dyspnea, headache, weakness
  - Severe:
    - MetHb $>60\%$
    - Confusion, seizures, death
- Diagnosis:
  - Co-oximetry: can accurately measure both MetHb and oxygen saturation levels
  - Pulse oximetry: cannot directly measure MetHb levels and may over- or underestimate the true oxygen saturation
  - "Chocolate" color of blood that does not change on exposure to air
- Treatment:
  - General supportive care and removal of inciting agent
  - Decontamination with GL followed by activated charcoal
  - Antidote:
    - Methylene blue:
      - Increases conversion of MetHb to Hb
      - Consider use in symptomatic patients
      - Dose 1–2 mg/kg IV over 5 minutes, repeat after 60 minutes
      - Contraindications:
        - Glucose-6-phosphate dehydrogenase deficiency
        - Renal failure
        - Failure to respond suggests cytochrome b5 reductase deficiency, glucose-6-phosphate dehydrogenase deficiency, or sulfhemoglobinemia

OPIOIDS

- Produce generalized depression of CNS via opioid receptor.
- Coingestions are common.

- Toxicity:
  - Severity depends on dose, drug type, and patient tolerance
  - Mild or moderate overdose:
    - Lethargy, miosis, hypotension, sinus bradycardia, diminished bowel sounds, flaccid muscles
  - Severe overdose:
    - Respiratory depression, apnea, coma
    - Death is usually a result of respiratory failure
  - Respiratory failure may be multifactorial:
    - Alveolar hypoventilation
    - Aspiration pneumonitis
    - Low pressure pulmonary edema:
      - Often presents after resuscitation
      - Idiopathic response
      - Complication of naloxone
  - Seizures are most likely to be seen after overdose with propoxyphene and meperidine
- Diagnosis:
  - Usually made on clinical grounds.
  - Rapid response to naloxone supports diagnosis but is neither sensitive nor specific.
  - Urine toxicology screening confirms opioid exposure.
  - Blood toxicology screening is more sensitive.
- Treatment:
  - Initial supportive measures
  - Naloxone is specific opioid antagonist:
    - Reverses sedation, hypotension, and respiratory depression
    - Administration:
      - Initial dose 0.2–0.4 mg IV
      - Repeat 1–2 mg IV if no response after 2–3 minutes to total dose of 10 mg
      - Half-life 45–90 minutes and may need to repeat every 20–60 minutes to maintain clinical response
      - Continuous infusion at 0.4–0.8 mg/h can be used
      - Side effects include pulmonary edema and seizures
    - In general, if no response after 10 mg opioid overdose can be ruled out
  - Supplemental oxygen and mechanical ventilation may be required to treat alveolar hypoventilation and hypoxemia
  - Decontamination:
    - GL (if oral intoxication), followed by
    - Activated charcoal
    - Time when GL useful; increased secondary to delayed gastric emptying
    - Ensure adequate airway protection prior to lavage or activated charcoal
  - Enhanced elimination: no role for HD, hemoperfusion, or forced diuresis secondary to large volume of distribution

ORGANOPHOSPHATES/CARBAMATE INSECTICIDES

- Widely used as insecticides in the United States.
- Organophosphates also used as nerve agents in chemical warfare.
- Exert toxicity by inhibiting acetylcholinesterase.
- Reversible (carbamates) or irreversible (organophosphates) inhibition of acetylcholinesterase causes the accumulation of acetylcholine at parasympathetic synapses leading to the cholinergic syndrome.
- Exposure is usually through the GI tract but substances can also be absorbed through the skin, conjunctiva, and respiratory tract.
- Exposure is usually accidental but occasionally with suicidal intent.
- Clinical features:
  - Symptoms are the result of overstimulation of muscarinic, nicotinic, and CNS receptors
  - Muscarinic: characterized by SLUDGE (**S**alivation, **L**acrimation, **U**rination, **D**iarrhea, **G**I cramps, and **E**mesis). Also blurred vision, miosis, bradycardia, and wheezing
  - Nicotinic: muscle fasciculations and weakness; severe overstimulation of nicotinic receptors results in hypertension, tachycardia, paresis, paralysis, and respiratory failure
  - CNS: organophosphates (not carbamates) enter the CNS and induce anxiety, confusion, seizures, psychosis, and ataxia
- Diagnosis:
  - Based on history of exposure and characteristic signs and symptoms
  - Cholinesterase activity:
    - Normal levels vary widely and do not correlate well with clinical symptoms
    - Severe intoxications: levels <20–50%
    - Serial postexposure levels may help confirm the diagnosis
- Treatment:
  - Initial supportive care with special attention to respiratory function secondary to risk of respiratory failure from wheezing, excess secretions, muscle weakness, and mental status changes
  - Take precaution to remove patient and staff from exposure from contaminated clothing and cleanse the skin and hair
  - Decontamination:
    - Activated charcoal
    - GL if immediately postingestion
  - Specific drugs and antidotes:
    - Atropine:
      - Indicated for all symptomatic patients
      - Competitively blocks acetylcholine at muscarinic receptors

- Dose required to achieve "atropinization" (mydriasis, dry mouth, increased heart rate) is highly variable:
  - Initial dose is 2 mg IV (6 mg if life threatening) followed by 2 mg every 15 minutes until atropinization
  - Large doses up to 100 mg/day may occasionally be required
- Pralidoxime:
  - Reverses muscarinic and nicotinic effects by reactivating phosphorylated cholinesterase enzyme and protects it from further inhibition prior to irreversible inactivation
  - Effectiveness best within first 6 hours but useful for 24–48 hours postexposure
  - Dosing:
    - Initial dose is 1–2 g IV over 10–20 minutes
    - Start continuous infusion (200–500 mg/h) titrated to effect
    - Duration dependent on half-life of toxin but may require >24 hours before tapering infusion while monitoring for signs or recurrent weakness
  - Generally not necessary for carbamate toxicity

PHENCYCLIDINE

- Dissociative anesthetic with properties similar to ketamine.
- Also known as "angel dust" and can be snorted, smoked, ingested orally, or injected IV.
- Coingestions with THC (delta-9-tetrahydrocannabinol), alcohol, and lysergic acid diethylamide (LSD) are common.
- Variable anticholinergic, opioid, dopaminergic, CNS stimulant, and alpha-adrenergic effects.
- Clinical presentation:
  - Mild intoxication: lethargy, euphoria, hallucinations, occasional bizarre or violent behavior, nystagmus: vertical and horizontal
  - Severe intoxication: hypertension +/– hypertensive crisis, rigidity, hyperthermia, tachycardia, diaphoresis, seizures, coma, rhabdomyolysis, acute renal failure, and apnea
- Diagnosis:
  - Suspect in patients with fluctuating behavior, sympathomimetic overstimulation, and nystagmus
  - Pinpoint pupils in an agitated patient is suggestive
  - Exposure is confirmed by urine toxicology screening
- Treatment:
  - Initial supportive measures
  - Decontamination:
    - No role for emesis or GL
    - Activated charcoal
  - No specific drugs or antidotes
  - Enhanced elimination not effective secondary to large volume of distribution, avoid urinary acidification
  - Violent or psychotic behavior:
    - Decrease stimulation
    - Haloperidol drug of choice
    - Can add a benzodiazepine
  - Severe hypertension:
    - Drug therapy if calming strategies fail
    - Nitroprusside or labetalol
    - Avoid beta-blockers alone; secondary to risk of unopposed alpha stimulation

SALICYLATES

- Common ingredients in prescription and nonprescription drugs.
- Pathophysiology:
  - Acetylsalicylic acid is converted to salicylic acid.
  - Salicylic acid is readily absorbed form stomach and small bowel.
  - Uncouples oxidative phosphorylation and interferes with Krebs cycle.
- Clinically features:
  - Acute:
    - Mild intoxication 150–200 mg/kg
    - Severe intoxication 300–500 mg/kg
    - Initially present with vomiting followed by hyperpnea, tinnitus, and lethargy
    - Respiratory alkalosis and metabolic acidosis
    - Severe intoxication can result in coma, seizures, hypoglycemia, hyperthermia, and pulmonary edema
  - Chronic:
    - Usually young children or elderly
    - Presentation nonspecific with confusion, dehydration, metabolic acidosis that may be attributed to other conditions
    - Cerebral and pulmonary edema more common
    - Toxicity seen at lower salicylate levels
- Diagnosis:
  - May be easy if history of acute ingestion
  - Arterial blood gas (ABG) is suggestive: respiratory alkalosis and metabolic acidosis
  - Salicylate levels:
    - Prognostic in acute intoxications
    - Measure serial levels
    - No clinical value
- Treatment:
  - Emergent and supportive care
  - Decontamination:

- Not indicated for chronic intoxications
- GL with activated charcoal
- Enhanced elimination:
  - Urinary alkalinization
  - HD:
    - Very effective to remove salicylate and correct acid-base and fluid abnormalities
    - Indications:
      - Serum level >120 mg/dL acutely
      - Serum level >100 mg/dL 6 hours postingestion
      - Refractory acidosis, coma, seizures, noncardiogenic pulmonary edema, volume overload, and renal failure
      - Symptomatic chronic intoxication with level >60 mg/dL
  - Hemoperfusion effective but does not address acid-base abnormalities
  - Multiple-dose activated charcoal is controversial
- Specific treatments:
  - Sodium bicarbonate:
    - Increase urinary elimination
    - Prevent acidemia which increases CNS salicylate levels
    - Goals of therapy:
      - Systemic pH 7.45–7.5
      - Urinary pH approximately 7–8
    - Avoid hypokalemia

SELECTIVE SEROTONIN REUPTAKE INHIBITORS (SEROTONIN SYNDROME)

- May become more common cause of overdose or intoxication secondary to increased popularity.
- Combination of a selective serotonin reuptake inhibitor (SSRI) with tryptophan, monamine oxidase (MAO) inhibitor, or other serotomimetic antidepressant can result in the serotonin syndrome and death.
- Pathophysiologic mechanism is presumed to be brain stem and spinal cord activation of 1A serotonin receptor.
- Long half-life may delay onset of symptoms.
- Clinical manifestations:
  - Can be mild, moderate, or severe
  - Mental status changes, restlessness, myoclonus, hyperreflexia, diaphoresis, shivering, tremor, flushing, fever, nausea, and diarrhea
  - Severe symptoms include DIC, seizures, coma, muscle rigidity, myoclonus, autonomic instability, orthostatic hypotension, and rhabdomyolysis
- Diagnosis:
  - Consider in any patient with history of depression, use of serotonergic drugs, and compatible clinical features at presentation
  - Blood and urine assays are not commonly available and not part of routine toxicology screen
- Treatment:
  - Stop suspected serotonergic agent and provide supportive care
  - Decontamination:
    - GL if 1 hour postingestion
    - Activated charcoal
  - Enhanced elimination techniques not effective
  - Specific drugs:
    - Serotonin antagonists have not been adequately evaluated
    - Chlorpromazine, diphenhydramine, and benzodiazepines have been used

THEOPHYLLINE

- Dimethyl xanthine used in management of obstructive lung disease.
- Low therapeutic index.
- Patient noncompliance, physician prescribing errors, and altered drug metabolism can result in toxicity.
- Intoxication:
  - Acute and chronic
  - Mild toxicity can occur within therapeutic range
  - Drug levels:
    - Toxicity usually when >25 mg/L
    - Seizure:
      - Acute 80–100 mg/L
      - Chronic 35–70 mg/L
    - Tachyarrhythmia 20–30 mg/L
    - Cardiovascular collapse >50 mg/L
  - Cardiovascular: tachycardia, supraventricular and ventricular arrhythmias, cardiovascular collapse
  - Neurologic: nervousness, insomnia, agitation, restlessness, headache, tremor, seizures
  - Metabolic: hypokalemia, hypomagnesemia, hyperglycemia, hypophosphatemia, hypercalcemia, respiratory acidosis
- Treatment:
  - Decontamination:
    - GL followed by activated charcoal
    - Emesis is contraindicated
  - Enhanced elimination:
    - Multiple-dose activated charcoal
    - Extracorporeal (see below):
      - Charcoal hemoperfusion
      - HD
  - Follow levels every 2–3 hours
  - Specific complications:
    - Seizure:
      - Benzodiazepines
      - Phenytoin may worsen seizures and should be avoided
      - Phenobarbital for refractory cases

- Hypotension:
  - Fluids and phenylephrine
- Arrhythmias:
  - Supraventricular tachycardia (SVT):
    - Best treated with β_1 cardioselective beta-blockers
    - Use caution in patients with obstructive lung disease and avoid if active bronchoconstriction present
    - Calcium channel blockers for sustained SVT
  - Ventricular:
    - Lidocaine or other appropriate agent
- Severe intoxication with life-threatening complications should be considered for extracorporal drug elimination:
  - Other indications include plasma level >100 mg/L in acute intoxication after initial charcoal therapy
  - Level >50 mg/L after chronic ingestion
  - 2 hours level >35 mg/L associated with clinical instability or high risk of adverse outcome and/or prolonged intoxication
  - High-risk characteristics include chronic intoxication, intolerance to charcoal or intractable vomiting, decreased theophylline metabolism (CHF, cirrhosis, severe hypoxemia), poor cardiovascular reserve, seizures, and respiratory failure

BIBLIOGRAPHY

Academy of Clinical Toxicology, European Association of Poisons Centres and Clinical Toxicologists. *J Toxicol Clin Toxicol* 1999;37:731–751.

Amirzadeh A, McCotter C. The intravenous use of oral acetylcysteine (Mucomyst) for the treatment of acetaminophen overdose. *Arch Intern Med* 2002;162:96–97.

Brent J, McMartin K, Phillips S, et al. Fomepizole for the treatment of ethylene glycol poisoning. *N Engl J Med* 1999;340: 832–838.

Corbridge T, Murray P, Mokhlesi B. Toxicology in adults. In: Hall JB, Schmidt GA, Wood LDH, eds., *Principles of Critical Care*, Chapter 102. New York, NY: McGraw-Hill; 2005:1499–1545.

Hall JB, Schmidt, GA, Wood LDH. *Principles of Critical Care*, 3rd ed. New York, NY: McGraw-Hill; 2005:1123–1136.

Litovitz TL, Klein-Schwartz W, White S, et al. 2000 annual report of the American Association of Poison Control Centers toxic exposure surveillance system. *Am J Emerg Med* 2001;19: 337–395.

Shannon M. Ingestion of toxic substances by children. *N Engl J Med* 2000;342:186–191.

Vale JA, Krenzelok EP, Barceloux GD, et al. Position statement and practice guidelines on the use of multi-dose activated charcoal in the treatment of acute poisoning. American. *N Engl J Med* 1999;37:731–740.

Vale JA. Position statement: gastric lavage. American Academy of Clinical Toxicology, European Association of Poison Centres and Clinical Toxicologists. *J Toxicol Clin Toxicol* 1997;35:711–719.

Weaver LK, Hopkins RO, Chan KJ, et al. Hyperbaric oxygen for acute carbon monoxide poisoning. *N Engl J Med* 2002;347: 1057–1067.

124 CHEMICAL WEAPONS

D. Kyle Hogarth

KEY POINTS

- Initial management of all chemical weapon victims is to protect YOURSELF with respirators and protective clothing.
- Nerve Agents work by inhibiting acetylcholinesterase. They can be odorless, but may smell like bitter almonds.
- Signs and Symptoms of Nerve Agents can be remembered using "SLUDGE and the Killer Bs" for muscarinic signs: Salivation, Lacrimation, Urination, Defecation, Gastroenteritis, Emesis, Bradycardia, Bronchorrhea, Bronchospasm. Nicotinic signs of nerve agents can be remembered using: "MTWHF": Mydriasis, Tachycardia, Weakness, Hypertension, Fasciculations.
- Atropine is used to treat the muscarinic effects of the agent: 2 mg IVP (1 mg for age 2–12, 0.5 mg for under 2), repeat q 5 min, titrate until effective in controlling symptoms. Average dose given is 6–15 mg.

MANAGEMENT

- Immediate management of all patients involves protecting yourself first. Ensure proper personal protective equipment (PPE), including respiratory protection with at least an organic vapor/P1 cartridge respirator. Higher exposures require pressure demand supplied air respirator and escape self-contained breathing apparatus (SCBA).
- Splash-protective chemical resistant suit and gloves/ boots should be worn by all people involved in the initial care/assessment.
- Remove the patient's clothing quickly and seal in plastic impervious bags and save for authorities.

- Wash the skin of the patient with shampoo and copious water. Rinse, soap, rinse, wait 1 minute, and repeat for 20 minutes. As always, follow basic life support and attend to the ABCs (airway, breathing, circulation) of emergency care and quickly obtain as much history as possible.
- Other immediate issues need to be attended to as well. Call Local Health Director, Police, Federal Bureau of Investigation (FBI), and hazardous materials (HAZMAT). All can be reached via 911. Also contact Poison Control (800-222-1222).
- Domestic Preparedness National Response Hotline (800-424-8802).
- Centers for Disease Control and Prevention (CDC) emergency response (770-488-7100).
- U.S. Army Chemical Casualty Care Handbook: http://ccc.apgea.army.mil.

TYPES OF AGENTS

NERVE AGENTS

- The G agents were synthesized in 1936 by Germany. The V agents were synthesized in the United Kingdom in 1952. Iraq used Sarin and Tabun against Iran and Iraqi Kurds between 1983 and 1988. Japan was victim of Sarin gas attack by Aum Shinrikyo Cult in 1994 and 1995.
- Types of nerve agents include: GA (Tabun), GB (Sarin), GD (Soman), GF, VX (methylphosphonothioic acid), and VR.
- Nerve agents are usually colorless and odorless, but may have a fruity smell like bitter almonds.
- They are all liquids, but Tabun, Sarin, and Soman have high volatility and easily become gas. These agents are usually absorbed via the respiratory system. VX and VR are usually absorbed dermally as they have a low volatility and tend to remain in liquid form.
- Each nerve agent essentially causes a syndrome of organophosphates toxicity as they are very potent acetylcholinesterase inhibitors.
- Each nerve agent has different characteristics in regards to ease of production, volatility, persistence, and onset of symptoms. For example, VX has a very low volatility, and therefore will persist in an environment for a very long time. It is also a liquid, while the others become gaseous at ambient temperature.

SIGNS AND SYMPTOMS

- Muscarinic signs of nerve agents can be remembered using "SLUDGE and the Killer Bs": Salivation, Lacrimation, Urination, Defecation, Gastroenteritis, Emesis, Bradycardia, Bronchorrhea, Bronchospasm.
- Nicotinic signs of nerve agents can be remembered using: "MTWHF": Mydriasis, Tachycardia, Weakness, Hypertension, Fasciculations.
- The nicotinic signs often predominate early in the course, but both can be found. Later, the muscarinic signs and symptoms predominate. Severe exposure can have both of the worst effects at the same time.
- Typical symptoms of moderate exposure to nerve agents include diffuse muscle cramping, especially abdominal muscles with nausea, vomiting, and occasionally diarrhea. Rhinorrhea and difficulty breathing often present, as well as sweating. Eye pain and frontal headache, as well as blurry vision are often present (of the 15 physicians secondarily exposed to Sarin vapors in Tokyo, 73% complained of dimmed vision). Tremors, palpitations, and fasciculations are often noted.
- Typical symptoms of high exposure to nerve agents include seizures and flaccid paralysis. Acute respiratory failure is the primary cause of death in acute poisonings with acetylcholinesterase inhibitors.
- Aerosol attack will give symptoms in seconds to minutes. Liquid attack (skin, conjunctival exposure) will give symptoms in minutes to hours. Head/neck exposure to liquid gives symptoms quicker than extremities, which is quicker than torso exposure. Oral ingestion can take hours (a study of volunteers who drank water with VX showed a 22% drop in cholinesterase activity after 400 μg/70 kg body weight 2–3 hours postingestion. A full stomach increased the absorption).

DIAGNOSTIC TESTS

- RBC or serum cholinesterase on whole blood sample is useful, but typically is a "send-out" lab. Sent in a heparinized green-top tube. The diagnosis is made clinically and with a good history and physical examination.

THERAPY

- Wash patient with 1 part household bleach, 9 parts water solution (0.5% sodium hypochlorite). The Sarin half-life in water is 5.4 hours: at pH 9, it's only 15 minutes.
- Atropine is used to treat the muscarinic effects of the agent: 2 mg IVP (1 mg for age 2–12, 0.5 mg for under 2), repeat q 5 min, titrate until effective in controlling symptoms. Average dose given is 6–15 mg.
- Pralidoxime chloride (2-PAM) can also be given, 600–1800 mg IM or 1 g IV over 20–30 minutes. This drug reacts with the nerve agent inhibited cholinesterase enzymes to remove the nerve agent from the enzyme. Timing is very important. Once the binding of the agent to the enzyme becomes irreversible, 2-PAM will not work. This is called "aging." Soman ages in <10 minutes, while VX takes several hours.
- Nebulized ipratropium may provide some benefit and can be attempted.

- Hemofiltration (4 hours) and hemoperfusion was used successfully in one patient in Tokyo during the Sarin attacks.

PROPHYLAXIS

- Pyridostigmine bromide, 30 mg tid, for up to 7 days can be taken. This was used in Operation Desert Storm. Half of the troops who took the drug noted mild abdominal symptoms (flatus, cramps, loose stools). Discontinuation rate of 0.07% of the 41,650 troops who took the drug.
- Fluoroakylpolyether and polytetrafluoroethylene, commonly called "SERPACWA" by the military (Skin Exposure Reduction Paste Against Chemical Warfare Agents) can also be applied to health workers after an attack. SERPACWA has been shown to decrease toxicity of sulfur mustard, VX, and Soman in animal studies.

BLISTER AGENTS

- First developed and used by the Germans in 1917 during World War I, but also used by the Italians against Ethiopia from 1935 to 1940. Egypt employed these agents in support of South Yemen during the Yemeni Civil War. Iranian soldiers attacked by the Iraqi army during the Iran-Iraq war (1983–1988) used blistering agents.
- Types of blister agents include: sulfur mustard (Yperite), nitrogen mustard, Lewisite, and phosgene oximine.

CHARACTERISTICS

- These agents are often odorless and colorless, depending on purity.
- An exposed patient's skin may smell of garlic, horseradish, or mustard.
- They can cause symptoms within minutes (Lewisite), but many don't cause symptoms for up to 12 hours (mustards).
- The agents are often nonfatal, but designed to incapacitate and to overutilize an opponent's resources and to hamper an ability to fight as the soldier takes precautions with gear/respirators.

SIGNS AND SYMPTOMS

- Blister agent victims describe their skin as burning, and pruritic. The skin is erythematous and develops thin walled blisters. They often have watery, swollen eyes. Many develop upper airway sloughing, with pulmonary edema and respiratory compromise.
- Mucosal irritation with lacrimation, conjunctival irritation, and erythema are present. Typically, patient will notice shortness of breath and experience nausea and vomiting.
- Can see neutropenia and sepsis, late in course, and often with sulfur mustard (of note, melphalan and cyclophosphamide are nitrogen mustards).

DIAGNOSTIC TESTS

- Patients will often have a distinct smell of garlic, horseradish, or mustard. Oily droplets present on the skin can be sent for testing.
- Urine can be sent for thiodiglycol (breakdown product of blistering agents). In animal studies and human volunteers, significant urine excretion of thiodiglycol occurred within 24 hours of exposure.
- Tissue biopsy can be obtained and samples sent to USAMRICD (United States Army Medical Research Institute of Chemical Defense) for analysis and confirmation.

TREATMENT

- Mustards have no antidote, and treatment is supportive.
- Patients should be managed similar to thermal bum patients, with careful attention to fluids, skin care, and need for antibiotics.
- Amifostine and some new analogues seem to offer prophylactic protection from the effects of mustards, but have no effect after exposure.
- For Lewisite exposure, British anti-Lewisite (Dimercaprol) given IM can help, but it is often not available. In animal studies, a parenteral combination of sodium thiosulfate (3 g/kg), vitamin E (20 mg/kg), and dexamethasone (8 mg/kg) improved survival and reduced organ damage after exposure to mustard gas.

CHOKING AGENTS

- These agents were developed and used during World War I. Phosgene was first used in 1915 and accounted for 80% of all chemical fatalities during the war. They work by primarily causing sudden, severe, massive pulmonary edema. Used by the Italians against Ethiopia in 1935–1940 and by the Japanese in China from 1937 to 1945 and in Yemen during 1963–1967 civil war.
- They are all in gas form and are heavier than air. They are typically odorless, but may smell of moldy or cut hay. They react with multiple different macromolecules in tissue to increase capillary permeability.
- Types of choking agents include: phosgene, diphosgene, chlorine, chloropicrin, oxides of nitrogen, and sulfur dioxide.

Signs and Symptoms

- Mucosal irritation with pulmonary infiltrates and pulmonary edema are seen.
- The patients note shortness of breath, chest tightness, wheezing, and laryngeal spasm.

Onset of Action

- Effects are seen from 1 to 24 hours after exposure, and rarely up to 72 hours.
- Typically, the patient may be asymptomatic for many hours after exposure.

Diagnostic Tests

- None.

Therapy

- No antidote. Management is supportive through control of secretions, oxygen supplementation, and positive end-expiratory pressure (PEEP) via mask ventilation or intubation.
- High-dose steroids for oxides of nitrogen agents may prevent the pulmonary edema, but this has not been proven in a clinical trial.
- Oral Zafirlukast 40–80 mg q12 for initial 48 hours and glutathione may lessen the respiratory damage after phosgene poisoning.

Bibliography

Ben Abraham R, Rudick V, Weinbroum AA. Practical guidelines for acute care of victims of bioterrorism: conventional injuries and concomitant nerve agent intoxication. *Anesthesiology* 2002;97(4):989–1004.

Davis KG, Aspera G. Exposure to liquid sulfur mustard. *Ann Emerg Med* 2001;37(6):653–6.

Evison D, Hinsley D, Rice P. Chemical weapons. *Bmj* 2002;324(7333):332–5.

Kadivar H, Adams SC. Treatment of chemical and biological warfare injuries: insights derived from the 1984 Iraqi attack on Majnoon Island. *Mil Med* 1991;156(4):171–7.

Leikin JB, Thomas RG, Walter FG, Klein R, Meislin HW. A review of nerve agent exposure for the critical care physician. *Crit Care Med* 2002;30(10):2346–54.

Munro NB, Watson AP, Ambrose KR, Griffin GD. Treating exposure to chemical warfare agents: implications for health care providers and community emergency planning. *Environ Health Perspect* 1990;98:205–15.

Vijayaraghavan R, Kumar P, Joshi U, et al. Prophylactic efficacy of amifostine and its analogues against sulphur mustard toxicity. *Toxicology* 2001;163(2–3):83–91.

White SM. Chemical and biological weapons. Implications for anaesthesia and intensive care. *Br J Anaesth* 2002;89(2):306–24.

ccc.apgea.army.mil/products/handbooks/books.htm. Accessed Feb 22, 2007. Free registration required.

125 ANAPHYLAXIS

Nina M. Patel

KEY POINTS

- Anaphylactic and anaphylactoid reactions are relatively rare, life-threatening events that are mediated largely by mast cell and basophil cell activation.
- Common triggers include antibiotics, contrast media, blood products, colloids, latex, envenomations, and severe food allergies.
- In most circumstances symptoms are immediate but on very rare occasion can be delayed up to several hours.
- Cardiovascular and respiratory instability are hallmarks, often preceded by a subjective sense of impending catastrophe.
- Mainstays of therapy include supportive management with oxygen, airway protection and maintenance, volume resuscitation, and epinephrine.
- Tryptase assay may help distinguish anaphylactic from anaphylactoid or other reactions.

EPIDEMIOLOGY

- No comprehensive studies of the incidence, prevalence, and morbidity of drug allergy and anaphylaxis in the general population have been performed.
- Anaphylaxis is estimated to occur in 1/5100 hospital admissions.
- Anaphylaxis occurs at a rate of 1/10,000 to 1/20,000 during anesthesia.
- Drugs (antibiotics, neuromuscular blocking agents [NMBA], or protamine commonly), radiocontrast media (RCM), blood products, colloids, latex, and preservatives are agents frequently involved in anaphylaxis in a hospital setting.
- Penicillin is the most common causative agent in anaphylaxis in humans.
- Anaphylaxis occurs in 1–2% of procedures involving RCM.
- The overall incidence of anaphylaxis is similar between men and women.

PATHOPHYSIOLOGY

- Anaphylaxis is a severe, acute systemic allergic reaction resulting from the binding of a foreign antigen to surface IgE on mast cells and/or basophils, with subsequent activation of these cells and release of chemical mediators.

- Anaphylactoid reactions have a similar clinical presentation (though sometimes less severe), but are not immune-mediated and result from direct drug or antigen activation of mast cells and basophils.
- The major known mediators of anaphylactic and anaphylactoid reactions are histamine, eosinophilic chemotactic factor of anaphylaxis (ECF-A), slow reacting substance of anaphylaxis (SRS-A), prostaglandins, platelet-activating factor (PAF), and kinins.
- Mediators of anaphylaxis induce an array of systemic physiologic perturbations, which include: decreased systemic vascular resistance, systemic vasodilation, increased capillary permeability, bronchospasm, mucosal edema, mucus secretion, and platelet aggregation.
- The aggregate effects of mediators of anaphylaxis are significant respiratory and cardiovascular compromise, often leading to shock, due to decreased effective plasma volume and systemic vasodilation.

CLINICAL FEATURES

- Symptoms arise within minutes of administration of the offending agent but can be delayed up to 2.5 hours. Five to twenty percent of patients experience biphasic anaphylaxis and will have recurrence of symptoms 1–8 hours after regression of the initial reaction.
- Patients with anaphylaxis often complain of an impending "sense of death."
- 30% of patients develop cardiovascular collapse and shock.
- Cardiovascular: Patients commonly complain of dizziness and exhibit tachycardia and hypotension. A number of ECG changes have been described, including nonspecific ST- and T-wave changes, multifocal premature ventricular contractions, electromechanical dissociation, asystole and ventricular fibrillation. Cardiac output is generally elevated, though some patients manifest myocardial depression as well as myocardial ischemia and chest pain.
- Respiratory: 50% of patients develop respiratory manifestations of anaphylaxis. Tachypnea, shortness of breath, wheezing, stridor, and chest tightness constitute the most common symptoms. Patients may exhibit a decline in forced expiratory volume in 1 second (FEV_1) and intubated patients may display an increase in peak airway pressures. Acute respiratory distress or asphyxiation can ensue due to severe bronchospasm (particularly in asthmatic patients) and bronchorrhea and/or severe laryngeal or glottic edema.
- Skin: Typical complaints are of pruritus, flushing, warmth, erythema, and minor edema. Rash, urticaria, and angioedema occur in 88% of individuals. Skin rash often resolves with antihistamine therapy. The degree of cutaneous involvement does not correlate with the extent of hemodynamic derangement. Cutaneous involvement is not requisite in establishing the diagnosis of anaphylaxis.
- Gastrointestinal: Patients may experience nausea, vomiting, diarrhea, abdominal pain, and cramping.
- Neurologic: Seizures have been described to occur very infrequently.
- Ophthalmologic: Excessive lacrimation and conjunctival injection.

DIFFERENTIAL DIAGNOSIS

- The diagnosis of anaphylaxis must be considered in any patient who develops hypotension in the operative or perioperative period.
- Vasovagal syncope, systemic mastocytosis, carcinoid syndrome, hereditary angioedema, pheochromocytoma, status asthmaticus, foreign body aspiration, scombroidosis, monosodium glutamate (MSG) syndrome, seizures, hyperventilation syndrome, and panic attacks constitute a few of the extensive number of syndromes which can produce clinical manifestations similar to anaphylaxis.
- The diagnosis of anaphylaxis rests upon a correlation in time between exposure to a known agent of anaphylactic or anaphylactoid reactions in concert with characteristic clinical features.
- Identification of the offending agent through allergy history, history of prior anaphylaxis, time frame to onset of symptoms, and route of administration of the putative causative agent is essential.
- Tryptase is a protease released during IgE-mediated mast cell activation. Tryptase levels >25 μg/L are suggestive of an immune rather than chemically mediated reaction. The sensitivity and specificity of tryptase in diagnosing anaphylaxis are 64% and 89.3%, respectively.
- Histamine levels are sometimes measured, but the highly labile nature of this molecule in plasma limits its clinical utility. The sensitivity and specificity of elevated plasma histamine levels (>9 nM) are 75% and 51%, respectively.
- If a potential causative agent is identified, skin prick, intradermal titration, RAST (radioallergoabsorbent test), and in rare cases, in vivo provocation, can be used to confirm the presence of IgE antibodies.

PREVENTION AND TREATMENT

- Extensive preoperative and preprocedure evaluation for history of allergic symptoms to NMBAs, hypnotics,

opioids, antibiotics, NSAIDs (nonsteroidal anti-inflammatory drugs), latex, RCM, blood products, colloids, or any other agents is imperative.
- Once an anaphylactic/anaphylactoid reaction has begun, a number of swiftly coordinated actions must ensue.
- Any and all suspected offending agents should be discontinued as well as any sedative or vasodepressor agents.
- A definitive airway should be established with administration of supplemental oxygen (100%). Aerosolized or inhaled β_2-adrenergic agents can be utilized additionally in patients with bronchospasm.
- Intravenous access should be secured with two large-bore (14- or 16-gauge) intravenous catheters.
- Epinephrine (IM) at 0.3–0.5 mL (1:1000) q 5-15 min to titration of effect is the principal therapy in patients with hypotension or severe bronchospasm due to its α_1-adrenergic, β_1- and β_2-adrenergic effects. In patients with life-threatening hypotension, epinephrine should be administered intravenously in cardiopulmonary resuscitation doses (0.01 mg/kg to max of 1 mg per dose).
- Intravascular volume expansion with crystalloid or colloid should be pursued aggressively. Persistent hypotension may require further support with continuous infusion of vasopressors such as epinephrine (1–2 μg/min) or norepinephrine (0.5–30 μg/min).
- Administration of antihistamines is considered a mainstay of therapy, though it is uncertain if these drugs have any potential to reverse the effects of histamine once it has been released. Recommended agents are diphenhydramine (1 mg/kg q 4-6 h) and cimetidine (4 mg/kg q 8 h).
- IV corticosteroids are recommended in patients with severe cardiopulmonary dysfunction and also to prevent biphasic anaphylactic reactions. A clear dose is not established. Methylprednisolone 125 mg IV q 6 h is a reasonable starting steroid regimen.

REFERENCES

The International Collaborative Study of Severe Anaphylaxis. An epidemiologic study of severe anaphylactic and anaphylactoid reactions among hospital patients: methods and overall risks. *Epidemiology* 1998;9:141–146.

Ellis AK, Day JH. Diagnosis and management of anaphylaxis. *CMAJ* 2003;169(4):307–312.

Fisher MM, Baldo BA. The incidence and clinical features of anaphylactic reactions during anesthesia in Australia. *Ann Fr Anesth Reanim* 1993;12:97–104.

Moss J, Mertes PM. Anaphylactic and anaphylactoid reactions. In: Hall JB, Schmidt GA, Woods LDH, eds., *Principles of Critical Care*, 3rd ed., Chapter 106. New York, NY: McGraw-Hill; 2005:1615–1626.

Mertes PM, Laxenaire M, Alla F, et al. Anaphylactic and anaphylactoid reactions occurring during anesthesia in France in 1999-2000. *Anesthesiology* 2003;99:536–545.

Neugut AI, Ghatak AT, Miller RL. Anaphylaxis in the United States. *Arch Intern Med* 2001;161:15–21.

O'Dowd LC, Zweiman B. Anaphylaxis in adults. Available at: <www.utdol.com/application/topic.asp?file=cc_medi/5448&type=A&selectedTitle=1~60>. Accessed 2006, Jan 19.

126 HYPOTHERMIA

Melanie L. Brown

KEY POINTS

- Most organ systems can withstand severe hypothermia with return of function if intervening insults such as hypoxia have not occurred.
- Cardiac arrhythmias are common during profound hypothermia and during the warming phase.
- The methods of rewarming the patient should be selected on the basis of the severity of the hypothermia.
- Volume resuscitation is most often required during rewarming.

OVERVIEW

- The body functions optimally at its normal temperature (36.2–38.2°C).
- In the unimpaired adult three compensatory mechanisms function to maintain normal body temperature:
  - Heat exchange with the environment
  - Change in metabolic rate
  - Behavioral responses
- Homeothermic responses to cold are regulated by the hypothalamus. The mechanisms of heat loss/exchange with the environment include the following:
  - Radiation
  - Conduction
  - Convection
  - Evaporation
- Hypothermia presentations range from the obvious cold water or winter exposures to the more subtle presentations such as an elderly person or drug intoxicated person with depressed mental status and those

TABLE 126-1 Causes of Hypothermia

Increased heat loss (environment, vasodilation, burns, cold infusion)
Decreased heat production (endocrine disorder, malnutrition)
Impaired peripheral regulation (peripheral neuropathy, diabetes, spinal cord transection)
Impaired central regulation (strokes, Parkinson disease, hypothalamic disorders, anorexia, drugs)
Other (sepsis, pancreatitis, uremia)

returning to the floor after a prolonged operative procedure (Table 126-1).
- Some sources have reported that 70% of the severe hypothermia cases result in death.

CLINICAL MANIFESTATIONS

SIGNS AND SYMPTOMS OF MILD HYPOTHERMIA

- Patient has core body temperature between 32.2 and 35°C (90–95°F)
- Awake
- Alert
- Hemodynamically stable
- Shivering

SIGNS AND SYMPTOMS OF MODERATE HYPOTHERMIA

- Patient has core temperature between 26.7 and 32.2°C (80–89°F)
- Dilated pupils
- Hemodynamic instability
- Prone to ventricular dysrhythmia
- Muscles are rigid
- Shivering ceases
- J or Osborne wave on ECG (Fig. 126-1)

SIGNS AND SYMPTOMS OF SEVERE HYPOTHERMIA

- Patient has core temperature <26.7°C (<80°F)
- Coma
- Poor muscle tone
- Apnea
- Asystole or frequent spontaneous fibrillation

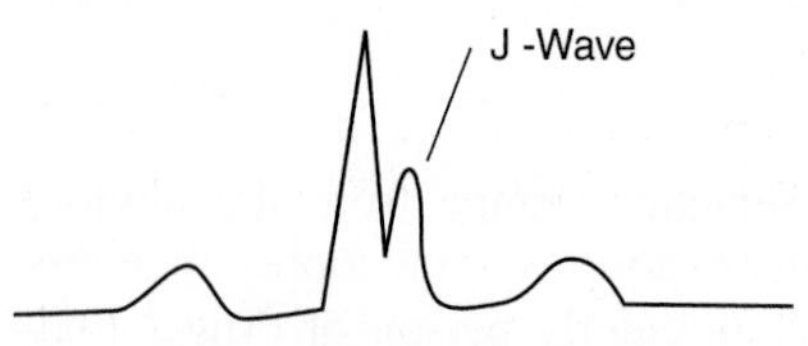

FIG. 126-1 ECG in hypothermia.

EFFECTS OF HYPOTHERMIA ON ORGAN SYSTEMS

- All organ systems are affected by hypothermia.
- To care for hypothermia, it is critical to understand the intravascular volume shifts during resuscitation, the cardiac physiology during hypothermia, and the effects on other organ systems.
- It is important to note that many of the secondary organ system derangements of hypothermia are corrected by rewarming and should be dealt with cautiously unless they are immediately life threatening.
- Conduction disturbances can be particularly refractory to treatment and are common particularly during the rewarming phase.
- As many as 80% of patients with moderate hypothermia have a J or Osborne wave. This wave is found on the ECG at the J point immediately following the QRS complex (Fig. 126-1).
- With worsening hypothermia QRS and ST lengthening occur.
  - Below 33°C, atrial fibrillation is common.
  - At 28°C the heart is particularly prone to ventricular fibrillation (VF). The VF can be precipitated by any irritation such as line placement or rewarming, and may be refractory to all treatments until the core body temperature reaches 30°C.
  - As the heart becomes increasingly more hypothermic, cardiac output decreases leading to eventual asystole. Asystole generally occurs below a core body temperature of 20°C.
- Cold can be protective to the brain in cases of ischemic, hypoxic, and traumatic injury.
- For each degree that body temperature decreases, cerebral blood flow (and metabolic rate) decreases by 7–10%.
  - At approximately 34°C, intellectual function is impaired.
  - Progressive somnolence occurs, leading to coma below 28°C.
  - Temperatures of <20°C are well tolerated by the brain.
  - Circulatory arrest at these temperatures has been tolerated for more than 1 hour without deficits on rewarming.
- Other effects of severe hypothermia include hyperglycemia, platelet dysfunction with coagulopathy, metabolic acidosis, hyperkalemia, and a brisk diuresis. These resolve with rewarming.

MANAGEMENT

- As always in an emergency situation, the first steps of treatment are: airway, breathing, and circulation.
- The patient should be removed from the cold environment and any cold/wet clothing should be removed.
- Treatment goals are to rewarm appropriately for level of hypothermia while anticipating any potential cardiac instability.
- Cardiopulmonary resuscitation (CPR) should be initiated for pulselessness unless body temperature is below 28°C.
- When the core temperature is more than 32°C, rewarming with blankets and warmed IV fluids (40–42°C) is the treatment of choice.
- When the body temperature is below 32°C, rewarming must be more aggressive.
- An arterial line will likely be necessary as the pulse ox will be unreliable. Blood gas interpretation should be done without blood gas temperature correction as regards acid-base balance.
- Adults have a low body surface area:mass ratio relative to children and conductive surface warming (e.g., blankets) may be ineffective at low temperatures. In this case, active core rewarming is required. Active core rewarming can be accomplished by a warm air circulating system (Bair hugger), body cavity warm water lavage with 40–42°C isotonic saline, heated countercurrent hemodialysis, and cardiopulmonary bypass.
- Volume resuscitation during rewarming is critical to preventing circulatory collapse.
- There is a higher incidence of ventricular arrhythmias as the patient is warmed from 28 to 32°C. Below 30°C, the arrhythmia will likely be refractory to all treatment.
- Core body temperatures of <25°C or a core temperature below 30°C with cardiac arrest are indications for extracorporeal membrane oxygenation (ECMO).
- The following therapies are ineffective or possibly dangerous: warm inspired air >60°C (can cause burns to airway epithelium), warm blankets (see above), warm water emersion (impractical in a resuscitation situation).
- Remember, death cannot be determined until resuscitation attempts fail at 35°C or above!

BIBLIOGRAPHY

Hanania NA, Zimmerman JL. Hypothermia. In: Hall JB, Schmidt GA, Wood LDH, eds., *Principles of Critical Care*, 3rd ed. New York, NY: McGraw-Hill; 2005: 1697–1686.

Oldham KT, Colombani PM, Foglia RP, et al. In: Brown M, Kahana M, eds., *Principles and Practice of Pediatric Surgery*, Chapter 29. Philadelphia, PA: Lippincott Williams & Wilkins; 2005: 473–480.

127 SEVERE HYPERTHERMIA

Nathan Sandbo

KEY POINTS

- Severe hyperthermia is defined as a core body temperature >40.0°C, which is not primarily due to the body's immunologic response to infection, but rather dysregulation of temperature homeostasis.
- Severe nonimmunologic hyperthermia is primarily defined by three syndromes: environmental hyperthermia, malignant hyperthermia, and NMS.
- CNS abnormalities in heatstroke may include inappropriate behavior, delirium, and confusion and may progress to seizures and coma.
- Management of heatstroke includes cooling the patient and administration of intravenous fluids for hypovolemia. Avoid use of vasopressor agents (alpha-agonists) for hypotension, as they inhibit normal cooling mechanisms.
- Heatstroke alone has caused over 7000 deaths in the United States in the past 20 years, and mortality can range up to 20%.
- For malignant hyperthermia, immediately give dantrolene IV push (2.5 mg/kg), repeating every 5 minutes until symptoms subside or maximal dose (10 mg/kg) has been reached. Dosing should be continued at 1 mg/kg every 4–6 hours for 36–48 hours.

PATHOPHYSIOLOGY

- Elevation in core body temperature is signaled to the preoptic nucleus of the anterior hypothalamus which in turn directs the body's physiologic response. This includes cutaneous vasodilation, decreased muscle tone, and increased sweating.
- Environmental hyperthermia results from the combination of elevated endogenous heat production and/or an inability to adequately unload heat due to high ambient temperatures with or without high humidity.

- Pharmacologic agents may predispose to the development of environmental hyperthermia via inhibition of normal adaptive responses to elevated body temperature.
  - Sympathomimetics (cocaine, amphetamine, ecstasy) increase heat production and may disrupt thermoregulation.
  - Anticholinergics (tricyclic antidepressants [TCAs], antihistamines, antipsychotics) inhibit sweating and disrupt hypothalamic function.
  - Ethanol, beta-blockers, dehydration, obesity, and head injury may all contribute to hyperthermia.
- Heatstroke is characterized by the presence of an acute phase inflammatory response that is characterized by the presence of elevated levels of circulating inflammatory cytokines, endothelial cell dysfunction, and activation of the clotting cascade.
- The combination of thermoregulatory dysfunction and systemic inflammatory response may lead to the development of life-threatening multisystem organ dysfunction.

• Malignant hyperthermia is a syndrome of hyperthermia, muscle contractions, and cardiovascular instability usually triggered by the administration of volatile anesthetics, such as halothane, or depolarizing paralytic agents, such as succinylcholine in a genetically susceptible host. In these patients, exposure to these agents leads to a marked intracellular calcium release from the sarcoplasmic reticulum in skeletal muscle, resulting in a hypermetabolic and hypercontractile state in skeletal muscle.

• Neuroleptic malignant syndrome (NMS) is an idiosyncratic reaction to the administration of neuroleptic drugs or withdrawal of dopaminergic drugs. It is characterized by hyperthermia, muscle rigidity, alteration in mental status, autonomic dysfunction, and rhabdomyolysis.

CLINICAL FEATURES

• Environmental hyperthermia:
- Heat injury is a spectrum of disease.
- Heat cramps are the mildest form, and are most often seen in younger individuals performing exertional activities in hot environments. Usually treated as an outpatient with oral hydration and relocation to a cool environment.
- Heat exhaustion is characterized by mildly elevated core temperature and systemic complaints (malaise, weakness, nausea), but does not include any severe central nervous system (CNS) dysfunction.
- Heatstroke is characterized by high body temperature (usually > 40°C and the presence of severe CNS dysfunction. Patients have a history of exposure to a heat load (internal or external).
- Two syndromes of heatstroke are: classical (nonexertional) and exertional.
  - Nonexertional heatstroke affects the elderly and chronically ill in the presence of sustained (days) heat stress as is seen in heat waves. Risk factors include immobility, social isolation, obesity, dehydration, and extremes of age.
  - Exertional heatstroke is typically seen in young, healthy individuals who undergo strenuous exercise in hot environments for a short period of time (military recruits, marathon runners).
- CNS abnormalities may include inappropriate behavior, delirium, and confusion and may progress to seizures and coma. Occasionally, cerebellar dysfunction or decerebrate posturing may be seen. Lumbar puncture may reveal increased protein, xanthochromia, and lymphocytic pleocytosis.
- Cardiovascular findings almost always include tachycardia and occasionally supraventricular tachycardias (SVTs). Peripheral vasodilation is usually present, and hypotension results if cardiac output cannot be augmented due to hypovolemia or myocardial dysfunction.
- Lab findings may include metabolic lactic acidosis from either hypoperfusion or sustained anaerobic metabolism by skeletal muscle (exertional hyperthermia), respiratory alkalosis secondary to hyperventilation, hypoglycemia, rhabdomyolysis, renal failure, hyper- or hypokalemia, leukocytosis, disseminated intravascular coagulation (DIC) (usually hours to days after presentation), and thrombocytopenia.

• Clinical signs of malignant hyperthermia usually present within 30 minutes of administration of anesthesia (succinylcholine or volatile inhaled anesthetics), but may be delayed up to 11 hours.
- Spectrum of disease from mild symptoms to fulminant crisis.
- Muscle rigidity is an early manifestation and often begins in extremities or chest with halothane, and in the jaw (masseter muscle) with succinylcholine.
- Capnography or arterial blood gas sampling may reveal elevated CO_2 levels due to elevated production, and is often the first manifestation of the syndrome noted during the induction of anesthesia.
- Pronounced, continuous rise in core temperature, without shivering is characteristic of the reaction, but may be a later finding.
- Tachycardia, hypertension, tachypnea, diaphoresis, and mottling of the skin often occur. As the syndrome progresses, metabolic acidosis, respiratory acidosis, ventricular arrhythmias, hypotension, and rhabdomyolysis may ensue. Rarely, the

syndrome can be characterized by rhabdomyolysis without fever.

- Neuroleptic malignant syndrome usually occurs 3–9 days after initiating a neuroleptic agent or changing the dose, and may last 1–3 weeks.
  - Majority of cases associated with high potency neuroleptics such as haloperidol and thiothixene. Estimated incidence is 0.2% of patients who receive neuroleptic agents.
  - Symptoms begin with mental status changes followed in sequence by muscle rigidity, hyperthermia, and autonomic dysfunction characterized by tachycardia, diaphoresis, blood pressure instability, and arrhythmias.
  - Changes in muscle tone usually include "lead pipe" rigidity or tremors. Other manifestations may include dysphagia, dysarthria, or dystonia. Altered mental status (agitation, coma) occurs in 75%.
  - Lab findings may include elevated creatine kinase (CK) and myoglobinuria, leukocytosis, and evidence of DIC.

DIAGNOSIS

- The diagnosis of a nonimmunologic hyperthermia syndrome should be in the differential of any febrile patient. The list of syndromes incorporating fever in association with mental status changes includes heatstroke, malignant hyperthermia, NMS, meningitis, drug overdose, thyroid storm, sepsis, toxic shock syndrome, and febrile delirium. The diagnosis of environmental hyperthermia, malignant hyperthermia, or NMS is established from the clinical history. Items suggesting infection, drug exposure, or environmental exposure allow for differentiation between fever-associated syndromes.
- Patients at risk for malignant hyperthermia often have a family history of complications from anesthesia. Screening for susceptibility is performed by muscle biopsy with caffeine-halothane contracture test.

TREATMENT

- Environmental hyperthermia:
  - Immediately cool with conductive (immersion in cool water, ice water soaks) or evaporative (fine mist spray and airflow). Other methods include peritoneal lavage, iced gastric lavage, and cardiopulmonary bypass, but none have been adequately tested in humans.
  - Place thermistor probe (esophageal or rectal) to continuously monitor core temperature. Cooling should be stopped at 38.0–38.8°C to prevent iatrogenic hypothermia.
  - Administer intravenous fluids for hypovolemia. Avoid use of vasopressor agents (alpha-agonists) for hypotension, as they inhibit normal cooling mechanisms.
  - Provide supplemental oxygen to all patients and definitive airway control with endotracheal intubation if clinically indicated.
  - If rhabdomyolysis is present, administer intravenous fluids to achieve urine outputs of 100–200 cc/h.
  - Consider invasive hemodynamic monitoring in patients with refractory hypotension or cardiac dysfunction.
  - Monitor for seizures and treat with benzodiazepines if needed.
  - Aggressive supportive therapy and rapid cooling results in >90% survival, with the majority of patients having complete resolution of neurologic dysfunction.
- Malignant hyperthermia:
  - Discontinue inciting drug, administer 100% O_2 to correct hypoxemia, IV fluids, and ventilatory support to correct respiratory acidosis.
  - Immediately give dantrolene IV push (2.5 mg/kg), repeating every 5 minutes until symptoms subside or maximal dose (10 mg/kg) has been reached. Dosing should be continued at 1 mg/kg every 4–6 hours for 36–48 hours.
  - Provide evaporative or conductive cooling if dantrolene is not fully effective.
  - Monitor for and treat rhabdomyolysis.
  - Mortality is now <10%, due to prompt recognition and treatment.
- NMS:
  - Admit to ICU and discontinue offending medication.
  - Control temperature, providing external cooling if needed.
  - Consider dantrolene and dopaminergic agonists (bromocriptine, amantadine, levodopa/carbidopa), although efficacy is not well established for either therapy.
  - Optimize intravascular volume, monitor and treat arrhythmias, ventilatory support if needed, and correct any metabolic derangements.

BIBLIOGRAPHY

Bouchama A, Knochel JP. Heat stroke. *N Engl J Med* 2002;346(25): 1978–1988.

Denborough M. Malignant hyperthermia. *Lancet* 1998;352: 1131–1136.

Hall JB, Schmidt GA, Wood LDH, eds. *Principles of Critical Care*, 2nd ed. New York, NY: McGraw-Hill; 1998: xxiv, 1767.

128 NEAR DROWNING

Melanie L. Brown

KEY POINTS

- Alcohol is a major contributing factor to drowning incidents in adults.
- Clinical consequences of drowning are usually secondary to hypoxic injury leading to multisystem dysfunction. Patients can suffer ARDS, brain injury, cardiac arrest, and acute renal failure.
- Even small amounts of aspirated water can lead to profound ventilation/perfusion mismatches.
- Initial management focuses on the ABCs with careful attention to C-spine stabilization as many drownings can be associated with diving accidents.

EPIDEMIOLOGY

- Males drown at five times the rate of females in the United States.
- Alcohol is a contributing factor in greater than half of the drowning incidents in adults.
- In scuba-related drowning incidents, entanglement or running out of oxygen are the two most common factors.

PATHOPHYSIOLOGY

- Most of the consequences of near drowning are secondary to asphyxia and multisystem hypoxic injury.
- Most drowning victims do not aspirate any of the drowning medium. This is likely secondary to reflex laryngospasm. Only 10–15% of near-drowning victims aspirate a small amount of fluid.
- Even a small amount of aspirated seawater or freshwater can cause ventilation perfusion mismatch and shunting which can lead to a more prolonged period of hypoxemia.
- Large amounts of fluid are often swallowed. This can lead to both electrolyte disturbances and vomiting with aspiration of stomach contents.

END-ORGAN EFFECTS

LUNG

- The presentation can be variable. Patient's presentation can vary from no complaints to florid pulmonary edema and acute respiratory distress syndrome (ARDS).
- Acute lung injury is usually due to the direct effect of aspiration of the drowning fluid or due to aspiration of gastric contents.
- Generally, the pulmonary edema is not cardiogenic in origin.
- X-ray appearance does not always correlate with clinical course and outcome.
- Management is similar to ARDS (see Chap. 35).

BRAIN

- Aggressive intracranial pressure (ICP) monitoring and management has shown no benefit for the near-drowning victim.
- Brain injury is secondary to the hypoxic insult (see Chap. 71).

HEART

- Supraventricular tachycardia can be seen secondary to hypoxemia and acidosis.
- Cardiac arrest is secondary to hypoxemia.
- The cardiac abnormalities are often responsive to cardiopulmonary resuscitation (CPR).

KIDNEY

- Renal insufficiency secondary to hypoxemia and acute tubular necrosis (ATN) can be seen.
- Rarely rhabdomyolysis and hemolysis with disseminated intravascular coagulation (DIC) can occur and can complicate existing renal failure.

GENERAL MANAGEMENT

- Follow the ABCs of acute care: airway, breathing, and circulation.
- Invasive blood pressure monitoring may be helpful in some cases.
- Sedatives and alcohol used by the patient may complicate sedation in the ICU.
- Causes of the near-drowning episode not related to entanglement or alcohol use need to be considered and ruled out quickly: cardiac arrhythmias, seizures, and subarachnoid hemorrhage are all possible contributing factors to a near-drowning episode.

- Injuries to the spine and skull may be present, especially in diving injuries.
- In acute near-drowning episodes in seawater or swimming pool water, antibiotics are not necessary. Prophylactic antibiotics do not improve morbidity or mortality.
- In the case of unexpected difficulty with mechanical ventilation, a bronchoscopy may be warranted to look for aspirated sand, gravel, or other debris.
- Experimental evidence suggests that routine steroid use does not improve outcome, but it has been reported that high-dose steroids might help near-drowning victims who present in pulmonary edema.

ADMISSION CRITERIA

- Patients should generally be admitted to the hospital if they present with the following things (noninclusive list):
    - Abnormal blood gas (gas exchange abnormalities are usually evident within 4–8 hours of the injury)
    - Abnormal chest x-ray
    - Any respiratory symptoms

PROGNOSIS

- 80% of near-drowning victim recover fully.
- Approximately 12% of near-drowning patients die.
- A lack of spontaneous respirations after resuscitation is associated with increased risk of death or severe neurologic impairment.
- Those who arrive to the hospital neurologically intact are likely to survive without neurologic sequelae. Outcome predictions are difficult if not impossible in the presence of hypothermia.

BIBLIOGRAPHY

Bove AA, Neuman T. Diving medicine. In: Murray JF, Nadel JA, eds., *Textbook of Respiratory Medicine*, 4th ed. Philadelphia, PA: W.B. Saunders; 2005:1869–1888.

Oldham KT, Colombani PM, Foglia RP, et al. In: Brown M, Kahana M, eds., *Principles and Practice of Pediatric Surgery*, Chapter 29. Philadelphia, PA: Lippincott Williams & Wilkins; 2005:473–480.

Piantadosi CA, Brown SD. Diving medicine and near drowning. In: Hall JB, Schmidt GA, Wood LDH, eds., *Principles of Critical Care*, 3rd ed. New York, NY: McGraw-Hill; 2005: 1693–1706.

129 CARBON MONOXIDE INTOXICATION

Michael A. Samara

KEY POINTS

- Carbon monoxide is the nonirritating, colorless, odorless, and tasteless gas produced by the incomplete combustion of hydrocarbons.
- CO intoxication is among the leading causes of poisoning death in the United States resulting in over 5000 fatalities each year. The vast majority of these are secondary to suicide attempts. Case fatality rates are highly variable (0–30%).
- Unintentional CO poisonings demonstrate seasonal and regional variation (peaking in winter months and in colder climates) and are primarily secondary to smoke inhalation.
    - Other causes include malfunctioning residential furnaces; poorly ventilated kerosene, wood, and charcoal heaters; and motor vehicle operation with insufficient ventilation.
    - Methylene chloride (an industrial solvent frequently found in paint remover) undergoes hepatic metabolism to CO and is a commonly overlooked cause of poisoning.
- Clinical presentations vary greatly.
    - During winter months, CO intoxication is important to consider in patients presenting with influenza-like signs/symptoms particularly when presenting in cohabitants.
    - CO intoxication should not be omitted from the differential diagnosis in cases of unexplained syncope.
- Neuropsychiatric derangements are the most common and best understood morbidities but CO intoxication can present with any complication of tissue hypoxia (e.g., myocardial infarction and bowel ischemia).

PATHOPHYSIOLOGY

- Carbon monoxide (CO) rapidly crosses the alveolar/capillary membrane. Absorption varies with ambient concentrations, minute ventilation, and the duration of exposure. CO elimination is primarily via the lung as an unchanged gas.
- CO's affinity for hemoglobin and other iron moieties is 200–250 times greater than that of oxygen.
    - In addition to functioning as a competitive inhibitor (effectively decreasing oxygen-carrying capacity), CO binding results in a conformational change in hemoglobin with a resultant left shift of the oxyhemoglobin

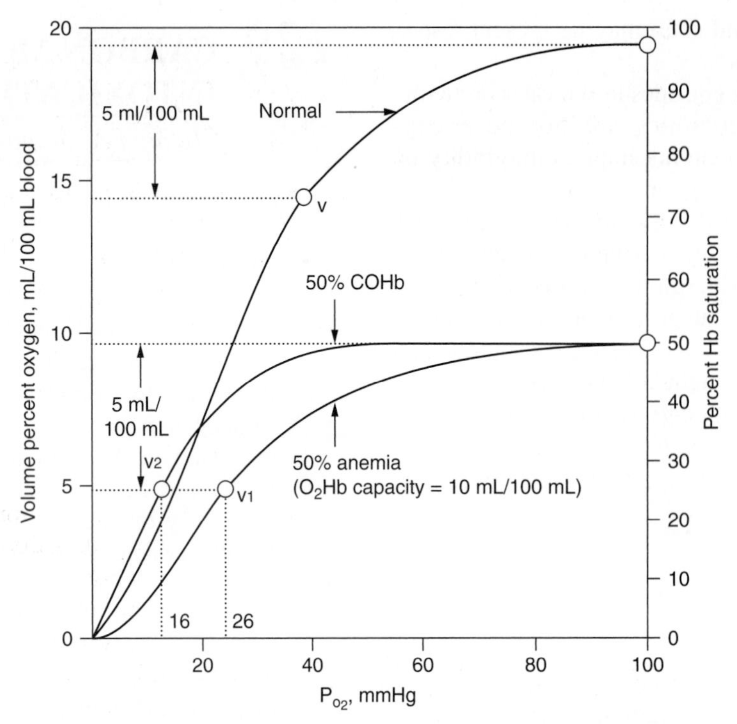

FIG. 129-1 Effect of HbCO on oxygen capacity and unloading. With a 50% reduction in hemoglobin both arterial and venous (v) oxygen content are reduced but the partial pressure at which hemoglobin is 50% saturated (P50) is unchanged. In subjects with 50% HbCO both oxygen content and the P50 are reduced.
SOURCE: Adapted from http://www.inchem.org/documents/ehc/ehc/ehc213.htm.

dissociation curve (decreased P50). This impaired release of O_2 is the principal mechanism by which CO intoxication results in cellular hypoxia (Fig. 129-1).
  - Binding to cardiac myoglobin results in myocardial depression and hypotension thereby exacerbating systemic tissue hypoxia.
- Non-hemoglobin-mediated toxicities (including deranged oxidative phosphorylation, lipid peroxygenation, and numerous effects on platelets, leukocytes, and endothelial cells) contribute to neurologic and cardiac sequelae.
- Pregnant woman pose a unique clinical challenge. The greater affinity of fetal hemoglobin for O_2 and the corresponding accentuated leftward shift in fetal carboxyhemoglobin (HbCO) results in greater sensitivity for the deleterious effects of CO in the fetus.

CLINICAL PRESENTATION

HISTORY

- While acute intoxications are readily apparent in the history (e.g., smoke inhalation and suicide attempts), the presentation of chronic intoxications can be quite subtle.

SYMPTOMS

- Severity of symptoms range from mild constitutional symptoms mimicking viral infection to respiratory depression, seizures, syncope, and coma.
- While many of the acute effects of CO intoxication vary with HbCO levels, the severity of most delayed effects has no clear correlation with HbCO levels.
- Nonlethal CO intoxication frequently presents with the nonspecific symptoms of a viral illness resulting in frequent misdiagnosis.
- Headache, dizziness, weakness, and nausea are the most common presenting complaints occurring in 91%, 77%, 53%, and 47% of patients, respectively.
- 10–30% of victims have no acute neurologic symptoms but present days to months later with a delayed neuropsychiatric syndrome (DNS) characterized by cognitive deficits, personality changes, movement disorders, and focal neurologic deficits. DNS may persist for 1 year or longer but in most cases resolves.
  - While DNS typically occurs within 28 days of exposure, case reports exist of presentations up to 240 days after apparent recovery from the acute exposure.

DIAGNOSIS

- In inadvertent intoxications the best diagnostic tool is a high clinical suspicion. The diagnosis is based on a suggestive history, physical examination, and HbCO measurements by co-oximetry.
- Signs
  - Tachycardia and tachypnea (as markers of impaired cellular oxygenation) are the most consistently found physical signs.
  - The classic findings of cherry-red lips, cyanosis, and retinal hemorrhages are rare and should not be relied upon for diagnosis.
  - More severe intoxications can result in severe lactic acidosis, ventricular arrhythmias, pulmonary edema, and myocardial ischemia.
- Laboratory
  - HbCO levels are important to obtain but may be misleading.
    - Serum levels of HbCO wane rapidly particularly if oxygen therapy has been initiated and therefore blood drawn in the field or ambient CO levels documented by emergency medical services (EMS)/fire department are helpful.
    - Chronic cigarette smokers may have baseline elevations in HbCO to as high as 10%.
    - HbCO must be measured with a spectrophotometer or co-oximeter.
      - HbCO absorbs light at the same wavelengths as oxyhemoglobin and as a result most commercially available pulse oximeters will overestimate the oxygen saturation (though a linear decline will occur).
      - The pulse oximetry gap (the difference between the oxygen saturation as determined by pulse oximetry and the directly measured saturation) is roughly equivalent to the HbCO.
  - Cardiac enzymes and ECG
    - Patients with underlying coronary artery disease may experience worsening symptoms with minimal levels of HbCO (5–10%).
    - Young, healthy patients with no preexisting cardiac disease may experience some myocardial stunning with high-level exposures.
  - Evaluation should also include basic chemistries, a complete blood count (to assess for concomitant anemia), an arterial blood gas (ABG), and a serum lactate level (to assess for ongoing tissue ischemia).
- Imaging
  - Except in their ability rule out structural causes of neuropsychiatric derangements imaging offers little to the evaluation in the acute setting.
  - Computed tomography (CT), magnetic resonance imaging (MRI), and positron emission tomography (PET) imaging however may demonstrate deep white matter abnormalities in patients with DNS.
- It is of the utmost importance to document initial neurologic/neuropsychiatric abnormalities. Dedicated screening batteries exist (e.g., the Carbon Monoxide Neuropsychological Screening Battery). The presence of these abnormalities correlates well with the occurrence and severity of DNS and should in part govern the decision of whether or not to treat with hyperbaric oxygen (HBO; see Chap. 130).

TREATMENT

- Management begins with immediate removal from the source and rapid initiation of the ABCs (airway, breathing, circulation) of basic life support.
- High flow 100% oxygen should be administered immediately and continued until HbCO levels are below 10% (2% in patients with significant cardiopulmonary comorbidities).
- Isocapnic hyperpnea (hyperventilation with O_2 containing ~5% CO_2) is an alternative initial treatment in the field and has been shown in dogs to double the rate of HbCO elimination without the development of hypocapnia.
- Patients who are comatose or have severe mental status changes with concern for airway compromise should be intubated without delay and ventilated with 100% oxygen.
- Continuous cardiac monitoring is essential.
- Once treatment is initiated it is important to consider the use of HBO.
  - The half-life of HbCO drops from 4–6 hours in patients breathing room air, to 40–80 minutes in patients breathing an FiO_2 of 1.0, and to only 15–30 minutes in patients breathing HBO.
  - Existing randomized-controlled trial (RCT) data are limited, however, some consensus for when to employ HBO is emerging:
    - Coma, any preceding period of unconsciousness, HbCO >40%, pregnancy with a HbCO level >15%, signs of cardiac ischemia or arrhythmia, history of coronary artery disease and HbCO >20%, and symptoms not resolving with normobaric O_2 after 4–6 hours.
  - HBO has demonstrated the most efficacy in reducing the risk of DNS when multiple sessions at 2–3 atm are used within 24 hours of the primary exposure.
  - If not available in your institution immediately notify the nearest HBO center for patients who are comatose or unstable. This information is available

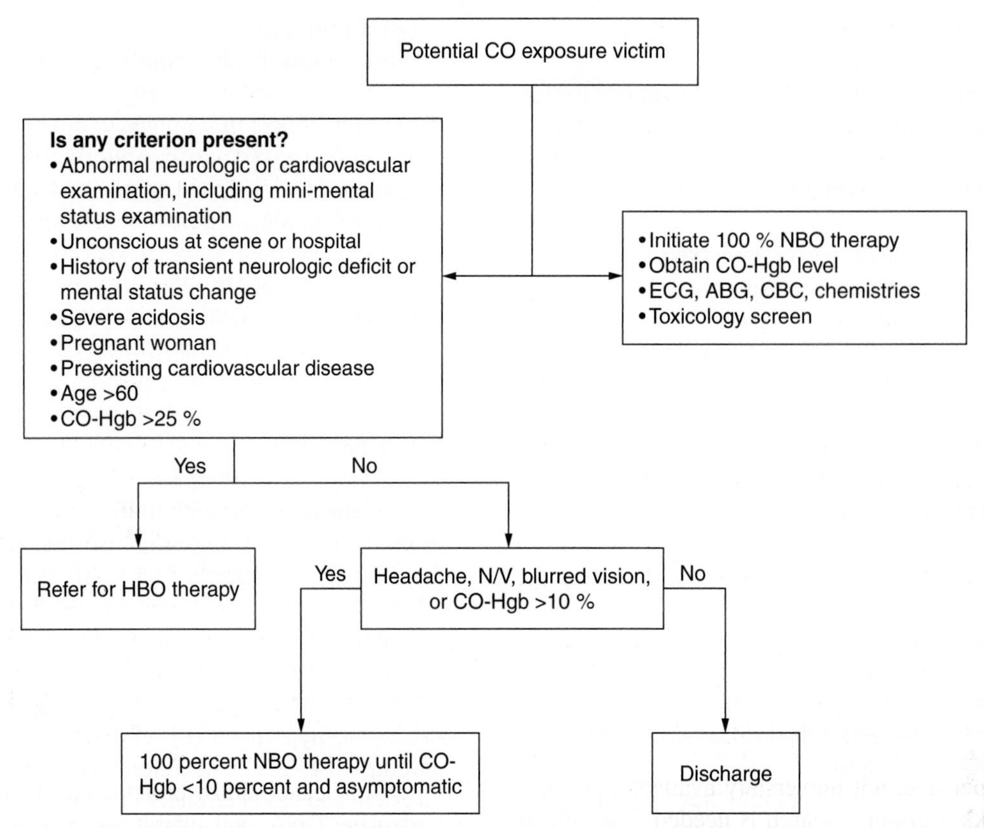

FIG. 129-2 Algorithm for using normobaric and HBO following CO exposure.
SOURCE: Adapted from O'Brien C, Manakar S. Carbon monoxide and smoke inhalation. In: Hanson CW, Lanken P, Manakar S, eds., The Intensive Care Manual. *Philadelphia, PA:* W.B. Saunders, in press; http://Wwddw.Uptodate.Com.

from Duke University's Divers Alert Network hotline (919) 684-2948.
- A sample decision tree for when to employ HBO (Fig. 129-2).

PREVENTION

- Safe operation of motor vehicles, residential furnaces, and portable heaters.
- CO detectors have repeatedly demonstrated their efficacy in minimizing unintentional exposures.

BIBLIOGRAPHY

Cardy P, Manaker S. Carbon monoxide poisoning. 2005. Available at: http://www.uptodateonline.com/application/topic.asp?file=cc_medi/25099&type=A&selectedTitle=1~14.

Ernst A, Zibrak J. Carbon monoxide poisoning. *N Engl J Med* 1998;339:1603–1608.

Kao LW, Nanagas KA. Carbon monoxide poisoning. *Emerg Med Clin North Am* 2004;22:985–1018.

Weaver L, Hopkins R, Chan JK, et al. Hyperbaric oxygen for acute carbon monoxide poisoning. *N Engl J Med* 2002;347:1057–1067.

130 HYPERBARIC OXYGEN THERAPY

May M. Lee

KEY POINTS

- Hyperbaric oxygen has been recommended and used for a wide variety of medical conditions with a varying evidence base. The paucity of randomized-controlled trials makes the efficacy of HBO in most diseases difficult to assess.
- HBO therapy is currently used for patients with severe CO poisoning, decompression sickness (DCS), and air

TABLE 130-1 Possible Uses for HBO Therapy

Air or gas embolism
CO poisoning
CO poisoning complicated by cyanide poisoning
Clostridial myositis and myonecrosis (gas gangrene)
Crush injury, compartment syndrome, and other acute traumatic ischemias
DCS
Enhancement of healing in selected problem wounds
Exceptional blood loss (anemia)
Intracranial abscess
Necrotizing soft-tissue infections
Osteomyelitis (refractory)
Delayed radiation injury (soft-tissue and bony necrosis)
Skin grafts and flaps (compromised)
Thermal burns

SOURCE: Adapted from http://www.UHMS.org.

embolism, and as adjunctive therapy for the prevention and treatment of osteoradionecrosis, clostridial myonecrosis, and compromised skin grafts and flaps.
- HBO therapy is the treatment of choice in severe anemia when transfusion is not an option because of the physiologic effect of arterial oxygen content.
- HBO is expensive, not universally available, and not without risks. Further research is needed to establish its efficacy and safety in other conditions.

BACKGROUND

- Hyperbaric oxygen (HBO) therapy is a unique intervention whose mechanism of action is not fully understood.
- It has been recommended for a wide range of medical conditions (Table 130-1), but with a paucity of randomized-controlled trials documenting its benefit.
- HBO is defined as a treatment in which a patient breathes 100% oxygen while in a chamber where the pressure is increased to greater than sea level (or 1 atmosphere, atm). This may occur in a single person chamber (monoplace) or multiplace chamber (may hold two or more people). Breathing 100% oxygen at 1 atm or exposing isolated parts of the body to 100% oxygen does not constitute HBO therapy.
- The Undersea and Hyperbaric Medical Society (UHMS) is the primary source of information for diving and hyperbaric medicine physiology. Many of the recommendations for the use of HBO come from this organization.

PHYSIOLOGY

- The effects of HBO are based on the biologic and physiologic effects of the gas laws ($PV = nRT$) and of hyperoxia on the tissues. Thus, HBO is most commonly used to treat situations of tissue hypoxia or conditions where gas bubbles obstruct blood flow, that is, decompression sickness (DCS) or gas embolism.
  - *Increased oxygen delivery*: Henry's law states that the amount of gas dissolved in a liquid or tissue is directly proportional to its partial pressure. Most oxygen carried by blood is bound to hemoglobin (CaO_2 = [1.39 × Hb (g/dL) × O_2 saturation (%) + 0.0031 × PaO_2]). That is, the proportion of oxygen carried in solution is increased at increased pressure. At 100% oxygen and 3 atm, arterial oxygen tensions can increase to 2000 mmHg (from 100 mmHg) and tissue oxygen tensions to around 500 mmHg (from 55 mmHg) allowing 60 mL of oxygen to be delivered per liter of blood (compared to 3 mL/L at 1 atm).
  - *Reduction of bubble size*: Boyle's law states that at a constant temperature, the volume of a gas is inversely proportional to the pressure. That is, the volume of a gas bubble at 3 atm is one-third that at sea level. Furthermore, bubble dissolution is accomplished by replacement of the gas inside the bubble with oxygen, which is swiftly metabolized by the tissues.
  - *Increased generation of oxygen free radicals*: Oxygen free radicals oxidize proteins and membrane lipids, damage DNA, and inhibit bacterial metabolic function. HBO alone is bactericidal for certain anaerobes, including *Clostridium perfringes*, and bacteriostatic for certain species of *Escherichia* and *Pseudomonas*.
  - *Improved wound healing*: Amplifies oxygen gradients along the periphery of ischemic wounds and promotes the oxygen-dependent collagen matrix formation needed for angiogenesis.
  - *Reduction in reperfusion injury*: Neutrophils have been implicated as the major culprit in reperfusion injury by adhering to the walls of ischemic vessels, releasing proteases and free radicals leading to pathologic vasoconstriction, and extensive tissue destruction. HBO has been shown to inhibit neutrophil adherence and postischemic vasoconstriction in ischemic rat tissue.
  - *Increased vasoconstriction*: Hyperoxia in normal tissues due to HBO causes quick and significant vasoconstriction, but with increased plasma oxygen carriage. Microvascular blood flow to ischemic tissue is actually improved by HBO. This vasoconstriction helps to reduce tissue edema, which contributes to the treatment of compartment syndromes and burns.
  - *Antagonism of carbon monoxide (CO)*: CO binds to hemoglobin at 200–250 times the affinity of oxygen. Carboxyhemoglobin causes a marked decrease in the oxygen-carrying capacity of blood and release of oxygen in tissue. HBO at 2.5 atm reduces the half-life of carboxyhemoglobin from 4 to 5 hours to 20 minutes or less in normal subjects.

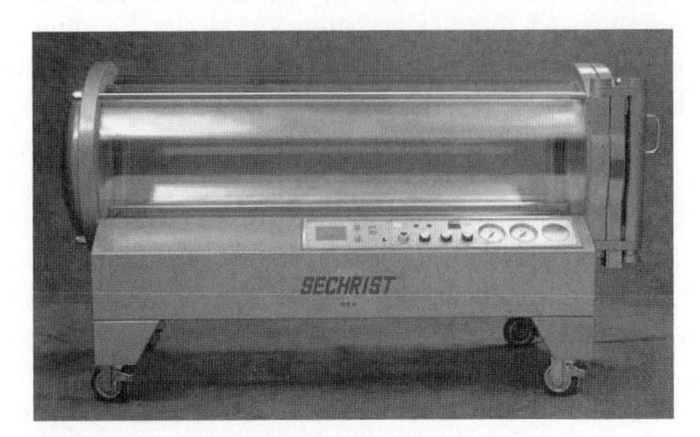

FIG. 130-1 Monoplace chamber.
SOURCE: Adapted from http://www.sechristind.com/.

ADMINISTRATION

- In order to be effective, HBO must be inhaled in the atmosphere or through an endotracheal tube in a monoplace chamber (Fig. 130-1), or through masks, tight-fitting hoods, or endotracheal tubes in a larger, multiplace chamber (Fig. 130-2).
- Monoplace chambers are used for the treatment of chronic medical conditions in stable patients. Multiplace chambers allow closer monitoring of critically ill patients.
- Chamber pressures are usually maintained between 2.5 and 3 atm and last 45–300 minutes depending on the indication.

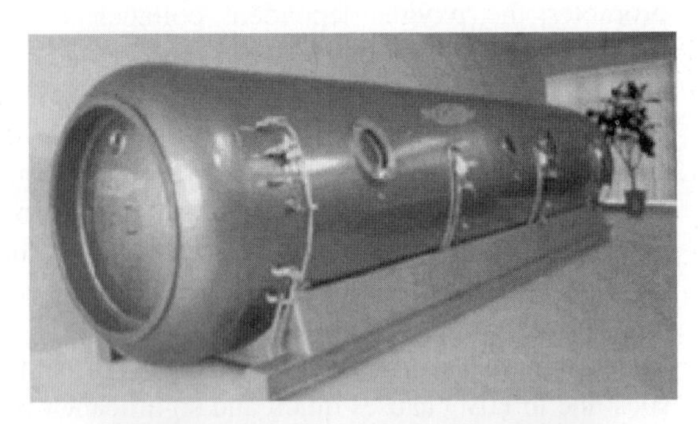

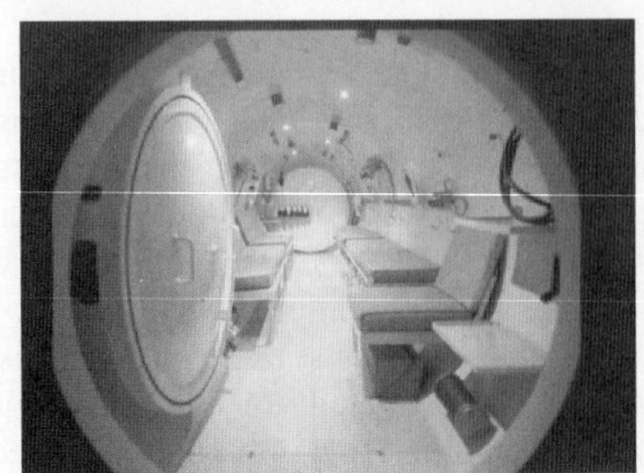

FIG. 130-2 Multiplace chambers.
SOURCE: Adapted from http://www.sechristind.com/.

- Typically, hyperbaric therapy is administered with pressurized oxygen or air.
- Critical care monitoring and treatment, including mechanical ventilation, should be readily available.

CLINICAL USES

CARBON MONOXIDE POISONING

- Carbon monoxide poisoning is the most common cause of death by poisoning in the United States. Severe poisoning is indicated by loss of consciousness (syncope, seizures, and coma), neurologic deficits, pulmonary edema, myocardial ischemia, and severe metabolic acidosis. In addition to the acute toxic effects, all victims of CO poisoning are at risk for delayed neuropsychological sequelae.
- The quality and results of clinical trials vary widely, but numerous nonrandomized studies show that HBO reverses both the acute and delayed effects of CO poisoning.
- HBO is not routine or recommended in patients with mild to moderate CO poisoning—treatment with 100% normobaric oxygen for 4–6 hours or until symptoms abate should be adequate.
- Many authorities favor the use of HBO in the presence of HbCO >40%, loss of consciousness, or in pregnant women with HbCO >20%, because the prognosis for these patients and exposed fetuses are sufficiently poor with normobaric oxygen treatment.
- Patients with severe CO poisoning should receive at least one treatment with HBO at 2.5–3 atm. Additional treatments may produce greater improvement in neuropsychological sequelae.

DECOMPRESSION SICKNESS

- Decompression sickness occurs mainly in recreational divers breathing compressed air who return to the surface too quickly, but can also affect aviators who ascend above 5500 m (altitude DCS).
- Bubble formation occurs when the partial pressure of nitrogen dissolved in tissue and blood exceed the ambient pressure. Bubbles can cause tissue deformation and vessel occlusion, impairing tissue perfusion and oxygenation. Biochemical effects at the blood-gas interface also cause endothelial damage, changes in hemostasis, and activation of leukocytes.
- DCS manifests a range of severity from self-limited rash to joint pain to paralysis, seizures, and even death.
- HBO is the definitive treatment for DCS, although no randomized-controlled trials have compared it to normobaric oxygen treatment.

- It is unclear whether the efficacy of HBO is due to reduction in bubble size and relief of local hypoxia or to the modulation of the pathologic effects mediated by bubbles in the tissues and vessels.
- Patients with DCS should undergo HBO treatment as soon as possible because a sharp decrease in the successful treatment of cerebral air emboli has been noted after a 4- to 5-hour delay.
- Patients should receive HBO at 2.5–3 atm for 2–4 hours, with repeated longer treatment as necessary until they are symptom free, or if there is no further clinical improvement.

ARTERIAL GAS EMBOLISM

- Gas embolism occurs when gas bubbles enter or form in the circulation. This can arise from pulmonary overinflation during a dive, mechanical ventilation, central venous catheter placement, hemodialysis, and other sources.
- There are few clinical trials of HBO treatment in gas embolism, but it is widely accepted as the only lifesaving treatment.
- Immediate therapy with HBO is typically at 2.5–3 atm for 2–4 hours with repeated treatments until no further clinical improvement is seen.

INFECTIONS

- *Clostridial myositis and myonecrosis*: The mainstay of treatment has always been immediate surgical decompression and excision and antimicrobials. Adjunctive HBO therapy is known to have antibacterial and antitoxin effects. There are many case reports and clinical series showing combined treatment can reduce the need for drastic surgery and amputation. The UHMS recommends three 90-minute sessions at 3 atm for the first 25 hours, followed by twice-daily treatments for 4–5 days until clinical improvement is seen.
- *Necrotizing fasciitis*: This rapidly progressive infection of the skin and underlying tissue has a very high mortality. Surgical debridement and antibiotics are conventional therapies. Animal studies have shown that HBO has a direct antibiotic effect, improves oxygen tension, leukocyte function, and bacterial clearance. HBO has been reported to improve mortality by two-thirds. Patients should receive twice-daily treatments for 90–120 minutes at 2–2.5 atm, reduced to once daily when the patient stabilizes. Further treatments may be given to reduce relapse.
- *Refractory osteomyelitis*: HBO is recommended in localized and diffuse osteomyelitis, particularly if there is vascular or immune compromise. HBO promotes the formation of oxygen-dependent collagen matrix needed for angiogenesis. It also directly and indirectly kills anaerobes and promotes oxygen-dependent osteoclastic resorption of necrotic bone. HBO's efficacy in osteomyelitis has been confirmed in animal studies. Treatment varies with severity, but it is recommended that HBO be given for 90–120 minutes daily at 2–2.5 atm in conjunction with debridement, antibiotics, and nutritional support.
- *Intracranial abscess*: In patients with severe infections, multiple, deep, or dominantly located abscesses, or who are immune compromised, poor surgical candidates, or resistant to conventional treatment, adjunctive HBO may be helpful. Clinical evidence is limited, but patients may be treated once or twice daily at 2–2.5 atm for 60–90 minutes. Success is determined by clinical and radiologic findings. The average number of treatments is 13.

COMPROMISED SKIN GRAFTS

- Skin grafts and reconstructive flaps may fail because of inadequate perfusion and hypoxia.
- A number of animal and human studies have shown improved survival of grafts with HBO. In skeletal microcirculation models, HBO significantly reduced endothelial leukocyte adherence and prevented with progressive vasoconstriction of reperfusion injury. Other mechanisms include fibroblast stimulation and collagen synthesis.
- HBO should be considered when a graft or flap must be placed over a capillary bed with poor circulation, in an irradiated field, and especially if a previous reconstruction in the same area was unsuccessful.
- Patients should receive twice daily treatments at 2–2.5 atm for 90–120 minutes reduced to once daily once the graft or flap has stabilized.

PROBLEM WOUNDS

- Problem wounds, especially diabetic foot infections and arterial insufficiency ulcers are among the most common conditions treated with HBO in the United States. Morbidity and mortality are high. HBO treatment has been shown to improve healing and limb salvage.
- HBO has been reported to enhance oxygenation, fibroblast proliferation, collagen synthesis, epithelialization, and neovascularization, increase bactericidal activity, and be toxic to anaerobes.
- A double-blind randomized-controlled trial in 2003 demonstrated improved healing and cost benefit with

adjunctive HBO treatment in diabetic ulcers compared to a placebo group receiving hyperbaric air, though the sample was small.
- HBO is very useful in the management of problem wounds by promoting limb preservation and speedier healing.
- Treatment at 2–2.5 atm for 90–120 minutes once or twice daily combined with grafts and infection control may be reasonable.

ANEMIA DUE TO EXCEPTIONAL BLOOD LOSS

- In hyperbaric conditions, the dissolved oxygen content in the blood can be sufficient to meet cellular and metabolic demands without the contribution of oxyhemoglobin.
- Hemorrhagic shock can be treated by HBO in patients for whom suitable blood is not available, or who refuse blood for religious or practical reasons.
- HBO is useful as a short-term temporizing measure, but it is inconvenient and expensive, and the risks of oxygen toxicity limit its treatment duration.
- It is recommended that patients be treated at up to 3 atm for 2- to 4-hour periods, three to four times a day until hypoxic symptoms have resolved and red blood cells have regenerated.

RADIATION-INDUCED TISSUE INJURY

- Radiation therapy impairs restorative cellular proliferation, causing decreased vascularity, local hypoxia, and eventually necrosis. This usually manifests itself as edema, ulceration, bone necrosis, poor wound healing, and increased risk of infections, which can persist for years after the initial insult. High doses of radiation can result in spontaneous radionecrosis.
- HBO increases vascular density and oxygenation in radiation-damaged tissues. Oxygen tension is increased to normal levels enabling fibroblast proliferation, collagen formation, angiogenesis at wound edges, and re-epithelization.
- Before HBO therapy was available, reconstruction of previously irradiated mandibular tissue in patients with oropharyngeal and other head and neck cancers were often unsuccessful with complications including osteonecrosis, soft-tissue radionecrosis, mucositis, dermatitis, and laryngeal radionecrosis found in 50–60% of patients. The use of HBO has increased success rates up to 93%.
- Successful treatment with HBO is also documented in other postradiation damage including chest wall necrosis, radiation-induced hemorrhagic cystitis, and central nervous system (CNS) radiation damage.
- There is extensive, though not conclusive, evidence for the use of HBO in radiation injury, particularly mandibular osteoradionecrosis.
- Current protocols for the prevention and treatment of osteoradionecrosis involve 30 preoperative HBO sessions at 2.4 atm for 90 minutes each, followed by 10 sessions postoperatively.

THERMAL BURNS

- The proposed mechanisms of benefit to burn wounds are decreased edema due to hyperoxic vasoconstriction, collagen formation, and improved bacterial killing.
- Some studies have shown that HBO improves healing time, hospitalization, and mortality compared to controls and reduces the need for grafting. However, other studies show no benefit.
- At this time, it is not clear that HBO confers any benefit when added to the usual care given to patients at burn centers.
- The UHMS recommends three sessions within 24 hours of injury and 90-minute treatments twice daily thereafter at 2–2.4 atm.

ACUTE CRUSH INJURIES

- In acute traumatic crush injuries, extravasation of intravascular fluid increases the diffusion difference from capillary to cell, producing progressive, self-perpetuating ischemia, edema, and inadequate healing.
- Surgical repair to maintain perfusion of tissues, blood replacement, and anticoagulation are the mainstays of management.
- HBO can improve tissue oxygen tension and increase plasma-based oxygenation and increasing erythrocyte deformability.
- Hyperoxic vasoconstriction resolves edema without impairing oxygen delivery and reverses the edema-ischemia cycle.
- HBO also antagonizes lipid peroxidation by free radicals thereby reducing reperfusion injury.
- Published research is limited, but a high-quality randomized-controlled trial in 1996 demonstrated significant improvements in healing with HBO.
- Patients should be treated within 4–6 hours of injury at 2–2.5 atm once daily for several days.

OTHER

- A number of other potential uses for HBO have been proposed, however remain poorly validated. Future indication for HBO are as disparate as malignant otitis media, sports injuries, traumatic brain or spinal cord injury, sickle cell disease, acute stroke, multiple sclerosis, tinnitus, sudden sensorineural hearing loss, the systemic inflammatory response syndrome, and acute myocardial infarction (MI). Further studies will need to be done before HBO can be endorsed for these potential indications.

COMPLICATIONS

- Hyperbaric oxygen therapy is safe when used according to standard protocols with oxygen pressures not exceeding 3 atm and with treatment sessions limited to 120 minutes. Some adverse effects may occur, however.
  - The most common side effect is reversible myopia, caused by either direct toxicity of oxygen to the lens or physical lens deformation. There is no evidence for increased cataract formation.
  - Middle ear and sinus barotraumas are preventable by equalization techniques or tympanostomy tubes, and otitis media can be prevented by pseudoephedrine. Inner ear barotrauma is extremely rare but tympanic rupture can result in permanent hearing loss, tinnitus, and vertigo.
  - Inhaling highly concentrated and pressurized oxygen may precipitate generalized seizures, but these are self-limited and cause no permanent damage. HBO has also been associated with hypoglycemia in some patients with diabetes. Hypoglycemia should be included in the differential for HBO-associated seizures.
  - Some patients have reversible tracheobronchial symptoms with repeated exposure to HBO: chest tightness, substernal burning, and cough, with reversible decrements in pulmonary function.
  - Critically ill patients who have required high concentrations of normobaric oxygen for a prolonged period who then undergo repeated exposure to HBO are at greater risk for toxic pulmonary effects.
  - Psychological side effects such as claustrophobia, especially in monoplace chambers, are common.
  - There is no evidence for stimulation of malignant growth with HBO therapy.
  - Clinical evidence does not support claims of fetal complications such as spina bifida or limb defects.

CONTRAINDICATIONS

- The only absolute contraindication to HBO therapy is untreated pneumothorax.
- Relative contraindications include obstructive lung disease, cardiac disease, impaired pressure equalization, upper respiratory or sinus infections, recent ear surgery or injury, fever, and claustrophobia.
- Patients with a history of seizure disorder, pneumothorax, or chest surgery are at highest risk for complications related to barotraumas or CNS oxygen toxicity.

COST

- On average, a single 90-minute HBO session can cost between $300 and $400.
- The cost for 30–40 sessions for the treatment of radionecrosis or problem wounds, therefore, can cost from $9000 to $16,000.

CONCLUSION

- Hyperbaric oxygen has been recommended and used for a wide variety of medical conditions with a varying evidence base. The paucity of randomized-controlled trials makes the efficacy of HBO in most diseases difficult to assess.
- The discovery of beneficial cellular and biochemical effects has strengthened the rationale for administering HBO as primary therapy in patients with severe CO poisoning, DCS, and air embolism, and as adjunctive therapy for the prevention and treatment of osteoradionecrosis, clostridial myonecrosis, and compromised skin grafts and flaps.
- The physiologic effect of HBO on arterial oxygen content makes this therapy the treatment of choice in severe anemia when transfusion is not an option.
- HBO is expensive, not universally available, and not without its risks. Further research is needed to establish its efficacy and safety in other conditions.

BIBLIOGRAPHY

Gill AL, Bell CN. Hyperbaric oxygen: its uses, mechanisms of action and outcomes. *QJM* 2004;97:385–395.

Leach RM, Rees PJ, Wilmhurst P. Hyperbaric oxygen therapy. *BMJ* 1998;317:1140–1143.

Tibbles PM, Edelsberg JS. Hyperbaric-oxygen therapy. *N Engl J Med* 1996;334:1642–1648.

Undersea and Hyperbaric Medical Society. Indications for Hyperbaric Oxygen Therapy. Available at: http://uhms.org/Indications/indications.htm. Accessed August 2005.

131 ACUTE ALCOHOL WITHDRAWAL

Brian Klausner

KEY POINTS

- Alcohol abuse is prevalent in hospitalized population, occurring in approximately 15–20% of patients.
- Alcohol withdrawal (AWD) symptoms can range from mild agitation to life-threatening seizures and delirium. Quick and adequate symptomatic control of AWD decreases associated mortality from approximately 10–15% to <1%.
- Benzodiazepines are the first-line agents used to treat withdrawal syndromes secondary to their cross-reactivity with alcohol and their rapid onset of action. Rapid and adequate control of agitation has been shown to decrease mortality and duration of symptoms.

PATHOPHYSIOLOGY

- Alcohol increases the binding of gamma-aminobutyric acid (GABA), an important inhibitory neurotransmitter, to its receptor while inhibiting the effects of the excitatory neurotransmitter, *N*-methyl-D-aspartate (NMDA), on its receptor. Over time, chronic exposure to alcohol will lead to a compensatory decrease in GABA receptor responsiveness and an upregulation of NMDA receptors. As a result, sudden abruption of alcohol intake in the chronic alcoholic leads to brain excitability and withdrawal symptoms. Benzodiazepines, which are the first-line agent for treatment, increase the affinity of GABA to $GABA_A$ receptors, helping to counteract the effects of alcohol withdrawal.
- With repeated detoxifications over time, there is believed to be a "kindling effect" where an increase in neuronal responsivity leads to worsening withdrawal symptoms for individual patients.

CLINICAL MANIFESTATIONS

- Symptoms of hyperexcitability range from mild to life-threatening and vary between patients and over time for individual patients.
- Table 131-1 list the DSM-IV (Diagnostic and Statistical Manual of Mental Disorders, Fourth Edition) diagnostic criteria for alcohol withdrawal, which include impairing symptoms of agitation and excitability that occur in the context of alcohol cessation after prolonged use that cannot be explained by other medical conditions. Alcohol withdrawal delirium (AWD), commonly known as delirium tremens (DTs) can be diagnosed when fluctuating changes in cognition and consciousness occurs in the setting of withdrawal symptoms.
- In general, minor withdrawal symptoms such as anxiety, agitation, tremulousness, nausea, anorexia, palpitations, and diaphoresis typically occur approximately 6–12 hours after the last drink, with more severe symptoms of hallucination (12–24 hours), tonic-clonic seizures (typically 24–48 hours but can occur within hours of cessation), and delirium (48–72 hours) occurring later.
- The Clinical Institute Withdrawal Assessment for Alcohol (CIWA-Ar) is a clinical scale used to assess severity of the 10 most common withdrawal phenomena and can be used to help guide treatment (see Fig. 131-1).

TABLE 131-1 DSM-IV Criteria for EtOH Withdrawal

a. Cessation of EtOH use that has been heavy and prolonged
b. Two or more of the following:
Autonomic hyperactivity
Increased hand tremor
Insomnia
Nausea and vomiting
Hallucinations
Psychomotor agitation
Grand mal seizures
c. The symptoms of part b cause distress and impairment
d. The symptoms of part b are not due to a medication

EVALUATION

- History: duration, amount, and type of alcohol use; any history of withdrawals, seizures, or other substance abuse.
- Physical: manifestations of liver disease, full neurologic examination, signs of trauma (alcoholics often present with evidence of falls or injuries). In the context of mental status changes, head trauma often must be ruled out as an etiology.
- Labs/imaging: liver function test, urine toxicology screen, basic metabolic panel identifying hypoglycemia as well as magnesium and phosphate deficiencies; possible head computed tomography (CT) and lumbar puncture (LP) if indicated in patients with seizures or delirium.

Clinical Institute Withdrawal Assessment of Alcohol Scale, Revised (CIWA-Ar)

Patient:________________ **Date:** ____________ **Time:** ____________ (24 hour clock, midnight = 00:00)

Pulse or heart rate, taken for one minute:________________ **Blood pressure:**______

NAUSEA AND VOMITING -- Ask "Do you feel sick to your stomach? Have you vomited?" Observation.
0 no nausea and no vomiting
1 mild nausea with no vomiting
2
3
4 intermittent nausea with dry heaves
5
6
7 constant nausea, frequent dry heaves and vomiting

TACTILE DISTURBANCES -- Ask "Have you any itching, pins and needles sensations, any burning, any numbness, or do you feel bugs crawling on or under your skin?" Observation.
0 none
1 very mild itching, pins and needles, burning or numbness
2 mild itching, pins and needles, burning or numbness
3 moderate itching, pins and needles, burning or numbness
4 moderately severe hallucinations
5 severe hallucinations
6 extremely severe hallucinations
7 continuous hallucinations

TREMOR -- Arms extended and fingers spread apart. Observation.
0 no tremor
1 not visible, but can be felt fingertip to fingertip
2
3
4 moderate, with patient's arms extended
5
6
7 severe, even with arms not extended

AUDITORY DISTURBANCES -- Ask "Are you more aware of sounds around you? Are they harsh? Do they frighten you? Are you hearing anything that is disturbing to you? Are you hearing things you know are not there?" Observation.
0 not present
1 very mild harshness or ability to frighten
2 mild harshness or ability to frighten
3 moderate harshness or ability to frighten
4 moderately severe hallucinations
5 severe hallucinations
6 extremely severe hallucinations
7 continuous hallucinations

PAROXYSMAL SWEATS -- Observation.
0 no sweat visible
1 barely perceptible sweating, palms moist
2
3
4 beads of sweat obvious on forehead
5
6
7 drenching sweats

VISUAL DISTURBANCES -- Ask "Does the light appear to be too bright? Is its color different? Does it hurt your eyes? Are you seeing anything that is disturbing to you? Are you seeing things you know are not there?" Observation.
0 not present
1 very mild sensitivity
2 mild sensitivity
3 moderate sensitivity
4 moderately severe hallucinations
5 severe hallucinations
6 extremely severe hallucinations
7 continuous hallucinations

ANXIETY -- Ask "Do you feel nervous?" Observation.
0 no anxiety, at ease
1 mild anxious
2
3
4 moderately anxious, or guarded, so anxiety is inferred
5
6
7 equivalent to acute panic states as seen in severe delirium or acute schizophrenic reactions

HEADACHE, FULLNESS IN HEAD -- Ask "Does your head feel different? Does it feel like there is a band around your head?" Do not rate for dizziness or lightheadedness. Otherwise, rate severity.
0 not present
1 very mild
2 mild
3 moderate
4 moderately severe
5 severe
6 very severe
7 extremely severe

FIG. 131-1 CIWA-Ar clinical scale.
SOURCE: Adapted from Sullivan JT, Sykora K, Schneiderman J, et al. Assessment of alcohol withdrawal: the revised Clinical Institute Withdrawal Assessment for Alcohol scale (CIWA-Ar). *Br J Addict* 1989;84:1353–1357.)

AGITATION -- Observation.
0 normal activity
1 somewhat more than normal activity
2
3
4 moderately fidgety and restless
5
6
7 paces back and forth during most of the interview, or constantly thrashes about

ORIENTATION AND CLOUDING OF SENSORIUM -- Ask "What day is this? Where are you? Who am I?"
0 oriented and can do serial additions
1 cannot do serial additions or is uncertain about date
2 disoriented for date by no more than 2 calendar days
3 disoriented for date by more than 2 calendar days
4 disoriented for place/or person

Total **CIWA-Ar** Score______
Rater's Initials______
Maximum Possible Score 67

The ***CIWA-Ar*** *is not* copyrighted and may be reproduced freely. This assessment for monitoring withdrawal symptoms requires approximately 5 minutes to administer. The maximum score is 67 (see instrument). Patients scoring less than 10 do not usually need additional medication for withdrawal.

FIG. 131-1 *(Continued)*

TREATMENT

- Goals of treatment: Alleviate and prevent progressions of symptoms; treat underlying comorbidities.
- Benzodiazepines are first-line agents due to their rapid absorption and cross-tolerance with alcohol. Meta-analysis demonstrates that treatment with benzodiazepines is associated with an improvement in mortality and duration of symptoms and with less side effects than neuroleptics.
- Studies have demonstrated that symptom-based treatment, where the CIWA score is calculated on an hourly basis and treatment is administered when scores are >8, is associated with a shorter treatment course (9 hours vs. 68 hours) and total dosage (100 mg vs. 425 mg of chlordiazepoxide) compared to fixed schedule regimens. Symptom-based treatment does require extensive monitoring.
  - Typical symptom-based treatment regimen: diazepam (Valium) 5–10 mg or lorazepam (Ativan) 1–4 mg IV q 1-2 h as needed to maintain light sedation or to keep CIWA-Ar scores below 8.
  - Fixed dose regimen: Chlordiazepoxide (Librium) 50 mg PO q 6 h for four doses followed by 25 mg PO q 6 h for eight doses; doses held for excessive somnolence or patient refusal. Additional doses of 25–100 mg doses given as needed hourly for CIWA scores >8.
- There are no randomized, control studies looking at long-acting versus shorter-acting benzodiazepines. Long-acting provide a smoother withdrawal course and are associated with less breakthrough symptoms and seizures. Short-acting may be preferred in elderly, patients with liver disease, or in patients who are expected to require prolonged sedation.
- Other agents: Neuroleptics, such as haloperidol, have been demonstrated to be inferior to benzodiazepines as first-line agents, but are often used as adjunct treatment to help control agitation and delirium. Beta-blockers can be used to help control blood pressure, tachycardia, and other symptoms of agitation, but must be used with caution as they can worsen delirium and mask withdrawal symptoms. Clonidine is also often used to treat the autonomic symptoms of withdrawal. Treatment with either clonidine or beta-blockers should be considered in patients with known coronary artery disease who might not be able to tolerate the cardiac autonomic strain of withdrawal.
- Supportive treatment: IV fluids with D_5NS, 100 mg IV thiamine (given before D_5NS to prevent the sudden onset or worsening of Wernicke encephalopathy that can occur with thiamine deficiency), folate 1 mg, multivitamins, replace electrolytes as needed (magnesium, potassium, and phosphate deficiencies are common in alcoholics).

ALCOHOL WITHDRAWAL DELIRIUM (DELIRIUM TREMENS)

- On the spectrum of clinical manifestations, AWD is the most severe and life-threatening, occurring in approximately 5% of withdrawal patients. AWD symptoms are typically first seen 48–72 hours after the last drink and tend to peak 5 days after cessation of alcohol. Risk factors for the development of AWD include history of prior episodes or withdrawal seizures, daily heavy alcohol use, concurrent medical illness, older age, abnormal liver tests, and severe withdrawal symptoms. All hospitalized patients undergoing alcohol detoxification should be monitored closely for evidence of AWD as the condition is associated with a high mortality and necessitates aggressive treatment. Any patient with clinical symptoms of AWD should be monitored in an ICU setting.

- In patients with AWD, it is essential to obtain quick and adequate control of agitation to a goal of light sedation, defined as either the patient being asleep but easily arousable, or awake but able to quickly fall asleep without stimulation. With benzodiazepine treatment, the mortality rate from AWD drops from approximately 10–15% to 0–1%.
    - Typical regimen: lorazepam 1–4 mg IV or diazepam 5–10 mg IV q 5-10 min as needed to control agitation and achieve light sedation, and then additional doses q 1-2 h as needed. Patients will often need high doses to reach treatment goals.
- In addition to the adjunct treatments listed above, propofol, a short-acting barbiturate, may be used in severe cases of delirium/agitation that is refractory to benzodiazepine treatment. Side effects of propofol include hypotension, hypertriglyceridemia, and risk of infection caused by the infusate medium. Patients require an artificial airway and mechanical ventilation in almost all cases.
- For withdrawal seizure, give 2 mg IV lorazepam; repeat dose for subsequent seizures; correct any electrolyte abnormalities or concurrent hypoglycemia. Consider other possible etiologies in patients with fever, history of trauma, focal seizures, or if their last drink was over 48 hours prior to presentation.
- Patients with seizures, severe impairment of consciousness, or who are at high risk for aspiration may require intubation for airway protection.
- Use physical restraints as needed for patient protection.
- Remember to monitor electrolytes and replace them as needed. Magnesium, phosphate, and potassium deficiencies commonly present in chronic alcoholics are often exacerbated during episodes of withdrawal as there is a shift of these electrolytes into the cells. Also, monitor closely for evidence of rhabdomyolysis which often occurs in the context of DTs.

BIBLIOGRAPHY

Al-Sanouri I, Dikin M, Soubani AO. Critical care aspects of alcohol abuse. *South Med J* 2005;98:372–381.

Bayard M, McIntyre J, Hill KR, et al. Alcohol withdrawal syndrome. *Am Fam Physician* 2004;69:1443–1450.

Lejoyeux M, Solomon J, Ades J. Benzodiazepine treatment for alcohol-dependent patients. *Alcohol Alcohol* 1998;33:563–575.

Mayo-Smith MF. Management of alcohol withdrawal delirium: an evidence-based practice guideline. *Arch Intern Med* 2004;164:1405–1412.

Saitz R. Individualized treatment for alcohol withdrawal: a randomized double-blind control trial. *JAMA* 1994;272:519–523.

Section 11
PROCEDURES IN THE ICU

132 CENTRAL VENOUS CATHETERIZATION

David R. Brush

KEY POINTS

- Careful consideration of the indication(s) for central line placement helps dictate correct catheter choice and site of cannulation.
- Patients with innate or iatrogenic coagulopathies should have their coagulopathy corrected before central venous catheter placement to reduce complications.
- Experience in the placement of central venous catheters results in a substantial decrease in the rate of complications. Proper supervision should be provided to trainees.
- When no longer needed, central venous catheters should be removed immediately to avoid long-term complications of infection and/or thrombosis.

INDICATIONS FOR CENTRAL LINE PLACEMENT

- To obtain measurements of central venous pressure (CVP) via subclavian or internal jugular cannulation. Femoral central venous catheters can be used to monitor intra-abdominal pressure.
- In preparation for the placement of pulmonary artery (PA) catheters.
- To provide rapid resuscitation with fluid or blood products.
- To provide medications such as chemotherapy, vasoactive drugs, and hyperalimentation that have the potential to cause phlebitis if not placed in central large veins.
- To perform hemodialysis or plasmapheresis.
- To sample central venous oxyhemoglobin saturation.
- For patients requiring frequent blood draws, or if peripheral access is unattainable.
- Cardiopulmonary resuscitation often calls for the emergent placement of a central venous catheter. Under these circumstances the femoral vein is most often cannulized due to ease of placement; however, breaks in sterile technique are common. When the patient is stabilized a new central line should be placed at another site using sterile technique and the femoral catheter should be removed. Any line placed emergently during a code situation should be considered nonsterile.
- Intracardiac pacing can be accomplished with subclavian and internal jugular venous catheters (Table 132-1).

GENERAL CONTRAINDICATIONS TO CENTRAL VENOUS CANNULATION

- Generally, patients with platelets $<50 \times 10^3/\mu L$, prothrombin time >1.5 times the normal limit, or activated partial thromboplastin time >2 times the normal limit are at increased risk of serious complications. Patients with blood coagulation disorders should have their derangements corrected prior to cannulation.
- For patients who have recently received therapeutic anticoagulation (e.g., heparin, low-molecular weight heparin, activated protein C, or tissue plasminogen activator), a proper amount of time should be given before proceeding with cannulation. The amount of time needed to wait will depend on the half-life of the medication.
- Uncooperative or delirious patients can be a significant barrier to safe placement of a central venous catheter. Short-acting parenteral benzodiazepines can be employed but should be used with extreme caution in patients with compromised cardiopulmonary or neurologic function.
- Physician inexperience with central venous cannulation is associated with increased mechanical and

TABLE 132-1 Indications for Central Venous Cannulation
Monitoring CVP or intra-abdominal pressure
Measuring central venous oxygen saturation
Placement of PA catheters
Extremely rapid fluid resuscitation
Hemodialysis
Plasmapheresis
Cardiopulmonary resuscitation
Administration of vasoactive drugs
Intracardiac pacing
Hyperalimentation
Administration of phlebitic medications (chemotherapy, potassium)
Inadequate peripheral access
Frequent phlebotomy

infectious complications. Close supervision is required. Inexperienced physicians in training should initially perform cannulations on sedated, mechanically ventilated patients and only with senior supervising physicians.

SITE CHOICE

- Generally, the subclavian vein is the preferred site for catheterization. It is associated with the lowest rates of catheter infection and thrombosis when compared to internal jugular and femoral cannulation. Aseptic techniques, combined with operator expertise and correct site selection can minimize complications associated with central line placement.
- In general, it is advisable to avoid sites with poor landmarks, anatomic defects, or recent surgery.
- If the patient is coagulopathic, consider femoral cannulation to avoid bleeding from a noncompressible vessel.
- Consider jugular or femoral catheter placement in patients requiring hemodialysis or plasmapheresis. This protects the subclavian veins for later placement of permanent catheters.
- If a PA catheter will be placed the preferred sites for the introducer catheter are the left subclavian vein or the right internal jugular due to the curved conformation of the PA catheter.
- Avoid subclavian and internal jugular cannulation in patients with severe refractory hypoxemia.
- Do not place more than one central catheter at a single site.
- Failed attempts for internal jugular or subclavian veins should not proceed to the contralateral side for new attempt until a chest x-ray (CXR) has been obtained and confirmed no pneumothorax complication.
- Avoid sites with superficial skin lesions and infections.
- Avoid placement in vessels with known or suspected thrombosis.

CATHETER SELECTION

SHORT, LARGE-BORE (8.5 F) INTRODUCER CATHETER

BENEFITS

- Flow is inversely related to resistance described by Poiseuille law: $R = (8\eta L/P\pi)r^4$, where η is fluid viscosity, L is catheter length, and r is the radius of the catheter lumen. Thus, short, large-bore (8.5 F) catheters are the catheter of choice for extremely rapid fluid resuscitation.
- Allows for introduction of a PA catheter through the sheath introducer.

DRAWBACKS

- Not designed for long-term use >72 hours.
- Associated with increased risk of air embolism.
- Using a PA catheter through the sheath introducer is associated with increased rates of catheter infection.
- Malfunction or accidental removal of the catheter by the patient can cause rapid exsanguination. Thus, only to be utilized in highly monitored settings such as in ICU.

LARGE-BORE, DOUBLE LUMEN CATHETERS (QUINTON)

BENEFITS

- Best suited for hemodialysis or plasmapheresis.

DRAWBACKS

- Slower rate of flow than an 8.5 F catheter due to decreased radius and increased catheter length.
- Can limit patient mobility.

TRIPLE LUMEN CATHETER

BENEFITS

- Allows for infusion of multiple agents.
- Can reduce the number of central venous catheters needed.

DRAWBACKS

- Should not be used for fluid resuscitation or dialysis due to high resistance and poor flow.
- A peripheral 16-gauge catheter can infuse fluids quicker than a central triple lumen.

PREPARATION FOR CATHETER PLACEMENT

- Obtain written informed consent for the procedure from the patient or the patient's surrogate. Consent

TABLE 132-2 Materials Necessary for Central Venous Catheter Placement

Clean bouffant cap to prevent hair falling on the field
Clean mask with face shield
Sterile gown
Sterile gloves
Sterile towels
Large sterile drape with fenestration for site of insertion
500 cc sterile 0.9% normal saline in sterile bowl
Chlorhexidine skin antiseptic
At least one 5 mL ampule of HCl 1% lidocaine
25-Gauge injection needle c/ 5 cc syringe for lidocaine
22-Gauge "finder" needle c/ 10 cc syringe
18-Gauge introducer needle c/ 10 cc syringe
Guidewire
Short catheter: 18-gauge over 20-gauge introducer
#11 scalpel
Tissue dilator
Indwelling central venous catheter
Central line clamp fastener
4 × 4 gauze pads
Suture: straight needle and 3-0 silk

should include discussion of the following risks: possible pneumothorax and need for tube thoracostomy, infection, bleeding, and thrombosis.

- Gather all materials necessary before proceeding with the procedure.
- Supervising physicians should employ all sterile protective barriers (e.g., gloves and gown) so they can quickly and safely assist during the procedure if needed.
- After employing sterile dress and gloves, arrange all sterile materials according to operator preference (Table 132-2).
- The catheter should always be examined under sterile conditions for defects and flushed with sterile saline to ensure proper function before placement.

INTERNAL JUGULAR CENTRAL VENOUS CATHETER PLACEMENT: CENTRAL APPROACH USING A MODIFIED SELDINGER TECHNIQUE

- Locate the apex of the triangle formed by the two bodies of the sternocleidomastoid muscle and their insertion points into the clavicle. The internal jugular vein, bound with the carotid artery in the carotid sheath, runs deep to the sternocleidomastoid muscle and emerges between the two heads of this muscle before passing deep to the clavicle to join the subclavian vein (Fig. 132-1A).
- Rotate the patient's head approximately 45° to the contralateral side and place the patient in Trendelenburg position. This will increase the size of the vein to be cannulated and will also reduce the risk of air embolism.
- Sterilize the area and apply all sterile barriers.
- Place the index and middle finger of the nondominant hand at the apex of the triangle directly over the carotid pulse. With the dominant hand, insert a 25-gauge needle with a syringe containing lidocaine just past the skin surface immediately lateral to the carotid pulse. Apply backpressure on the plunger, assuring there is no blood return, then deliver lidocaine to create a wheal at the skin surface.
- While applying gentle backpressure to the syringe, advance the needle slowly in the direction of the ipsilateral nipple, stopping frequently to deliver lidocaine until sufficient anesthesia has been applied.
- Obtain a 22-gauge "finder" needle and an empty 10 cc syringe. Continue to hold fingers over the carotid pulse to help avoid puncturing the carotid artery. Advance the needle and syringe along the same track, lateral to the carotid pulse toward the ipsilateral nipple at an angle of 20° to the skin surface. Draw back the syringe during advancement to create negative pressure within the syringe.
- The internal jugular vein is often located close to the skin surface, so there is rarely a need to advance needle more than 2 cm. When the vein is located, venous blood will flow easily into the syringe.
- If the first pass is unsuccessful, withdraw the needle close to the skin surface and redirect the needle more medially on the next advancement.
- When the finder needle successfully locates the vein, note the angle and depth of the needle.
- Withdraw the needle and insert an 18-gauge introducer needle and 10 cc syringe along the same path, using the previous technique.
- When venous blood flow is again demonstrated, hold the 18-gauge needle steady in place and remove the syringe.
- Feed the guidewire through the 18-gauge introducer needle. If the guidewire does not feed easily, remove the wire and use the syringe to reconfirm blood flow. Reposition the needle if needed.
- When the guidewire is in place, remove the 18-gauge introducer needle over the wire.
- Guide an 18-gauge short tip intravenous catheter over the guidewire. When the catheter is hubbed at the proximal end, hold the catheter in place and withdraw the wire entirely. Attach a transducer tube to the catheter, and confirm venous pressure and venous waveform. If venous access is confirmed, reintroduce the guidewire to its previous position and remove the 18-gauge catheter over the wire. If arterial puncture is suspected, do not reintroduce the guidewire. Instead, remove the 18-gauge catheter and apply direct pressure for 15 minutes. This additional step of confirming a

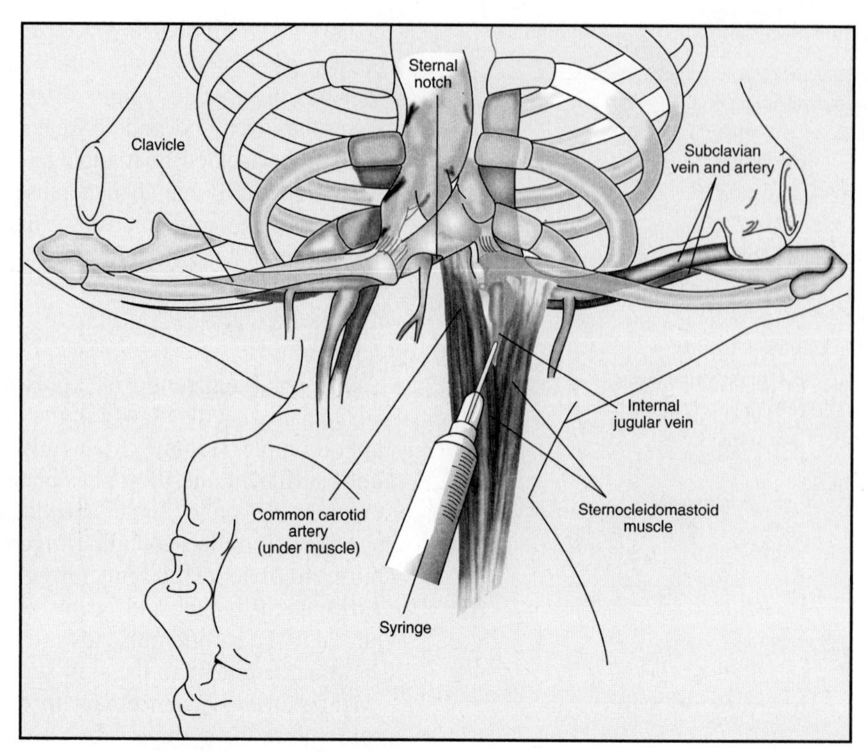

FIG. 132-1 A Internal jugular placement.
SOURCE: McGee DC, Gould MK. Preventing complications of central venous catheterization. *N Engl J Med* 2003;348:1123–1133.

venous pressure waveform has been shown to dramatically reduce the incidence of accidental dilation and cannulation of arteries.

- Once venous access has been confirmed, proceed to cannulation. While holding the wire, insert the #11 blade along the wire to reduce skin tension. Next feed the tissue dilator over the wire, withdraw the wire tip from the dilator and advance the dilator to the hub. Once this is complete, immediately remove the tissue dilator over the wire and apply sterile 4 × 4 gauze pads with pressure to reduce bleeding.
- Introduce the central venous catheter over the guidewire, again withdraw the tip of the wire so it is not inadvertently pushed into the patient, then advance the catheter to a length that approximates the catheter tip placement in the correct position in the superior vena cava (SVC). It is better to overestimate the length needed, as the catheter can always be further withdrawn in a sterile fashion, but obviously cannot be further advanced.
- Remove the guidewire, leaving the central venous catheter in place. With a 5 cc syringe and 0.9% normal saline, ensure that each port for the central line draws blood and flushes appropriately.
- Reapply lidocaine below skin surface at the selected suture site. Suture the catheter in place, and apply appropriate sterile dressing.
- Order a CXR to check for complications and to confirm proper placement of the catheter tip 2–4 cm above the junction of the SVC and atria.

SUBCLAVIAN CENTRAL VENOUS CATHETER PLACEMENT: INFRACLAVICULAR MIDDLE APPROACH USING A MODIFIED SELDINGER TECHNIQUE

- The subclavian vein lies directly underneath the clavicle and begins where the axillary vein crosses the lateral border of the first rib. The anterior scalene muscle separates the subclavian vein from the subclavian artery, with the artery posterior (Fig. 132-1B).
- Rotate the patient's head approximately 45° to the contralateral side and place the patient in Trendelenburg position.
- Place a small towel vertically between the patient's shoulder blades to widen the sternoclavicular angle.
- Identify landmarks by locating the midpoint of the clavicle and the sternal notch. The finder needle will be guided a few centimeters caudal to the midclavicular point angled parallel with the table and toward the sternal notch.

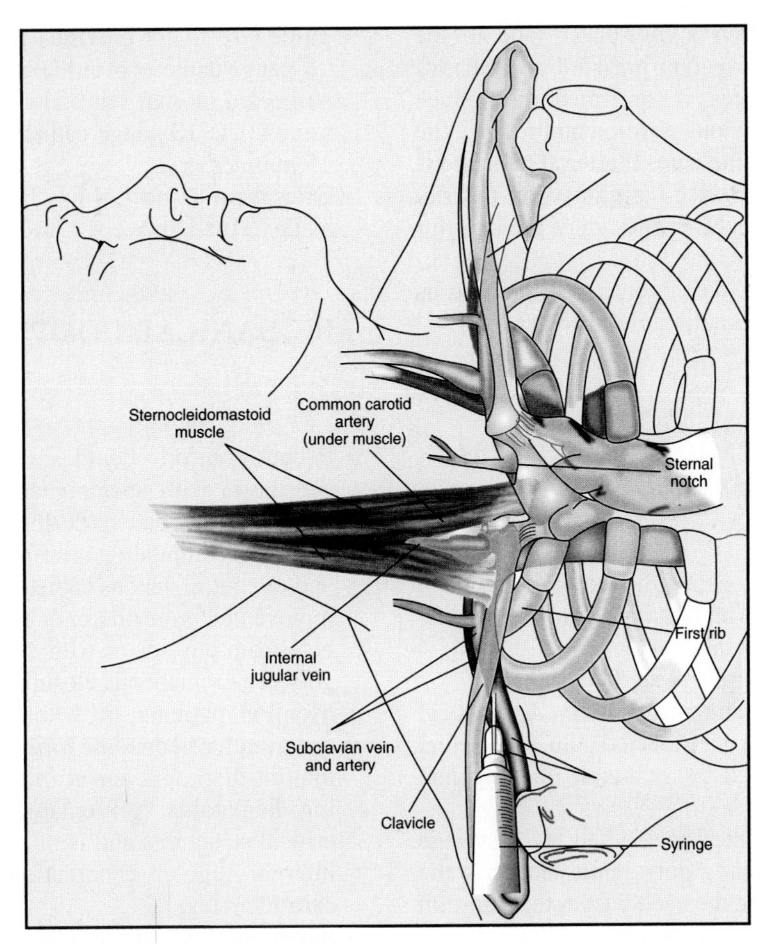

FIG. 132-1 B Subclavian placement.

- Sterilize the area and apply all sterile barriers.
- Apply local anesthesia to the area in the expected path described above. When the clavicle is encountered, provide ample anesthesia to the periosteum.
- Obtain a 22-gauge "finder" needle and 10 cc syringe c/ 5 cc of normal saline. Apply gentle suction to the syringe while advancing the needle from the insertion point inferior to the midclavicular point toward the sternal notch at an angle parallel with the examining table. The needle should encounter the clavicle around the junction between the middle and medial thirds.
- While keeping the needle and syringe parallel with the table, apply gentle downward pressure. While slightly withdrawing and advancing the needle, carefully guide the needle inferiorly along the clavicular surface until the needle passes just under the inferior surface of the clavicle.
- Advance the needle under the clavicle slowly applying gentle backpressure. When the subclavian vein is located, venous blood will flow easily into the syringe. If this first pass is not successful, withdraw the needle from under the clavicle and change the angle slightly toward the patient's head before readvancing.
- The internal jugular vein is often located close to the skin, so there is rarely a need to advance the entire length of the needle.
- When the finder needle successfully locates the vein, note the angle and depth of the needle.
- Withdraw the needle and insert an 18-gauge introducer needle and 10 cc syringe along the same path, using the previous technique.
- When venous blood flow is again demonstrated, hold the 18-gauge needle steady in place and remove the syringe.
- Feed the guidewire through the 18-gauge introducer needle. If the guidewire does not feed easily, remove the wire and use the syringe to reconfirm blood flow and reposition the needle if needed.
- When the guidewire is in place, remove the 18-gauge introducer needle over the wire.
- Guide an 18-gauge short tip intravenous catheter over the guidewire. When the catheter is hubbed at the proximal end, hold the catheter in place and withdraw

the wire entirely. Attach a transducer tube to the catheter, and confirm venous pressure and venous pulsation. If venous access if confirmed, reintroduce the guidewire to its previous position and remove the 18-gauge catheter over the wire. If arterial puncture is suspected, do not reintroduce the guidewire. Instead, remove the 18-gauge catheter and apply pressure for 15 minutes.
- Once venous access has been confirmed, proceed as described above for internal jugular catheter.

FEMORAL CENTRAL VENOUS CATHETER PLACEMENT: APPROACH USING A MODIFIED SELDINGER TECHNIQUE

- Identify landmarks by locating the femoral artery and the inguinal ligament. The femoral vein lies immediately medial to the femoral artery.
- Sterilize the area and apply all sterile barriers.
- With one hand, locate the femoral artery. Apply local anesthesia to the area in the expected path, just medial to the femoral artery 2–3 cm below the inguinal ligament.
- Obtain a 22-gauge "finder" needle and 10 cc syringe with 5 cc of normal saline Apply gentle suction to the syringe while advancing the needle from the insertion point toward the inguinal ligament parallel with the arterial pulse at an angle approximately 20° from the skin surface.
- When the vein is located, venous blood will flow easily into the syringe. Note the angle and depth of the needle.
- Withdraw the needle and insert an 18-gauge introducer needle and 10 cc syringe along the same path, using the previous technique.
- When venous blood flow is again demonstrated, hold the 18-gauge needle in place and remove the syringe.
- Feed the guidewire through the 18-gauge introducer needle. One hand should be holding the guidewire at all times to prevent guidewire embolization. If the guidewire does not feed easily, remove the wire and use the syringe to reposition the needle and reconfirm blood flow.
- When the guidewire is in place, remove the 18-gauge introducer needle over the wire.
- Guide an 18-gauge short tip intravenous catheter over the guidewire. When the catheter is hubbed at the proximal end, hold the catheter in place and withdraw the wire entirely. Attach a transducer tube to the catheter, and confirm venous pressure and venous pulsation. If venous access is confirmed, reintroduce the guidewire to its previous position and remove the 18-gauge catheter over the wire. If arterial puncture is suspected, do not reintroduce the guidewire. Instead, remove the 18-gauge catheter and apply pressure for 15 minutes.
- Once venous access has been confirmed, proceed as described above for internal jugular cathater.

MECHANICAL COMPLICATIONS

GENERAL

- Patient comfort should always be a concern. Local anesthesia with agents such as lidocaine should be used for every patient during every procedure.
- If arterial cannulation is suspected after tissue dilation and/or central venous catheter has been placed, do not remove the tissue dilator or catheter. Call for emergent help from physicians with experience in vascular surgery or percutaneous closure.
- Monitor patients in whom arterial puncture has occurred for hematoma formation. Patients with coagulation disorders are at increased risk. An expanding hematoma can enlarge to compress adjacent critical structures and is of particular concern during internal jugular cannulation with damage to the carotid artery.
- Symptoms of air embolism include acute mental status changes and hypotension. Occasionally, a "cogwheel" murmur can be auscultated. If air embolism is suspected the patient should immediately be placed in a Trendelenburg left decubitus position. Provide 100% oxygen to increase the rate of resorption. Skilled operators should attempt to aspirate the embolized air if the catheter is in the heart.
- Guidewire and catheter embolization can be largely prevented though vigilance. Catheters with any malfunction or irregularity on inspection should never be placed. Also, catheters should be removed with extreme care. During cannulation, the operator should always maintain visual control of the guidewire. If the guidewire slips into the catheter during catheter placement immediately clamp the catheter at the base and attempt to remove the catheter and wire as a single unit. Vascular surgery should be contacted immediately should embolization of a guidewire occur.
- Catheter tip misplacement is not uncommon. Catheters advanced past the SVC into or near the right atrium increase the risk for arrhythmias. This should be promptly corrected by withdrawing the catheter the appropriate length and resecuring the catheter. Occasionally, the catheter will advance into

TABLE 132-3 Mechanical Complications

General
Pain
Bleeding
Hematoma
Arterial puncture
Air embolism
Guidewire or catheter embolization
Catheter tip misplacement
Complications associated with subclavian and internal jugular
Pneumothorax
Arrhythmia
Hemothorax
Mediastinal hematoma
Cardiac tamponade
Myocardial or central vein perforation
Thoracic duct injury
Complications from femoral cannulation
Retroperitoneal hematoma

an unintended vein (e.g., subclavian catheter with tip in the internal jugular). Repositioning can be attempted with the use of a guidewire and placement of a new catheter (Table 132-3).

SUBCLAVIAN AND INTERNAL JUGULAR CANNULATION

- Pneumothorax after cannulation can occur with both subclavian and internal jugular cannulation, but is more common with the subclavian approach. Severity of the pneumothorax can range from small and asymptomatic to rapid and catastrophic. CXR should always be ordered after cannulation and inspected for pneumothorax. Treatment can range from supportive care to thoracostomy and chest tube insertion depending on the magnitude and rate of onset.
- Careful insertion at the internal jugular site with attention to not insert the needle "deep" can often prevent pneumothorax. A frequent mistake junior operators make is to "hub" the large-bore needle while attempting to find the vein.
- Myocardial or central vein perforation occurs infrequently and can manifest as a mediastinal hematoma or pericardial effusion. Hemothorax is suggested by symptoms similar to a pneumothorax and new effusion on CXR. If the perforation is above the pericardium a wide mediastinum may be seen on CXR.
- Thoracic duct laceration is a rare complication of left internal jugular placement.

FEMORAL CANNULATION

- Arterial puncture or laceration is not uncommon during femoral cannulation.
- The formation of a retroperitoneal hematoma should be considered in patients with clinical or laboratory evidence of blood loss after femoral cannulation. Treatment in most cases involves correcting deficits in coagulation and supportive care.

REDUCING MECHANICAL COMPLICATIONS

- Experience: Physicians who have performed more than 50 cannulations have half the mechanical complication rate of physicians with 50 or less.
- Ultrasound guidance has been shown to increase cannulation success rates and reduce mechanical complications.
- The risk of mechanical complications increases sixfold after the third unsuccessful pass of the needle. The operator should seek assistance if this third attempt fails.
- Arterial damage during central venous catheter placement can be minimized by confirming venous blood pressure and pulsation via short 18-gauge single lumen catheter connected transducing tubing before dilation over the guidewire.
- The chance of air embolism can be reduced substantially by maintaining a closed system during catheter placement. Needles should not be employed without being attached to syringes filled with sterile saline. All catheters should be promptly closed to air when not in use.
- The use of soft catheters and slow introduction of the catheter can reduce the risk of myocardial or central vein perforation.

CATHETER-RELATED THROMBOSIS

- Considered a common long-term complication of central vein cannulation.
- More common in femoral cannulation and least common with subclavian cannulation.
- Should be suspected when clinical signs and symptoms of venous stasis are present corresponding anatomically with the path of the catheter. Also can be indicated by catheter occlusion or compromise.
- Confirmed by ultrasonography, computed tomography (CT) scan with contrast, or contrast venogram.
- Treatment is anticoagulation for deep vein thrombosis and removal of the catheter.

CATHETER-RELATED INFECTIONS

HISTORY AND CLINICAL DIAGNOSIS

- Catheter-related infection should always be considered for patients demonstrating signs of infection or sepsis without a confirmed source and who have a central venous catheter in place for ≥3 days.
- Any signs of infection around the exit site demands prompt removal of the catheter regardless of the presence or absence of other signs or symptoms. A new site should be chosen for a new catheter and empiric antibiotics should be provided.
- Resolution of signs and symptoms of infection 24–48 hours after catheter removal suggests the presence of a catheter-related infection regardless of culture results in the absence of other sources for infection.

LABORATORY DIAGNOSIS

- Laboratory evidence of systemic infection or sepsis.
- Obtain two peripheral blood cultures to identify the presence of bacteremia. Blood cultures should not be drawn though the catheter due to greater opportunity for contamination.
- Positive peripheral blood cultures with organisms associated with central venous catheter infection (e.g., *Staphylococcus epidermis*) should raise concerns for catheter-related infection.
- Strong clinical suspicion alone is enough to prompt initiation of antibiotics and catheter removal.

MANAGEMENT

- Initiate empiric parenteral antibiotics that provide adequate coverage for *S. epidermis* and *S. aureus*. Broader empiric coverage should be initiated for immunocompromised patients.
- Once antibiotics have been provided, and if there are no signs of infection at the exit site, the catheter can be changed over a guidewire and the tip sent for culture. All uncuffed catheters should be changed over guidewire, replaced at a new site, or discontinued.
    - A positive catheter tip culture with >15 colony forming units (CFU): the catheter placed over the guidewire should be removed and a catheter and new site should be chosen.
    - If the catheter tip culture is negative or with <15 CFU: the replaced catheter can remain. Attempt to identify another infectious source.
- Monitor surveillance cultures for resolution of bacteremia after proper management. Persistent bacteremia should prompt investigation into additional causes of infection.

PREVENTION

- Quality assurance and continuing education should be provided for standardization of aseptic care.
- Avoid placing catheters in the femoral area as it will be difficult to maintain aseptic conditions.
- Oral or parenteral antibiotics have not been shown to reduce incidence of catheter infections in adults.
- Routine line changes do not prevent catheter-related infection and increase mechanical complications due to multiple procedures.

BIBLIOGRAPHY

Centers for Disease Control and Prevention. Guidelines for the Prevention of Intravascular Catheter-Related Infections. *MMWR* 2002;51(RR-10):1–29.

Mansfield PF, Hohn DC, Fornage BD, et al. Complications and failures of subclavian-vein catheterization. *N Engl J Med* 1994;331:1735–1738.

McConville J, Kress JP. Intravascular devices, Chapter 12. In: Hall JB, Schmidt GA, Wood LH, eds., *Principals of Critical Care*, New York, NY: McGraw-Hill; 2005:131–138.

McGee DC, Gould MK. Preventing complications of central venous catheterization. *N Engl J Med* 2003;348:1123–1133.

Merrer J, De Jonghe B, Golliot F, et al. Complications of femoral and subclavian venous catheterization in critically ill patients: a randomized controlled trial. *JAMA* 2001;286: 700–707.

Sznajder JI, Zveibil FR, Bitterman H, et al. Central vein catheterization: failure and complication rates by three percutaneous approaches. *Arch Intern Med* 1986;146:259–261.

133 PULMONARY ARTERY CATHETER INSERTION

Jennifer Sauk

KEY POINTS

- Recent randomized trials have not demonstrated benefit to large patient populations receiving monitoring with the PAC, but there may be patients who require this intervention.

- Serious complications from insertion are rare but problems with recording artifact or misinterpretation of data are common.
- While specific cardiac disorders can often be diagnosed or strongly suspected on the basis of the waveforms obtained by PAC, the right atrial pressure (RAP) and pulmonary artery wedge pressure (PCWP) are in and of themselves poor predictors of ventricular preload and response to fluid resuscitation.

OBJECTIVES

- Understand indications for pulmonary artery catheter (PAC) insertion.
- Understand preparation of the patient and the catheter prior to the procedure.
- Understand the anatomy pertinent to PAC insertion.
- Be aware of potential complications associated with the procedure.
- Understand pulmonary artery waveforms.
- Be aware of the hemodynamic calculations which can be derived from PAC data.

INTRODUCTION

- A PAC, also known as a Swan-Ganz catheter, is a balloon-tipped, four- or five-lumen polyvinyl chloride catheter that can yield important hemodynamic data such as pressures in the chambers of the right heart, cardiac output (CO), and the pulmonary capillary wedge pressure (PCWP), which reflects left atrial pressure. Blood can also be sampled from the pulmonary artery using this technique (Table 133-1; Fig. 133-1).

INDICATIONS AND CONTRAINDICATIONS

- Much controversy exists regarding the use of the PAC. Multiple studies suggest that large-scale, protocol-driven trials would better define the role of the PAC.

TABLE 133-1 Hemodynamic Information That can be Derived From PAC

DERIVED VALUE	NORMAL PARAMETER
CO = VO_2 (mL/min)/(10 × (CaO_2 – CvO_2))	5 L/min
CI = CO/BSA (m^2)	2–4 L/min/m^2
SVR = (MAP – RAP) × 80/CO	900–1200 dyne-sec/cm^5
PVR = (PAP – PCWP) × 80/CO	120–200 dyne-sec/cm^5

ABBREVIATIONS: VO_2, oxygen consumption; CvO_2, mixed venous oxygen saturation; CaO_2, arterial oxygen saturation; CI, cardiac index; BSA, body surface area; SVR, systemic vascular resistance; MAP, mean arterial pressure; PVR, pulmonary vascular resistance; PAP, pulmonary artery pressure.

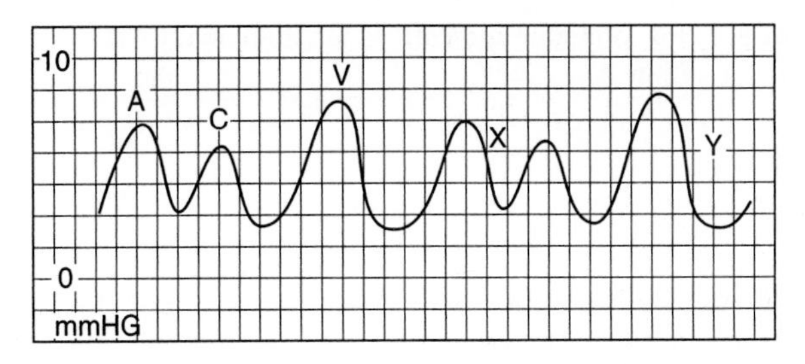

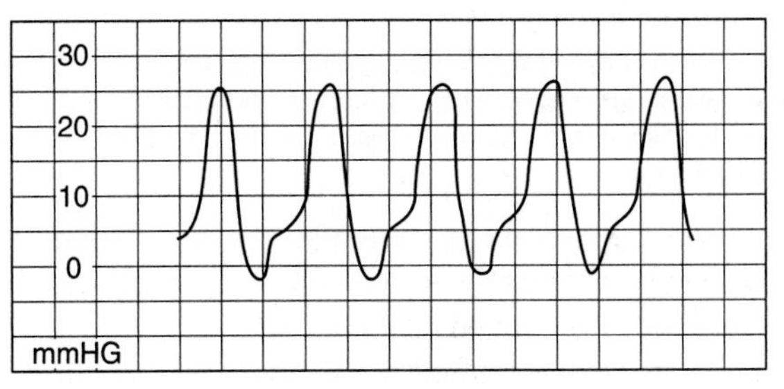

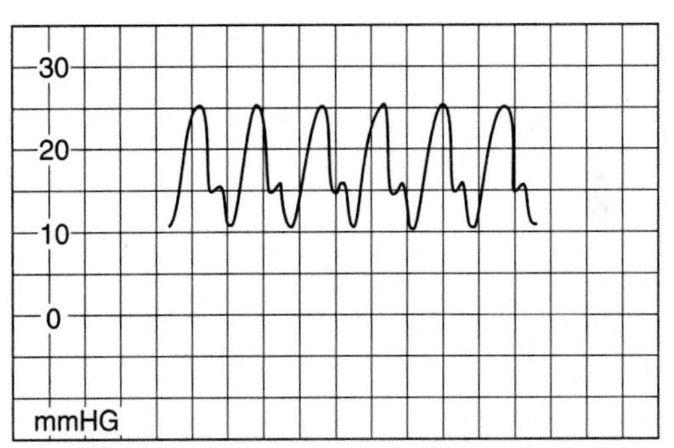

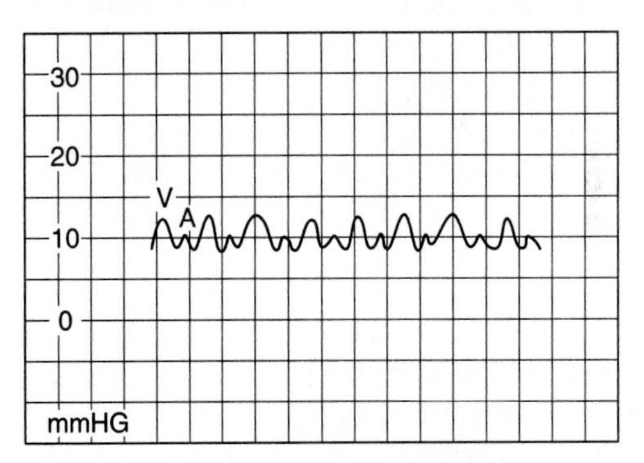

FIG. 133-1 Important hemodynamic waveforms to recognize via PAC. (A) RAP tracing. Normal: 2–8 mmHg; A = atrial contraction; C = tricuspid valve closure; V = atrial filling. (B) Right ventricular pressure tracing. Normal: 20–30/2–8 mmHg. Be aware of ventricular ectopy while in the right ventricle. (C) PAP tracing. Normal: 20–30/8–15 mmHg. Monitored by distal port of PAC. Dicrotic notch: represents closure of pulmonary valve. PA diastolic approximates PAWP if no lung disease or mitral valve disease. (D) PCWP tracing: (approx. left atrial pressure). Normal: 5–12 mmHg (mean). Since no valves between pulmonary artery and mitral valve, PAWP approximates left atrial pressure, or left ventricular end-diastolic pressure (LVEDP). A waves = atrial contraction; V waves = atrial filling.

TABLE 133-2 Possible Indications for Pulmonary Artery Catheterization
Shock
Oliguric renal failure
Pulmonary disorders
Pulmonary hypertension
Pulmonary edema
Lactic acidemia
Cardiac disorders
Myocardial infarction (MI)—Catheter Consensus Conference justified use in MI complicated by cardiogenic shock, right ventricular infarction, or ventricular septal defect (VSD)/papillary muscle rupture
Trauma

Large studies have not demonstrated a beneficial effect with the use of PAC. However, PACs may be useful in cases where hemodynamic data are needed to establish a diagnosis or assist in management (Tables 133-2 and 133-3; Fig. 133-2).

METHODS

PREPARATION

- Discuss risk: benefit of procedure with patient and obtain written informed consent.
- Obtain all necessary equipment before the procedure (Table 133-4).
- Insert an introducer catheter as described in Chapter 132.

FLOTATION OF PULMONARY ARTERY CATHETER

- Flush all catheter lumens with saline.
- Connect distal lumen to pressure transducer.
- Check balloon for proper inflation by injecting 1.5 cc of air and looking for symmetry of balloon and absence of leaks by immersing balloon in bowl of sterile saline. Deflate balloon.
- Place PAC into PAC introducer and advance slowly to 20 cm mark.
- Inflate balloon with 1.5 cc of air.
- Maintain inflation with balloon lock.
- After inflation, advance catheter slowly to allow blood flow to direct catheter through cardiac chambers. If you meet resistance before reaching the pulmonary artery, deflate the balloon, pull back, reinflate, and attempt advancement. (See Table 133-5 for use of PAC ports)

TABLE 133-3 Contraindications to Pulmonary Artery Catheterization
Tricuspid or pulmonary valve stenosis
Prosthetic tricuspid or pulmonary valve
Right atrial or right ventricular mass
Cyanotic heart disease
Latex allergy
Complete left bundle branch block
Conduction abnormalities
Anticoagulation
IJ cannulation: previous carotid surgery
SVC obstruction

TABLE 133-4 Materials Needed for PAC
Other materials needed
Sterile drapes
Bouffant
Sterile gown
Sterile gloves
Sterile saline
Hexidine
1% lidocaine
Needles
25 gauge for lidocaine injection
21 gauge attached to 5 cc syringe as finder needle
18 gauge with catheter hub attached to 10 cc syringe used to pass through
Seldinger J-wire
Scalpel
Vessel dilator
PAC introducer—9 F catheter
PAC catheter (described to the left)
Transducer pressure tubing
Suture

TABLE 133-5 Ports needed for PAC
PAC ports (refer to Fig. 133-2)
Proximal port
CVP monitoring since in SVC/RA
Inject thermodilution fluid or dye dilution for CO monitoring
Intravenous fluid (IVF) injection
Distal port
Monitor pressure waveforms during passage of the catheter
Assess PAPs when balloon inflated
Sample mixed venous blood
Never can be used for medication infusion
Thermistor port
Connects to CO monitor
Thermistor wire within measures blood temperature to estimate CO
Balloon port
<1 cm from tip of catheter
Inflates with air 0.8–1.5 cc

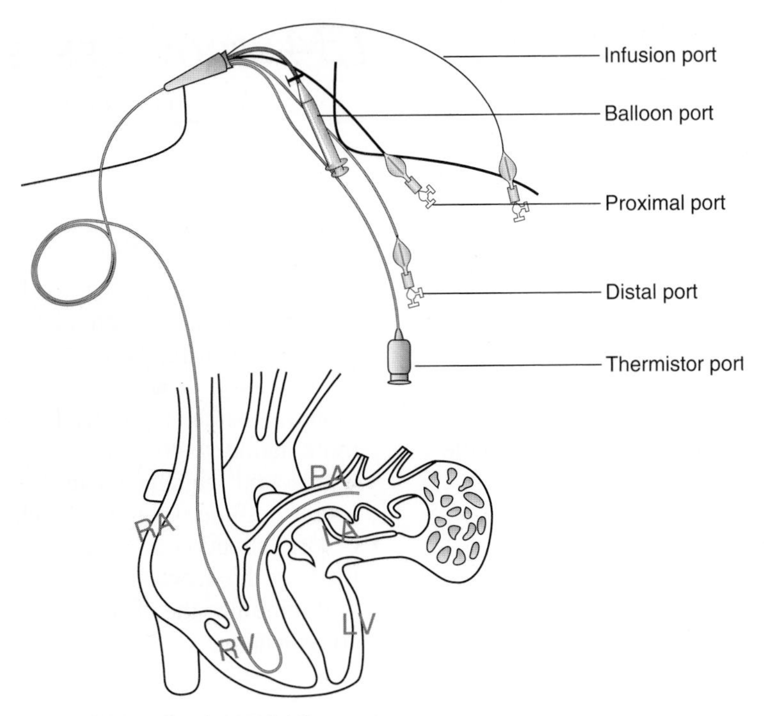

FIG. 133-2 Five-lumen PAC.

- Observe pressure waveforms to determine catheter location (Figs. 133-1B and C, 133-2, 133-3).
- Advance catheter until inflated balloon wedges (does not move further) and observe fall in mean pressure. Confirm placement with balloon deflation and observance of PA tracing. Reinflate and observe "PCWP" tracings.
- Attach sterile sheath to introducer.
- Obtain chest x-ray to confirm placement of PA catheter.
- Appropriate damping of pressure transducer to ensure adequate waveform readings >rapid flush test: opening flush valve produces high pressures in normally patent system. Close valve and observe rapid fall in pressure before returning to PA wave.
- Calibration of PA catheter: open transducer to atmospheric pressure while at the level of the left atrium.
- Once measurements are obtained, deflate the balloon and secure PA catheter in the introducer hub.

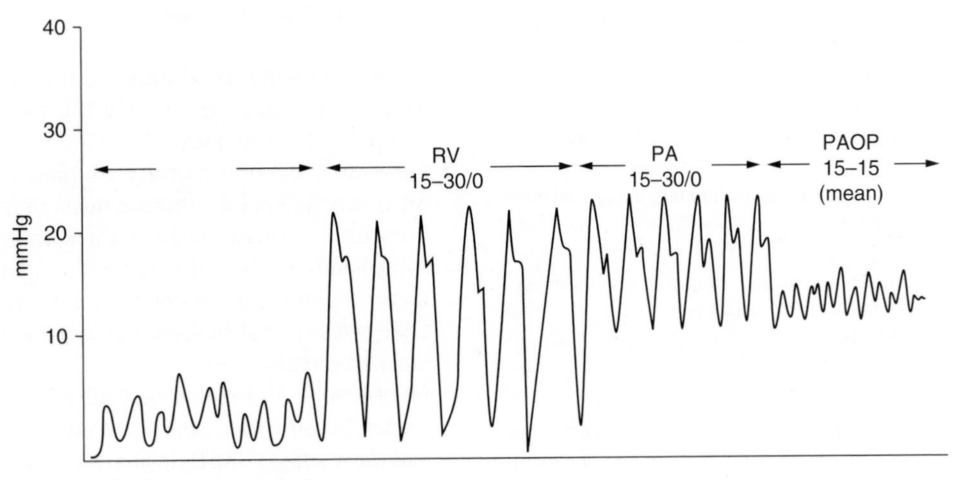

FIG. 133-3 PA catheter waveforms.

COMPLICATIONS

INTRODUCTION OF CENTRAL VENOUS CATHETER

- Pneumothorax 0.3–4.5%
- Arterial puncture 1.1–13%
- Air embolism 0.5%

FLOTATION OF PULMONARY ARTERY CATHETER

- Transient arrhythmia 4.7–68.9%
- Complete heart block (in patients with left bundle branch block) 0–8.5%
- Pulmonary artery rupture 0.1–1.5%
- Pulmonary artery infarction 0.1–5.6%
- Catheter knotting

MAINTENANCE

- Similar to risks of central venous catheterization.
  - Catheter-related infection 0.7–11.4%
  - Thrombosis (higher after 36 hours of catheterization) 0.5–66.7%

BIBLIOGRAPHY

Clinical competence in hemodynamic monitoring. A statement for physicians from the ACP/ACC/AHA Task Force on Clinical Privileges in Cardiology. *J Am Coll Cardiol* 1990;15:1460–1464.

Connors AF Jr, Speroff T, Dawson NV, et al. The effectiveness of right heart catheterization in the initial care of critically ill patients. SUPPORT Investigators. *JAMA* 1996;276:889–897.

Gore JM, Goldberg RJ, Spodick DH, et al. A community-wide assessment of the use of pulmonary artery catheters in patients with acute myocardial infarction. *Chest* 1987;92:721–727.

Leatherman JW, Marini JJ. Clinical use of the pulmonary artery catheter, Chapter 13. In: Hall JB, Schmidt GA, Wood LH, eds., *Principals of Critical Care.* New York, NY: McGraw-Hill; 2005: 139–163.

Pinsky MR, Vincent JL. Let us use the pulmonary artery catheter correctly and only when we need it. *Crit Care Med* 2005;33: 1119–1122.

Pulmonary Artery Catheter Consensus conference: consensus statement. *Crit Care Med* 1997;25:910–925.

Ryan TJ, Antman EM, Brooks NH, et al. 1999 Update: ACC/AHA guidelines for the management of patients with acute myocardial infarction. A report of the American College of Cardiology/American Heart Association Task Force on Practice Guidelines (Committee on Management of Acute Myocardial Infarction). *J Am Coll Cardiol* 1999;34:890–911.

134 THORACENTESIS

Adam P. Ronan

KEY POINTS

- Pleural effusions may be divided broadly into transudates and exudates, with relatively simple chemistries guiding this distinction.
- Identification of an empyema or complex parapneumonic effusion should lead to early consideration of more definitive drainage.
- Ultrasound guidance can be extremely useful in acquiring fluid when it is loculated.
- Careful attention to correcting coagulopathy and performing thoracentesis at the upper margin of the rib will minimize the chance of significant bleeding as a complication.

PATHOPHYSIOLOGY

- A pleural effusion is a collection of fluid in the pleural cavity of which there are two broad categories:
  - *Transudative effusions*: Form when there is an imbalance between hydrostatic and oncotic pressures (e.g., increased hydrostatic pressure in the form of high pulmonary capillary wedge pressures due to congestive heart failure (CHF) or decreased oncotic pressure due to cirrhosis or nephrotic syndrome).
  - *Exudative effusions*: Form when there is an increase in capillary permeability due to inflammation or when there is a decrease in lymphatic drainage of the pleural space (e.g., infection, malignancy, or autoimmune disorders).

INDICATIONS

- To obtain pleural fluid for diagnostic purposes.
- Therapeutic purposes to give the patient relief from symptomatic effusions.
- Generally, all noncritically ill patients with pleural effusions will need a thoracentesis unless the effusion is extremely small (<10 mm thick on lateral decubitus x-ray) and the clinical diagnosis is obvious (e.g., viral pleurisy), or if the patient has a definitive diagnosis of CHF with typical failures and is responding appropriately to therapy.
- In critically ill patients, not all effusions need to be tapped because the cause of the effusion is often known and the results of the fluid analysis would not alter therapy. In addition, coagulopathies and cardiopulmonary

TABLE 134-1 ICU Indications for Thoracentesis

GENERALLY NEED	GENERALLY DO NOT NEED
Effusion due to infection near pleura	CHF
(pulmonary, upper abdomen, mediastinal)	Postesophageal sclerotherapy
High-grade systemic sepsis	Known malignancy diagnosis
Suspected malignancy	Hepatic hydrothorax
Vasculitis	Peritoneal dialysis
Pancreatitis	Uremia
Drug-induced	Central line complication (noninfectious) PE

instability increases the risk for serious complication (see Table 134-1).

RELATIVE CONTRAINDICATIONS

- Patient unable to cooperate
- Coagulation abnormalities or thrombocytopenia
- Patient on mechanical ventilation (greater risk for developing a tension pneumothorax or persistent air leak)
- Patient with severe cough or hiccups
- Bullous emphysema near site of effusion

COMPLICATIONS

- Pneumothorax
- Infection or empyema
- Localized bleeding or hemothorax
- Re-expansion pulmonary edema (if >1.5 L drained)
- Diaphragm injury
- Puncture of visceral organs (spleen or liver)
- Bronchopleural fistula
- Nerve injury

EQUIPMENT

- Adjustable table
- Skin cleansing materials (e.g., chlorhexidine solution)
- 25-Gauge needle, and a 20–22-gauge needle that is 1.5 in. long (longer for obese patients)
- Thoracentesis needle/catheter, or, if a such a catheter is not available, a 14–18-gauge needle and clamp may be used
- Scalpel
- Three-way stopcock
- Sterile drainage tube
- Fluid collection container (vacuum container or collection bag)
- 12 cc syringe for anesthetization and larger syringe (30–50 cc) for fluid withdrawal
- 1% lidocaine
- Sterile gloves, sterile gown, sterile drape, mask, and eye protection
- Appropriate containers for laboratory tests

PROCEDURE

PREPARE PATIENT

- Obtain informed consent: letting the patient or responsible party know the potential complications which include pneumothorax, hemothorax, infection, and pulmonary edema from re-expansion.
- If the patient is able, sit him/her straight upright on the edge of the bed. (If the patient is unable to sit up in this position, there are alternative approaches described below.)

SELECT AND PREPARE SITE

- Identify the level of the effusion by gentle percussion or ultrasound guidance.
- If the effusion is smaller than 10 mm on lateral decubitus x-ray, or, if there is a concern that the effusion is loculated (not freely moveable on lateral decubitus x-ray), use ultrasound guidance to locate the effusion.
- Identify and mark the site for needle insertion:
  - On the posterior thoracic wall, 5–10 cm lateral to the spine, along the midscapular line.
  - 1 to 2 intercostal spaces below the superior margin of dullness on percussion, thus overlying the effusion (or as marked by ultrasound guidance).
  - Overlying the middle of a rib just below the selected intercostals space. One will not aim the needle at the intercostal space during insertion but at the middle of the rib. (The neurovascular bundle runs along the inferior aspect of the rib, and, by directing the needle into the midrib, this will be avoided).
  - Alternative approaches in ICU patients: If the patient must remain supine, the effusion can be confirmed by ultrasound marking and a catheter can be inserted into the midaxillary or posterior axillary lines in the 4th or 5th intercostal spaces. If the patient can tolerate some elevation, the patient's weight can be supported by the hospital bed as the head of the bed is elevated, and the effusion can then be approached by the midaxillary or posterior axillary line. Another option is to have the patient in a lateral decubitus position (with the effusion side down), with the head of the bed elevated, and the effusion can be tapped by a posterior approach.

- Cleanse the skin with the appropriate antiseptic solution.
- Tape a fenestrated sterile drape on the patient's back with only a small area of skin exposed for the procedure.

ANESTHETIZE THE SITE AND ADVANCE THE NEEDLE INTO THE EFFUSION

- Anesthetize the superficial dermis with the 1% lidocaine using the 25-gauge needle inserted at a close angle to the skin (<30°) to form a superficial weal about 1 cm in diameter.
- Anesthetize the deeper structures using the 20–22-gauge needle. Advance this needle perpendicular to the skin surface aiming directly at the middle of the rib. Remember to aspirate before each injection of the lidocaine to avoid injecting the anesthetic intravascularly. Maintain a negative pressure within the syringe as you advance the needle forward.
- Advance the needle until it hits the rib. Be sure to anesthetize the periosteum. Slowly "walk" the needle up the rib until it slides over the superior margin of the rib, thus avoiding the neurovascular bundle running in the inferior margin. Continue gently advancing the needle anesthetizing along the way—aspirating then injecting lidocaine—until you are through the intercostal muscles and finally the pleura itself.
- Stop advancing the needle once you aspirate fluid. This is a sign that the needle has been introduced into the pleural cavity. Before removing the needle, observe the depth and angle of the needle, as this will be the same route you will take the larger thoracentesis needle/catheter. You may consider placing a clamp on the needle flush with the skin prior to withdrawing the needle to mark the depth of needle insertion.

INSERTING THORACENTESIS DEVICE AND REMOVING FLUID

- If you are using a thoracentesis catheter, then use the scalpel to make a small nick into the skin to aid the insertion of the catheter/needle.
- Attach the thoracentesis catheter/needle to the three-way stopcock and large (30–50 cc) syringe. Make sure the stopcock position only allows flow between the needle and syringe, and is closed to the 3rd hub.
- Insert the thoracentesis catheter/needle into the puncture following the same path as before, "walking" over the superior rib margin, remembering to maintain negative pressure in the syringe the entire time.
- When pleural fluid is aspirated, hold the needle in place and carefully advance the catheter into the pleural space. Withdraw the needle. Remember to never advance the needle back into the catheter.
- If you are using a 14–18-gauge needle and no catheter, then once the needle has been introduced into the pleural cavity, place a clamp on the needle at the level of the skin to keep the needle from slipping further into the cavity.
- Attach the side arm of the three-way stopcock to the drainage tubing and remove up to 1.5 L of fluid. Avoid removing more than 1.5 L at any one time as this may lead to re-expansion pulmonary edema and there is a greater risk of pneumothorax.
- When finished removing the fluid, have the patient Valsalva or hum while withdrawing the catheter.

POSTPROCEDURE

- Place bandage on site.
- Order necessary laboratory tests for fluid.
- Obtain an upright chest x-ray to check for pneumothorax or signs of hemothorax if patient symptomatic or if procedure done in high-risk setting (critically ill patients).

LABORATORY ANALYSIS

- Send samples of the pleural effusion to the laboratory for the following studies:
  - Total protein
  - Lactate dehydrogenase (LDH)
  - Cell count and differential
  - Gram's stain and culture
  - Glucose
  - Others dictated by clinical suspicion:
    - pH if infection, collagen vascular disease, or esophageal rupture suspected
    - Cytology if malignancy suspected
    - Hematocrit (Hct) if effusion bloody
    - Amylase if pancreatitis or esophageal rupture suspected
    - Acid fast smear if tuberculosis (TB) suspected
    - Rheumatoid factor (RF) or antinuclear antibody (ANA) if collagen vascular disease suspected
    - Triglycerides and cholesterol if chylothorax suspected

EXUDATES VERSUS TRANSUDATES

- *Light criteria*: Used to differentiate exudates from transudates, these criteria are 98% sensitive and 83% specific. If *any* of the following are true, then the effusion is likely an *exudate* (see Tables 134-2 and 134-3):

TABLE 134-2 Summary of General Characteristics of Exudates vs. Transudates

PARAMETER	EXUDATE	TRANSUDATE
TP_{eff}/TP_{serum}	>0.5	<0.5
LDH_{eff}/LDH_{serum}	>0.6	<0.6
TP (g/dL)	>3.0	<3.0
LDH (IU/L)	>200	<200
Cholesterol (mg/dL)	>45	<45
Glucose	<60 in complicated parapneumonic effusions, RA, esophageal rupture, and some malignancies	≈Serum
pH	<7.3 in TB, complicated parapneumonic effusions, RA, esophageal rupture	≈7.4
WBC	>1000	<1000
Appearance	Serosanguinous, bloody, turbid, or purulent	Clear to straw colored

- ◦ Ratio of effusion total protein to serum total protein >0.5 (TP_{eff}/TP_{serum} >0.5) or
- ◦ Ratio of effusion LDH to serum LDH >0.6 (LDH_{eff}/LDH_{serum} >0.6) or
- ◦ Effusion LDH greater than two-thirds of the upper limit of normal serum LDH

DIFFERENTIAL DIAGNOSIS FOR EXUDATES

- Bacterial pneumonia (parapneumonic effusions and empyema)
- Viral pneumonia (usually small)
- Other pulmonary infections (TB, fungal, parasites)
- Intraperitoneal or retroperitoneal infections
- Malignancy (primary lung, mesothelioma, metastases)
- Pulmonary embolism (75% are exudates)
- Collagen vascular disease (systemic lupus erythematosus [SLE], rheumatoid arthritis [RA], dermatomyositis)
- Pancreatitis

TABLE 134-3 General Characteristics of Pleural Fluid

	APPEARANCE	WBC	RBC	GLUCOSE	PH	OTHER
Exudates						
Uncomplicated parapneumonic	Turbid	Moderate to elevated, ↑ polys	<5000	>40	>7.2	Negative Gram's stain, LDH <1000
Complicated parapneumonic	Turbid or purulent	Elevated (>10,000) ↑ polys	<5000	<40	<7.2	Usually positive Gram's stain, LDH >1000; need complete drainage
Empyema	Purulent	Elevated (20,000–100,000) ↑ polys	<5000	<40	<7.0	Positive Gram's stain, LDH >1000; need complete drainage
TB	Serosanguinous	<10,000 ↑ lymphs	5000–10,000	<40–110	>7.2	Protein >4, + AFB, ADA>70
Malignancy	Turbid or bloody	Variable (usually <10,000) ↑ lymphs	Up to 100,000 Hct 1–20	<40–110	>7.2	+ Cytology
RA	Green or turbid	Variable	<1000	<60	7.2–7.3	↑ RF
PE	Straw or bloody	Variable (often elevated)	Up to 100,000 Hct 1–20	>60	≈Serum	May be transudate
Pancreatitis	Turbid or serosanguinous	Variable (often elevated) ↑ polys	<10,000	>60	≈Serum	Left-sided, ↑ amylase
Esophageal rupture	Turbid or bloody	Variable (often elevated)	<10,000	40–70	<7	Left-sided, ↑ amylase
Transudates						
CHF	Clear or straw colored	<1000 lymphs	<5000	≈Serum	≈Serum	Most common type; usually bilateral; may become exudative after aggressive diuresis
Cirrhosis	Clear or straw colored	<1000	<5000	≈Serum	≈Serum	Right-sided; often massive
Nephrotic syndrome or hypoproteinemia	Clear or straw colored	<1000	<5000	≈Serum	≈Serum	Usually bilateral, small, asymptomatic

ABBREVIATIONS: AFB, acid fast bacilli; ADA, adenosine deaminase; RA, rheumatoid arthritis; PE, pulmonary embolism.

- Drug reactions (nitrofurantoin, methysergide, practolol)
- Asbestosis
- Dressler syndrome
- Lymphatic disease/thoracic duct damage (if chylothorax: expect triglycerides >110)
- Intra-abdominal abscess
- Esophageal rupture
- Uremia
- Sarcoid
- Iatrogenic causes

DIFFERENTIAL DIAGNOSIS FOR TRANSUDATES

- CHF
- Cirrhosis
- Nephrotic syndrome
- Hypoproteinemia
- Pulmonary embolism (25% are transudates)
- Peritoneal dialysis
- Superior vena caval obstruction
- Urinary obstruction (urinothorax)
- Atelectasis
- Myxedema

BIBLIOGRAPHY

Kruse JA. Thoracentesis. In: Kruse JA, Fink MP, Carlson RW, eds., *Saunders Manual of Critical Care.* Philadelphia, PA: W.B. Saunders; 2003: 719–721.

Light RW. A new classification of parapneumonic effusions and empyema. *Chest* 1995;108:299–301.

Light RW. Pleural effusion. *N Engl J Med* 2002;346:1971–1977.

Schmidt GA. Special problems in the ICU. In: Hall JB, Schmidt GA, Wood LDH, eds., *Principles of Critical Care*, 2nd ed. New York, NY: McGraw-Hill; 1998:1466–1467.

135 PERICARDIOCENTESIS

J. Matthew Brennan

KEY POINTS

- The most common etiologies of pericardial effusions include infection (viral, bacterial, TB), malignancy, uremia, postinfarction inflammatory response, collagen vascular disease, radiation, traumatic, iatrogenic, and idiopathic.
- Bacterial, tuberculous, fungal, HIV-associated infections, malignancy, and hemorrhage are the most likely to lead to cardiac tamponade.
- 80% of patients treated with pericardiocentesis require no further drainage for effusions. However, 62% of malignant effusions redevelop within 7 days. The treatment of recurrent pericardial effusions involves surgical or balloon pericardiotomy.
- Cardiac tamponade can be diagnosed by physical examination. However, ultrasound and right heart catheterization (RHC) assessment is helpful in most cases.
- On physical examination, the presence of pulsus paradoxus (change in systolic blood pressure >10 mmHg with inspiration), the loss of the "y" descent on the venous waveform, as well as the triad of hypotension, increased jugular venous pressure, and clear lungs are suggestive of cardiac tamponade.
- Ultrasound criterion of tamponade include early diastolic collapse of the right ventricle (specific) and right atrium (sensitive), decrease in transmitral E wave >25% with inspiration, and decrease in tricuspid E wave >40% with inspiration.
- When RHC is performed in patients with cardiac tamponade, high (10–30 mmHg) and equalized (within 4 mmHg) right atrial, RV middiastolic, pulmonary artery diastolic, and pulmonary capillary wedge pressures are found.

DIAGNOSTIC TESTS

- No consensus exists regarding the appropriate, cost-effective workup for pericardial fluid samples. However, the following have been suggested as high yield in effusions of unknown etiology:
    - Specific gravity
    - Protein content
    - White blood cell count with differential
    - Gram's stain
    - Bacterial, fungal, tuberculosis (TB) cultures
    - Acid fast bacilli (AFB) stain
    - Adenosine deaminase (ADA)
    - Cytology with pathology review
- Consider carcinoembryonic antigen (CEA), bilirubin, and cholesterol (mostly found in traumatic, neoplastic obstruction, or severe hypothyroidism) as other lower yield tests.

PREPARATION

- A transthoracic echocardiogram (TTE) on the day of the procedure has been shown to decrease complications.

For greatest safety, anterior and posterior echo-free space should be ≥10 mm. Intraprocedural echo guidance has been recommended with small and regional effusions.
- In the nonemergent situation, combining right heart catheterization (RHC) and pericardiocentesis leads to the highest yield workup. Approximately 40% of medical patients with tamponade also have coexisting causes of increased right atrial pressures diagnosed on RHC.
- Computed tomography (CT) fluoroscopy guidance is another option that some institutions utilize.

PROCEDURE

- Performance of this procedure in the cardiac cath lab allows for RHC monitoring, fluoroscopic guidance, and intrapericardial pressure monitoring which can increase the diagnostic yield and safety of the procedure. However, in the emergent situation, time constraints often make this option impractical.
- Continuous ECG monitoring is recommended throughout the procedure.
- The attachment of an ECG lead to the puncture needle is losing favor secondary to the cumbersome nature of the technique and possible accidental arrhythmias, which may be induced by improperly grounded leads.
- Several approaches exist; however, the most widely used is the subcostal approach.

SUBCOSTAL APPROACH

- Place the patient at a 45° angle.
- Sterilize the subxiphoid area.
- 0.5 cm inferior to the xiphoid process, inject 1–2 cc 1% lidocaine.
- Using an 18-gauge, thin-walled needle puncture the skin 0.5 cm inferior to the right costoxiphoid angle, directing the needle posteriorly (perpendicular to the skin) until below the costal margin (~1 cm).
- Holding the syringe with your dominant hand, walk the needle under the xiphoid process while applying downward pressure to the needle shaft with your nondominant hand and directing the needle cephalad toward the patient's left shoulder.
- Alternate aspirating and injecting small amounts of 1% lidocaine as the needle is advanced until the pericardial space is entered or ST elevations are seen on the ECG; if ST elevations are noted, withdraw the needle and begin again.
- When the pericardial space is entered, aspirate a small amount of fluid (2–3 cc) to ensure proper needle placement.
- Advance a floppy tip guidewire through the needle into the pericardial space.
- Remove the needle over the wire, leaving the wire in place.
- Advance a pig-tailed catheter over the wire and into the pericardial space, keeping control of the wire at all times. When properly placed, the catheter should wrap around the contour of the heart.
- Remove the wire, leaving the catheter in place.
- Aspirate pericardial fluid in no more than 1 L aliquots. Often, a hemodynamic response will be seen with aspiration of relatively small amounts of fluid (depending on the chronicity of the fluid accumulation).

BLOOD VERSUS PERICARDIAL FLUID

- If the fluid aspirate appears hemorrhagic, place a few drop of fluid on a sponge. Pericardial fluid typically will leave a lighter stain than blood. Alternatively, place ~5 cc on the sterile drape and wait ~30 seconds; if the fluid clots, it is blood—likely from a traumatic tap; if it does not clot, it is likely pericardial fluid. Remember, the pericardium has intrinsic fibrinolytic activity, which prevents clotting; however, rapid hemorrhage into the pericardium can overcome this fibrinolytic effect.

POSTPROCEDURE CATHETER CARE

- Fill the catheter with heparin or urokinase.
- Leave the catheter in place for 24–48 hours, flushing q 1 h.
- Repeat TTE 24 hours postprocedure to determine extent of fluid reaccumulation, if any.

COMPLICATIONS

- Coronary artery laceration
- Left ventricular (LV) puncture (very rarely leads to significant bleeding)
- Right ventricular (RV) puncture (more bleeding than the LV, but rarely serious)
  - Look for an injury current on the ECG (ST elevation) in cases of LV or RV puncture
- Arrhythmia (induced by myocardial irritation from the puncture needle, guidewire, or pig-tailed catheter)
- Puncture of the lung, liver, or stomach
- Pneumopericardium
- Pericarditis
- Acute LV failure with pulmonary edema (rare, but increased risk if >1 L fluid removed)
- Acute RV dilation (rare)

BIBLIOGRAPHY

Allen KB, Faber LP, Warren WH, et al. Pericardial effusion: subxiphoid pericardiotomy versus percutaneous catheter drainage. *Ann Thorac Surg* 1999;67:437–440.

Appleton PA, Hatle LK, Popp RL. Cardiac tamponade and pericardial effusion: respiratory variation and transvalvular flow velocities studied by Doppler echocardiography. *J Am Coll Cardiol* 1988;11:1020–1030.

Chow WH, Chow TC, Yip AS, et al. Inoue balloon pericardiotomy for patients with recurrent pericardial effusion. *Angiology* 1996;47:57–60.

Corey GR, Campbell PT, van Trigt P, et al. Etiology of large pericardial effusions. *Am J Med* 1993;95:209–213.

Fowler N, Gabel M, Buncher CR. Cardiac tamponade: a comparison of right versus left heart compression. *J Am Coll Cardiol* 1988;12:187–193.

Krikorian JG, Hancock EW. Pericardiocentesis. *Am J Med* 1978;65:808–814.

Laham RJ, Cohen DJ, Kuntz RE, et al. Pericardial effusion in patients with cancer: outcomes with contemporary management strategies. *Heart* 1996;75:67–71.

Lewinter MM, Kabbani S. Pericardial disease. In: Braunwald E, Zipes DP, Libby P, et al., eds., *Braunwald's Heart Disease: A Textbook of Cardiovascular Medicine*, 7th ed. Philadelphia, PA: W.B. Saunders; 2005: 1757–1780.

Lorell BH, Grossman W. Profile in constrictive pericarditis, restrictive cardiomyopathy, and cardiac tamponade. In: Baim DS, Grossman W, eds., *Grossman's Cardiac Catheterization, Angiography, and Intervention*, 6th ed. Philadelphia, PA: Lippincott Williams & Wilkins; 2000.

Sagrista-Sauleda J, Merce J, Permamyer-Miralda G, et al. Clinical clues to the causes of large pericardial effusions. *Am J Med* 2000;109:95–101.

Shabetai R. Technique of pericardiocentesis. Available at: http://www.uptodateonline.com/application/topic.asp?file=myoperic/7479&type=A&selectedTitle=1~16. Accessed September 1, 2005.

Zayas R, Auguita M, Torres F, et al. Incidence of specific etiology and role of methods for specific etiologic diagnosis of primary acute pericarditis. *Am J Cardiol* 1995;75:378–382.

136 EMERGENT SURGICAL AIRWAY

Kristopher M. McDonough

KEY POINTS

- Emergent surgical airways remain an important component of the algorithms to be applied to patients with evolving respiratory failure requiring mechanical support.
- While the majority of patients with respiratory failure will be managed with noninvasive mask ventilation or translaryngeal intubation, on occasion an emergent airway will be required.
- While all care providers attending to critically ill patients cannot be expected to accrue a large experience with emergent surgical airways, the potential need for such an intervention should be considered when appropriate and each institution should provide the means for staff and equipment to perform this intervention to be assembled in a timely way.

BACKGROUND

- Emergent and nonemergent surgical airways are some of the oldest surgeries documented. They were practiced as early as 3000 B.C. in Egypt and India. They were popularized in Western medicine during the nineteenth century when diphtheria and its resultant upper airway obstruction were epidemic. The surgical airway saw a re-emergence in the early twentieth century when its champion, Chevalier Jackson, advocated its application for a variety of conditions.
- Currently, there are a variety of techniques used to introduce an artificial airway. For the purposes of this chapter, cricothyroidotomy and tracheostomy will be discussed in detail, as will be their emergent indications.
- Recall that there are a variety of *chronic* conditions that necessitate or are improved by the placement of a surgical airway. These are, by far, the majority of the cases in which surgical airways are used.
- When an acute airway compromise arises, requiring the placement of an artificial airway, endotracheal intubation is possible and preferable in approximately 97% of cases. As such, endotracheal intubation should always be the first choice for establishment of an airway.
- Nevertheless, the placement of a surgical airway has its indications, and in roughly 3% of airway emergencies, is the procedure of choice.

ANATOMY

- An understanding of the regional anatomy of the larynx and the trachea is essential to understanding the procedure and its indications. For reference please see Fig. 136-1.
- Recall that the airway is lined and supported by a number of cartilaginous rings. The first of these is the most identifiable anatomic landmark in the neck, the thyroid cartilage. The thyroid cartilage contains and protects most of the larynx including both the false and true vocal cords.

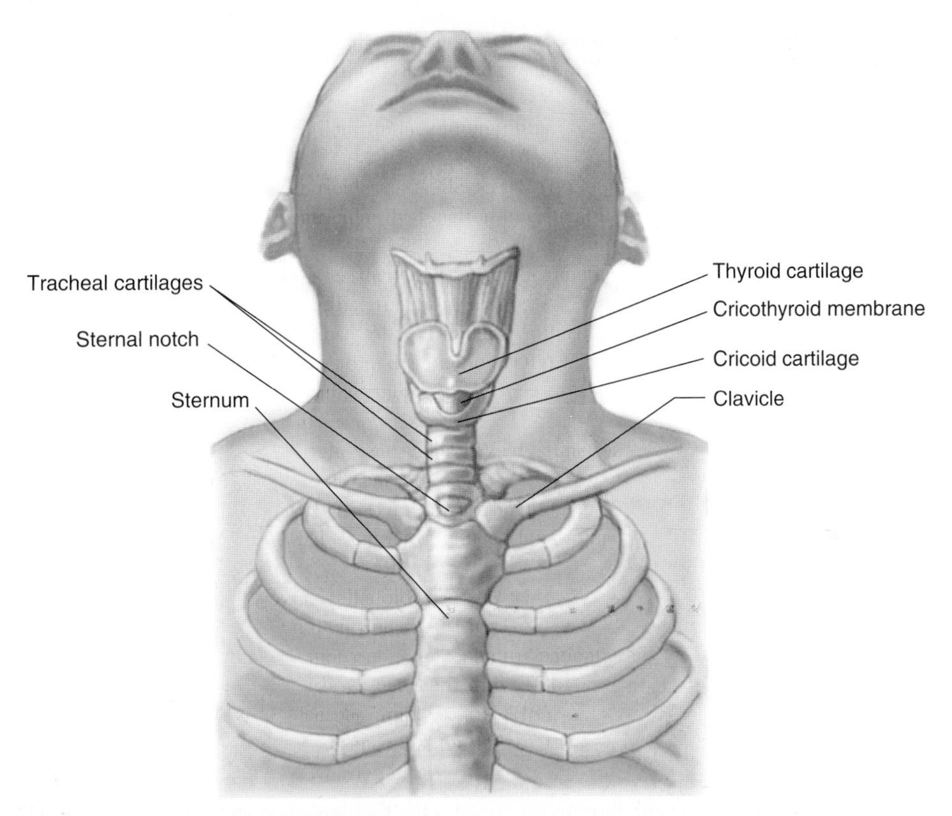

FIG. 136-1 Anatomy of the larynx and sternal region.

- Immediately inferior to the thyroid cartilage is the cricoid cartilage. It should be palpable in most patients, except for the very obese, and defines the inferior aspect of the larynx. The fibrous structure between the cricoid and thyroid cartilages is known as the cricothyroid membrane.
- Below the larynx, the trachea begins. Cartilage rings surrounding the trachea are numbered (e.g., first tracheal cartilage, second tracheal cartilage, and so on).
- Below the thyroid cartilage the airway should be largely free of interior structures to the level of the branching into the right and left main stem bronchi, known as the carina. This is important because surgical airways are largely indicated in cases were there is obstruction at the level of the larynx or above.
- Overlying the larynx are the thyroid gland, its arterial supply, and several nerves, including the recurrent laryngeal nerve, which supplies the muscles of the vocal cords.

PROCEDURES

- Generally, someone with extensive experience, especially in emergent situations, should perform these procedures. This lessens the chance of poor outcome, as well as decreasing the risk of both early and late complications.
- Cricothyroidotomy is an incision made in the cricothyroid membrane. This procedure requires an identification of the relevant anatomic structures. This is the most common method for establishment of the surgical airway in the emergent setting.
- Tracheostomy is the classic surgical airway, and in the past the most commonly used in emergent situations. It is no longer the procedure of choice, however, as it is time-consuming, requires more expertise, and is associated with twice as many complications in the emergent setting. There are some emergency situations where tracheostomy may be considered the procedure of choice, as described in Indications below. The standard site for tracheostomy is between the second and third tracheal cartilages.
- The process of placing an airway via both cricothyroidotomy and tracheostomy is summarized in Table 136-1.

INDICATIONS

- In general, indications for emergent surgical airway placement are the same as those for any airway

TABLE 136-1 Surgical Procedure for Placement of an Airway

CRICOTHYROIDOTOMY	TRACHEOSTOMY
1. Position—neck should be hyperextended with the head supported by the table	1. Position—neck should be hyperextended with the head supported by the table
2. Stabilization—the nondominant hand stabilizes the laryngeal cartilage with the index finger in the superior notch and the thumb and forefinger laterally	2. Cutaneous incision—is made 1–2 cm below the cricoid cartilage in the triangle formed by the heads of the sternocleidomastoid muscles and the cricoid cartilage
3. Cutaneous incision—is made in either a horizontal or vertical direction depending on landmark identification, skill of the surgeon, and desire for future cosmetic appearance	3. Dissection—is performed to identify and separate strap muscles, transect the thyroid isthmus, and, if necessary, identify and avoid the recurrent laryngeal nerves
4. Cricothyroid incision—is made as a horizontal stab incision performed with the knife directed slightly cephalad to avoid injury to the posterior tracheal wall	4. Tracheal incision—is made into the membrane between the 2nd to 3rd or 3rd to 4th tracheal cartilage with a midline division (not horizontal stab). The incision should not be more than 5 mm
5. Dilatation—is summarized by "Once in, stay in." The blade should be replaced by a dilator or hemostat before withdrawing	5. Cannulation—is performed using a tube that is approximately 50–75% of the diameter of the trachea, placed at a 90° angle and rotated caudally
6. Insertion—an appropriate-sized (usually 6 mm) tracheostomy, endotracheal, or special cricothyroidotomy tube is inserted	6. Confirmation—of air and suction should be performed
7. Confirmation—of air flow and suction should be performed	7. Fixation—is performed using tracheal sutures and around the neck straps
8. Fixation—is assured with skin sutures, tape, or other means	

placement, but in the circumstance that endotracheal intubation is not possible, or should not be performed.

- A list of indications for surgical airway is found in Table 136-2. In general, cricothyroidotomy is the procedure of choice for urgent and emergent situations, as noted above.
- Emergent tracheostomy should probably only be performed if: (1) cricothyroidotomy fails; (2) the urgent high-grade obstruction requiring airway is found at the level of, or inferior to the site of cricothyroidotomy; (3) massive neck swelling precludes identification of necessary landmarks; or (4) other laryngeal injury is so great that cricothyroidotomy is impossible.
- Notably, tracheostomy is the preferred procedure in a patient with *chronic* need for a surgical airway.
- If tracheostomy rather than cricothyroidotomy is required for the emergent case, there are recent data in a variety of situations (especially traumatic injury) suggesting that "high" tracheostomy should be performed percutaneously. High percutaneous tracheostomy placement is performed via needle into the membrane between the first and second tracheal cartilages. This procedure, by most accounts, is not yet universally accepted though it may be in the future as experience grows.

COMPLICATIONS

- Even in the most experienced hands, emergency surgical airways are associated with a high degree of complications. Most studies report composite complication rates ranging from 18 to 32% for cricothyroidotomy. Emergent tracheostomy is associated with an even higher risk of poor outcome.

TABLE 136-2 Indications for Emergent Surgical Airway Placement

INDICATION	REASON
1. Failed intubation	Regardless of the reason, failure to intubate (especially repeatedly) in a patient who needs emergent airway placement is always an indication for surgical airway.
2. Upper airway obstruction	For purposes of classification, think of this as a "tube" problem. The tube can be blocked by anything in it, outside of it, or the tube can block itself. As an example: obstruction can come from inside the airway (aspirated foreign body), from the walls of the airway (laryngeal edema from angiotensin-converting enzyme [ACE] inhibitors), or from external compression (traumatic cervical spine injury).
3. Cervical fracture/neck trauma	Compromise of the cervical spine and structures supporting the head and neck may lead to compromise of the upper airway. In addition, cervical fracture may predispose a patient to traumatic intubation and its attendant complications.
4. Facial or nasal trauma	As these conditions lead to a high likelihood of disruption of the normal anatomy of the naso- and oropharynx, intubation is difficult or impossible.
5. Endotracheal tube laryngeal injury	Though this could be contained within #2 above, however, it deserves its own category. Recall that this type of condition often occurs when failed or difficult intubation is combined with any of the other indications listed. Airway compromise can be from tissue, blood, or edema.

- Adverse outcomes are often due to the poor conditions surrounding most emergencies. An especially common complicating factor is massive neck swelling obscuring the thyroid cartilage.
- Complications range from minor to major or life threatening, but more often fall toward the severe end. This is largely due to the dire conditions in which we find these patients.
- Complications can be grouped into those that occur early, or immediate, and those that occur late.
- Possible complications include: subcutaneous or mediastinal emphysema, pneumothorax (especially common with tracheostomy), hemorrhage, tube occlusion from debris, tube misplacement (see below), infection of the site, tracheobronchopulmonary infection, tracheobrachiocephalic artery fistula, and tracheal or subglottic stenosis.
- Tube misplacement may occur in a variety of locations. It is the only complication more common in cricothyroidotomy. Tube misplacement can result in a fatal loss of airway control.
- Approximately one-third of malpositioning occurs when the tube is placed into the pretracheal tissue. In addition, the tube may commonly be passed upward into the pharynx rather than downward into the trachea. More rarely, the tube may be placed into the thyroid cartilage itself, into the pharynx, or even into the esophagus.
- Complications are summarized in Table 136-3.

TABLE 136-3 Complications of Emergent Surgical Airway

EARLY COMPLICATION	LATE COMPLICATION
Hemorrhage	Pneumonia
Pneumothorax (unilateral or bilateral)	Paratracheal abscess
Tube misplacement	Stomal infection
Posterior wall or other tissue ulceration	Tube occlusion
Subcutaneous or mediastinal emphysema	Tracheoesophageal fistula
Tube occlusion	Tracheobrachiocephalic artery fistula
	Tracheomalacia
	Tracheostenosis/subglottic stenosis

BIBLIOGRAPHY

Ben-Nun A, Altman E, Best LA. Emergency percutaneous tracheostomy in trauma patients: an early experience. *Ann Thorac Surg* 2004;77:1045–1047.

Gysin C, Dulguerov P, Guyot JP, et al. Percutaneous versus surgical tracheostomy—a double-blind randomized trial. *Ann Surg* 1999;230:708–714.

Lewis RJ. Tracheostomies: indications, timing, and complications. *Clin Chest Med* 1992;13:137–147.

Vukmir RB, Grenvik A, Lindholm CE. Surgical airway, cricothyroidotomy, and tracheotomy: procedures, complications, and outcome. In: Ayers SM, ed., *Textbook of Critical Care,* 3rd ed. Philadelphia, PA: W.B. Saunders; 1995: 724–734.

Section 12
GENERAL ISSUES IN THE ICU

137 INFECTION CONTROL IN THE ICU

Vidya Krishnan

KEY POINTS

- Nosocomial infections (NI) represent a huge burden to patients and the health care system.
- The incidence of many NIs can be reduced by relatively simple means—hand-washing, upright positioning during feeding, strict barrier control for invasive catheter placement—but compliance with such routine measures requires constant effort.
- Tracking the microbiologic flora of the ICU can help guide empiric antibiotic use.

EPIDEMIOLOGY

- Nosocomial infections afflict 5–35% of patients admitted to ICUs, and contribute to increased mortality, length of ICU and hospital stay, and medical care costs.
- More than 80% of NIs are caused by the following: ventilator-associated pneumonia (VAP), catheter-related bloodstream infections (BSI), surgical site infections, and urinary catheter-related infections.

AIMS OF INFECTION CONTROL IN THE INTENSIVE CARE UNIT

- The primary goal of infection control is to prevent cross-contamination and to control potential sources of pathogens that could be transmitted between patients and from health care workers to patients.
- Another important goal is to direct appropriate use of surgical antibiotic prophylaxis or empirical therapy among vulnerable patient groups.
- When the source of the NI is identified, the implementation of specifically targeted measures against various types of NIs is critical.
- Infection control also entails curtailing the emergence of antibiotic-resistant microorganisms.

RISK FACTORS FOR INFECTION

- The greater the severity of underlying illness, the greater the chance for the patient to develop an infection. Scoring systems, such as APACHE II/III, have been used, but the consistency of these scores in predicting NIs has been limited.
- Prolonged length of stay in the hospital predicts increased severity of illness and increases the opportunity for infection.
- The use of interventions that are common in the ICU, including mechanical ventilation and vascular access, increases the risk of infection.
- Understaffing of nurses and overcrowding in the ICU (both resulting in high patient:nurse ratios) have both been shown to increase NIs. Reasons for these findings include lower compliance with hand hygiene and increased colonization pressure.
- Use of multiple-dose vials for medications may promote cross-contamination. Multidose vials of medications have been independently associated with *Enterobacter cloacae* carriage.
- Immunosuppression of patients, including neutropenia, HIV, medications, and burn patients, results in higher rates of infection.

INFECTION PREVENTION AND CONTROL

- Hand hygiene. Hand hygiene by health care workers is the simplest intervention that has the greatest potential of reducing NIs. Surveillance studies have shown that the hands of over 75% of ICU health care workers carry infectious organisms, including gram-negative bacilli and *Candida* spp. Alternative hand hygiene agents (e.g., chlorhexidine gluconate) reduce hand contamination more than hand-washing alone. Alcohol-based treatments cause less skin drying and damage and take less time to perform, resulting in increased compliance.

- Isolation of patients. The isolation practices recommended by the Health Care Infection Control Practices Advisory Committee (HICPAC), which are also available online at http:www.cdc.gov/ncidod/hip/isolat/isolat.htm, are summarized in Table 137-1.
- Restriction of antibiotic use:
  - Rational use of antibiotics. One of the critical factors that are associated with outcome is time to appropriate antibiotic therapy, resulting in frequent use of broad-spectrum of antibiotics in the management of critically ill patients. It is necessary, however, to readdress the choice of antibiotics often, and narrow the spectrum as possible. Antibiotic prescription should be guided by a thorough, systematic approach.
    - Is infection confirmed or likely to be present in the patient?
    - What is the infectious disease occurring in the patient?
    - Have diagnostic studies (such as blood cultures, tissue biopsy, or noninvasive radiologic imaging techniques) been performed to confirm the presence or persistence of infection?
  - Prevention of wound infection. The use of antibiotics for wound infection prevention has been well established prior to surgical procedures.
  - Prevention of bacterial endocarditis. The use of antibiotics for prevention of bacterial endocarditis has not been well established by clinical trials. Nonetheless, antibiotic prophylaxis is recommended for patients with valvulopathy (congenital or acquired) or prosthetic valves (bioprosthetic and homograft valves) prior to certain procedures. The 1997 updated recommendations from the American Heart Association for prevention of infectious endocarditis, which are available online at the American Heart Association Web site (http://216.185.112.5/presenter.jhtml?identifier=1729), are summarized in Table 137-2.
  - Topical antibiotics for sterile sites or clean skin wounds. With the exception of sulfonamide creams in the management of burn patients, all other methods of topical antibiotic application (endotracheal nonabsorbable antibiotics, urinary bladder instillation of antibiotics, antibiotic creams for skin wounds) have been ineffective, due to ineffective prophylaxis of infection, development of resistance, and/or superinfection.
  - Selective decontamination of the digestive tract (SDD). Because evidence of effectiveness in reducing morbidity and mortality is lacking, this method is not recommended.

TABLE 137-1 Diseases With Transmission-Based Precautions and Recommended Barrier Protection

PRECAUTION	DISEASE*	BARRIER
Standard universal	All	Gloves (for all anticipated contact with body fluid) Gown, mask, eye protection recommended, if possible splash or spray of body fluid
Airborne precautions	Measles, VZV, TB, viral hemorrhagic fever	Mask (N-95 standard certified-mask 170)
Droplet precautions	Meningitis, pneumonia, epiglottitis, sepsis (*Neisseria meningitidis*, *Haemophilus influenzae*, diphtheria, *Mycoplasma pneumoniae*, *Pertussis*, group A *Streptococcus*) Serious viral infections (adenovirus, influenza, mumps, parvovirus B19, rubella)	Mask Eye protection
Contact precautions	Resistant bacteria (MRSA, VRE, multiresistant pseudomonal strains) Enteric infections (*C. difficile*) Respiratory and enteral infections in young children (syncytial virus, rotavirus, parainfluenza) Highly contagious skin infections (diphtheria, HSV, impetigo, uncovered abscess, pediculosis, scabies, staphylococcal furunculosis, VZV) Viral hemorrhagic fever	Gloves Gown

ABBREVIATIONS: VZV, varicella zoster virus; TB, tuberculosis; MRSA, methicillin-resistant *Staphylococcus aureus*; VRE, vancomycin-resistant enterococcus; HSV, herpes simplex virus.

*Includes common diseases, but not an exhaustive list.

SOURCE: Adapted from Garner JS. Guideline for isolation precautions in hospitals: the Hospital Infection Control Practices Advisory Committee. *Infect Control Hosp Epidemiol* 1996;17:53–80.

TABLE 137-2 Prophylaxis of Infectious Endocarditis

CARDIAC CONDITIONS BY RISK OF INFECTIOUS ENDOCARDITIS	PROCEDURES FOR WHICH INFECTIOUS ENDOCARDITIS PROPHYLAXIS IS RECOMMENDED
High-risk category:	Endocarditis prophylaxis recommended:
Prosthetic cardiac valves, including bioprosthetic and homograft valves	Dental procedures*
Previous bacterial endocarditis	Respiratory tract
Complex cyanotic congenital heart disease (e.g., single ventricle states, transposition of the great arteries, and tetralogy of Fallot)	Tonsillectomy and/or adenoidectomy
Surgically constructed systemic pulmonary shunts or conduits	Surgeries involving respiratory mucosa
	Bronchoscopy with a rigid scope
	Gastrointestinal tract†
	Sclerotherapy for esophageal varices
	Esophageal stricture dilation
	ERCP with biliary obstruction
	Biliary tract surgery
	Surgeries that involve intestinal mucosa
	Genitourinary tract
	Prostatic surgery
	Cystoscopy
	Urethral dilation
Moderate-risk category:	Endocarditis prophylaxis not recommended:
Most other congenital cardiac malformations (other than above and below)	Respiratory tract
Acquired valvular dysfunction (e.g., rheumatic heart disease)	Endotracheal intubation
Hypertrophic cardiomyopathy	Bronchoscopy with a flexible scope
MVP with valvular regurgitation and/or thickened leaflets	Tympanostomy tube insertion
	Gastrointestinal tract
	Transesophageal echocardiography
	Endoscopy with or without biopsy
	Genitourinary tract
	Vaginal hysterectomy
	Vaginal delivery
	Cesarean section
	In uninfected tissue:
	Urethral catheterization
	Uterine dilatation and curettage
	Therapeutic abortion
	Sterilization procedures
	Intrauterine devices insertion/removal
	Other
	Cardiac catheterization
	Implanted cardiac pacemakers, implanted defibrillators, and coronary stents
	Incision/biopsy of surgically scrubbed skin
	Circumcision
Negligible-risk category (no greater risk than the general population)—endocarditis prophylaxis not recommended:	
Isolated secundum atrial septal defect	
Surgical repair of atrial septal defect, ventricular septal defect, or patent ductus arteriosus (without residua beyond 6 months)	
Previous coronary artery bypass graft surgery	
MVP without valvular regurgitation	
Physiologic, functional, or innocent murmurs	
Previous Kawasaki disease without valvular dysfunction	
Previous rheumatic fever without valvular dysfunction	
Cardiac pacemakers (intravascular and epicardial) and implanted defibrillators	

ABBREVIATIONS: MVP, mitral valve prolapse; ERCP, endoscopic retrograde cholangiopancreatogram.
*Refer to source article for detailed description of procedures.
†Prophylaxis is recommended for high-risk patients; it is optional for medium-risk patients.
SOURCE: Adapted from Adnan Dajani AS, Taubert KA, Wilson W, et al. Prevention of bacterial endocarditis. *JAMA* 1997;277:1794–1801.

- Surveillance programs should be designed to monitor the rates of NIs, and detect the emergence of resistant or unusual infectious organisms. Successful surveillance programs require the teamwork of physicians, nurses, and epidemiologists. A comprehensive surveillance strategy requires both patient-directed (epidemiologic surveillance of resistant or unusual organisms) and environment-directed (administrative surveillance of health care workers, patients, and medical equipment) interventions.

- Specific measures of intervention are warranted when the source of the NI is identified. One universal measure that will reduce NIs is the liberation of the patient from unnecessary devices and interventions. Examples of other targeted measures include the following:
    - BSI secondary to vascular access are the most common type of ICU NI. Practices that reduce catheter-related BSIs include consideration of the best insertion site, observation of maximal barrier precautions during insertion of the catheter, use of chlorhexidine gluconate for insertion site skin antisepsis, and use of antimicrobial-impregnated or antibiotic-coated catheters (particularly when patient risk is high or catheter use is expected to be at least 1 week).
    - VAP is associated with significant morbidity and mortality. Noninvasive ventilation should be used when appropriate, since the risk of VAP is considerably less with this intervention. Preventive strategies to reduce the incidence of VAP include orotracheal (nonnasal) route of intubation, semirecumbent patient positioning, subglottic secretion suctioning, optimal use of sedation (to reduce the duration of mechanical ventilation), avoidance of large gastric volumes, and promotion of patient oral hygiene (e.g., chlorhexidine mouth rinse). Prophylactic antibiotics have not been shown to prevent VAP, but are being considered in high-risk patient subsets (e.g., neutropenia, HIV infection, and postabdominal surgery). Once VAP is confirmed or suspected, the implementation of a rotating antibiotic schedule may reduce the emergence of antibiotic-resistant organisms.
    - Urinary tract infections (UTIs) develop in 5% of patients with a urinary catheter per day of catheterization. Interventions that can reduce the risk of catheter-related bacteriuria include use of suprapubic or condom catheters (instead of urethral catheters), and aseptic catheter insertion and maintenance.
    - *Clostridium difficile* colitis is common among patients receiving antibiotics. Restriction of antibiotic use and hand hygiene are the cornerstones in prevention of *C. difficile* colitis.

BIBLIOGRAPHY

Adnan Dajani AS, Taubert KA, Wilson W, et al. Prevention of bacterial endocarditis. *JAMA* 1997;277:1794–1801.

Dodek P, Keenan S, Cook D, et al. Evidence-based clinical practice guideline for the prevention of ventilator-associated pneumonia. *Ann Intern Med* 2004;141:305–313.

Doebbeling BN, Stanley GL, Sheetz CT, et al. Comparative efficacy of alternative hand-washing agents in reducing nosocomial infections in intensive care units. *N Engl J Med* 1992;327:88–93.

Eggimann P, Pittet D. Infection control in the ICU. *Chest* 2001;120:2059–2093.

Garner JS. Guideline for isolation precautions in hospitals: the Hospital Infection Control Practices Advisory Committee. *Infect Control Hosp Epidemiol* 1996;17:53–80.

Mangram AJ, Horan TC, Pearson ML, et al. Guideline for prevention of surgical site infection, 1999. Centers for Disease Control and Prevention (CDC). Hospital Infection Control Practices Advisory Committee. *Am J Infect Control* 1999;27:97–132.

Pittet D, Mourouga P, Perneger TV. Members of the Infection Control Program. Compliance with handwashing in a teaching hospital. *Ann Intern Med* 1999;130:126–130.

Rubinson L, Diette GB. Best practices for insertion of central venous catheters in intensive-care units to prevent catheter-related bloodstream infections. *J Lab Clin Med* 2004;143:5–13.

Saint S, Lipsky BA. Preventing catheter-related bacteriuria: should we? Can we? How? *Arch Intern Med* 1999;159:800–808.

138 TRANSPORTING THE CRITICALLY ILL

Joseph Levitt

KEY POINTS

- The goals of the transport of the critically ill patient should include provision of all necessary monitoring and emergent interventions to minimize risk during this transition period.
- Each transport should weigh the risks and benefits of moving the patient.
- While the physician sending the patient is responsible for making the essential on-site evaluation of the patient and determining the patient's stability, guidance from more specialized centers receiving the patient should be sought as well.

BACKGROUND

- The movement of any critically ill or injured patient is not without hazard. Though these patients may be considered "stable," their physiologic reserve is often limited. Even minor adverse physiologic changes in these patients during transport may cascade into life-threatening complications. Rates of complications or serious physiologic derangements during intrahospital transport have been reported as high as 45–75%.

- Transfers may be between hospitals (via ambulance, helicopter, or airplane), within the hospital (from the emergency department, to the operating rooms or radiology), or simply between beds, gurneys, and so forth. While each situation has unique features to address, they all share potential hazards.
- In an effort to reduce patient risks, recommendations have been published by the Transfer Guidelines Task Force Committee of the Society of Critical Care Medicine, the American College of Critical Care Medicine, and the American Association of Critical Care Nurses.

INTERHOSPITAL TRANSFERS

- Transfers from an emergency department are regulated under the Emergency Medical Treatment and Active Labor Act (EMTALA). While this act does not specifically address other interfacility transfers, its guidelines are generally applicable.
- When transferring between hospitals, utilizing appropriately trained and experienced personnel to plan and carry out the transfer is recommended. Direct physician-to-physician contact and detailed communication between receiving and accepting facilities is required.
- Federal law also has implications for receiving institutions. Hospitals with specialized services may not refuse to accept an appropriate transfer if they have the capacity to treat the individual.
- A receiving hospital cannot refuse to accept the transfer of a patient who is unstable or has an emergency medical condition if they have the capacity and ability to care for a patient.
- Excluding variation in road and weather conditions, ambulances are generally the fastest mode of transport for distances under 25 miles, with helicopters fastest between 25 and 150 miles, and airplanes preferred for distances beyond 150 miles.

PLANNING

- Careful assessment of risks and benefits should be performed prior to deciding to attempt transfer with consideration of alternatives when the risks are significant.
- For unstable patients, it may be preferable for diagnostic studies (e.g., substituting portable ultrasound and x-ray for a computed tomography [CT] scan) and therapeutic or surgical procedures to be done at the bedside in the ICU.
- When deteriorating status requires transfer to a more acute care setting, assessment of the pace of deterioration and benefit of speed of transfer must be weighed against delaying transfer while attempting to stabilize the patient.
- Prior to all transfers, a brief assessment of the patient and anticipation of potential complication is necessary to ensure proper planning.
- Appropriate transport personnel and equipment should be arranged prior to transfer.

AIRWAY

- Maintaining a patent airway and adequate oxygenation and ventilation is the highest priority of any transfer.
- Patients with significant respiratory distress, especially those receiving active therapy (noninvasive positive pressure ventilation, heliox, continuous nebulizers) which may not be possible during transfer, should be intubated prior to transfer, even if they may not otherwise require it.
- For intubated patients, position and security of the endotracheal tube should be confirmed prior to transfer. Particular attention must be paid to not dislodging or advancing the tube. While ventilation can be performed with either a manual bag-valve-mask or portable ventilator, studies suggest portable ventilators provide more constant and reliable ventilation.
- For patients requiring high levels of supplemental oxygen, sufficient oxygen supply to last the duration of transfer, including unexpected delays must be confirmed prior to departure.
- When patients require high levels of positive end-expiratory pressure (PEEP), a bag-valve-mask or portable ventilator capable of providing similar PEEP levels should be used. For extremely unstable patients, demonstrating adequate oxygenation and hemodynamic stability during 10–15 minutes of manual bagging or being connected to the portable ventilator prior to transfer may be prudent.

CIRCULATION

- Securing an adequate vascular access is a necessity prior to transfer of patients with unstable circulations.
- Large-bore peripheral IVs are more prone to being displaced during transfer and are not appropriate for infusing many vasoactive medication.
- Transferring physicians should consider placing a central venous catheter (CVC) in any patient whose circulation may require infusion of fluids or vasoactive medications during transfer.

- All nonessential medications should be discontinued prior to during transfer to minimize risk of disrupting delivery of essential medication. Paralytics and sedatives may be given by IV bolus during transport rather than by continuous infusion.

MEDICAL PERSONNEL

- The Transfer Guidelines Task recommended that all critical care transports, both intrahospital and interhospital, should be performed by dedicated, specially trained transport teams.
- The guidelines recommend that all transported critically ill patients be accompanied by a minimum of two people, one of which should be a critical care nurse. They suggest that an accompanying physician is necessary only for unstable patients.
- Physician presence during transfers has been shown to reduce complications.

EQUIPMENT

- Critically ill or injured patients require real-time monitoring. Pulse oximetry and ECG monitoring can provide continuous oxygenation and cardiac assessment. The blood pressure can be measured using an automatic noninvasive blood pressure device if continuous measurements via arterial line are not indicated.
- Suitable transport monitors and equipment are portable, durable, lightweight, and battery powered. Audible and visible alarms for monitors, infusion pumps, and ventilators are required.
- Transport equipment should be compatible with the lines, fittings, and power outlets at the destination unit or in the transport vehicle. All transport equipment should fit into elevators and transport vehicles, while leaving enough room for transport personnel to function.
- Transport personnel should familiarize themselves with all equipment and an adequate supply of medication and battery charge for infusion pumps should be confirmed prior to transfer.

BIBLIOGRAPHY

Blumen IJ, Thomas F, Williams DH. Transportation of the critically ill patient. In: Hall JB, Schmidt GA, Wood LDH, eds., *Principles of Critical Care*, 3rd ed. New York, NY: McGraw-Hill; 2005: 79–92.

Guidelines for the transfer of critically ill patients. Guidelines Committee of the American College of Critical Care Medicine; Society of Critical Care Medicine and American Association of Critical-Care Nurses Transfer Guidelines Task Force. *Crit Care Med* 1993;21:931–937.

Smith JM. EMTALA basics: what medical professionals need to know. Emergency Medical Treatment and Active Labor Act. *J Natl Med Assoc* 2002;94:426–429.

139 TELEMEDICINE AND THE EICU

Jeremy Leventhal

KEY POINTS

- Current technology makes possible the import of much of the bedside and hospital data concerning critically ill patients to a central location for physician assessment.
- In theory, telemedicine would distribute a limited resource (the critical care physician) over a large patient population, particularly during time periods when direct physician coverage was not available to the ICU.
- Further assessment will be needed to know if this approach to care helps achieve the goals of standardized care practices, enhanced operating effectiveness, and improved patient outcomes.

BACKGROUND

- Since the birth of intensive care medicine in the 1950s, a growing demand has arisen for its heavily monitored setting.
- The advent of therapeutic modalities that include dialysis and mechanical ventilation have resulted in the prolongation of lives that would surely have been lost in the past.
- With the increased use of intensive care units (ICU) in hospitals, efforts of researchers have been directed at ways to decrease the mortality rates amongst the aggregate of unstable patients who normally populate an ICU.
- In 2000, the Institute of Medicine published a report citing that between 44,000 and 98,000 deaths have been the result of medical errors. Because of the acuity of a critically ill patient, the ICU is vulnerable

to errors that will result in poor outcomes. A successful effort to curb the amount of medical errors in the ICU will surely result in a consequent decrease in mortality.
- The role of the physicians making decisions in the ICU has come into close scrutiny. Large purchasers of health care in the United States formed the Leapfrog group in 1998. Its purpose was to find ways to increase the safety and value of health care delivered in this country. One of its many recommendations involved physician staffing in the ICU.
- The Leapfrog group hypothesized that by having certified intensivists more closely involved in the care of the patients in the ICU, mortality could be decreased by as much as 10%. The Leapfrog group has predicted this intervention alone to result in the prevention of as many as 50,000 deaths a year.

DATA

- A study in the Journal of the American Medical Association supported this hypothesis. The *JAMA* study identified 26 individual studies which were then used to compare alternative staffing strategies in the ICU. The unit physician staffing was grouped into staffing categories as either low-intensity or high-intensity.
  - The low intensity group had either no staffing by an intensivist or elective staffing only.
  - The high-intensity group involved having either a mandatory consultation by an intensivist, or having care given in a closed unit where all the care was directed by intensivists.
  - The high-intensity staffing categories were found to be associated with a decreased mortality in the ICU as well as overall hospital mortality (61% and 71%, respectively).
- A 2000 paper in *JAMA* commented that intensivists were providing only 37% of care in the ICU.
- Furthermore, the same study in *JAMA* found that the percentage of patients receiving high-intensity coverage by intensivists is as low as 10%.
- There are approximately 5500 intensivists now practicing in the United States. With increasing admissions to ICUs, the demand for these subspecialists will surely increase. The supply, however, is not projected to increase accordingly.
- The paper in *JAMA* projects this short supply to result in a shortfall in intensivist hours by 22% in 2020 and increase to 35% in 2030. A creative solution to staffing ICUs with the limited supply of intensivists available as well as designing systems that will help decrease medical errors needed to be found.

THE eICU OR "TELEMEDICINE"

- In attempting to address the increased needs medical advances have placed on the ICUs, the notion of an electronic ICU (eICU) and telemedicine have arisen. The notion of an eICU incorporates telemedicine.
- A *Critical Care Medicine* 2001 article on the subject defined telemedicine as "the use of medical information exchanged from one site to another via electronic communication for health and education of the patient or health care provider and for the purpose of improving health care." Put simply, telemedicine allows physicians in remote locations to take in active role in evaluating and guiding the care of patients in the ICU. The location of the practitioner can include his/her home.
- What makes the eICU a true innovation is not just the way it makes better use of a limited amount of intensivists with telemedicine. Rather, the eICU refers to a model that uses both the 24-hour decision-making capability of a remote intensivist in conjunction with a multidisciplinary team. This team benefits from the preventive strategies, early computerized clinical alarms, evidence-based medicine derived from previous outcomes data, and 24-hour access to an intensivist's clinical expertise and provides superior care to the patient.
- The eICU model incorporates intensivists, housestaff, nurses, physician's assistants, respiratory therapists, health care administrators, and information technologists in providing care to its patients.
  - The intensivist can interact with members of the team on-site by use of teleconferencing.
  - This can allow for observation of the patient as well as supervision of procedures performed on the patient.
  - The teleconferencing can be used for interactions amongst the staff and even for family interactions.
- Furthermore, the eICU works with data (lab values, imaging), smart alarms, and computerized order entry to potentially decrease the amount of medical errors.
- Outcome research can be automatically generated by the data followed on the computer in order to constantly upgrade the quality of care provided by an institution. The data are immediately available to the multidisciplinary team for interpretation and subsequent action.
- This availability, along with smart alarms that would bring to attention concerning labs/vital signs, would help handle or even prevent complications such as pneumonia, cerebral vascular accidents, and myocardial infarctions. The amount of time that this eICU paradigm would need to be in place depends on how often a specific hospital is adequately staffed with intensivists.
- eICUs can be linked to provide support to multiple ICUs. For academic centers the amount of time where eICU coverage is needed could be as little as 12 hours,

whereas more rural locations might require the eICU model all the time to ensure the highest level of care.

- A study published in 2000 in *Critical Care Medicine* journal supports the use of eICUs.
  - The design was a triple-cohort study that took place in the surgical ICU of an academically affiliated community hospital where intensivist consultations were available, but not on-site.
  - The outcomes from the intervention time were compared to outcomes from two separate periods of equal time in the same ICU.
  - Camera and data transmission equipment were installed in both the ICUs as well as the intensivists' homes.
  - The intensivists all provided care exclusively from their homes through teleconferencing with housestaff and nursing.
- The study examined three different 16-week periods. During only one of these periods was the telemedicine intervention enacted. During the other 16-week periods, intensivists reviewed the charts to aid with triage. If the need was there, they would act as consultants (~30%) or assist in the management (5–10%).
  - Data were gathered on ICU and hospital mortality rates, complication rates, length of ICU stay, and length of hospital stay.
  - Throughout the intervention period, the intensivist involved would formulate a plan while teleconferencing with the on-site housestaff.
  - Physiologic data from bedside monitors were reviewed throughout the day, approximately every 2 hours except for the period between midnight and 6 in the morning.
  - An intensivist was available 24 hours a day.
  - The intensivists never actually physically examined the patients.
- The results:
  - Severity-adjusted ICU mortality, in comparison to the two baseline periods, decreased by 68% and 46%.
  - Rates of complications decreased by 44% and 50%.
  - ICU length of stay decreased by 34% and 30%.
- The eICU is a fairly recent but increasingly necessary response to adapting our ICUs to the inadequate supply of intensivists while attempting to actuate previously proven methods of achieving improved outcomes in the ICU.

BIBLIOGRAPHY

Angus D, Kelley M, Schmitz R, et al. Caring for the critically ill patient. Current and projected workforce requirements for the care of the critically ill and patients with pulmonary disease. *JAMA* 2000;284:2762–2770.

Celi LA, Hassan E, Marquardt C, et al. The eICU: it's not just telemedicine. *Crit Care Med* 2001;29(Suppl):N183–N189.

Pronovost PJ, Angus DC, Darman T, et al. Physician staffing patterns and clinical outcomes in critically ill patients. A systematic review. *JAMA* 2002;288:2151–2162.

Rosenfeld B, Dorman T, Breslow M, et al. Intensive care unit telemedicine: alternate paradigm for providing continuous intensivist care. *Crit Care Med* 2000;28:3925–3931.

140 WITHHOLDING AND WITHDRAWING LIFE-SUSTAINING THERAPY AND ADMINISTERING PALLIATIVE CARE

Steven Q. Davis

KEY POINTS

- Most patients who die in the intensive care unit will do so after conscious decisions are made to shift goals from cure to palliative care.
- Ideally, agreement will be achieved among patients, families, and care providers that further restorative care would not be beneficial when such decisions are made.
- Accordingly, palliative care is an essential part of critical care management, and the skill set to support patients and families through this difficult process should be part of all critical care physicians' training and clinical expertise.

DEFINITION

- Withholding and withdrawing life-sustaining therapy or life support is a process by which various medical interventions either are not given to or are taken away from patients with the expectation that they will die from their underlying illnesses.
- When applied to patients who are brain dead, life support should more appropriately be referred to as organ support.
- Palliative care is the prevention or treatment of pain, dyspnea, anxiety, and other kinds of suffering in dying patients. It represents an attitude that includes open communication between all caregivers and patients and their surrogates and acknowledgement of the emotional needs of all involved.

ETHICAL ASPECTS

- A decision to withdraw a treatment is equivalent to not initiating it, particularly since starting a therapy may be necessary to evaluate the patient's condition.
- There are no ethical or moral differences between categories of treatment (cardiopulmonary resuscitation [CPR], mechanical ventilation, vasoactive medications, nutrition, and so forth).
- The indefinite maintenance of a patient in a persistent vegetative state raises ethical concerns both for the patient's dignity and appropriate health care resource utilization.
- The wishes of an informed adult patient with decision-making capacity should be the primary consideration in treatment decisions.
- The patient's needs during this process are to receive adequate pain control, avoid prolongation of death, achieve a sense of control over the dying process, and to strengthen relationships with loved ones.
- The family's needs are to be with the dying loved one, to be helpful to them, to be informed of changes in the patient's condition, to understand therapy, to be assured of the patient's comfort, and to be comforted themselves, to express their emotions, to be assured that their decisions were correct, to find meaning in the death of the loved one, and to be fed and rested through the dying process of their loved one.
- The critical care team's needs are to establish consensus regarding the goals and strategies for providing palliative care, to gain skills and knowledge in palliative care, to be supported by their institution and to have opportunities for bereavement after the patient dies.

LEGAL ASPECTS

- Withholding and withdrawing care are justified by the principles of informed consent and informed refusal, both of which are derived from the patient's right of self-determination.
- All American courts recognize a competent adult's right to refuse life-sustaining care.
- When a patient is unable to make decisions for himself or herself, courts recognize the authority of a surrogate decision maker. However, the standards used to decide whether care will be withheld or withdrawn vary by jurisdiction.
- The U.S. Supreme Court has described the distinction between assisted suicide and withdrawal or withholding of care. "When a patient refuses life-sustaining medical treatment, he dies from an underlying fatal disease or pathology; but if a patient ingests lethal medication prescribed by a physician, he is killed by that medication."
- The principle of double effect allows that medications that relieve pain and suffering (analgesics and sedatives) are permissible even if they may have the unintended consequence of hastening death. The positive, morally acceptable reason (limiting pain and suffering) must be the reason for using the therapy that could produce an undesirable consequence.

CLINICAL ASPECTS

- In various surveys of intensive care units in the United States, withholding or withdrawal of support was involved in 75–90% of deaths.
- Prior to meeting with the patient or surrogate, all involved caregivers, including the primary service and any consultants, must arrive at a consensus. Otherwise, the patient or family is very likely to be confused and angered by the lack of consensus.
- Generally, surrogate decision makers eventually agree with a physician recommending withdrawal or withholding of care. Effective and frequent communication with the surrogate is essential. A care provider must be ready for the surrogate to not accept the decision and have a plan, usually involving the transfer of care for the patient to another provider.
- While individual items may be discussed with the patient or surrogate (CPR, mechanical ventilation, vasoactive drugs, and so forth), it is preferable to present these items more generally and grouped together as interventions that will not benefit the patient and will most likely cause harm or prolong death.
- Most families are not equipped to pick from a menu of options to decide which therapies to withhold. Also, this may create the impression that some of the options may benefit the patient, making the decision far more difficult to make.
- Adequate and aggressive sedation and analgesia are an absolute requirement. In one study, prior to withholding care patients received approximately 3 mg/h of morphine and 2 mg/h of diazepam. After withholding and withdrawal of support, this increased to approximately 11 mg/h of morphine and 10 mg/h of diazepam.
- If a family is unable to reach a decision due to dissension within the family, they must appoint one member of the family to act as a spokesperson and to make decisions for the group. When this happens, it is crucial to have meetings that involve as many members of the family as possible, so that everyone starts with the same information about the patient's clinical condition.

- The patient and family should be assured that care will be withdrawn expeditiously, with the primary concern for the patient's comfort.
- Extubation may be considered, but changing the ventilator to a FiO_2 of 21% with no positive end-expiratory pressure (PEEP) may be sufficient to provide comfort and prevent gasping for air. Enough sedation and analgesia must be used no matter what changes are made to the ventilator.

BIBLIOGRAPHY

Luce JM. Withholding and withdrawing life-sustaining therapy and administering palliative care. In: Hall JB, Schmidt GA, Wood LDH, eds., *Principles of Critical Care*, 3rd ed. New York, NY: McGraw-Hill; 2005: 201–206.

INDEX

D

R

T